Recent Progress in Pulmonary Medicine

Recent Progress in Pulmonary Medicine

Edited by Lily Hartman

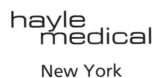

New York

Hayle Medical,
750 Third Avenue, 9th Floor,
New York, NY 10017, USA

Visit us on the World Wide Web at:
www.haylemedical.com

© Hayle Medical, 2019

This book contains information obtained from authentic and highly regarded sources. Copyright for all individual chapters remain with the respective authors as indicated. All chapters are published with permission under the Creative Commons Attribution License or equivalent. A wide variety of references are listed. Permission and sources are indicated; for detailed attributions, please refer to the permissions page and list of contributors. Reasonable efforts have been made to publish reliable data and information, but the authors, editors and publisher cannot assume any responsibility for the validity of all materials or the consequences of their use.

ISBN: 978-1-63241-752-7

Trademark Notice: Registered trademark of products or corporate names are used only for explanation and identification without intent to infringe.

Cataloging-in-Publication Data

Recent progress in pulmonary medicine / edited by Lily Hartman.
   p. cm.
Includes bibliographical references and index.
ISBN 978-1-63241-752-7
1. Lungs--Diseases. 2. Respiratory organs--Diseases.
3. Respiratory infections. I. Hartman, Lily.
RC756 .R43 2019
616.24--dc23

Table of Contents

Preface IX

Chapter 1 **Pathogenesis, imaging and clinical characteristics of CF and non-CF bronchiectasis** 1
Jürgen Schäfer, Matthias Griese, Ravishankar Chandrasekaran, Sanjay H. Chotirmall and Dominik Hartl

Chapter 2 **Earlier smoking after waking and the risk of asthma** 12
Arielle S. Selya, Sunita Thapa and Gaurav Mehta

Chapter 3 **Geographic variation in the aetiology, epidemiology and microbiology of bronchiectasis** 18
Ravishankar Chandrasekaran, Micheál Mac Aogáin, James D. Chalmers, Stuart J. Elborn and Sanjay H. Chotirmall

Chapter 4 **Global lung function initiative 2012 reference values for spirometry in Asian Americans** 32
Jingzhou Zhang, Xiao Hu, Xinlun Tian and Kai-Feng Xu

Chapter 5 **Asthma exacerbations in a subtropical area and the role of respiratory viruses** 41
Lusmaia Damaceno Camargo Costa, Paulo Augusto Moreira Camargos, Paul L. P. Brand, Fabíola Souza Fiaccadori, Menira Borges de Lima Dias e Souza, Divina das Dôres de Paula Cardoso, Ítalo de Araújo Castro, Ruth Minamisava and Paulo Sérgio Sucasas da Costa

Chapter 6 **The lung microbiome in children with HIV-bronchiectasis** 47
Refiloe Masekela, Solize Vosloo, Stephanus N. Venter, Wilhelm Z. de Beer and Robin J. Green

Chapter 7 **Latent class analysis to define radiological subgroups in pulmonary nontuberculous mycobacterial disease** 57
Steven A. Cowman, Joseph Jacob, Sayed Obaidee, R. Andres Floto, Robert Wilson, Charles S. Haworth and Michael R. Loebinger

Chapter 8 **Pulmonary arterial hypertension in Latin America: epidemiological data from local Studies** 65
Ana Beatriz Valverde, Juliana M. Soares, Karynna P. Viana, Bruna Gomes, Claudia Soares and Rogerio Souza

Chapter 9 **Comorbidities and COPD severity in a clinic-based cohort** 73
Chantal Raherison, El-Hassane Ouaalaya, Alain Bernady, Julien Casteigt, Cecilia Nocent-Eijnani, Laurent Falque, Frédéric Le Guillou, Laurent Nguyen, Annaig Ozier and Mathieu Molimard

Chapter 10	**Delayed isolation of smear-positive pulmonary tuberculosis patients in a Japanese acute care hospital**	82
	Sho Nishiguchi, Shusaku Tomiyama, Izumi Kitagawa and Yasuharu Tokuda	
Chapter 11	**"The missing ingredient": the patient perspective of health related quality of life in bronchiectasis**	89
	Emily K. Dudgeon, Megan Crichton and James D. Chalmers	
Chapter 12	**Characterization, localization and comparison of c-Kit+ lung cells in never smokers and smokers with and without COPD**	98
	Alejandra López-Giraldo, Tamara Cruz, Laureano Molins, Ángela Guirao, Adela Saco, Sandra Cuerpo, Josep Ramirez, Álvar Agustí and Rosa Faner	
Chapter 13	**Effectiveness of a standardized electronic admission order set for acute exacerbation of chronic obstructive pulmonary disease**	105
	Sachin R. Pendharkar, Maria B. Ospina, Danielle A. Southern, Naushad Hirani, Jim Graham, Peter Faris, Mohit Bhutani, Richard Leigh, Christopher H. Mody and Michael K. Stickland	
Chapter 14	**Patient information, education and self-management in bronchiectasis: facilitating improvements to optimise health outcomes**	113
	Katy L. M. Hester, Julia Newton, Tim Rapley and Anthony De Soyza	
Chapter 15	**"Velcro-type" crackles predict specific radiologic features of fibrotic interstitial lung disease**	122
	Giacomo Sgalla, Simon L. F. Walsh, Nicola Sverzellati, Sophie Fletcher, Stefania Cerri, Borislav Dimitrov, Dragana Nikolic, Anna Barney, Fabrizio Pancaldi, Luca Larcher, Fabrizio Luppi, Mark G. Jones, Donna Davies and Luca Richeldi	
Chapter 16	**Profiling non-tuberculous mycobacteria in an Asian setting: characteristics and clinical outcomes of hospitalized patients**	129
	Albert Y. H. Lim, Sanjay H. Chotirmall, Eric T. K. Fok, Akash Verma, Partha P. De, Soon Keng Goh, Ser Hon Puah, Daryl E. L. Goh and John A. Abisheganaden	
Chapter 17	**Anti-IL-5 therapy in patients with severe eosinophilic asthma – clinical efficacy and possible criteria for treatment response**	135
	Nora Drick, Benjamin Seeliger, Tobias Welte, Jan Fuge and Hendrik Suhling	
Chapter 18	**A modified risk score in one-year survival rate assessment of group 1 pulmonary arterial hypertension**	144
	Wei Xiong, Yunfeng Zhao, Mei Xu, Bigyan Pudasaini, Xuejun Guo and Jinming Liu	
Chapter 19	**Real-world treatment patterns for patients 80 years and older with early lung cancer: a nationwide claims study**	154
	Kyungjong Lee, Hye Ok Kim, Hee Kyoung Choi and Gi Hyeon Seo	
Chapter 20	**Impact of multidrug-resistant bacteria on outcome in patients with prolonged weaning**	160
	Johannes Bickenbach, Daniel Schöneis, Gernot Marx, Nikolaus Marx, Sebastian Lemmen and Michael Dreher	

Chapter 21	**The long-term rate of change in lung function in urban professional firefighters** 168	
	Flynn Slattery, Kylie Johnston, Catherine Paquet, Hunter Bennett and Alan Crockett	
Chapter 22	**Albuminuria in patients with chronic obstructive pulmonary disease**.................................... 188	
	Festo K. Shayo and Janet Lutale	
Chapter 23	**Adherence to inhaled therapy and its impact on chronic obstructive pulmonary disease (COPD)**.. 195	
	Magdalena Humenberger, Andreas Horner, Anna Labek, Bernhard Kaiser, Rupert Frechinger, Constanze Brock, Petra Lichtenberger and Bernd Lamprecht	
Chapter 24	**Solid part size is an important predictor of nodal metastasis in lung cancer with a subsolid tumor**.. 201	
	Jun Yeun Cho, Cho Sun Leem, Youlim Kim, Eun Sun Kim, Sang Hoon Lee, Yeon Joo Lee, Jong Sun Park, Young-Jae Cho, Jae Ho Lee, Choon-Taek Lee and Ho Il Yoon	
Chapter 25	**Epidemiology of pulmonary disease due to nontuberculous mycobacteria**............................207	
	Yaoju Tan, Biyi Su, Wei Shu, Xingshan Cai, Shaojia Kuang, Haobin Kuang, Jianxiong Liu and Yu Pang	
Chapter 26	**Intratracheal administration of adipose derived mesenchymal stem cells alleviates chronic asthma in a mouse model**.. 214	
	Ranran Dai, Youchao Yu, Guofeng Yan, Xiaoxia Hou, Yingmeng Ni and Guochao Shi	
Chapter 27	**Change in the prevalence asthma, rhinitis and respiratory symptom over a 20 year period: associations to year of birth, life style and sleep related symptoms**........................... 223	
	Christer Janson, Ane Johannessen, Karl Franklin, Cecilie Svanes, Linus Schiöler, Andrei Malinovschi, Thorarinn Gislason, Bryndis Benediktsdottir, Vivi Schlünssen, Rain Jõgi, Deborah Jarvis and Eva Lindberg	
Chapter 28	**Erlotinib versus gefitinib for brain metastases in Asian patients with exon 19 EGFR-mutant lung adenocarcinoma: a retrospective, multicenter study**........................... 231	
	Ye Jiang, Jing Zhang, Juanjuan Huang, Bo Xu, Ning Li, Lei Cao and Mingdong Zhao	
Chapter 29	**Lymphatic vessel density as a prognostic indicator in Asian NSCLC patients**...................... 238	
	Shuanglan Xu, Jiao Yang, Shuangyan Xu, Yun Zhu, Chunfang Zhang, Liqiong Liu, Hao Liu, Yunlong Dong, Zhaowei Teng and Xiqian Xing	

Permissions

List of Contributors

Index

Preface

Every book is initially just a concept; it takes months of research and hard work to give it the final shape in which the readers receive it. In its early stages, this book also went through rigorous reviewing. The notable contributions made by experts from across the globe were first molded into patterned chapters and then arranged in a sensibly sequential manner to bring out the best results.

Pulmonology is the branch of science and medicine, which is concerned with the disorders related to the respiratory tract. It is a sub-field of internal medicine. Some common disorders associated with the respiratory tract include common cold, pulmonary embolism, asthma, sinusitis, pneumonia, pharyngitis and tuberculosis. Auscultation for unusual breath sounds and percussion of the lung fields for dullness or hyper-resonance, pulmonary function tests, chest X-rays and CT scans are common ways to diagnose respiratory diseases. Inhalers are considered effective in the treatment of asthma. Other treatment methods include oxygen therapy and mechanical ventilation. Pulmonary medicine is an upcoming field of medicine that has undergone rapid development over the past few decades. The various advancements in pulmonology are glanced at and their applications as well as ramifications are looked at in detail. As this field is emerging at a rapid pace, the contents of this book will help the readers understand the modern concepts and applications of the subject.

It has been my immense pleasure to be a part of this project and to contribute my years of learning in such a meaningful form. I would like to take this opportunity to thank all the people who have been associated with the completion of this book at any step.

Editor

Pathogenesis, imaging and clinical characteristics of CF and non-CF bronchiectasis

Jürgen Schäfer[1*], Matthias Griese[2], Ravishankar Chandrasekaran[3], Sanjay H. Chotirmall[3] and Dominik Hartl[4,5]

Abstract

Bronchiectasis is a common feature of severe inherited and acquired pulmonary disease conditions. Among inherited diseases, cystic fibrosis (CF) is the major disorder associated with bronchiectasis, while acquired conditions frequently featuring bronchiectasis include post-infective bronchiectasis and chronic obstructive pulmonary disease (COPD). Mechanistically, bronchiectasis is driven by a complex interplay of inflammation and infection with neutrophilic inflammation playing a predominant role. The clinical characterization and management of bronchiectasis should involve a precise diagnostic workup, tailored therapeutic strategies and pulmonary imaging that has become an essential tool for the diagnosis and follow-up of bronchiectasis. Prospective future studies are required to optimize the diagnostic and therapeutic management of bronchiectasis, particularly in heterogeneous non-CF bronchiectasis populations.

Background

Bronchiectasis is a condition in which an area of the bronchial lumen is permanently and abnormally widened, with accompanying infection. Bronchiectasis is found in a variety of pulmonary diseases, both genetically caused and acquired, such as severe pulmonary infections and cystic fibrosis (CF), but is also a feature of Kartagener syndrome, chronic obstructive pulmonary diseases (COPD), alpha 1-antitrypsin deficiency, asthma, or primary immunodeficiencies [1–3]. Bronchietasis is caused by long-term excessive inflammatory damage to the airways, which results in tissue breakdown, enlargement of the affected airways and the key clinical symptoms of chronic productive cough and shortness of breath. Globally, in up to half of all cases the cause cannot be identified (idiopathic). Those cases together with several other known aetiologies such as post-infectious and allergic hypersensitivity collectively fall under the category 'non-cystic fibrosis' (non-CF) bronchiectasis [4]. Here we discuss the key features of both CF and non-CF related bronchiectasis with respect to their pathogenesis, imaging and clinical management.

* Correspondence: Juergen.Schaefer@med.uni-tuebingen.de
[1]Department of Radiology, Division of Pediatric Radiology, University of Tübingen, Tübingen, Germany
Full list of author information is available at the end of the article

Pathogenesis of bronchiectasis formation

Bronchiectasis mechanistically results from chronic inflammatory microenvironments that trigger airway tissue breakdown. In both CF and non-CF bronchiectasis, the complex interplay between infection and inflammation feeds a pro-inflammatory vicious circle that progressively drives the generation of bronchiectasis and the destruction of the pulmonary architecture [5]. Inflammatory immune cells (mainly activated macrophages and neutrophils) represent the major infiltrating population in disease conditions associated with bronchiectasis and contribute significantly to tissue damage and bronchiectasis generation through the release of their harmful cellular ingredients. Particularly, cell-derived proteases and reactive oxygen species represent key mediators in the degradation and destruction of extracellular pulmonary tissue components, leading to bronchiectasis formation. The precise early immune-mediated mechanisms that trigger and maintain the formation of bronchiectasis remain yet incompletely understood. Regulated immune homeostasis seems to be essential since both immune deficiencies as well as hyper-active immune responses are associated with bronchiectasis. Particularly, the protease-antiprotease imbalance [6, 7], as found in CF and COPD airways, is considered as key pathogenic component in degrading extracellular matrix. Mutations in the cystic fibrosis transmembrane conductance regulator (CFTR) gene are causative for CF lung disease and drive the earliest pathogenic events in epithelial cells that ultimately lead to the genesis of bronchiectasis. Also beyond CF lung disease, CFTR-related cellular mechanisms regulating mucociliary clearance have been involved in cigarette smoke-induced COPD [8].

In the following two sections, we will focus on the microbiological (a) and immunological/inflammatory (b) findings associated with the pathogenesis of bronchiectasis.

Microbiology

Pseudomonas aeruginosa is a common and dominant pathogen found in the airways of both CF and non-CF bronchiectasis patients [9–13]. Chronic infection has been associated with more severe decline in lung function [14–19], increased hospitalizations [20, 21], frequent exacerbations [22] and disease severity [23, 24]. Although clinical manifestations between the two settings vary, their core airway microbiota is largely analogous [25]. Along with *Pseudomonas*, bacteria belonging to other genera such as *Haemophilus, Streptococcus, Staphylococcus, Veillonella, Prevotella* and *Achromobacter* also make up the core microbiota observed in bronchiectasis [9, 26, 27]. Interestingly, *P. aeruginosa* and *H. influenzae* have been described to competitively inhibit each other, which in turn alters the core microbiota in the non-CF bronchiectasis airway [28]. Non-tuberculous mycobacteria (NTM) form another significant group of pathogens colonizing CF and non-CF airways [29–31]. *Mycobacterium avium complex* (MAC) and *Mycobacterium abscessus* are most frequently isolated in CF [32, 33] with high rates of multi-drug resistance in these species making them notoriously difficult to treat [34]. NTM belonging to the MAC group are also highly prevalent in non-CF bronchiectasis with a female preponderance [35, 36]. This group of organisms are surprisingly poorly associated with disease severity and exacerbations in the non-CF setting when compared to *Pseudomonas* [37, 38]. In contrast for CF patients, MAC and *M. abscessus* are often associated with an aggressive and accelerated lung function decline [39–42]. Interestingly, bacterial populations do not drastically change between stable and exacerbation states in bronchiectasis. However, viral load has been positively correlated with exacerbations in both CF and non-CF bronchiectasis patients. Infection with viruses belonging to the *coronavirus, rhinovirus* and *influenza A/B* virus families are frequently detected during exacerbations of bronchiectasis [43–45]. Whether the occurrence of such viruses, forming part of the airway 'virome' in bronchiectasis, are a cause or consequence of exacerbations remains to be elucidated [43, 46]. Most attention towards understanding the microbiome in bronchiectasis is directed at the bacteriome. Although fungi are frequently isolated from the same airways, the role of the pulmonary mycobiome in the pathogenesis of these disease states remains largely elusive [47–49]. Filamentous fungi belonging to the genus *Aspergillus* are frequently isolated fungal organisms in sputum samples from CF patients [50, 51]. Among the different species of *Aspergillus*, *A. fumigatus* is the most common chronic colonizer in CF [47, 52] Allergic bronchopulmonary aspergillosis (ABPA), an allergic *Aspergillus*-associated disease, is a frequent co-morbidity in CF [53], while *Aspergillus* colonization and sensitization has also been independently correlated with lung function declines and radiological severity in CF [54–56]. Only a single study to date has shown that fungi belonging to the *Aspergillus spp.* and *Candida albicans* are also identifiable in the airways of non-CF bronchiectasis patients [57]. Importantly, in a study of severe asthma patients, *Aspergillus* fumigatus sensitization has also been associated with poorer lung function and an increased incidence of bronchiectasis, a likely cause and consequence for this anatomical airway distortion [58, 59]. Among yeasts, *Candida spp.* are frequent colonizers of the bronchiectatic airways [47, 57, 60]. Isolation of *Candida albicans* from such airways is shown to be a predictor for frequent hospital-exacerbations and declines in lung function [61]. Compared to bacteria, our present understanding of fungal pathogenesis in the context of both CF and non-CF bronchiectasis remains limited and further work is required to determine their prevalence, colonization frequency, host-pathogen interaction and risk factor profile in this key patient group.

Immunology & inflammation

Neutrophil-dominant inflammation is a key feature of bronchiectasis. Sputum neutrophils are higher in bronchiectasis patients versus healthy controls and this correlates with an increased disease severity [62–64]. Both interleukin-8 (IL-8) and leukotriene-B4 (LTB4) are key chemo-attractants required for migration and infiltration of neutrophils into bronchiectatic airways [65]. High systemic IL-8 levels are detectable in individuals with bronchiectasis [66–68]. Antibacterial neutrophil responses (such as reactive oxygen species (ROS) formation) are activated through the IL-8-CXCR1 axis, but proteolytic cleavage mediated by neutrophil elastase (NE), which itself is associated with exacerbations and lung function decline in bronchiectasis, impairs antibacterial neutrophil functions [69, 70]. Uncontrolled NE activity, as found in CF airways, causes further respiratory tissue damage through degradation of extracellular proteins (such as surfactant proteins [71–73]) and cellular surface receptors (such as complement receptors [74]); high NE levels correlating with disease severity and poorer lung function are described in both CF and non-CF bronchiectasis settings

[75, 76]. In this context, CXCR receptor antagonists are hypothesized to inhibit neutrophil airway influx and have been shown to be effective in modulating the inflammatory state in bronchiectasis [77, 78]. Airway neutrophils in CF illustrate an impaired phagocytic ability [79]. This is in line with the observation that CF neutrophils have an impaired ROS production, a critical mediator of antimicrobial host defense [80]. Neutrophils defective in their oxidative abilities obtained from non-CF bronchiectasis patients were poorer at bacterial killing when compared to those of healthy controls [81]. Serine proteases are also important neutrophil derived products, released in response to TNF-α signalling. They degrade proteoglycans in the respiratory epithelium subsequently inducing airway damage [82]. In bronchiectasis, activated airway neutrophils secrete an abundance of human neutrophil peptides (HNPs), which have been described to inhibit their phagocytic ability. Importantly, high concentrations of HNPs are detected in both CF and non-CF airways, which in turn may contribute to the decreased phagocytic abilities and higher rates of infection described in both conditions [83]. Poorer clearance of neutrophils by alveolar macrophages further augments the inflammatory state in bronchiectasis [63]. Eosinophils contribute to tissue injury in CF and the presence of eosinophil cationic protein (ECP) heralds the cell activation state. ECP levels are elevated both in the airway and systemically in bronchiectasis [84–86]. Other eosinophilic markers including eosinophil protein X and peroxidase follow a similar pattern and like ECP contribute to poorer pulmonary function [87]. Importantly, eosinophilic granule release in CF may be triggered by NE illustrating the cross-granulocyte talk that occurs in the setting of bronchiectasis [88]. T-cells constitute another key component of the inflammatory response in bronchiectasis [89]. In CF, high T-helper 2 (Th2) [90, 91] and Th17 [91] responses are observed. Th2 cytokines such as IL-4, - 13 and TARC/CCL17 are correlated with a decreased pulmonary function in CF-*Pseudomonas*-colonized patients. Th17 cells, neutrophils and NKT cells are found in abundance in all-cause bronchiectasis compared to healthy controls [92]. While high Th17 infiltrates independently associate with poorer lung function in CF [93], activation of Th17 antigen-specific pathways have been described in non-CF bronchiectasis [94]. IL-17, a central mediator of the Th17 pathway lacks correlation with bronchiectasis disease phenotypes suggestive of the more prominent role that neutrophil-mediated inflammation likely plays in the pathogenesis of bronchiectasis [94]. Both CD8+ T cells and NKT that express pro-inflammatory IFN-γ and TNF-α have been described in paediatric bronchiectasis [95]. Common pro-inflammatory markers such as TNF-α, IL-8, NE and matrix metalloproteinases − 2, − 8 and − 9 (MMP2, MMP8 and MMP9), are all elevated in bronchiectasis with the latter two indicative of a poorer prognostic outcome [96–100]. A seminal study in CF children identified the key risk factors for bronchiectasis: Sly et al. (2013) showed that elevated airway neutrophil elastase activity was major risk factor and predicted bronchiectasis development [101, 102]. Bacterial load in non-CF bronchiectasis has been correlated with increases in airway (NE, IL-8, IL-1β and TNF-α) and systemic (ICAM-1, E-selectin) derived inflammatory markers, phenomena confirmed in vitro using bronchial epithelial cell lines treated with sputum from bronchiectasis patients [103, 104]. Exacerbations of both CF and non-CF bronchiectasis increases inflammation irrespective of bacterial, viral or fungal causation [43, 105, 106]. Interestingly, sTREM-1 a novel inflammatory marker described in a variety of pulmonary disease states including COPD, has also been identified in children with both CF- and HIV-related bronchiectasis although concentrations in the latter setting are highest. High sTREM-1 levels correlate closely with lung function decline and future studies should explore sTREM-1 levels in bronchiectasis of other aetiologies to better understand its role in the pathogenesis of bronchiectasis [107]. Vitamin-D deficiency, observed in CF [108, 109] is associated with increased bacterial infection, exacerbations and poorer lung function [110–112]. This is corroborated in non-CF bronchiectasis where it indicates disease severity and associates with more infection, bacterial colonization, airway inflammation and consequently frequent exacerbations [113].

Clinical characteristics and management of bronchiectasis

Bronchietasis patients are clinically characterized by sputum production (upon exercise or spontaneously) leading to productive coughing with mucopurulent masses of yellowish, greenish or brown sputum in the morning or over the day. However, bronchiectasis are mainly detected at time points when irreversible structural damage has already been done to the airway architecture. Bronchiectasis initially may be reversible in children, later probably not. Major genetic diseases associated with bronchiectasis include CF, primary ciliary dyskinesia (PCD, Kartagener syndrome), alpha 1-antitrypsin deficiency, primary immunodeficiencies or other rare disorders like Williams-Campbell syndrome and Marfan syndrome. Major acquired causes are severe bacterial infections (*Tuberculosis*, *Staphylococcus*, *Klebsiella* and others) or postinfectious bronchiolitis obliterans. Notably, also fungal infections can lead to bronchiectasis, particularly ABPA, as a chronic Th2-driven *Aspergillus fumigatus*-caused pulmonary condition. Based on this, it is essential in the clinical work-up of patients featuring bronchiectasis to screen for these congenital and acquired conditions in order to tailor appropriate treatments and to attenuate disease progression. In a preventive manner, it is key in the above mentioned conditions to diagnose and monitor for pulmonary symptoms and structural changes (using pulmonary function testing and high-resolution computed tomography, HRCT) to avoid established bronchiectasis-related disease. To this end, it is helpful to follow a concept that has been introduced previously to classify forms of bronchitis in children [114–116]. An acute bronchitis, usually triggered by a viral infection, resolves within days or one to two weeks. Sometimes – for many reasons of which most are unknown – symptoms do not resolve spontaneously, but persist. This state is called protracted bacterial bronchitis (PBB). While PBB has been initially established for pediatrics, current publications have discussed and transferred this concept to adults {Birring, 2015 #16382;Gibson, 2010 #16381;Martin, 2015 #16380}. PBB is further differentiated into various forms, depending on the tools used to diagnose it [114, 115]. PBB can be further characterized based on different stratifiers:

- PBB-microbiologic ("PBB-micro"): (1) presence of chronic wet cough (> 4 weeks), (2) respiratory bacterial pathogens growing in sputum or BAL at density of a single bacterial specifies > 10^4 colony-forming units/ml, and (3) cough resolves following a 2-week course of an appropriate oral antibiotic (usually amoxicillin-clavulanate)
- PBB-clinical: (1) presence of chronic wet cough (> 4 weeks), (2) absence of symptoms or signs of other causes of wet or productive cough, (3) cough resolves following a 2-week course of an appropriate oral antibiotic (usually amoxicillin-clavulanate)
- PBB-extended: as above, but cough resolves only after 4 weeks of antibiotics
- PBB-recurrent: > 3 episodes of PBB per year

Based on this concept, it is believed that, if left untreated, a fraction of PBBs will progress to chronic suppurative lung disease (CSLD) with radiologically confirmed bronchiectasis (Fig. 1). CSLD differs from bronchiectasis only by lacking the radiographic signs of bronchiectasis on HRCT scans. Clinically, CSLD is diagnosed in children whose chronic wet cough does not resolve with oral antibiotics and in whom other causes are excluded [117, 118]. Although not proven formally for all causes of bronchiectasis, the sequence of progression from PBB over CSLD to bronchiectasis is highly likely, but needs to be substantiated with prospective studies. Of interest is the recent finding that otherwise healthy children with PBB, children with bronchiectasis, and children with CF shared similar core airway microbiota patterns, with *H. influenzae* making the greatest contribution to the observed similarity, while the microbiota in adults with CF and bronchiectasis were significantly different [25]. The authors concluded that chronic airway infections starts similarly with defective airway clearance, but over time with intervention and host factors, i.e. the underlying cause, progressively diverge.

The prevalence of bronchiectasis in children with CF has recently been assessed in studies conducted by the Australian Respiratory Early Surveillance Team for Cystic Fibrosis (AREST CF) and others. Although 50–70% of CF patients have CT-defined bronchiectasis by 3 to 5 years of age [119], most young children have isolated, i.e. localized disease, with only the mildest severity of lung abnormalities and lobar disease extent that is well below 50% [120–122]. On the other hand, it is clear that

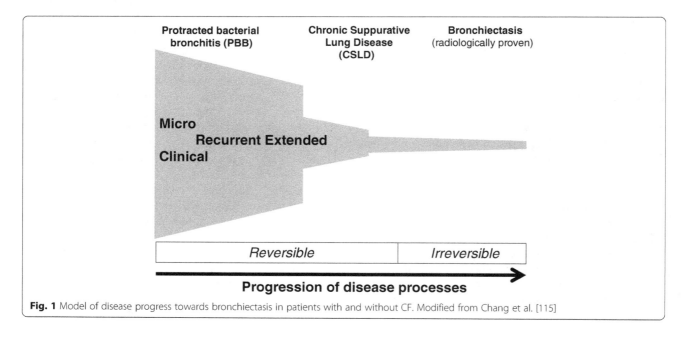

Fig. 1 Model of disease progress towards bronchiectasis in patients with and without CF. Modified from Chang et al. [115]

once established, bronchiectasis persists and/or progresses despite current optimized standard-of-care therapies in about 75% of young children [121, 122]. Currently great effort is undertaken to close the diagnostic gap from 0 to about 5 years of age, to non-invasively assess the extent of lung disease. The PRAGMA-CF score was developed as a sensitive and reproducible outcome measure for assessing the extent of lung disease in very young children with CF [123]. Moreover, the lung clearance index is a measure of ventilation distribution obtained by the multiple-breath washout technique. Several studies have shown its sensitivity to airway disease in CF and other bronchial diseases [124, 125]. However, in infants with CF, lung clearance index was insensitive to structural disease, as assessed by PRAGMA scoring [126]. In preschool and school-age children with CF's lung clearance index correlated with total disease extent. Of interest, it had good positive predictive value of about 85%, but a poor negative predictive value of 55% to detect bronchiectasis. Therefore, lung clearance index may be a good surveillance tool to monitor structural lung disease up to school-age in CF [126]. In an effort to identify the preceding-stages of bronchiectasis in CF children by using at least four consecutive biennial volumetric CTs, areas with bronchiectasis on CT scans were marked, further analyzed and associated to potential pre-stages, which were mucus plugging (18%), airway wall thickening (2%) or atelectasis/consolidation in 1% [127].

The basic clinical management of bronchiectasis includes tailored antimicrobial therapy and airway clearance techniques. The latter include mucolytics, such as hypertonic saline and rhDNA, as well as chest physiotherapy and vigorous physical sporting activities. In PBB, oral antibiotics for 2 weeks up to several months have been described to be helpful. Antibiotics commonly used in the clinics include amoxicillin, amoxicillin-clavulanate or second generation cephalosporins. Particularly in patients with CF, gram-negative organisms are treated with inhaled tobramycin, colistin, actreonam or levofloxacin as well as oral inhibitors of gyrases, i.e. ciprofloxacin. The duration of treatment should be guided by symptoms; goal is a symptom-free patient. This can be mostly achieved in young children or patients in the stages of PBB, CSLD and the early stages of bronchiectasis. More specific treatment strategies in bronchiectasis depend on the underlying etiology and include protein augmentation (alpha 1-antitrypsin deficiency), anti-allergic approaches (asthma/ABPA) and/or immunoglobulin substitution (immunodeficiencies).

Imaging of bronchiectasis in CF lung disease

Detection and characterization of bronchiectasis are the domain of thin-section computed tomography (CT). High-resolution CT (HRCT) with 0.6 to 1.5 mm slice thickness serves as a reference standard for imaging. However, pulmonary MRI has gained interest due to the possibility of functional imaging without radiation burden. Moreover, new technical developments overcome the limitations of low MR-signal and low spatial resolution. In CF, standardized reporting using scores or automated quantification are essential requisites to measure and track findings, particularly when results focus on risk stratification. In this context, bronchiectasis is one of the important imaging markers and generally correlates with clinical outcome.

Imaging characteristics of bronchiectasis

Bronchiectasis is defined as irreversible dilation of bronchi in cylindrical, varicose, or a more cystic morphological appearance. In CF, it is often associated with mucus plugging, bronchial wall thickening, and small airway disease [128, 129]. The radiological evaluation of bronchiectasis is based on definition published in the terms for thoracic imaging of the Fleischner Society [130]: *"Morphologic criteria on thin-section CT scans include bronchial dilatation with respect to the accompanying pulmonary artery (signet ring sign), lack of tapering of bronchi, and identification of bronchi within 1 cm of the pleural surface."* The so-called signet ring sign is the primary sign for bronchiectasis representing a ring-shaped opacity, whereas the smaller adjacent artery stays for the signet. According to this concept, the extent of bronchial dilation can be quantified using the ratio between bronchi and vessels [128], an approach challenged by a recent pediatric study [131]. On HRCT, the bronchial tree is only visible up to the 6-8th generation [130]. CT findings like the tree-in-bud sign and centrilobular opacity are linked to small airway disease with dilation and inflammation of the ronchiole or mucus plugging in its periphery (Fig. 2) [130]. There are differences in CF bronchiectasis depending on pancreas insufficiency (PI), with PI patients illustrating more severe bronchiectasis [132]. Primary ciliary dyskinesia (PCD) patients have similar CT scores as pancreatic-sufficient (PS) CF patients, but in contrast to CF, no correlation between structural change and clinical parameters has been detected in a previous study [133]. However, recent studies in adult PCD patient cohorts indicate that CT findings relate to lung function changes [134, 135]. There are no clear identifiers of pre-bronchiectasis in imaging. However, mucus plugging has been shown to be a common precursor in CF [127].

Imaging can illustrate lung damage even when lung function (such as forced expiratory volume in 1 s, FEV1) is normal [128, 136, 137] (Fig. 3). In contrast to imaging, pulmonary function tests (PFT) are challenging in young children. A complementary role with lung clearance index (LCI) has been described [138]. Regarding the

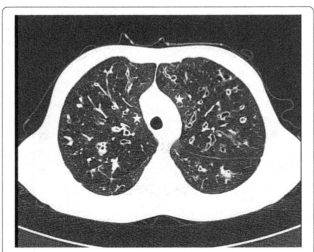

Fig. 2 15 y/o male, CF-patient, FEV$_1$ predicted 45%. Thin-section HR-reconstruction from MDCT (effective dose of 1.5 mSv). Severe bronchiectasis is visible. Note also dilated bronchi within the periphery of the lung. Air trapping is noted, only in central parenchyma, the CT attenuation appears normal (asterisks)

evaluation of the presence and extent of bronchiectasis, CT imaging is accepted as the most sensitive and reproducible modality to date. Using new generation dual source multidetector CT (MDCT) maintaining subsecond acquisition of the whole lung breathing and pulsation artifacts are negligible even in young children and no sedation is needed [139, 140]. Finally, using spectral beam shaping and iterative reconstruction algorithms, ultralow-dose pediatric chest CT can be realized with an effective dose below 0.3 mSv [139]. These conditions, therefore, challenge the routine use of MRI. On the other hand, there are a couple of reasons supporting MRI. The radiation burden of routinely performed volumetric chest CT may be many times higher than that of a third generation of dual source CT recently published. Incremental HRCT with significant gaps lowers the dose but also diagnostic performance and leads to more motion artifact in the pediatric population [141]. Estimated risk of radiation-induced cancer from a pediatric chest CT is small but not negligible, particularly in cases of repeated exposure [142, 143]. MRI has no side effects by radiation enabling long-term surveillance of lung damage. The overall diagnostic performance by scores evaluation of MRI in direct comparison to CT is good to excellent [144–146] (Fig. 4). Moreover, apart from polarized 3+ Helium imaging, functional imaging can be easily implemented using perfusion or ventilation weighted standard proton MRI that assesses small airway disease [146–149] (Fig. 5).

Clinical value

Standardized reporting of cross-sectional imaging by scoring systems is suitable for several reasons: (a) to assess and to quantify individual progression of lung damage in comparison or complementary to lung function testing, (b) to use total or partial score values as endpoints for interventional studies, and (c) to establish predictive imaging biomarkers. Most CT scoring systems use a semiquantitative scale for the extent and severity of specific findings either based on lobe, involved bronchopulmonary segments, or using an overlay grid [128, 129, 150]. According to the disease-specific prevalence from the imaging

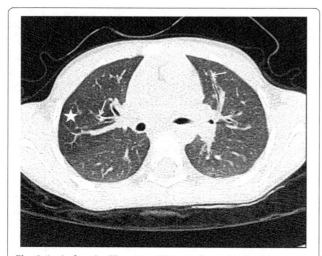

Fig. 3 6 y/o female CF-patient, FEV$_1$ predicted 105%. Thin-section HR-reconstruction from MDCT (effective dose of 1 mSv). Mild bronchiectasis, bronchial wall thickening (arrows) and mosaic attenuation (asterisk) are visible

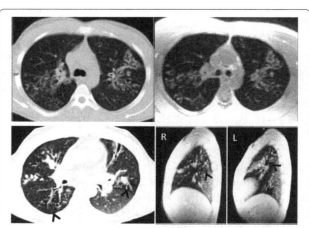

Fig. 4 29 y/o male CF-patient, FEV1 predicted 67%. Left side CT, right side MRI at the same day. Upper row, transverse thin-section images from 3D acquisition in breath hold (CT and MRI). Note, despite lower resolution and signal to noise a similar depiction of bronchiectasis is possible. Lower row, expiration images (transverse CT and saggital MRI). In both modalities focal air trapping within the same lung region is demonstrated (arrow heads)

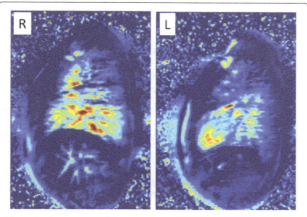

Fig. 5 Perfusion map of same patient as in fig. 4 using the noninvasive arterial-spin-labeling technique without contrast media application. The relevant perfusion differences between upper and lower lung regions correlate with morphological damage and air trapping

abnormalities, sub-scores for bronchiectasis and bronchial wall thickening are more heavily weighted (1, 2). Inter-observer and intra-observer agreement of the common CT scores has shown to be good to excellent [128, 129]. Comparable reproducibility has also been found for MRI using CT or MR-specific adapted scoring systems in small numbers of studies [144, 148]. For semiautomatic evaluation of bronchi dimension excellent inter-observer agreement has been found particularly for the bronchial lumen [151]. On the other hand, mucus can obscure or mimic bronchial wall thickening. Apart from reproducibility, the weighting of abnormalities within the scores, and validation are even more challenging and related to the purpose and the use of score (e.g. interventional or clinical study). As aforementioned imaging is more sensitive than FEV1 particularly in mild disease, and, in assessment of disease progression [128, 136, 137, 152]. In this context scoring of bronchiectasis particularly in the lung periphery is important [137], whereas air trapping, mosaic perfusion, and mucus plugging seem to be more sensitive markers than CT or MRI which detect effects of interventions [153, 154]. The role of bronchiectasis as a robust predictive marker has been shown in several longitudinal observations [150, 155–159]. The extent of bronchiectasis at baseline can predict the number of respiratory tract exacerbations (RTE) [155–158], and the change of the subscore in a two year follow up is strongly associated with numbers of RTEs where FEV1 did not provide value [156]. This has been similarly described for a decade long observational study [158]. In an older study, a maximum combined score for bronchiectasis and emphysema on HRCT was indicative of a poorer prognosis [159]. In a recent study of patients with severe lung disease awaiting lung transplantation, the combined score of bronchiectasis, bronchial wall thickening, mucus, and consolidation was associated with mortality [150].

Conclusions

Bronchiectasis is a heterogeneous and complex condition and remains a challenge for both diagnostic and therapeutic strategies. While pathomechanisms in the pulmonary compartment share commonalities from a microbiological and immunological perspective, clinical implications and treatment approaches remain challenging and individualized, depending on the underlying disease and the infection status. High-resolution imaging has revolutionized the diagnosis and monitoring of bronchiectasis and will further pave the way for a more precise understanding of disease pathogenesis and treatment response in the future. Therapeutically, lessons learned from the well-known phenotype of CF bronchiectasis are increasingly transferred to the multifaceted genotype and phenotype of non-CF bronchiectasis. Airway infections are treated with inhaled and systemic antibiotics. Mucus clearance can be improved by inhaled therapies and chest physiotherapy, whereas specific anti-inflammatory approaches have still not been clinically established. Prospective future studies are urgently needed to optimize the diagnostic and therapeutic management of bronchiectasis, particularly in children with non-CF bronchiectasis, an indication with a high unmet medical need.

Funding
This research has been supported by the Singapore Ministry of Health's National Medical Research Council under its Transition Award (NMRC/TA/0048/2016) (S.H.C). The funding had no impact on the writing of the manuscript.

Authors' contributions
JS wrote large parts of the manuscript and created most of the Figs. 2 3 4 and 5. MG, RC and SC wrote major parts of the manuscript and created Fig. 1. DH supervised the whole process and wrote major parts of the manuscript. All authors read and approved the final manuscript.

Competing interests
Sanjay Chotirmall is a member of the editorial board (Section Editor). Dominik Hartl has an affiliation with University of Tübingen and Roche Basel (I3-DTA, pRED). All other authors declare that they have no competing interests.

Author details
[1]Department of Radiology, Division of Pediatric Radiology, University of Tübingen, Tübingen, Germany. [2]Children's Hospital, University of Munich, Munich, Germany. [3]Lee Kong Chian School of Medicine, Nanyang Technological University, Singapore, Singapore. [4]Department of Pediatrics I, University of Tübingen, Tübingen, Germany. [5]Roche Pharma Research & Early Development (pRED), Immunology, Inflammation and Infectious Diseases (I3) Discovery and Translational Area, Roche Innovation Center, Basel, Switzerland.

References

1. Chalmers JD, Aliberti S, Blasi F. Management of bronchiectasis in adults. Eur Respir J. 2015;45(5):1446–62.
2. Sidhu MK, Mandal P, Hill AT. Bronchiectasis: an update on current pharmacotherapy and future perspectives. Expert Opin Pharmacother. 2014; 15(4):505–25.
3. McShane PJ, Naureckas ET, Tino G, Strek ME. Non-cystic fibrosis bronchiectasis. Am J Respir Crit Care Med. 2013;188(6):647–56.
4. Boyton RJ, Altmann DM. Bronchiectasis: current concepts in pathogenesis, immunology, and microbiology. Annu Rev Pathol. 2016;11:523–54.
5. Moulton BC, Barker AF. Pathogenesis of bronchiectasis. Clin Chest Med. 2012;33(2):211–7.
6. Stockley RA. Neutrophils and protease/antiprotease imbalance. Am J Respir Crit Care Med. 1999;160(5 Pt 2):S49–52.
7. Taggart CC, Greene CM, Carroll TP, O'Neill SJ, McElvaney NG. Elastolytic proteases: inflammation resolution and dysregulation in chronic infective lung disease. Am J Respir Crit Care Med. 2005;171(10):1070–6.
8. Rab A, Rowe SM, Raju SV, Bebok Z, Matalon S, Collawn JF. Cigarette smoke and CFTR: implications in the pathogenesis of COPD. Am J Physiol Lung Cell Mol Physiol. 2013;305(8):L530–41.
9. Moran Losada P, Chouvarine P, Dorda M, Hedtfeld S, Mielke S, Schulz A, Wiehlmann L, Tummler B: The cystic fibrosis lower airways microbial metagenome. ERJ Open Res. 2016;2(2):96–115.
10. Bacci G, Paganin P, Lopez L, Vanni C, Dalmastri C, Cantale C, Daddiego L, Perrotta G, Dolce D, Morelli P et al: Pyrosequencing unveils cystic fibrosis lung microbiome differences associated with a severe lung function decline. 2016, 11(6):e0156807.
11. King PT, Holdsworth SR, Freezer NJ, Villanueva E, Holmes PW. Microbiologic follow-up study in adult bronchiectasis. Respir Med. 2007;101(8):1633–8.
12. Kapur N, Grimwood K, Masters IB, Morris PS, Chang AB. Lower airway microbiology and cellularity in children with newly diagnosed non-CF bronchiectasis. Pediatr Pulmonol. 2012;47(3):300–7.
13. Grimwood K. The pathogenesis of Pseudomonas aeruginosa lung infections in cystic fibrosis. J Paediatr Child Health. 1992;28(1):4–11.
14. Evans SA, Turner SM, Bosch BJ, Hardy CC, Woodhead MA. Lung function in bronchiectasis: the influence of Pseudomonas aeruginosa. Eur Respir J. 1996;9(8):1601–4.
15. Davies G, Wells AU, Doffman S, Watanabe S, Wilson R. The effect of Pseudomonas aeruginosa on pulmonary function in patients with bronchiectasis. Eur Respir J. 2006;28(5):974–9.
16. Hector A, Kirn T, Ralhan A, Graepler-Mainka U, Berenbrinker S, Riethmueller J, Hogardt M, Wagner M, Pfleger A, Autenrieth I, et al. Microbial colonization and lung function in adolescents with cystic fibrosis. J Cystic Fibros. 2016; 15(3):340–9.
17. Konstan MW, Wagener JS, Vandevanter DR, Pasta DJ, Yegin A, Rasouliyan L, Morgan WJ. Risk factors for rate of decline in FEV1 in adults with cystic fibrosis. J Cystic Fibros. 2012;11(4):405–11.
18. Ren CL, Konstan MW, Yegin A, Rasouliyan L, Trzaskoma B, Morgan WJ, Regelmann W. Multiple antibiotic-resistant Pseudomonas aeruginosa and lung function decline in patients with cystic fibrosis. J Cystic Fibros. 2012; 11(4):293–9.
19. Harun SN, Wainwright C, Klein K, Hennig S: A systematic review of studies examining the rate of lung function decline in patients with cystic fibrosis. Paediatr Respir Rev. 2016;20:55–66.
20. McDonnell MJ, Jary HR, Perry A, MacFarlane JG, Hester KL, Small T, Molyneux C, Perry JD, Walton KE, De Soyza A. Non cystic fibrosis bronchiectasis: a longitudinal retrospective observational cohort study of Pseudomonas persistence and resistance. Respir Med. 2015;109(6):716–26.
21. Emerson J, Rosenfeld M, McNamara S, Ramsey B, Gibson RL. Pseudomonas aeruginosa and other predictors of mortality and morbidity in young children with cystic fibrosis. Pediatr Pulmonol. 2002;34(2):91–100.
22. Rogers GB, Zain NM, Bruce KD, Burr LD, Chen AC, Rivett DW, McGuckin MA, Serisier DJ. A novel microbiota stratification system predicts future exacerbations in bronchiectasis. Ann Am Thorac Soc. 2014;11(4):496–503.
23. Chalmers JD, Goeminne P, Aliberti S, McDonnell MJ, Lonni S, Davidson J, Poppelwell L, Salih W, Pesci A, Dupont LJ, et al. The bronchiectasis severity index. An international derivation and validation study. Am J Respir Crit Care Med. 2014;189(5):576–85.
24. Martinez-Garcia MA, de Gracia J, Vendrell Relat M, Giron RM, Maiz Carro L, de la Rosa CD, Olveira C. Multidimensional approach to non-cystic fibrosis bronchiectasis: the FACED score. Eur Respir J. 2014;43(5):1357–67.
25. van der Gast CJ, Cuthbertson L, Rogers GB, Pope C, Marsh RL, Redding GJ, Bruce KD, Chang AB, Hoffman LR. Three clinically distinct chronic pediatric airway infections share a common core microbiota. Ann Am Thorac Soc. 2014;11(7):1039–48.
26. Rogers GB, van der Gast CJ, Cuthbertson L, Thomson SK, Bruce KD, Martin ML, Serisier DJ. Clinical measures of disease in adult non-CF bronchiectasis correlate with airway microbiota composition. Thorax. 2013;68(8):731–7.
27. Tunney MM, Einarsson GG, Wei L, Drain M, Klem ER, Cardwell C, Ennis M, Boucher RC, Wolfgang MC, Elborn JS. Lung microbiota and bacterial abundance in patients with bronchiectasis when clinically stable and during exacerbation. Am J Respir Crit Care Med. 2013;187(10):1118–26.
28. Rogers GB, van der Gast CJ, Serisier DJ. Predominant pathogen competition and core microbiota divergence in chronic airway infection. Isme j. 2015; 9(1):217–25.
29. Fowler SJ, French J, Screaton NJ, Foweraker J, Condliffe A, Haworth CS, Exley AR, Bilton D. Nontuberculous mycobacteria in bronchiectasis: prevalence and patient characteristics. Eur Respir J. 2006;28(6):1204–10.
30. Chu H, Zhao L, Xiao H, Zhang Z, Zhang J, Gui T, Gong S, Xu L, Sun X. Prevalence of nontuberculous mycobacteria in patients with bronchiectasis: a meta-analysis. Arch Med Sci. 2014;10(4):661–8.
31. Viviani L, Harrison MJ, Zolin A, Haworth CS, Floto RA. Epidemiology of nontuberculous mycobacteria (NTM) amongst individuals with cystic fibrosis (CF). J Cystic Fibros. 2016;15(5):619–23.
32. Roux AL, Catherinot E, Ripoll F, Soismier N, Macheras E, Ravilly S, Bellis G, Vibet MA, Le Roux E, Lemonnier L, et al. Multicenter study of prevalence of nontuberculous mycobacteria in patients with cystic fibrosis in France. J Clin Microbiol. 2009;47(12):4124–8.
33. Seddon P, Fidler K, Raman S, Wyatt H, Ruiz G, Elston C, Perrin F, Gyi K, Bilton D, Drobniewski F, et al. Prevalence of nontuberculous mycobacteria in cystic fibrosis clinics, United Kingdom, 2009. Emerg Infect Dis. 2013;19(7):1128–30.
34. Candido PH, Nunes Lde S, Marques EA, Folescu TW, Coelho FS, de Moura VC, da Silva MG, Gomes KM, Lourenco MC, Aguiar FS, et al. Multidrug-resistant nontuberculous mycobacteria isolated from cystic fibrosis patients. J Clin Microbiol. 2014;52(8):2990–7.
35. Mirsaeidi M, Hadid W, Ericsoussi B, Rodgers D, Sadikot RT. Non-tuberculous mycobacterial disease is common in patients with non-cystic fibrosis bronchiectasis. Int J Infect Dis. 2013;17(11):e1000–4.
36. Wickremasinghe M, Ozerovitch LJ, Davies G, Wodehouse T, Chadwick MV, Abdallah S, Shah P, Wilson R. Non-tuberculous mycobacteria in patients with bronchiectasis. Thorax. 2005;60(12):1045–51.
37. Faverio P, Stainer A, Bonaiti G, Zucchetti SC, Simonetta E, Lapadula G, Marruchella A, Gori A, Blasi F, Codecasa L et al: Characterizing Non-Tuberculous Mycobacteria Infection in Bronchiectasis. Int J Mol Sci. 2016;17(11):1913–18.
38. Maiz L, Giron R, Olveira C, Vendrell M, Nieto R, Martinez-Garcia MA. Prevalence and factors associated with nontuberculous mycobacteria in non-cystic fibrosis bronchiectasis: a multicenter observational study. BMC Infect Dis. 2016;16(1):437.
39. Esther CR Jr, Esserman DA, Gilligan P, Kerr A, Noone PG. Chronic Mycobacterium abscessus infection and lung function decline in cystic fibrosis. J Cystic Fibros. 2010;9(2):117–23.
40. Martiniano SL, Nick JA. Nontuberculous mycobacterial infections in cystic fibrosis. Clin Chest Med. 2015;36(1):101–15.
41. Qvist T, Taylor-Robinson D, Waldmann E, Olesen HV, Hansen CR, Mathiesen IH, Hoiby N, Katzenstein TL, Smyth RL, Diggle PJ, et al. Comparing the harmful effects of nontuberculous mycobacteria and gram negative bacteria on lung function in patients with cystic fibrosis. J Cystic Fibros. 2016;15(3):380–5.
42. Mussaffi H, Rivlin J, Shalit I, Ephros M, Blau H. Nontuberculous mycobacteria in cystic fibrosis associated with allergic bronchopulmonary aspergillosis and steroid therapy. Eur Respir J. 2005;25(2):324–8.
43. Gao YH, Guan WJ, Xu G, Lin ZY, Tang Y, Lin ZM, Gao Y, Li HM, Zhong NS, Zhang GJ, et al. The role of viral infection in pulmonary exacerbations of bronchiectasis in adults: a prospective study. Chest. 2015;147(6):1635–43.
44. Wat D, Gelder C, Hibbitts S, Cafferty F, Bowler I, Pierrepoint M, Evans R, Doull I. The role of respiratory viruses in cystic fibrosis. J Cystic Fibros. 2008; 7(4):320–8.
45. Kieninger E, Singer F, Tapparel C, Alves MP, Latzin P, Tan HL, Bossley C, Casaulta C, Bush A, Davies JC, et al. High rhinovirus burden in lower airways of children with cystic fibrosis. Chest. 2013;143(3):782–90.
46. Kapur N, Mackay IM, Sloots TP, Masters IB, Chang AB. Respiratory viruses in

47. Chotirmall SH, McElvaney NG. Fungi in the cystic fibrosis lung: bystanders or pathogens? Int J Biochem Cell Biol. 2014;52:161–73.
48. Moss RB. Fungi in cystic fibrosis and non-cystic fibrosis bronchiectasis. Semin Respir Crit Care Med. 2015;36(2):207–16.
49. Knutsen AP, Bush RK, Demain JG, Denning DW, Dixit A, Fairs A, Greenberger PA, Kariuki B, Kita H, Kurup VP, et al. Fungi and allergic lower respiratory tract diseases. J Allergy Clin Immunol. 2012;129(2):280–91. quiz 292-283
50. Sudfeld CR, Dasenbrook EC, Merz WG, Carroll KC, Boyle MP. Prevalence and risk factors for recovery of filamentous fungi in individuals with cystic fibrosis. J Cystic Fibros. 2010;9(2):110–6.
51. Cimon B, Symoens F, Zouhair R, Chabasse D, Nolard N, Defontaine A, Bouchara JP. Molecular epidemiology of airway colonisation by aspergillus fumigatus in cystic fibrosis patients. J Med Microbiol. 2001;50(4):367–74.
52. Cimon B, Zouhair R, Symoens F, Carrere J, Chabasse D, Bouchara JP. Aspergillus terreus in a cystic fibrosis clinic: environmental distribution and patient colonization pattern. J Hosp Infect. 2003;53(1):81–2.
53. Chotirmall SH, Al-Alawi M, Mirkovic B, Lavelle G, Logan PM, Greene CM, McElvaney NG. Aspergillus-associated airway disease, inflammation, and the innate immune response. Biomed Res Int. 2013;2013:723129.
54. Kraemer R, Delosea N, Ballinari P, Gallati S, Crameri R. Effect of allergic bronchopulmonary aspergillosis on lung function in children with cystic fibrosis. Am J Respir Crit Care Med. 2006;174(11):1211–20.
55. Wojnarowski C, Eichler I, Gartner C, Gotz M, Renner S, Koller DY, Frischer T. Sensitization to aspergillus fumigatus and lung function in children with cystic fibrosis. Am J Respir Crit Care Med. 1997;155(6):1902–7.
56. McMahon MA, Chotirmall SH, McCullagh B, Branagan P, McElvaney NG, Logan PM. Radiological abnormalities associated with aspergillus colonization in a cystic fibrosis population. Eur J Radiol. 2012;81(3):e197–202.
57. Maiz L, Vendrell M, Olveira C, Giron R, Nieto R, Martinez-Garcia MA. Prevalence and factors associated with isolation of aspergillus and Candida from sputum in patients with non-cystic fibrosis bronchiectasis. Respiration. 2015;89(5):396–403.
58. Menzies D, Holmes L, McCumesky G, Prys-Picard C, Niven R. Aspergillus sensitization is associated with airflow limitation and bronchiectasis in severe asthma. Allergy. 2011;66(5):679–85.
59. Fairs A, Agbetile J, Hargadon B, Bourne M, Monteiro WR, Brightling CE, Bradding P, Green RH, Mutalithas K, Desai D, et al. IgE sensitization to aspergillus fumigatus is associated with reduced lung function in asthma. Am J Respir Crit Care Med. 2010;182(11):1362–8.
60. Chotirmall SH, Greene CM, McElvaney NG. Candida species in cystic fibrosis: a road less travelled. Med Mycol. 2010;48(Suppl 1):S114–24.
61. Chotirmall SH, O'Donoghue E, Bennett K, Gunaratnam C, O'Neill SJ, McElvaney NG. Sputum Candida albicans presages FEV(1) decline and hospital-treated exacerbations in cystic fibrosis. Chest. 2010;138(5):1186–95.
62. Dente FL, Bilotta M, Bartoli ML, Bacci E, Cianchetti S, Latorre M, Malagrino L, Nieri D, Roggi MA, Vagaggini B, et al. Neutrophilic bronchial inflammation correlates with clinical and functional findings in patients with noncystic fibrosis bronchiectasis. Mediat Inflamm. 2015;2015:642503.
63. Watt AP, Brown V, Courtney J, Kelly M, Garske L, Elborn JS, Ennis M. Neutrophil apoptosis, proinflammatory mediators and cell counts in bronchiectasis. Thorax. 2004;59(3):231–6.
64. Wilson CB, Jones PW, O'Leary CJ, Hansell DM, Dowling RB, Cole PJ, Wilson R. Systemic markers of inflammation in stable bronchiectasis. Eur Respir J. 1998;12(4):820–4.
65. Mikami M, Llewellyn-Jones CG, Bayley D, Hill SL, Stockley RA. The chemotactic activity of sputum from patients with bronchiectasis. Am J Respir Crit Care Med. 1998;157(3 Pt 1):723–8.
66. Dean TP, Dai Y, Shute JK, Church MK, Warner JO. Interleukin-8 concentrations are elevated in bronchoalveolar lavage, sputum, and sera of children with cystic fibrosis. Pediatr Res. 1993;34(2):159–61.
67. Armstrong DS, Grimwood K, Carlin JB, Carzino R, Gutierrez JP, Hull J, Olinsky A, Phelan EM, Robertson CF, Phelan PD. Lower airway inflammation in infants and young children with cystic fibrosis. Am J Respir Crit Care Med. 1997;156(4 Pt 1):1197–204.
68. Ayhan G, Tas D, Yilmaz I, Okutan O, Demirer E, Ayten O, Kartaloglu Z. Relation between inflammatory cytokine levels in serum and bronchoalveolar lavage fluid and gene polymorphism in young adult patients with bronchiectasis. J Thorac Dis. 2014;6(6):684–93.
69. Hartl D, Latzin P, Hordijk P, Marcos V, Rudolph C, Woischnik M, Krauss-Etschmann S, Koller B, Reinhardt D, Roscher AA, et al. Cleavage of CXCR1 on neutrophils disables bacterial killing in cystic fibrosis lung disease. Nat Med. 2007;13(12):1423–30.
70. Chalmers JD, Moffitt KL, Suarez-Cuartin G, Sibila O, Finch S, Furrie E, Dicker A, Wrobel K, Elborn JS, Walker B et al: Neutrophil Elastase Activity is Associated with Exacerbations and Lung Function Decline in Bronchiectasis. American journal of respiratory and critical care medicine 2016.
71. Hartl D, Griese M. Surfactant protein D in human lung diseases. Eur J Clin Investig. 2006;36(6):423–35.
72. von Bredow C, Birrer P, Griese M. Surfactant protein a and other bronchoalveolar lavage fluid proteins are altered in cystic fibrosis. Eur Respir J. 2001;17(4):716–22.
73. von Bredow C, Wiesener A, Griese M. Proteolysis of surfactant protein D by cystic fibrosis relevant proteases. Lung. 2003;181(2):79–88.
74. Hartl D, Gaggar A, Bruscia E, Hector A, Marcos V, Jung A, Greene C, McElvaney G, Mall M, Doring G. Innate immunity in cystic fibrosis lung disease. J Cystic Fibros. 2012;11(5):363–82.
75. Tsang KW, Chan K, Ho P, Zheng L, Ooi GC, Ho JC, Lam W. Sputum elastase in steady-state bronchiectasis. Chest. 2000;117(2):420–6.
76. Mayer-Hamblett N, Aitken ML, Accurso FJ, Kronmal RA, Konstan MW, Burns JL, Sagel SD, Ramsey BW. Association between pulmonary function and sputum biomarkers in cystic fibrosis. Am J Respir Crit Care Med. 2007;175(8):822–8.
77. De Soyza A, Pavord I, Elborn JS, Smith D, Wray H, Puu M, Larsson B, Stockley R. A randomised, placebo-controlled study of the CXCR2 antagonist AZD5069 in bronchiectasis. Eur Respir J. 2015;46(4):1021–32.
78. Planaguma A, Domenech T, Pont M, Calama E, Garcia-Gonzalez V, Lopez R, Auli M, Lopez M, Fonquerna S, Ramos I, et al. Combined anti CXC receptors 1 and 2 therapy is a promising anti-inflammatory treatment for respiratory diseases by reducing neutrophil migration and activation. Pulm Pharmacol Ther. 2015;34:37–45.
79. Morris MR, Doull IJ, Dewitt S, Hallett MB. Reduced iC3b-mediated phagocytotic capacity of pulmonary neutrophils in cystic fibrosis. Clin Exp Immunol. 2005;142(1):68–75.
80. Houston N, Stewart N, Smith DS, Bell SC, Champion AC, Reid DW. Sputum neutrophils in cystic fibrosis patients display a reduced respiratory burst. J Cystic Fibros. 2013;12(4):352–62.
81. King P, Bennett-Wood V, Hutchinson P, Robins-Browne R, Holmes P, Freezer N, Holdsworth S. Bactericidal activity of neutrophils with reduced oxidative burst from adults with bronchiectasis. APMIS. 2009;117(2):133–9.
82. Shum DK, Chan SC, Ip MS. Neutrophil-mediated degradation of lung proteoglycans: stimulation by tumor necrosis factor-alpha in sputum of patients with bronchiectasis. Am J Respir Crit Care Med. 2000;162(5):1925–31.
83. Voglis S, Quinn K, Tullis E, Liu M, Henriques M, Zubrinich C, Penuelas O, Chan H, Silverman F, Cherepanov V, et al. Human neutrophil peptides and phagocytic deficiency in bronchiectatic lungs. Am J Respir Crit Care Med. 2009;180(2):159–66.
84. Koller DY, Gotz M, Eichler I, Urbanek R. Eosinophilic activation in cystic fibrosis. Thorax. 1994;49(5):496–9.
85. Koller DY, Urbanek R, Gotz M. Increased degranulation of eosinophil and neutrophil granulocytes in cystic fibrosis. Am J Respir Crit Care Med. 1995;152(2):629–33.
86. Kroegel C, Schuler M, Forster M, Braun R, Grahmann PR. Evidence for eosinophil activation in bronchiectasis unrelated to cystic fibrosis and bronchopulmonary aspergillosis: discrepancy between blood eosinophil counts and serum eosinophil cationic protein levels. Thorax. 1998;53(6):498–500.
87. Koller DY, Nilsson M, Enander I, Venge P, Eichler I. Serum eosinophil cationic protein, eosinophil protein X and eosinophil peroxidase in relation to pulmonary function in cystic fibrosis. Clin Exp Allergy. 1998;28(2):241–8.
88. Liu H, Lazarus SC, Caughey GH, Fahy JV. Neutrophil elastase and elastase-rich cystic fibrosis sputum degranulate human eosinophils in vitro. Am J Phys. 1999;276(1 Pt 1):L28–34.
89. Silva JR, Jones JA, Cole PJ, Poulter LW. The immunological component of the cellular inflammatory infiltrate in bronchiectasis. Thorax. 1989;44(8):668–73.
90. Hartl D, Griese M, Kappler M, Zissel G, Reinhardt D, Rebhan C, Schendel DJ, Krauss-Etschmann S. Pulmonary T(H)2 response in Pseudomonas aeruginosa-infected patients with cystic fibrosis. J Allergy Clin Immunol. 2006;117(1):204–11.

91. Tiringer K, Treis A, Fucik P, Gona M, Gruber S, Renner S, Dehlink E, Nachbaur E, Horak F, Jaksch P, et al. A Th17- and Th2-skewed cytokine profile in cystic fibrosis lungs represents a potential risk factor for Pseudomonas aeruginosa infection. Am J Respir Crit Care Med. 2013;187(6):621–9.
92. Tan HL, Regamey N, Brown S, Bush A, Lloyd CM, Davies JC. The Th17 pathway in cystic fibrosis lung disease. Am J Respir Crit Care Med. 2011;184(2):252–8.
93. Mulcahy EM, Hudson JB, Beggs SA, Reid DW, Roddam LF, Cooley MA. High peripheral blood th17 percent associated with poor lung function in cystic fibrosis. PLoS One. 2015;10(3):e0120912.
94. Chen AC, Martin ML, Lourie R, Rogers GB, Burr LD, Hasnain SZ, Bowler SD, McGuckin MA, Serisier DJ. Adult non-cystic fibrosis bronchiectasis is characterised by airway luminal Th17 pathway activation. PLoS One. 2015;10(3):e0119325.
95. Hodge G, Upham JW, Chang AB, Baines KJ, Yerkovich ST, Pizzutto SJ, Hodge S. Increased peripheral blood pro-inflammatory/cytotoxic lymphocytes in children with bronchiectasis. PLoS One. 2015;10(8):e0133695.
96. Bergin DA, Hurley K, Mehta A, Cox S, Ryan D, O'Neill SJ, Reeves EP, McElvaney NG. Airway inflammatory markers in individuals with cystic fibrosis and non-cystic fibrosis bronchiectasis. J Inflamm Res. 2013;6:1–11.
97. Guan WJ, Gao YH, Xu G, Lin ZY, Tang Y, Gu YY, Liu GH, Li HM, Chen RC, Zhong NS. Sputum matrix metalloproteinase-8 and -9 and tissue inhibitor of metalloproteinase-1 in bronchiectasis: clinical correlates and prognostic implications. Respirology. 2015;20(7):1073–81.
98. Guran T, Ersu R, Karadag B, Akpinar IN, Demirel GY, Hekim N, Dagli E. Association between inflammatory markers in induced sputum and clinical characteristics in children with non-cystic fibrosis bronchiectasis. Pediatr Pulmonol. 2007;42(4):362–9.
99. Patel IS, Vlahos I, Wilkinson TM, Lloyd-Owen SJ, Donaldson GC, Wilks M, Reznek RH, Wedzicha JA. Bronchiectasis, exacerbation indices, and inflammation in chronic obstructive pulmonary disease. Am J Respir Crit Care Med. 2004;170(4):400–7.
100. Osika E, Cavaillon JM, Chadelat K, Boule M, Fitting C, Tournier G, Clement A. Distinct sputum cytokine profiles in cystic fibrosis and other chronic inflammatory airway disease. Eur Respir J. 1999;14(2):339–46.
101. Sly PD, Gangell CL, Chen L, Ware RS, Ranganathan S, Mott LS, Murray CP, Stick SM. Risk factors for bronchiectasis in children with cystic fibrosis. N Engl J Med. 2013;368(21):1963–70.
102. Sly PD, Brennan S, Gangell C, de Klerk N, Murray C, Mott L, Stick SM, Robinson PJ, Robertson CF, Ranganathan SC. Lung disease at diagnosis in infants with cystic fibrosis detected by newborn screening. Am J Respir Crit Care Med. 2009;180(2):146–52.
103. Chalmers JD, Smith MP, McHugh BJ, Doherty C, Govan JR, Hill AT. Short- and long-term antibiotic treatment reduces airway and systemic inflammation in non-cystic fibrosis bronchiectasis. Am J Respir Crit Care Med. 2012;186(7):657–65.
104. Angrill J, Agusti C, De Celis R, Filella X, Rano A, Elena M, De La Bellacasa JP, Xaubet A, Torres A. Bronchial inflammation and colonization in patients with clinically stable bronchiectasis. Am J Respir Crit Care Med. 2001;164(9):1628–32.
105. Guan WJ, Gao YH, Xu G, Lin ZY, Tang Y, Li HM, Lin ZM, Jiang M, Zheng JP, Chen RC, et al. Inflammatory responses, spirometry, and quality of life in subjects with bronchiectasis exacerbations. Respir Care. 2015;60(8):1180–9.
106. Brill SE, Patel AR, Singh R, Mackay AJ, Brown JS, Hurst JR. Lung function, symptoms and inflammation during exacerbations of non-cystic fibrosis bronchiectasis: a prospective observational cohort study. Respir Res. 2015;16:16.
107. Masekela R, Anderson R, de Boeck K, Vreys M, Steel HC, Olurunju S, Green RJ. Expression of soluble triggering receptor expressed on myeloid cells-1 in childhood CF and non-CF bronchiectasis. Pediatr Pulmonol. 2015;50(4):333–9.
108. Hall WB, Sparks AA, Aris RM. Vitamin d deficiency in cystic fibrosis. Int J Endocrinol. 2010;2010:218691.
109. Rovner AJ, Stallings VA, Schall JI, Leonard MB, Zemel BS. Vitamin D insufficiency in children, adolescents, and young adults with cystic fibrosis despite routine oral supplementation. Am J Clin Nutr. 2007;86(6):1694–9.
110. Simoneau T, Bazzaz O, Sawicki GS, Gordon C. Vitamin D status in children with cystic fibrosis. Associations with inflammation and bacterial colonization. Ann Am Thorac Soc. 2014;11(2):205–10.
111. Sexauer WP, Hadeh A, Ohman-Strickland PA, Zanni RL, Varlotta L, Holsclaw D, Fiel S, Graff GR, Atlas A, Bisberg D, et al. Vitamin D deficiency is associated with pulmonary dysfunction in cystic fibrosis. J Cystic Fibros. 2015;14(4):497–506.
112. McCauley LA, Thomas W, Laguna TA, Regelmann WE, Moran A, Polgreen LE. Vitamin D deficiency is associated with pulmonary exacerbations in children with cystic fibrosis. Ann Am Thorac Soc. 2014;11(2):198–204.
113. Chalmers JD, McHugh BJ, Docherty C, Govan JR, Hill AT. Vitamin-D deficiency is associated with chronic bacterial colonisation and disease severity in bronchiectasis. Thorax. 2013;68(1):39–47.
114. Wurzel DF, Marchant JM, Yerkovich ST, Upham JW, Petsky HL, Smith-Vaughan H, Masters B, Buntain H, Chang AB. Protracted bacterial bronchitis in children: natural history and risk factors for bronchiectasis. Chest. 2016;150(5):1101–8.
115. Chang AB, Upham JW, Masters IB, Redding GR, Gibson PG, Marchant JM, Grimwood K. Protracted bacterial bronchitis: the last decade and the road ahead. Pediatr Pulmonol. 2016;51(3):225–42.
116. Wurzel DF, Marchant JM, Yerkovich ST, Upham JW, Mackay IM, Masters IB, Chang AB. Prospective characterization of protracted bacterial bronchitis in children. Chest. 2014;145(6):1271–8.
117. Goyal V, Grimwood K, Marchant JM, Masters IB, Chang AB. Paediatric chronic suppurative lung disease: clinical characteristics and outcomes. Eur J Pediatr. 2016;175(8):1077–84.
118. Goyal V, Grimwood K, Marchant J, Masters IB, Chang AB. Pediatric bronchiectasis: no longer an orphan disease. Pediatr Pulmonol. 2016;51(5):450–69.
119. Stick SM, Brennan S, Murray C, Douglas T, von Ungern-Sternberg BS, Garratt LW, Gangell CL, De Klerk N, Linnane B, Ranganathan S, et al. Bronchiectasis in infants and preschool children diagnosed with cystic fibrosis after newborn screening. J Pediatr. 2009;155(5):623–U652.
120. Thia LP, Calder A, Stocks J, Bush A, Owens CM, Wallis C, Young C, Sullivan Y, Wade A, McEwan A, et al. Is chest CT useful in newborn screened infants with cystic fibrosis at 1 year of age? Thorax. 2014;69(4):320–7.
121. Mott LS, Park J, Gangell CL, de Klerk NH, Sly PD, Murray CP, Stick SM, Australian Respiratory Early Surveillance Team for Cystic Fibrosis Study G. Distribution of early structural lung changes due to cystic fibrosis detected with chest computed tomography. J Pediatr. 2013;163(1):243–8. e241-243
122. Mott LS, Park J, Murray CP, Gangell CL, de Klerk NH, Robinson PJ, Robertson CF, Ranganathan SC, Sly PD, Stick SM, et al. Progression of early structural lung disease in young children with cystic fibrosis assessed using CT. Thorax. 2012;67(6):509–16.
123. Rosenow T, Oudraad MC, Murray CP, Turkovic L, Kuo W, de Bruijne M, Ranganathan SC, Tiddens HA, Stick SM, Australian respiratory early surveillance team for cystic F. PRAGMA-CF. a quantitative structural lung disease computed tomography outcome in young children with cystic fibrosis. Am J Respir Crit Care Med. 2015;191(10):1158–65.
124. Kent L, Reix P, Innes JA, Zielen S, Le Bourgeois M, Braggion C, Lever S, Arets HG, Brownlee K, Bradley JM, et al. Lung clearance index: evidence for use in clinical trials in cystic fibrosis. J Cystic Fibros. 2014;13(2):123–38.
125. Fuchs SI, Gappa M. Lung clearance index: clinical and research applications in children. Paediatr Respir Rev. 2011;12(4):264–70.
126. Ramsey KA, Rosenow T, Turkovic L, Skoric B, Banton G, Adams AM, Simpson SJ, Murray C, Ranganathan SC, Stick SM, et al. Lung clearance index and structural lung disease on computed tomography in early cystic fibrosis. Am J Respir Crit Care Med. 2016;193(1):60–7.
127. Tepper LA, Caudri D, Rovira AP, Tiddens HA, de Bruijne M. The development of bronchiectasis on chest computed tomography in children with cystic fibrosis: can pre-stages be identified? Eur Radiol. 2016;26(12):4563–9.
128. Brody AS, Klein JS, Molina PL, Quan J, Bean JA, Wilmott RW. High-resolution computed tomography in young patients with cystic fibrosis: distribution of abnormalities and correlation with pulmonary function tests. J Pediatr. 2004;145(1):32–8.
129. de Jong PA, Ottink MD, Robben SG, Lequin MH, Hop WC, Hendriks JJ, Pare PD, Tiddens HA. Pulmonary disease assessment in cystic fibrosis: comparison of CT scoring systems and value of bronchial and arterial dimension measurements. Radiology. 2004;231(2):434–9.
130. Hansell DM, Bankier AA, MacMahon H, McLoud TC, Muller NL, Remy J. Fleischner society: glossary of terms for thoracic imaging. Radiology. 2008;246(3):697–722.
131. Kapur N, Masel JP, Watson D, Masters IB, Chang AB. Bronchoarterial ratio on high-resolution CT scan of the chest in children without pulmonary pathology: need to redefine bronchial dilatation. Chest. 2011;139(6):1445–50.

132. Simanovsky N, Cohen-Cymberknoh M, Shoseyov D, Gileles-Hillel A, Wilschanski M, Kerem E, Hiller N. Differences in the pattern of structural abnormalities on CT scan in patients with cystic fibrosis and pancreatic sufficiency or insufficiency. Chest. 2013;144(1):208–14.
133. Cohen-Cymberknoh M, Simanovsky N, Hiller N, Gileles Hillel A, Shoseyov D, Kerem E. Differences in disease expression between primary ciliary dyskinesia and cystic fibrosis with and without pancreatic insufficiency. Chest. 2014;145(4):738–44.
134. Frija-Masson J, Bassinet L, Honore I, Dufeu N, Housset B, Coste A, Papon JF, Escudier E, Burgel PR, Maitre B. Clinical characteristics, functional respiratory decline and follow-up in adult patients with primary ciliary dyskinesia. Thorax. 2017;72(2):154–60.
135. Shah A, Shoemark A, SJ MN, Bhaludin B, Rogers A, Bilton D, Hansell DM, Wilson R, Loebinger MR. A longitudinal study characterising a large adult primary ciliary dyskinesia population. Eur Respir J. 2016;48(2):441–50.
136. Bonnel AS, Song SM, Kesavarju K, Newaskar M, Paxton CJ, Bloch DA, Moss RB, Robinson TE. Quantitative air-trapping analysis in children with mild cystic fibrosis lung disease. Pediatr Pulmonol. 2004;38(5):396–405.
137. de Jong PA, Lindblad A, Rubin L, Hop WC, de Jongste JC, Brink M, Tiddens HA. Progression of lung disease on computed tomography and pulmonary function tests in children and adults with cystic fibrosis. Thorax. 2006;61(1):80–5.
138. Owens CM, Aurora P, Stanojevic S, Bush A, Wade A, Oliver C, Calder A, Price J, Carr SB, Shankar A, et al. Lung clearance index and HRCT are complementary markers of lung abnormalities in young children with CF. Thorax. 2011;66(6):481–8.
139. Weis M, Henzler T, Nance JW Jr, Haubenreisser H, Meyer M, Sudarski S, Schoenberg SO, Neff KW, Hagelstein C. Radiation dose comparison between 70 kVp and 100 kVp with spectral beam shaping for non-contrast-enhanced pediatric chest computed tomography: a prospective randomized controlled study. Investig Radiol. 2016;
140. Tsiflikas I, Thomas C, Ketelsen D, Seitz G, Warmann S, Claussen CD, Schafer JF. High-pitch computed tomography of the lung in pediatric patients: an intraindividual comparison of image quality and radiation dose to conventional 64-MDCT. RoFo. 2014;186(6):585–90.
141. Bastos M, Lee EY, Strauss KJ, Zurakowski D, Tracy DA, Boiselle PM. Motion artifact on high-resolution CT images of pediatric patients: comparison of volumetric and axial CT methods. AJR Am J Roentgenol. 2009;193(5):1414–8.
142. Journy NM, Lee C, Harbron RW, McHugh K, Pearce MS, Berrington de Gonzalez A. projected cancer risks potentially related to past, current, and future practices in paediatric CT in the United Kingdom, 1990-2020. Br J Cancer. 2017;116(1):109–16.
143. Niemann T, Colas L, Roser HW, Santangelo T, Faivre JB, Remy J, Remy-Jardin M, Bremerich J. Estimated risk of radiation-induced cancer from paediatric chest CT: two-year cohort study. Pediatr Radiol. 2015;45(3):329–36.
144. Roach DJ, Cremillieux Y, Fleck RJ, Brody AS, Serai SD, Szczesniak RD, Kerlakian S, Clancy JP, Woods JC. Ultrashort Echo-time magnetic resonance imaging is a sensitive method for the evaluation of early cystic fibrosis lung disease. Ann Am Thorac Soc. 2016;13(11):1923–31.
145. Sileo C, Corvol H, Boelle PY, Blondiaux E, Clement A, Ducou Le Pointe H. HRCT and MRI of the lung in children with cystic fibrosis: comparison of different scoring systems. J Cystic Fibros. 2014;13(2):198–204.
146. Teufel M, Ketelsen D, Fleischer S, Martirosian P, Graebler-Mainka U, Stern M, Claussen CD, Schick F, Schaefer JF. Comparison between high-resolution CT and MRI using a very short echo time in patients with cystic fibrosis with extra focus on mosaic attenuation. Respiration. 2013;86(4):302–11.
147. Bauman G, Puderbach M, Heimann T, Kopp-Schneider A, Fritzsching E, Mall MA, Eichinger M. Validation of Fourier decomposition MRI with dynamic contrast-enhanced MRI using visual and automated scoring of pulmonary perfusion in young cystic fibrosis patients. Eur J Radiol. 2013;82(12):2371–7.
148. Eichinger M, Optazaite DE, Kopp-Schneider A, Hintze C, Biederer J, Niemann A, Mall MA, Wielputz MO, Kauczor HU, Puderbach M. Morphologic and functional scoring of cystic fibrosis lung disease using MRI. Eur J Radiol. 2012;81(6):1321–9.
149. Schraml C, Schwenzer NF, Martirosian P, Boss A, Schick F, Schafer S, Stern M, Claussen CD, Schafer JF. Non-invasive pulmonary perfusion assessment in young patients with cystic fibrosis using an arterial spin labeling MR technique at 1.5 T. Magma. 2012;25(2):155–62.
150. Loeve M, Hop WC, de Bruijne M, van Hal PT, Robinson P, Aitken ML, Dodd JD, Tiddens HA. Chest computed tomography scores are predictive of survival in patients with cystic fibrosis awaiting lung transplantation. Am J Respir Crit Care Med. 2012;185(10):1096–103.
151. Martinez TM, Llapur CJ, Williams TH, Coates C, Gunderman R, Cohen MD, Howenstine MS, Saba O, Coxson HO, Tepper RS. High-resolution computed tomography imaging of airway disease in infants with cystic fibrosis. Am J Respir Crit Care Med. 2005;172(9):1133–8.
152. de Jong PA, Nakano Y, Hop WC, Long FR, Coxson HO, Pare PD, Tiddens HA. Changes in airway dimensions on computed tomography scans of children with cystic fibrosis. Am J Respir Crit Care Med. 2005;172(2):218–24.
153. Robinson TE, Goris ML, Zhu HJ, Chen X, Bhise P, Sheikh F, Moss RB. Dornase alfa reduces air trapping in children with mild cystic fibrosis lung disease: a quantitative analysis. Chest. 2005;128(4):2327–35.
154. Wielputz MO, Puderbach M, Kopp-Schneider A, Stahl M, Fritzsching E, Sommerburg O, Ley S, Sumkauskaite M, Biederer J, Kauczor HU, et al. Magnetic resonance imaging detects changes in structure and perfusion, and response to therapy in early cystic fibrosis lung disease. Am J Respir Crit Care Med. 2014;189(8):956–65.
155. Bortoluzzi CF, Volpi S, D'Orazio C, Tiddens HA, Loeve M, Tridello G, Assael BM. Bronchiectases at early chest computed tomography in children with cystic fibrosis are associated with increased risk of subsequent pulmonary exacerbations and chronic pseudomonas infection. J Cystic Fibros. 2014;13(5):564–71.
156. Brody AS, Sucharew H, Campbell JD, Millard SP, Molina PL, Klein JS, Quan J. Computed tomography correlates with pulmonary exacerbations in children with cystic fibrosis. Am J Respir Crit Care Med. 2005;172(9):1128–32.
157. Loeve M, Gerbrands K, Hop WC, Rosenfeld M, Hartmann IC, Tiddens HA. Bronchiectasis and pulmonary exacerbations in children and young adults with cystic fibrosis. Chest. 2011;140(1):178–85.
158. Sanders DB, Li Z, Brody AS. Chest computed tomography predicts the frequency of pulmonary exacerbations in children with cystic fibrosis. Ann Am Thorac Soc. 2015;12(1):64–9.
159. Logan PM, O'Laoide RM, Mulherin D, O'Mahony S, FitzGerald MX, Masterson JB. High resolution computed tomography in cystic fibrosis: correlation with pulmonary function and assessment of prognostic value. Ir J Med Sci. 1996;165(1):27–31.

Earlier smoking after waking and the risk of asthma

Arielle S. Selya[1*], Sunita Thapa[1,2] and Gaurav Mehta[1]

Abstract

Background: Recent research shows that nicotine dependence conveys additional health risks above and beyond smoking *behavior*. The current study examines whether smoking within 5 min of waking, an indicator of nicotine dependence, is independently associated with asthma outcomes.

Methods: Data were drawn from five pooled cross-sectional waves (2005–14) of NHANES, and the final sample consisted of $N = 4081$ current adult smokers. Weighted logistic regressions were run examining the relationship between smoking within 5 min of waking and outcomes of lifetime asthma, past-year asthma, and having had an asthma attack in the past year. Control variables included demographics, smoking behavior, family history of asthma, depression, obesity, and secondhand smoking exposure.

Results: After adjusting for smoking behavior, smoking within 5 min was associated with an approximately 50% increase in the odds of lifetime asthma ($OR = 1.46$, $p = .008$) and past-year asthma ($OR = 1.47$, $p = .024$), respectively. After additionally adjusting for demographics and other asthma risk factors, smoking within 5 min of waking was associated with a four-fold increase in the odds of lifetime asthma ($OR = 4.05$, $p = .015$).

Conclusions: Smoking within 5 min of waking, an indicator of nicotine dependence, is associated with a significantly increased risk of lifetime asthma in smokers. These findings could be utilized in refining risk assessment of asthma among smokers.

Keywords: Asthma, Cigarettes, Nicotine dependence, Smoking, Time to first cigarette

Background

Asthma is a highly disabling but treatable disease, which consists of chronic airway inflammation and episodes of acute exacerbations in response to certain stimuli. Several risk factors for asthma have been identified, and a notable avoidable risk factor is cigarette smoking [1]. However, most existing research does not distinguish between nicotine dependence (ND), a psychological construct capturing the addiction to nicotine, and smoking *behavior*. Traditionally, smoking behavior and ND were largely considered synonymous; however, recent research has increasingly highlighted the importance of distinguishing between them. ND is a psychological construct capturing addiction to smoking, and this is to some extent separable from smoking behavior itself. For example, adolescent smokers often develop ND at low, even non-daily levels of smoking [2–4], and this predicts future smoking behavior even after accounting for prior smoking behavior [3, 5, 6], while other demographic groups show very low ND despite heavy smoking behavior [2]. Moreover, ND poses a higher risk than does smoking behavior alone for several other smoking-related health outcomes, including lung cancer [7, 8], larynx cancer [9], head and neck cancer [10], and chronic obstructive pulmonary disease (COPD) [11, 12]. A limited number of studies reported that asthma significantly increases the risk of both smoking behavior and ND [13, 14]; however, the association between asthma and ND was not assessed *independently* of smoking behavior. Thus, very little is

* Correspondence: arielle.selya@med.und.edu
[1]Master of Public Health Program, Department of Population Health, University of North Dakota, 1301 North Columbia Rd. Stop 9037, Grand Forks, ND 58202, USA
Full list of author information is available at the end of the article

known about whether higher ND is associated with increased risk of asthma, over and above smoking behavior.

The current study tests the novel hypothesis that smoking within 5 min of waking, a version of time to first cigarette (TTFC) which is a strong and reliable indicator of ND [15, 16], is associated with a greater risk of asthma even after accounting for lifetime smoking history. Data are pooled across five consecutive, cross-sectional waves (2005–06, 2007–08, 2009–10, 2011–12, and 2013–14) of the National Health and Nutrition Examination Survey (NHANES) survey, and include current adult smokers. Though causality cannot be established here, data were restricted to those who initiated smoking prior to developing asthma, in order to ensure a temporal relationship that is at least *consistent with* smoking as a causal factor in the development or exacerbation of asthma. The relationships between smoking within 5 min after waking and binary outcomes of 1) lifetime asthma, 2) past-year asthma, and 3) having had an asthma attack in the past year were examined using weighted logistic regressions. Control variables included smoking behavior (past-month cigarettes per day (CPD) and years of smoking duration), demographic characteristics (age, race/ethnicity, and gender), and other risk factors for asthma (obesity, family history of asthma, depression, and secondhand smoke exposure).

Methods
Study sample
This study utilized data from five cross-sectional waves (2005–06, 2007–08, 2009–10, 2011–12, and 2013–14) of NHANES, a publicly available, nationally-representative survey conducted by the Centers for Disease Control. NHANES is a nationally representative sample of the non-institutionalized civilian U.S. population that is conducted on an ongoing, semiannual basis since 1999. NHANES consists of an extensive questionnaire on medical conditions, health-related behaviors and risk factors, and a subcomponent involving physical examination and laboratory tests. Since complete smoking behavior and ND information was available only from current smokers 20 years or older, participants younger than 20 or who did not report being a current smoker were excluded from all analyses. Additionally, among participants who reported having had asthma at some point in their lifetime, those who developed asthma prior to initiating smoking were also excluded. The final analytic sample includes $N = 4081$ current adult smokers.

Measures
Asthma outcomes were examined with three binary variables: self-reported lifetime asthma ("Has a doctor or other health professional ever told you that you have asthma?"); and among those who said yes, self-reported past-year asthma ("Do you still have asthma?"), and having reported at least one asthma attack in the past year ("During the past 12 months, have you had an episode of asthma or an asthma attack?"). Additionally, self-reported age of asthma diagnosis ("How old were you when first told you had asthma?") was used to determine exclusion from the final study sample: participants were excluded if age of asthma diagnosis was younger than the self-reported age of first regular smoking.

Smoking within 5 min after waking was derived from self-reported time to first cigarette (TTFC), perhaps the best single-item measure of ND [15, 16], which was asked using the question "How soon after waking up do you smoke?" In order to ensure sufficient group sizes in the current sample, the four original response categories were dichotomized into ≤5 (high dependence) vs. > 5 min (low to moderate dependence), consistent with other recent research [17].

Control variables included current smoking behavior (self-reported cigarettes per day (CPD) in the past 30 days) and lifetime smoking behavior (years of smoking duration, calculated by subtracting self-reported age of first regular smoking from age at questionnaire), in accordance with recent recommendations for controlling for smoking behavior [18] .

Additionally, demographic characteristics included age, sex, and race/ethnicity. Race/ethnicity was self-reported as "non-Hispanic white," "non-Hispanic black," "Mexican-American," "other Hispanic," and "other;" for the current analyses, "Mexican-American" and "other Hispanic" were combined into a single category, and participants reporting "other" were excluded from analyses due to small sample size ($N = 220$).

Other risk factors for asthma were used as potential confounding variables, and included self-reported family history of asthma, depression (derived from 10 items based on the DSM-5 criteria), obesity (measured in the physical examination component of NHANES), and secondhand smoke exposure (SHS; dichotomized into any vs. no self-reported exposure to cigarette smoke at home and in the workplace).

Statistical analysis
Weighted logistic regression was used in accordance with NHANES Analytic Guidelines [19] using R statistical software and its "survey" package to examine outcomes of lifetime asthma, past-year asthma, and having had an asthma attack in the past year. Weighted regressions take into account NHANES' complex sampling design to produce results that are representative of the larger U.S. noninstitutionalized civilian population, rather than the particular NHANES sample. The outcomes were each examined as a function of smoking within 5 min after waking. For each outcome, three models of

varying complexity were run: 1) an unadjusted model; 2) a model adjusted for smoking behavior (past-month CPD and years of smoking duration); and 3) a model additionally adjusted for other risk factors for asthma (family history of asthma, depression, obesity), demographic characteristics (age, race/ethnicity, and sex), and interactions of TTFC with a) secondhand smoke exposure [20, 21] and b) sex [22]. Missing data on variables were handled by listwise deletion.

Results

Table 1 shows descriptive statistics separately for those who smoke within 5 min of waking ($N = 1290$) and those who smoke after 5 min of waking ($N = 2791$). Those who reported smoking within 5 min of waking were approximately 1.5 times as likely to report having asthma at some time in their lives, 1.5 times as likely to report still having asthma in the past year, and 1.7 times as likely to report having had an asthma attack in the past year. Additionally, those who smoked within 5 min after waking reported heavier past-month smoking, and a longer lifetime smoking duration.

Weighted regression analyses of varying complexity are presented in Table 2. At the unadjusted level, smoking within 5 min of waking was associated with higher odds of lifetime and past-year asthma, as well as of a past-year asthma attack. When adjusting for current and lifetime smoking behavior, smoking within 5 min of waking was associated with an approximately 47% increase in the odds of lifetime asthma, and a 46% increase in the odds of past-years asthma. Finally, when also adjusting for demographic characteristics and other risk factors for asthma, smoking within 5 min of waking remained independently associated with lifetime asthma, such that those who smoke within 5 min of waking have approximately four times the odds of reporting lifetime asthma. Secondhand smoke exposure significantly moderated this relationship, such that SHS exposure slightly weakened the effect of smoking within 5 min after waking. Finally, there was a trend between smoking within 5 min of waking with both past-year asthma and having had an asthma attack in the past year. Unweighted regressions are presented in Additional file 1: Table S1.

Significant interactions were also found between smoking within 5 min of waking and secondhand smoke exposure in the fully-adjusted model for both lifetime and past-year asthma (Table 2). This indicates significant moderation, such that the odds of asthma for those with both risk factors (smoking within 5 min of waking and being exposed to second hand smoke) are lower than would be expected based on their respective independent OR's. Similarly, an additional interaction between smoking within 5 min of waking and sex was found only for outcomes of past-year asthma, such that being male and smoking within 5 min of waking results in a *higher* risk of past-year asthma than would be expected by the respective independent OR's of these variables.

Table 1 Descriptive statistics of sample

Measure	Smoking within 5 min of waking ($N = 1290$)	Smoking after 5 min of waking ($N = 2791$)	p
Lifetime asthma	**150, 11.6%**	**210, 7.5%**	**<.001**
Past-year asthma	**115, 9.0%**	**153, 5.5%**	**<.001**
Past-year asthma attack	**60, 4.8%**	**82, 3.0%**	**.006**
Cigarettes per day	**20.0, 1.0–25.0**	**10, 6.0–20.0**	**<.001**
Smoking duration	**29.5, 18.0–40.0**	**28, 15.0–40.0**	**.001**
Age	46.0, 35.0–56.0	46.0, 33.0–59.0	.969
Sex			.753
Female	561, 43.5%	1230, 44.1%	
Male	729, 56.5%	1561, 55.9%	
Race			**<.001**
White	**812, 63.0%**	**1541, 55.2%**	
Black	**352, 27.3%**	**698, 25.1%**	
Hispanic	**126, 9.8%**	**552, 19.8%**	
Depression	**261, 23.5%**	**388, 16.0%**	**<.001**
Obesity	371, 30.4%	817, 30.8%	.843
Family history of asthma	**324, 25.8%**	**575, 21.1%**	**.001**
Secondhand smoking	**895, 92.8%**	**1460, 75.9%**	**<.001**

Categorical variables are presented as N, valid percentage, and continuous variables are presented as median, interquartile range. p-values are based on chi-square tests for categorical variables, and Wilcoxon signed-rank tests for continuous variables. Bold: $p < .05$

Table 2 Weighted regression results of smoking within 5 min of waking on asthma outcomes

Model	Covariate	Outcome		
		Lifetime Asthma	Past-Year Asthma	Past-Year Asthma Attack
		OR (95% CI) p-value	OR (95% CI) p-value	OR (95% CI) p value
Unadjusted	Smoking within 5 min. (vs. > 5 min.)	**1.71 (1.26–2.31)** **p = .001**	**1.72 (1.22–2.43)** **p = .003**	**1.66 (1.04–2.67)** **p = .038**
Adjusted for smoking behavior[a]	Smoking within 5 min. (vs. > 5 min.)	**1.47 (1.11–1.93)** **p = .008**	**1.46 (1.06–2.01)** **p = .024**	1.31 (0.82–2.09) p = .268
Adjusted for smoking[a] and other covariates[b]	Smoking within 5 min. (vs. > 5 min.)	**4.05 (1.35–12.14)** **p = .015**	3.95 (0.93–16.84) p = .069	5.45 (0.85–34.88) p = .079
	Smoking within 5 min x SHS	**0.23 (0.08–0.71)** **p = .014**	**0.20 (0.04–0.90)** **p = .041**	0.18 (0.02–1.31) p = .096
	Smoking within 5 min x sex	–	**3.21 (1.56–6.64)** **p = .003**	–

Results are presented as odds ratio (95% confidence interval), p-value. Boldface indicates statistical significance (p < .05)
[a] Smoking covariates: cigarettes per day and years of smoking duration
[b] Other covariates: depression, obesity, family history of asthma, secondhand smoke exposure (SHS), age, sex, race/ethnicity, and interactions of smoking within 5 min with secondhand smoke exposure and sex. Interaction terms are only included in the model if p < .10

Discussion

This study presents the novel finding that smoking sooner after waking, a reliable indicator for ND, is independently associated with a heightened risk of lifetime and recent asthma outcomes among a nationally representative sample of current adult smokers, over and above current and lifetime smoking behavior. Notably, the association with lifetime asthma remained significant after also adjusting for demographic characteristics and other risk factors for asthma, such that those who smoke within 5 min of waking are at an approximately four-fold risk of reporting asthma at some point in their lives.

The relationships between smoking within 5 min of waking with outcomes of past-year asthma and past-year asthma attacks were not significant after adjusting for current and lifetime smoking behavior, demographics, and other risk factors for asthma. Considering that active smoking has been shown to aggravate inflammation and hypersensitivity of the airways [23], we had expected to find that smoking within 5 min of waking to be associated with past-year asthma outcomes as well. However, the relationship did show a trend (p < .10), which suggests that this negative finding may reflect low statistical power due to a relatively small analytic sample given the complexity of the fully-adjusted model. This possibility is bolstered by the fact that smoking within 5 min was associated with both past-year asthma and past-year asthma attacks at the bivariate level, and with past-year asthma after adjusting only for current and lifetime smoking behavior. Future studies using larger sample sizes and/or prospective data are needed to more rigorously evaluate whether indicators of ND are associated with concurrent asthma outcomes and the exacerbation of asthma symptoms.

It is noteworthy that the strength of the relationship between smoking within 5 min and asthma was stronger *after* adjusting for covariates, relative to the unadjusted model and the model adjusted only for smoking behavior. Including the interaction terms of smoking within 5 min with secondhand smoke exposure and with sex were critical in explaining this increase; excluding these significant interactions resulted in substantially lower and even nonsignificant OR's (data not shown). The significance of these interaction terms indicate important moderation of the relationship between time to first cigarette in the morning and asthma. In the case of sex, the current findings align with sex difference in the relationship between ND and asthma [22]; though differences in the statistical models prevent a direct comparison with the current findings. In the case of secondhand smoke exposure, this confirms previous research showing that those exposed to secondhand smoke have more severe ND [20, 21]. Taken together with the current findings, this suggests ND as a possible mechanism for why secondhand smoke exposure increases the risk of asthma. Future research is needed to disentangle the complex relationship between secondhand smoke exposure, ND, and asthma, including ND as a possible mediator.

Two potential explanations may underlie the current findings that smoking within 5 min of waking is associated with a heightened four-fold risk of asthma. Asthma involves inflammation and hypersensitivity of airways which could be a result of persistent irritation by the components of cigarette smoke [23]. Given that smokers can moderate their nicotine intake by altering their smoking style [24, 25], more dependent smokers may inhale more deeply and take more puffs per cigarette [26, 27]. If dependent smokers (as indicated by smoking within 5 min of waking) routinely extract more nicotine, and incidentally more smoke and tars from each cigarette, this may raise the risk of increased inflammatory mediators and bronchiolar damage. This could explain the significantly higher risk of lifetime asthma among such smokers. In this explanation, the effect of ND on asthma would be fully mediated through nuanced smoking style rather than the number of cigarettes consumed.

A second potential explanation could be that the relationship between ND and asthma may be the result of a common genetic predisposition. Genetic pathways have been identified that increase the risk of both ND and COPD [28, 29] as well as ND and lung cancer [30–32]. Though no such common genetic risk is currently known for ND and asthma, independent genetic risk factors have been identified for both ND [33–36] and asthma [37–39]. Future genetic studies examining potential *common* genetic links are warranted to test this potential explanation.

Strengths and limitations
Strengths of this study include its novelty in establishing an association between smoking within 5 min of waking, a symptom of ND, and lifetime asthma. Additionally, the use of data from the large, nationally-representative NHANES survey increase the generalizability of our findings to current adult smokers in the US. The current study extends the existing literature in important ways by demonstrating a novel link between smoking within 5 min of waking, an indicator of ND, and asthma outcomes.

Limitations of the current study should be taken into account. First, due to the use of cross-sectional data, temporality and causation cannot be examined. This is especially important considering that asthma often develops in children who have not yet initiated smoking; however, the current study reduced this limitation by excluding participants whose asthma preceded smoking initiation. Second, the results are limited to the accuracy of self-reported variables. It is possible that some diagnoses of asthma are other types of pulmonary disorders such as chronic obstructive pulmonary disease, bronchitis, etc. However, the wording of the question ("have you ever been told by a doctor or health professional…") reduces the likelihood of an incorrect diagnoses. Nevertheless, follow-up research is necessary to replicate these findings using clinical diagnosis rather than self-report. Third, the measurement of ND in NHANES is restricted to a single question (i.e. TTFC) to current smokers; this prevents an examination of ND among ex-smokers or passive smokers and excludes other aspects of the multi-dimensional construct of ND. Finally, the current study is intended as a preliminary examination of a novel association, and future research is needed to more rigorously test the relationship between ND and asthma outcomes.

Conclusions
The current preliminary findings report a novel association between smoking within 5 min of waking, an indicator of ND, and lifetime occurrence of asthma. That is, among smokers with similar smoking histories, those who are more "addicted" as indicated by sooner smoking after waking have an approximately four-fold risk of having asthma at some time in their lives, independently of smoking behavior and other risk factors for asthma. This novel finding has important potential implications for treating smokers suffering from asthma. In particular, if the current preliminary findings are corroborated and extended in future research, healthcare professionals could screen smokers based on how soon they smoke after waking in order to more accurately assess their risk for asthma, among other health outcomes. Through more detailed risk assessment of smokers, closer monitoring and increased support for smoking cessation for those at risk for asthma, we could ultimately reduce the disease burden associated with asthma.

Abbreviations
COPD: Chronic Obstructive Pulmonary Disease; CPD: Cigarettes per Day; IDeA: Institutional Development Award; ND: Nicotine Dependence; NHANES: National Health and Nutrition Examination Survey; OR: Odds Ratio; SHS: Second Hand Smoke; TTFC: Time to First Cigarette

Funding
This work was supported by an Institutional Development Award (IDeA) from the National Institute of General Medical Sciences of the National Institutes of Health under grant number P20GM103442 to Dr. Donald Sens, Department of Pathology, School of Medicine & Health Sciences at the University of North Dakota, Grand Forks, ND. The funding agency was not involved in the design of the study, data collection, analysis, interpretation, or writing of this manuscript.

Authors' contributions
AS, ST and GM performed data analysis and drafted the manuscript. AS conceived and designed the study, supervised the data analysis, interpreted the data, and drafted parts of the manuscript. All authors contributed to manuscript revisions and approved the final version of this article.

Competing interests
The authors declare that they have no competing interests.

Author details
[1]Master of Public Health Program, Department of Population Health, University of North Dakota, 1301 North Columbia Rd. Stop 9037, Grand Forks, ND 58202, USA. [2]Department of Public Policy, Vanderbilt University School of Medicine, 2525 West End Ave, Suite 1200, Nashville, TN 37203, USA.

References

1. Siroux V, Pin I, Oryszczyn MP, Le Moual N, Kauffmann F. Relationships of active smoking to asthma and asthma severity in the EGEA study. Epidemiological study on the genetics and environment of asthma. Eur Respir J. 2000;15(3):470–7.
2. Kandel DB, Chen K. Extent of smoking and nicotine dependence in the United States: 1991-1993. Nicotine Tob Res. 2000;2(3):263–74.
3. DiFranza JR, Savageau JA, Rigotti NA, Fletcher K, Ockene JK, McNeill AD, Coleman M, Wood C. Development of symptoms of tobacco dependence in youths: 30 month follow up data from the DANDY study. Tob Control. 2002;11(3):228–35.
4. O'Loughlin J, DiFranza J, Tyndale RF, Meshefedjian G, McMillan-Davey E, Clarke PB, Hanley J, Paradis G. Nicotine-dependence symptoms are associated with smoking frequency in adolescents. Am J Prev Med. 2003;25(3):219–25.
5. Dierker L, Hedeker D, Rose J, Selya A, Mermelstein R. Early emerging nicotine dependence symptoms in adolescence predict daily smoking in young adulthood. Drug Alcohol Depend. 2015;151:267–71.
6. Dierker L, Mermelstein R. Early emerging nicotine-dependence symptoms: a signal of propensity for chronic smoking behavior in adolescents. J Pediatr. 2010;156(5):818–22.
7. Muscat JE, Ahn K, Richie JP Jr, Stellman SD. Nicotine dependence phenotype and lung cancer risk. Cancer. 2011;117(23):5370–6.
8. Kunze U, Scholer E, Schoberberger R, Dittrich C, Aigner K, Bolcskei P, Groman E. Lung cancer risk measured by the Fagerstrom test for nicotine dependence? Nicotine Tob Res. 2007;9(5):625–6.
9. Muscat JE, Liu HP, Livelsberger C, Richie JP Jr, Stellman SD. The nicotine dependence phenotype, time to first cigarette, and larynx cancer risk. Cancer Causes Control. 2012;23(3):497–503.
10. Muscat JE, Ahn K, Richie JP Jr, Stellman SD. Nicotine dependence phenotype, time to first cigarette, and risk of head and neck cancer. Cancer. 2011;117(23):5377–82.
11. Guertin KA, Gu F, Wacholder S, Freedman ND, Panagiotou OA, Reyes-Guzman C, Caporaso NE. Time to first morning cigarette and risk of chronic obstructive pulmonary disease: smokers in the PLCO Cancer screening trial. PLoS One. 2015;10(5):e0125973.
12. Selya AS, Oancea SC, Thapa S. Time to first cigarette, a proxy of nicotine dependence, increases the risk of pulmonary impairment, independently of current and lifetime smoking behavior. Nicotine Tob Res. 2016;18(6):1431–9.
13. McLeish AC, Cougle JR, Zvolensky MJ. Asthma and cigarette smoking in a representative sample of adults. J Health Psychol. 2011;16(4):643–52.
14. Van De Ven MO, van Zundert RM, Engels RC. Effects of asthma on nicotine dependence development and smoking cessation attempts in adolescence. J Asthma. 2013;50(3):250–9.
15. Fagerstrom K. Time to first cigarette; the best single indicator of tobacco dependence? Monaldi Arch Chest Dis. 2003;59(1):91–4.
16. Transdisciplinary Tobacco Use Research Center (TTURC) Tobacco Dependence Phenotype Workgroup, Baker TB, Piper ME, DE MC, Bolt DM, Smith SS, Kim SY, Colby S, Conti D, Giovino GA, et al. Time to first cigarette in the morning as an index of ability to quit smoking: implications for nicotine dependence. Nicotine Tob Res. 2007;9(Suppl 4):S555–70.
17. Khaled SM, Bulloch AG, Williams JV, Lavorato DH, Patten SB. Major depression is a risk factor for shorter time to first cigarette irrespective of the number of cigarettes smoked per day: evidence from a National Population Health Survey. Nicotine Tob Res. 2011;13(11):1059–67.
18. Peto J. That the effects of smoking should be measured in pack-years: misconceptions 4. Br J Cancer. 2012;107(3):406–7.
19. Mirel LB, Mohadjer LK, Dohrmann SM, Clark J, Burt VL, Johnson CL, Curtin LR. National Health and nutrition examination survey: estimation procedures. Vital Health Stat 2. 2007-2010;2013(159):1–17.
20. Okoli CT, Browning S, Rayens MK, Hahn EJ. Secondhand tobacco smoke exposure, nicotine dependence, and smoking cessation. Public Health Nurs. 2008;25(1):46–56.
21. Okoli CT, Kodet J. A systematic review of secondhand tobacco smoke exposure and smoking behaviors: smoking status, susceptibility, initiation, dependence, and cessation. Addict Behav. 2015;47:22–32.
22. Guo SE, Ratner PA, Okoli CT, Johnson JL. The gender-specific association between asthma and the need to smoke tobacco. Heart Lung. 2014;43(1):77–83.
23. Stapleton M, Howard-Thompson A, George C, Hoover RM, Self TH. Smoking and asthma. J Am Board Fam Med. 2011;24(3):313–22.
24. Kassel JD, Greenstein JE, Evatt DP, Wardle MC, Yates MC, Veilleux JC, Eissenberg T. Smoking topography in response to denicotinized and high-yield nicotine cigarettes in adolescent smokers. J Adolesc Health. 2007;40(1):54–60.
25. Veilleux JC, Kassel JD, Heinz AJ, Braun A, Wardle MC, Greenstein J, Evatt DP, Conrad M. Predictors and sequelae of smoking topography over the course of a single cigarette in adolescent light smokers. J Adolesc Health. 2011;48(2):176–81.
26. Jiménez-Ruiz CA, Miravitlles M, Sobradillo V, Gabriel R, Viejo JL, Masa JF, Fernández-Fau L, Villasante C. Can cumulative tobacco consumption, FTND score, and carbon monoxide concentration in expired air be predictors of chronic obstructive pulmonary disease? Nicotine Tob Res. 2004;6(4):649–53.
27. Kim DK, Hersh CP, Washko GR, Hokanson JE, Lynch DA, Newell JD, Murphy JR, Crapo JD, Silverman EK. Epidemiology, radiology, and genetics of nicotine dependence in COPD. Respir Res. 2011;12(1):9.
28. Galvan A, Dragani TA. Nicotine dependence may link the 15q25 locus to lung cancer risk. Carcinog. 2010;31(3):331–3.
29. Kaur-Knudsen D, Nordestgaard BG, Bojesen SE. CHRNA3 genotype, nicotine dependence, lung function and disease in the general population. Eur Respir J. 2012;40(6):1538–44.
30. MacQueen DA, Heckman BW, Blank MD, Van Rensburg KJ, Park JY, Drobes DJ, Evans DE. Variation in the α 5 nicotinic acetylcholine receptor subunit gene predicts cigarette smoking intensity as a function of nicotine content. Pharmacogenomics J. 2014;14(1):70–6.
31. Strasser AA, Benowitz NL, Pinto AG, Tang KZ, Hecht SS, Carmella SG, Tyndale RF, Lerman CE. Nicotine metabolite ratio predicts smoking topography and carcinogen biomarker level. Cancer Epidemiol Biomark Prev. 2011;20(2):234–8.
32. Strasser AA, Malaiyandi V, Hoffmann E, Tyndale RF, Lerman C. An association of CYP2A6 genotype and smoking topography. Nicotine Tob Res. 2007;9(4):511–8.
33. Bierut L, Stitzel J, Wang J, Hinrichs A, Grucza R, Xuei X, Saccone N, Saccone S, Bertelsen S, Fox L, et al. Variants in nicotinic receptors and risk for nicotine dependence. Am J Psychiatry. 2008;165(9):1163–71.
34. Yang J, Wang S, Yang Z, Hodgkinson CA, Iarikova P, Ma JZ, Payne TJ, Goldman D, Li MD. The contribution of rare and common variants in 30 genes to risk nicotine dependence. Mol Psychiatry. 2014;20(11):1467–78.
35. Bidwell LC, McGeary JE, Gray JC, Palmer RHC, Knopik VS, MacKillop J. NCAM1-TTC12-ANKK1-DRD2 variants and smoking motives as intermediate phenotypes for nicotine dependence. Psychopharmacol. 2015;232(7):1177–86.
36. Haberstick BC, Timberlake D, Ehringer MA, Lessem JM, Hopfer CJ, Smolen A, Hewitt JK. Genes, time to first cigarette and nicotine dependence in a general population sample of young adults. Addiction. 2007;102(4):655–65.
37. Postma DS, Bleecker ER, Amelung PJ, Holroyd KJ, Xu J, Panhuysen CIM, Meyers DA, Levitt RC. Genetic susceptibility to asthma — bronchial Hyperresponsiveness Coinherited with a major gene for atopy. N Engl J Med. 1995;333(14):894–900.
38. Zhang Y, Moffatt MF, Cookson WOC. Genetic and genomic approaches to asthma: new insights for the origins. Curr Opin Pulm Med. 2012;18(1):6–13.
39. Wan YI, Shrine NRG, Soler Artigas M, Wain LV, Blakey JD, Moffatt MF, Bush A, Chung KF, Cookson WOCM, Strachan DP, et al. Genome-wide association study to identify genetic determinants of severe asthma. Thorax. 2012;67(9):762–8.

Geographic variation in the aetiology, epidemiology and microbiology of bronchiectasis

Ravishankar Chandrasekaran[1], Micheál Mac Aogáin[1], James D. Chalmers[2], Stuart J. Elborn[3,4] and Sanjay H. Chotirmall[1*]

Abstract

Bronchiectasis is a disease associated with chronic progressive and irreversible dilatation of the bronchi and is characterised by chronic infection and associated inflammation. The prevalence of bronchiectasis is age-related and there is some geographical variation in incidence, prevalence and clinical features. Most bronchiectasis is reported to be idiopathic however post-infectious aetiologies dominate across Asia especially secondary to tuberculosis. Most focus to date has been on the study of airway bacteria, both as colonisers and causes of exacerbations. Modern molecular technologies including next generation sequencing (NGS) have become invaluable tools to identify microorganisms directly from sputum and which are difficult to culture using traditional agar based methods. These have provided important insight into our understanding of emerging pathogens in the airways of people with bronchiectasis and the geographical differences that occur. The contribution of the lung microbiome, its ethnic variation, and subsequent roles in disease progression and response to therapy across geographic regions warrant further investigation. This review summarises the known geographical differences in the aetiology, epidemiology and microbiology of bronchiectasis. Further, we highlight the opportunities offered by emerging molecular technologies such as -omics to further dissect out important ethnic differences in the prognosis and management of bronchiectasis.

Keywords: Bronchiectasis, Microbiome, Mycobiome, *Pseudomonas aeruginosa*, Fungi, *Aspergillus spp.*

Background

Bronchiectasis is a major chronic pulmonary disease characterised by infection, inflammation and a permanent, irreversible dilatation of the bronchial wall. The interaction of chronic infection, exacerbations and inflammation drive a vicious cycle resulting in lung injury to the bronchi and lung parenchyma. This model proposed by Cole is not well understood in terms of the underlying biology but includes deficits in mucociliary clearance and innate and adaptive immunity (Fig. 1). There is amplification of injury processes following anatomical damage to the bronchi leading to progressive worsening of pulmonary physiology and symptoms with associated increase in exacerbations [1]. The host immune response to infection is primarily neutrophilic and neutrophil derived proteases are deleterious and result in further pulmonary damage amplifying a recurrent cycle [2] (Fig. 1).

Literature search strategy

A PUBMED review of all articles mentioning the keyword "bronchiectasis" in combination with "epidemiology" or "microbiology" published between 1997 and 2017 was performed. As bronchiectasis in Cystic Fibrosis (CF) represents a separate disease entity in its own right, retrieved articles dealing exclusively with CF-associated bronchiectasis were excluded, as were original articles without radiological confirmation of bronchiectasis. Studies of both adult and paediatric populations were considered and appropriately included.

* Correspondence: schotirmall@ntu.edu.sg
[1]Lee Kong Chian School of Medicine, Nanyang Technological University, Clinical Sciences Building, 11 Mandalay Road, Singapore 308232, Singapore
Full list of author information is available at the end of the article

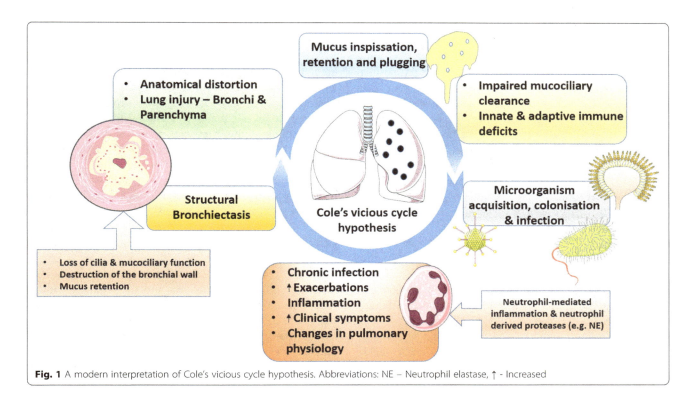

Fig. 1 A modern interpretation of Cole's vicious cycle hypothesis. Abbreviations: NE – Neutrophil elastase, ↑ - Increased

Ageing and its impact on bronchiectasis

Bronchiectasis is an age-associated disease [3]. A marked increase in prevalence, particularly of severe disease is observed in the elderly [4]. The global shift in ageing will continue to influence the burden of bronchiectasis, its disease epidemiology and implications for the healthcare systems that provide therapy [5]. In many chronic lung diseases there is an age-related increased prevalence given the multifactorial impact of the aging process on respiratory physiology. Physiological change including decreased diaphragm strength, reduced breathing efficiency and vital capacity (VC) coupled to increases in residual volume (RV) all have important influences on the diagnosis and interpretation of pulmonary function testing (PFTs) across a variety of respiratory pathologies as described by our group and others [6–8]. The diminution of swallowing reflexes and increased prevalence of GORD in the elderly may contribute to the development of bronchiectasis due to subclinical microaspiration including the nasopharyngeal microbiota [9]. Elderly people have more severe disease and atypical presentation with poorer outcomes compared to younger cohorts [10]. Age-associated disease manifestations also correlate closely with variation in immune and microbiome signatures that are associated with the ageing process itself [11, 12]. The immune system, and potentially the microbiome, also undergoes its own change with age, a process incompletely understood, termed 'immunosenescence' [13, 14]. Although immunosenescence influences a variety of respiratory disease states, little is known about its effects on bronchiectasis [15]. Nevertheless, associations between lung function decline, infection and age suggest that immunosenecence and potentially bronchiectasis pathogenesis are likely interrelated [16]. Immunosuppression due to leukaemias and their treatment are also interestingly associated with bronchiectasis, a relevant observation for elderly populations [17]. Age-associated pathways including WNT signalling, mTOR and Toll-like receptors (TLRs) all have possible roles in COPD and IPF pathogenesis and could explain age-associated severity in bronchiectasis. Telomere dysfunction and senescence associated pathways have been described in explants studied from patients with bronchiectasis [18]. As such, this represents an important area of future interest and research [19–21].

Geographic variation in the aetiology of bronchiectasis
Bronchiectasis in children vs adults

A increased risk of non-CF bronchiectasis is observed at the extremes of age with children under 5 years and adults over 75 years of age at greatest risk of disease [22]. Particular aetiologies and clinical manifestations are observed in childhood bronchiectasis, which more frequently includes primary and secondary immunodeficiency, ciliary dyskinesia, congenital malformations, bronchiolitis obliterans and skeletal disease [23]. As with adult bronchiectasis, infection is highly associated with disease and those with childhood bronchiectasis are at increased risks of more severe disease in later life [24]. While the most striking incidence of childhood bronchiectasis is seen in indigenous populations including Maori and Pacific Islanders of New Zealand, Australian aboriginal and Alaskan native children, increasing rates have also been observed outside these at risk populations [25]. It is difficult from the current literature to discern if the broader global shifts in bronchiectasis prevalence are due to 'true' changes in our understanding of aetiology, including that in childhood or alternatively a better awareness of the disease, a development of more recent times.

Bronchiectasis in Europe
Cystic fibrosis (CF), caused by dysfunction or absence of the Cystic Fibrosis Transmembrane Conductor Regulator protein (CFTR) genetically predisposes those affected to bronchiectasis; but this condition is most prevalent in Caucasian populations and is less commonly encountered in Asians. In Europe, North America, Australian and New Zealand, neonatal screening is widely available and most people with CF are diagnosed soon after birth. The majority of non-CF bronchiectasis in studies reported from Europe, Australia and the USA have no identifiable aetiology and is labelled idiopathic [3, 26]. As infection is crucial in the pathophysiology of bronchiectasis, it is unsurprising that post-infection bronchiectasis is the most commonly identifiable cause for disease development. Infection with *Mycobacterium tuberculosis*, non-tuberculosis mycobacteria (NTM), childhood *Bordetella pertussis* (whooping cough) and viruses including influenza, measles and adenovirus, have all been implicated in post-infection bronchiectasis states. It is however, in many such cases, difficult to be certain of this aetiology because of recall bias from events often many decades in the past. Importantly, COPD, asthma, connective tissue disease and immunodeficiency are all noted as important potential contributing factors among European patients [3, 27]. Gender seems to additionally exert an effect on particular aetiologies with males more likely to exhibit COPD and females more likely to exhibit asthma-related aetiologies [3]. European patients with COPD also tended to be older while immunodeficiency, ciliary dysfunction and irritable bowel disease (IBD) were all observed in younger patients [3]. The co-morbidities seen most commonly in Europe include COPD, asthma and IBD; all representing independent mortality risk factors in those with non-CF bronchiectasis [27]. COPD-associated bronchiectasis is a leading cause in Europe [3, 28–30] with allergic reactions to fungi belonging to the genus *Aspergillus* (Allergic bronchopulmonary aspergillosis - ABPA) particularly notable in United Kingdom (UK) based cohorts [28, 31, 32].

Bronchiectasis in the Americas
Bronchiectasis caused by immune-related mechanisms including autoimmunity, immunodeficiencies and hematologic malignancies were identified as predominant aetiologies in the United States [33]. This work demonstrates a low rate of idiopathic bronchiectasis and importantly reveals that systematic evaluation may identify an aetiology in a high proportion of cases suggested by an earlier UK study [31]. In the US, immune dysfunction was frequently associated with bronchiectasis including that among stem-cell transplant recipients who suffered graft versus host disease [33]. Outside of indigenous Canadian cohorts, where high rates of childhood bronchiectasis are reported, data on aetiology of adult Canadian non-CF bronchiectasis is rather limited and the precise nature of aetiology in this country is largely uncertain [34, 35]. In Latin America aetiology is, like elsewhere, driven by infection and influenced by infectious disease epidemiology such as that in endemic TB regions or against backdrops of higher rates of pertussis and measles which in turn relate to the lower vaccine uptake rates. Higher rates of pneumonia and tuberculosis in childhood are also likely key contributing factors to bronchiectasis in this region [36].

Bronchiectasis in the Asia-Pacific region
The true prevalence of bronchiectasis in communities in the Asia-Pacific region is largely unknown and should be considered a potential diagnosis in all populations. Important aetiologies of bronchiectasis seen in other regions including immunodeficiency syndromes such as, common variable immunodeficiency, secondary immunoglobulin disorders (frequently drug related) and mucociliary defects including primary ciliary dyskinesia, chronic aspiration, autoimmune/connective tissue diseases, particularly rheumatoid arthritis, and ABPA are described and in some cases result in a delayed diagnoses. In Japan, a less studied inflammatory disease, sinobronchial syndrome is documented in many cases of bronchiectasis [37].

While geographic variation in bronchiectasis aetiology is described, selection or referral biases, and, the extent of testing to seek a diagnosis of bronchiectasis in individual patients may have resulted in the observed patterns in the populations reported. Figure 2 illustrates the existing literature of available studies focused on bronchiectasis aetiology based on geography.

Geographic variation in the epidemiology of bronchiectasis
Bronchiectasis in children vs adults
The most striking variation in bronchiectasis epidemiology is observed among indigenous children of Australia, Alaska, Canada and New Zealand [34, 35, 38–40]. Here, paediatric populations exhibit exceptionally high rates

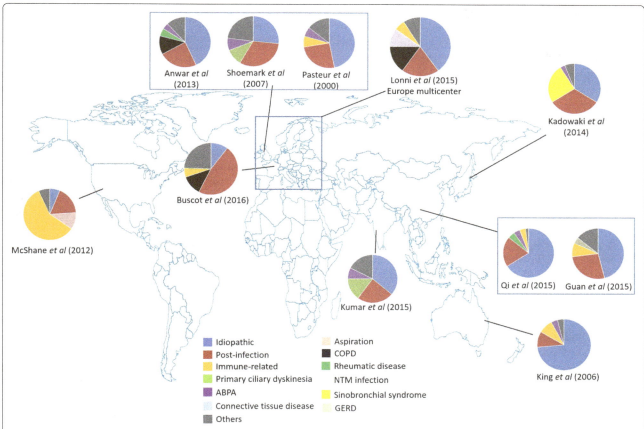

Fig. 2 Predominant aetiologies across different geographic regions and ethnic populations. The individual pie charts indicate the top aetiologies (top 4 or 5) in each cohort. Abbreviations: ABPA – Allergic Broncho-Pulmonary Aspergillosis, COPD – Chronic Obstructive Pulmonary Disorder, NTM – Non-Tuberculosis Mycobacteria, GERD – Gastro-Esophageal Reflux Disease

compared to non-indigenous groups with infant or childhood pneumonia cited as the primary cause in many cases. These combined observations point to the contribution of genetic predisposition, early childhood infection and overall lower socio-economic status as important features in pathogenesis particularly among specific indigenous populations [25]. Considering the Pacific region; a high incidence is observed in children under 15 years of age in New Zealand and substantial differences noted within their indigenous ethnic groups and across their geographic regions [41]. Most paediatric bronchiectasis in New Zealand is idiopathic with predominant chronic *Haemophilus influenzae* infection which in turn associates with reduced lung function [42]. Bronchiectasis in children is also associated with high rates of hospital admission particularly in Australian aboriginal children. This latter group have one of the highest reported prevalence rates of bronchiectasis (14.7 per 1000) worldwide [43, 44]. In separate work, Alaskan native children are described to have extremely high rates of bronchiectasis compared to other populations and, in most of these individuals, infant or childhood pneumonia is the primary cause of disease [38–40]. All the aforementioned patient groups are clearly enriched by disease occurrence, an important feature that offers the opportunity for research to better understand the roles and interaction of genetic predisposition and early childhood infection to the subsequent development of bronchiectasis.

Bronchiectasis in Europe

Incidence and prevalence rates of bronchiectasis in the UK have increased annually from 2004 and are associated with significant mortality [4]. Studies from the UK's North East ($n = 189$) illustrate that occurrence of idiopathic bronchiectasis is high and that those identified with post-infective aetiology developed the condition earlier in life [28]. In contrast, a Greek study ($n = 277$) demonstrated that prior tuberculosis, pertussis, measles and pneumonia were the leading causes of bronchiectasis [45]. A retrospective study from Nice in southern France ($n = 311$) similarly described high rates of post-infectious (mainly post-tuberculous) bronchiectasis [29]. Despite these country-based reports, a large multicentre dataset ($n = 1258$) collated from across Europe (Monza, Italy; Dundee and Newcastle, UK; Leuven,

Belgium; Barcelona, Spain; Athens, Greece and Galway, Ireland) illustrated that most patients have idiopathic disease. Among identifiable causes of bronchiectasis, post-infectious did however remain the commonest. Interestingly in this large dataset, COPD-related bronchiectasis was associated with a higher Bronchiectasis severity index (BSI) [3].

In Germany (2005–2011) the prevalence of bronchiectasis was 67 cases per 100,000; associated with concomitant increases in hospital admissions and an increased incidence with age [46, 47]. A large population based study in Catalonia (north-eastern Spain) similarly found high prevalence (36.2 cases per 10,000) and incidence rates (4.81 cases per 10,000). In contrast to other global datasets, the prevalence and incidence of bronchiectasis in this study was highest in older males [48]. A larger multicentre study in Spain however showed contrasting results with higher prevalence in females and elevated rates of post-infectious disease [30]. Of interest, greater hospital admissions and treatment costs per patient in Spain were inversely related to bronchiectasis where it was the primary diagnosis but increased when identified as a secondary diagnosis clearly highlighting a need for focus on earlier diagnosis [49]. Northern European countries such as Finland interestingly report a lower incidence of bronchiectasis compared to worldwide estimates. This is also accompanied by lower hospitalisation and mortality rates from the disease [50, 51]. Overall, these data clearly illustrate the changing and variation in epidemiology and aetiology of bronchiectasis even within Europe which in turn contrasts to that in the Americas and Asian sub-continents.

Bronchiectasis in the Americas

Seitz et al. (2012) reported an annual increase of 8.7% in the prevalence of bronchiectasis in the US with a higher prevalence in Asian Americans when compared to European and African Americans. This was based on thoracic computed tomography (CT) scans [52]. Similar increases in bronchiectasis incidence was described between 2009 and 2013 with high rates in women and the elderly [53]. McShane et al. (2012) further illustrated that ethnicity was one of the major contributing factors for the observed aetiological differences in disease, an important consideration for clinicians in an increasingly multi-ethnic resident population across different countries. Rheumatoid Arthritis (RA) was interestingly a common aetiology in African Americans and hematologic malignancies more common in European Americans in this study. Subsequent work also supports the association between hematologic malignancy and bronchiectasis while the role of connective tissue disorders is also corroborated by several investigations [17, 54]. The first report from the US bronchiectasis research registry was recently published and characterised 1826 patients. Its results concurred with others and illustrated a higher occurrence in women. Within the analysed cohort, a higher prevalence of the disease was described in European Americans [55]. The status of bronchiectasis as a largely under-studied disease is further reflected by the relative lack of prevalence data from Canada, the Caribbean and South America, where further studies are warranted.

Bronchiectasis in the Asia-Pacific region

In the Asian subcontinent, considerable gaps in our understanding of bronchiectasis epidemiology continue to exist. No comprehensive prevalence datasets for either China or India are currently available however work is currently ongoing to address this. There are sporadic regional reports available that provide some insight into bronchiectasis in this highly affected region.

A recent pan-Indian study ($n = 680$) identified post-infection (41%) to be the primary cause for bronchiectasis with post-tuberculous disease identified as the predominant aetiology (29.8%), whilst ABPA is the most common cause after this and identified in 12% of Indian cases [56]. An aetiological study across different ethnicities in the Guangzhou region of mainland China ($n = 148$) identified idiopathic bronchiectasis (45%) as the most common cause with the high rates of disease related to post-infection (27%) also noted [57]. Among the Han population of mainland China ($n = 476$), rates of idiopathic bronchiectasis (66%) are even more striking and followed by post-tuberculosis as the most prevalent aetiologies observed (16%) [58].These Chinese studies illustrate that whilst post-tuberculous bronchiectasis remains important in Asia, idiopathic bronchiectasis is also highly prevalent. In a small study from Hong Kong ($n = 100$), idiopathic disease dominates (82%) and patients with bronchiectasis are mainly female with high hospitalisation and mortality rates; 21.9 cases per 100,000 and 2.7 cases per 100,000 respectively [59, 60].

In contrast to China however, work from Thailand ($n = 50$) indicates that post-infection related bronchiectasis and specifically post-tuberculosis associated disease was commonest. Similarly, a high prevalence of post-infectious bronchiectasis was reported in Indian children ($n = 80$) followed by primary ciliary dyskinesia and ABPA [61, 62]. A high prevalence of bronchiectasis is reported in South Korea ($n = 1409$) and in one particular study of respiratory patients, 9% were deemed to have bronchiectasis with higher prevalence in females [63].

A variety of reasons may be put forward to explain the outlined epidemiological differences in bronchiectasis that exist across Europe, the Americas and the Asia-Pacific. For example, tuberculosis is rare in more developed countries when compared to the Asia-Pacific or

Africa potentially explaining the high frequencies of post-tuberculous disease found in these regions. Potential genetic predisposition to bronchiectasis may account for the increased disease prevalence in indigenous communities in the Asia-Pacific region. The influence of the environment and its accompanying climate may also influence microorganisms and/or pathogens that affect the bronchiectasis airway. Hence, we next outline geographic variations in the airway microbiology in bronchiectasis which in itself may account for some of the observed differences in epidemiological patterns of disease.

Geographic variation in the microbiology of bronchiectasis
The Bacteriome
Pseudomonas aeruginosa and *H. influenzae* are the most common bacteria detected in bronchiectasis airways globally although proportions vary among the different populations [45, 64]. Other bacterial genera described in bronchiectasis airways include *Streptococcus*, *Prevotella*, *Veillonella* and *Staphylococcus* [65–67]. *P. aeruginosa* is associated with poorer pulmonary function, higher hospitalisation rates and greater morbidity and mortality compared to *H. influenzae* [68–78].

Non-tuberculosis mycobacteria (NTM) are another important group of organisms that frequently infect the airway in adult bronchiectasis. Bronchiectasis and NTM are highly associated pulmonary diseases with airway distortion predisposing to NTM infection [79, 80]. While NTM is isolated from the bronchiectasis airway and clearly associates with poorer outcomes and more aggressive disease in most cases (largely dependent on the species involved), in some studies, it interestingly has been associated with a milder phenotype, less severe disease, lower exacerbations and better pulmonary function [81, 82]. NTM colonisation in common with *P. aeruginosa* is more frequent in older patients with gender preponderance for postmenopausal women and a lower prevalence is observed in paediatric populations [82–85]. *Mycobacterium avium complex* (MAC) is generally the most common form affecting bronchiectasis patients although geographic variation exists [80, 82, 84, 86].

The bronchiectasis bacteriome in children vs adults
Studies in children focused on bronchiectasis microbiology highlight *H. influenzae* as the most prevalent sputum organism (30–83%) from work originating in New Zealand. Of note, *P. aeruginosa* largely considered an airway organism affecting adults was described in up to 4% of children with bronchiectasis with *S. pneumoniae* (5–14%) and *M. catarrhalis* (2–8%) also described [41, 42, 85]. Several studies, some using bronchoalveolar lavage (BAL) from indigenous children in Northern Australia, showed marked similarity for their microbiology compared to the New Zealand datasets except that none of the children in this latter work were *P. aeruginosa* positive [87, 88]. When compared to European paediatric data from the UK and Ireland; children were found to have similar dichotomy between *H. influenzae* and *P. aeruginosa* in the airway and also high detection of *S. pneumoniae* [89–91]. There are however some notable intra-country differences in geographic patterns for *P. aeruginosa*: low levels in Newcastle compared to higher levels in London (5% versus 11% respectively) which contrasts to *M. catarrhalis* where occurrence in Newcastle is higher than that in London [90, 91]. Such differences may reflect differing referral patterns or presence of specialist clinics at particular centres but nonetheless serve to highlight the spectrum of disease heterogeneity seen in children. When evaluated against data from an adult bronchiectasis population in the UK, expectedly higher rates of *P. aeruginosa* (49%) are observed compared to the paediatric cohorts [70]. Taken together, these observations suggest that variation in paediatric bronchiectasis microbiology may be more complex than that in adults and illustrate within-country differences in addition to geographic and continental variation.

The bronchiectasis bacteriome in Europe
In European studies of the bacteriome in adult bronchiectasis, data combining Spanish and Scottish datasets illustrate equal proportions of *H. influenzae* and *P. aeruginosa* with *E.coli* interestingly isolated from a tenth of the studied cohort [92]. Separate work from Greece, Belgium and France concur with other European studies detecting high rates of airway *P. aeruginosa* and *H. influenzae* but low NTM [29, 45, 47, 93]. An important study, using 16 s rRNA sequencing from Northern Ireland showed that change to bacterial communities in the bronchiectasis airways may not in fact be a driver for exacerbations however a trend toward lower microbial diversity was described. In terms of relative abundance, *Haemophilus spp.* dominates *Pseudomonas spp.* in stable patients and post-antibiotic treatment, a mild increase in anaerobic bacteria is seen with a corresponding decrease in aerobes [94]. In contrast however, other 16 s rRNA datasets assessing both the stable and exacerbation states found that *P. aeruginosa* was the commonest organism in both categories [65]. More recent studies, also from the UK, have reaffirmed the important original observations that changes from a stable to exacerbation state involves more than a simple alteration in the bronchiectasis airway bacteriome [67]. While it may be too early to speculate on specific patterns of microbes and an association to exacerbations, data in support of this hypothesis is the observation (from pyrosequencing UK datasets) that an inverse relationship does exist between

airway abundance of *P. aeruginosa* and *H. influenzae* in the bronchiectasis airway and that specific microbial patterns do associate with the exacerbation state [71]. Sequencing approaches have also interestingly shown that long-term erythromycin treatment adversely affects *H. influenzae*-dominant patients by increasing the relative abundance of *P. aeruginosa* [66, 95].

The bronchiectasis bacteriome in the Americas

Varying rates of colonisation by *P. aeruginosa* are described across varied ethnic groups in the US with Hispanic Americans having the highest rates, followed by European Americans and African Americans [33]. In more recent data from the US Bronchiectasis research registry (n = 1826) however, NTM were found to be most frequent (54%) with MAC followed by *M. abscessus* and *M. chelonae* being the commonest isolated NTM species. *P. aeruginosa* was described in one-third and *S. aureus* in one-eighth of patients with colonisation by either of these species less in patients affected by NTM. Patients with detectable NTM also developed bronchiectasis later and were predominantly female [55]. Studies from Europe have found similar discordance between NTM and these other bacteria in the bronchiectasis airways [96]. Of note, however, is the ascertainment bias in the US bronchiectasis research registry: many are tertiary referral centres with NTM referral patterns potentially skewing the reported data. It is likely that the US does however have more NTM-associated disease overall in comparison to other geographic regions however the current available datasets don't permit us to definitively establish this.

The bronchiectasis bacteriome in the Asia-pacific region

In Asia, similar patterns, in both the ethnic Han population from Shandong province (eastern China) and the southern Chinese city of Guangzhou are observed with predominance of *P. aeruginosa* and *H. influenzae* with colonisation rates of the former stable across the different bronchiectasis aetiologies identified in these populations. NTM rates unlike the US were low in Chinese studies [57, 58]. Prospective work from Thailand found similar patterns to that described in China although in this population *Klebsiella pneumoniae* was detected in equal proportions to *H. influenzae* [61]. South Korea has a different distribution with high NTM (44.5%), similar to that of the US and lower rates of *P. aeruginosa* (18.1%). Like the Thai patients, South Koreans also had a significant prevalence of *K. pneumoniae* [97]. While geographically close; work from Japan however reports *P. aeruginosa* as the predominant airway bacteria (24%) closely followed by only moderate levels of NTM (19%) [37]. Interestingly, in the Pacific region, specifically central and southern Australia; reported rates of *H. influenzae* (36–81%) compared to *P. aeruginosa* (7–26%) are higher with very low occurrences of NTM (1–2%) [88, 98, 99].

A higher mean relative abundance of *Haemophilus spp.* compared to *Pseudomonas spp.* was reported in an Australian study. The authors propose a bacteriome based patient stratification system to predict exacerbations in bronchiectasis. In this system, patients with an airway bacteriome dominated by *P. aeruginosa* or *Veillonella spp.* experience higher rates of future exacerbations compared to patients whose airways are dominated by *H. influenzae* [100]. In addition, *H. influenzae* dominant individuals experience milder disease in contrast to *P. aeruginosa* which may be attributed to competitive exclusion between the organisms [101]. While interesting, these observations are importantly derived from datasets from the BLESS trial that assessed patients with a history of at least two exacerbations per year. Therefore, these identified patterns were based on comparisons between 'very frequent' to 'less frequent' exacerbators and lacked assessment against non-exacerbators.

While culture based detection of airway bacteria is routinely used in bronchiectasis, next-generation sequencing (NGS) approaches are being used in research as a faster and more robust alternative for identifying airway pathogens [65, 66, 102]. Such culture-independent sequencing methodologies have been applied in bronchiectasis and identify a greater degree of airway microbial diversity (Table 1) [103, 104]. These methods are not yet appropriate for clinical use because of the challenges in bioinformatic analysis and standardisation. This will be efficiently computerised in the coming years and facilitate clinical translation. In spite of the increasing exploration of the bacteriome using such technological advances, exploration of viral and fungal residents of the lung and their association with bronchiectasis has lagged behind. While the small number of available studies limits our understanding of viral and fungal contributions to bronchiectasis and their geographic variability, we nonetheless review below their currently understood respective contributions and the evidence supporting their clinical association with bronchiectasis.

The Virome

Our current understanding of the virome in bronchiectasis is limited and most studies of viruses in bronchiectasis are rarely assessed compared to the baseline presence of viruses in healthy individuals. Recent work however has suggested a role for viruses in exacerbations of bronchiectasis where bacterial density and diversity remains stable during exacerbations [94]. Early work from the US and Canada were the first to report viral infection, specifically Influenza B and adenovirus in bronchiectasis, respectively [105, 106]. More recently, work from China (Guangzhou) reports coronavirus, rhinovirus

Table 1 Predominant pathogens identified in bronchiectasis cohort studies

Method			Population	Sample size	Predominant pathogens (by sequencing)	Predominant pathogens (by culture)	Ref
Sputum culture	BAL culture	16S rRNA sequencing					
✓			Adult	$n = 123$	N.A.	P. aeruginosa H. influenzae M. avium intracellulare S. pneumoniae S. aureus	[128]
✓			Adult	$n = 100$	N.A.	P. aeruginosa H. influenzae S. pneumoniae S. aureus M. catarrhalis	[74]
✓			Adult	$n = 193$	N.A.	H. influenzae P. aeruginosa M. catarrhalis S. pneumoniae S. aureus A. fumigatus	[32]
✓			Adult	$n = 155$	N.A.	H. influenzae P. aeruginosa S. pneumoniae M. catarrhalis S. aureus	[70]
✓	✓		Adult	$n = 77$	N.A.	H. influenzae S. pneumoniae P. aeruginosa	[129]
	✓		Children	$n = 113$	N.A	NTHi S. pneumoniae M. catarrhalis S. aureus P. aeruginosa	[88]
✓			Adult	$n = 89$	N.A.	H. influenzae P. aeruginosa M. catarrhalis S. pneumoniae S. aureus Aspergillus spp. M. avium complex	[69]
		✓	Adult	$n = 11$	P. aeruginosa Prevotella spp. Streptococcus spp. Haemophilus spp	N.A.	[65]
		✓	Adult	$n = 41$	H. influenzae P. aeruginosa S. pneumoniae S. aureus M. catarrhalis	N.A.	[66]
✓		✓	Adult	$n = 70$	Pseudomonadaceae Pasteurellaceae Streptococcaceae	P. aeruginosa H. influenzae	[71]
✓		✓	Adult	Culture: Stable: $n = 40$ Exacerbation : $n = 11$ Sequencing: Stable: $n = 10$ Exacerbation : $n = 19$	Haemophilus spp. Pseudomonas spp. Streptococcus spp. Achromobacter spp	**Stable patients:** P. aeruginosa H. influenzae Prevotella spp. Veillonella spp. **Exacerbation patients:** P. aeruginosa H. influenzae S. pneumoniae Methicillin-resistant S. aureus	[94]

Table 1 Predominant pathogens identified in bronchiectasis cohort studies (Continued)

Method			Population	Sample size	Predominant pathogens (by sequencing)	Predominant pathogens (by culture)	Ref
Sputum culture	BAL culture	16S rRNA sequencing					
✓		✓	Adult	Stable $n = 76$, $n = 64/76$ patients followed-up during exacerbation.	Hemophilus spp. Pseudomonas spp. Streptococcus spp.	P. aeruginosa S. aureus H. influenzae	[67]

The list order of pathogens corresponds to frequency of identification. Abbreviations: P. aeruginosa – Pseudomonas aeruginosa, NTM – Non-Tuberculosis Mycobacteria, H.influenzae – Haemophilus influenzae, NTHi – Non-typeable Haemophilus influenzae, C. albicans – Candida albicans, S. pneumoniae – Streptococcus pneumoniae, S. aureus – Staphylococcus aureus, M. catarrhalis – Moraxella catarrhalis, A. fumigatus – Aspergillus fumigatus, M. avium – Mycobacterium avium

and influenza A and B detection during exacerbations which is associated with concomitant increases in both airway and systemic inflammation (IL-1β; IL-6) [107]. Systemic and airway TNF-α was also elevated in virus positive exacerbations [107]. Interesting work from Australian indigenous children similarly illustrates an increased viral detection, particularly rhinoviruses during exacerbations. Children positive for virus during an exacerbation are also more likely to be hospitalised [108]. These data however do not elucidate whether viruses are a cause or consequence of exacerbations, an area for future investigation. Despite this, recent work from both Europe and the Asia-Pacific has indicated a potential role for human T-lymphotropic virus type 1 (HTLV-1) mediated inflammation in the causation of bronchiectasis [109, 110]. A separate New Zealand based study similarly proposed adenovirus infection as a potential cause of post-infectious bronchiectasis (Fig. 3) [111].

The Mycobiome

Our knowledge of the pulmonary mycobiome is less well characterised and although technically challenging, may provide new insight into its potential role in bronchiectasis. Fungi, a separate kingdom of organisms with more

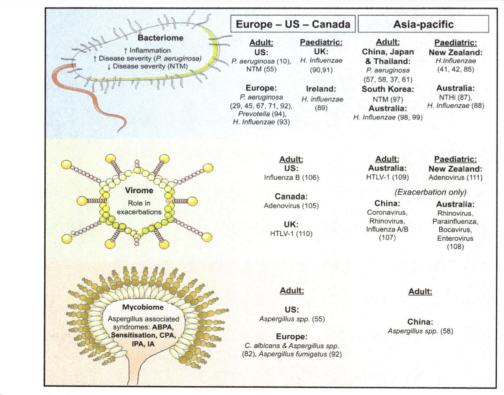

Fig. 3 Differences in the microbiome between Europe, the US and the Asia-Pacific by sputum culture illustrating the predominant organisms in stable states and viruses only during exacerbations. The bacteriome contributes to host inflammation and disease severity, the virome in exacerbations and the mycobiome is an understudied group with potential clinical impact. Abbreviations: US – United States, UK – United Kingdom, P. aeruginosa – Pseudomonas aeruginosa, NTM – Non-Tuberculosis Mycobacteria, H.influenzae – Haemophilus influenzae, NTHi – Non-typeable Haemophilus influenzae, HTLV-1 – Human T-Lymphotropic Virus type 1, C. albicans – Candida albicans, ABPA – Allergic Broncho-Pulmonary Aspergillosis, CPA – Chronic Pulmonary Aspergillosis, IPA – Invasive Pulmonary Aspergillosis, IA – Invasive Aspergillosis ↑ - Increased, ↓ - Decreased

than 1.5 million estimated species requires dedicated study in bronchiectasis where anatomical distortion to the airways predisposes patients to both acquisition and colonisation by fungi [103, 112–115]. Those belonging to the Ascomycota phyla (e.g. Aspergillus *spp.*) form spores and through inhalation, on a daily basis, thousands of fungal spores have access to the airways [103]. Dependant on the underlying state of host immunity, disease can result and, manifestations range from allergic (in immune hyper-reactivity) to invasive (in severe immunodeficiency). Such disease variation is best characterised by *Aspergillus*-associated syndromes outlined in Fig. 3. Allergic bronchopulmonary aspergillosis (ABPA) is a recognised aetiological factor for the occurrence of bronchiectasis while sensitisation increases the incidence of bronchiectasis in asthmatics [116–119].

In addition to *Aspergillus*, *Candida spp.* represents another fungal genus of potential importance, one routinely cultured from airway samples. Importantly, *Candida spp.* are abundant in the oral cavity even of healthy individuals and hence whether they represent genuine respiratory colonisers and/or pathogens in bronchiectasis remains uncertain [120].

A great paucity of data exist specifically assessing fungi in the airways of patients with bronchiectasis. Most studies of bronchiectasis don't specifically include dedicated fungal culture and most published reports are based on their incidental detection. As documented by recently published 'research priorities in bronchiectasis' from the EMBARC collaboration, work addressing fungi is both necessary and of importance in bronchiectasis [121]. A Spanish study reports that *Aspergillus* and *Candida spp.* together contribute the highest proportion of fungi isolated by culture from the bronchiectasis airway. Within the *Aspergillus* genus, *A. fumigatus* is the most common coloniser and other filamentous fungi such as *Penicillium*, *Scedosporium* and *Fusarium* are less frequently seen. Critically, chronic antibiotic use in this work was associated with prolonged colonisation by these fungi [82]. Data from the US bronchiectasis research registry (n = 1826) reports an incidence of 19% of *Aspergillus spp.* in their population [55] Two separate studies from the UK illustrate that *A. fumigatus* colonisation and/or sensitisation is positively correlated with NTM occurrence. The co-existence of chronic pulmonary aspergillosis and NTM infection predicts mortality in bronchiectasis [122, 123]. Culture-based identification, part of the routine diagnostic microbiology work up in bronchiectasis is inefficient for fungal detection because most fungal species do not grow on common laboratory media [124]. To overcome this, work employing next-generation sequencing (NGS) such as targeted amplicon sequencing and whole-genome shotgun metagenomics may reveal the true diversity of fungal microorganisms within the microbiome that may colonise and contribute to pulmonary pathology in bronchiectasis and as such should be a focus for future work [103, 104, 125]. Figure 3 summarises the 'microbiome' in bronchiectasis that consists of the 'bacteriome', 'virome' and 'mycobiome' where based on country, the predominant organism has been identified and geographical differences outlined between Europe, the US and the Asia-Pacific. Findings relating to adult and paediatric populations are also indicated.

Geographic variation in clinical bronchiectasis phenotypes

Studies assessing clinical phenotypes in bronchiectasis are lacking. The most extensive study to date included 1145 patients across five databases in Europe and identified four distinct phenotypes: severe *Pseudomonas* infection (16%), other chronic infections (24%), daily sputum production without colonisation (33%) and dry bronchiectasis (27%) [126]. This contrasted with a single reported Asian analysis from China where 148 patients were assessed [127]. Again, four different groups were identified but the only commonality was a severe group with post-infective bronchiectasis and the presence of airway *Pseudomonas*. Other key groups from the Chinese study included mild idiopathic disease in young patients, severe idiopathic disease of late-onset and moderate disease in the elderly. A third study focused solely on the Spanish national database of 468 patients again identified the presence of airway *Pseudomonas* as a separate clinical phenotype [30]. In this setting, it was characterised by severe disease, chronic infection, airflow obstruction and severe exacerbations in elderly men. Geographic variation in bronchiectasis phenotypes is likely very relevant for our understanding of disease pathogenesis according to region and requires further and more detailed study. Importantly, while results from the various cluster studies in bronchiectasis may represent true geographic variation in disease, they are limited by the quality and quantity of data put into the clustering process itself and, has largely remained uncontrolled for referral bias. An overwhelming message across all three studies is that clinical data alone was poor at identifying meaningful patient 'clusters' providing a strong argument for alternative approaches including use of "omics" for patient stratification. Perhaps targeted therapeutic approaches in the future, applicable to specific regions and populations may become relevant as we start to decipher the drivers of varying endotypes of disease.

Conclusion

As the incidence and prevalence rates of bronchiectasis continue to increase with global ageing, it can no longer be considered an 'orphan' respiratory disease. Despite its documented economic burden, effects on quality of life, and social implications, bronchiectasis is a relatively neglected pulmonary disease. Further investment and research are now required, that which focuses on ethnic variations and accounts for geographical differences to permit a more 'personalised' approach to its diagnosis, management and understanding of prognosis across countries. The recommendations for research priorities in bronchiectasis by the European Multicentre Bronchiectasis Audit and Research Collaboration (EMBARC) stresses the importance of large cohort studies to better understand the varying aetiologies that drive the disease across different populations. Elucidating differences in less studied organisms including fungi and viruses are also highlighted and research focus in these key areas would improve our understanding of disease while permitting a more personalised therapeutic approach perhaps varied by geographic region [121].

Differences in the aetiology, epidemiology and microbiology of bronchiectasis can be observed across countries and continents and may influence the observed clinical phenotypes, which in turn likely influences treatment and outcomes. Studies targeting geographic regions where a paucity of data exists including Asia, Africa and South America are now necessary. If effective treatment approaches are to be realised in bronchiectasis – a condition for which no licenced therapies currently exist – success will likely depend on more targeted approaches that acknowledge the marked geographic variability associated with this heterogeneous disease.

Abbreviations
ABPA: Allergic Broncho-Pulmonary Aspergillosis; *B. pertussis*: *Bordetella pertussis*; BAL: Broncho-Alveolar Lavage; BLESS: Bronchiectasis and Low-Dose Erythromycin Study; BSI: Bronchiectasis Severity Index; CF: Cystic Fibrosis; CFTR: Cystic Fibrosis Transmembrane Conductor Regulator protein; COPD: Chronic Obstructive Pulmonary Disease; CT: Computed Tomography; *E.coli*: *Escherichia coli*;; EMBARC: European Multicentre Bronchiectasis Audit and Research Collaboration; *H. influenza*: *Haemophilus influenza*; HTLV-1: Human T-Lymphotropic Virus type 1; IL: Interleukin; IPF: Idiopathic Pulmonary Fibrosis; *K. pneumoniae*: *Klebsiella pneumoniae*; *M. abscessus*: *Mycobacterium abscessus*; *M. catarrhalis*: *Moraxella catarrhalis*; *M. chelonae*: *Mycobacterium chelonae*; *M. tuberculosis*: *Mycobacterium tuberculosis*; MAC: *Mycobacterium avium complex*; mTOR: Mechanistic Target Of Rapamycin; NGS: Next Generation Sequencing; NTM: Non-Tuberculosis mycobacteria; *P. aeruginosa*: *Pseudomonas aeruginosa*; PFTs: Pulmonary Function Testing; RA: Rheumatoid Arthritis; RNA: Ribo-Nucleic Acid; rRNA: Ribosomal RNA; RV: Residual Volume; *S. aureus*: *Staphylococcus aureus*; *S. pneumoniae*: *Streptococcus pneumoniae*; spp.: Species; TLR: Toll-Like Receptors; UK: United Kingdom; US: United States; USA: United States of America; VC: Vital Capacity

Funding
This research is supported by the Singapore Ministry of Health's National Medical Research Council under its Transition Award (NMRC/TA/0048/2016) (S.H.C) and the Lee Kong Chian School of Medicine, Nanyang Technological University Start-Up Grant (S.H.C). The funding bodies had no role in the design of the study and collection, analysis, and interpretation of data in writing the manuscript.

Authors' contributions
RC, MMA, JC, JSE and SHC all contributed to conception, drafting, writing and final approval of the manuscript.

Competing interests
Dr. Chotirmall is a section editor for BMC pulmonary medicine. The authors declare that they have no competing interest.

Author details
[1]Lee Kong Chian School of Medicine, Nanyang Technological University, Clinical Sciences Building, 11 Mandalay Road, Singapore 308232, Singapore. [2]Division of Molecular and Clinical Medicine, School of Medicine, Ninewells Hospital and Medical School, Dundee, UK. [3]Imperial College and Royal Brompton Hospital, London, UK. [4]Queen's University Belfast, Belfast, UK.

1. Barker AF. Bronchiectasis. N Engl J Med. 2002;346(18):1383–93.
2. Cole PJ. Inflammation: a two-edged sword–the model of bronchiectasis. Eur J Respir Dis Suppl. 1986;147:6–15.
3. Lonni S, Chalmers JD, Goeminne PC, McDonnell MJ, Dimakou K, De Soyza A, Polverino E, Van de Kerkhove C, Rutherford R, Davison J, et al. Etiology of non-cystic fibrosis bronchiectasis in adults and its correlation to disease severity. Ann Am Thorac Soc. 2015;12(12):1764–70.
4. Quint JK, Millett ER, Joshi M, Navaratnam V, Thomas SL, Hurst JR, Smeeth L, Brown JS. Changes in the incidence, prevalence and mortality of bronchiectasis in the UK from 2004 to 2013: a population-based cohort study. Eur Respir J. 2016;47(1):186–93.
5. Bongaarts J. Human population growth and the demographic transition. Philos Trans R Soc Lond Ser B Biol Sci. 2009;364(1532):2985–90.
6. Chotirmall SH, Watts M, Branagan P, Donegan CF, Moore A, McElvaney NG. Diagnosis and management of asthma in older adults. J Am Geriatr Soc. 2009;57(5):901–9.
7. Al-Alawi M, Hassan T, Chotirmall SH. Advances in the diagnosis and management of asthma in older adults. Am J Med. 2014;127(5):370–8.
8. Bom AT, Pinto AM. Allergic respiratory diseases in the elderly. Respir Med. 2009;103(11):1614–22.
9. Kikawada M, Iwamoto T, Takasaki M. Aspiration and infection in the elderly: epidemiology, diagnosis and management. Drugs Aging. 2005;22(2):115–30.
10. Gavazzi G, Krause KH. Ageing and infection. Lancet Infect Dis. 2002;2(11):659–66.
11. Chotirmall SH, Burke CM. Aging and the microbiome: implications for asthma in the elderly? Expert Rev Respir Med. 2015;9(2):125–8.
12. Chotirmall SH, Gellatly SL, Budden KF, Mac Aogain M, Shukla SD, Wood DL, Hugenholtz P, Pethe K, Hansbro PM. Microbiomes in respiratory health and disease: an Asia-Pacific perspective. Respirology (Carlton, Vic). 2017;22(2):240–50.
13. Linton PJ, Dorshkind K. Age-related changes in lymphocyte development and function. Nat Immunol. 2004;5(2):133–9.
14. Castelo-Branco C, Soveral I. The immune system and aging: a review. Gynecol Endocrinol. 2014;30(1):16–22.
15. Murray MA, Chotirmall SH. The impact of Immunosenescence on pulmonary disease. Mediat Inflamm. 2015;2015:692546.
16. Kvell K, Pongracz JE. Immunosenescence and the ageing lung. In: Bueno V, Lord JM, Jackson TA, editors. The ageing immune system and health. Cham: Springer International Publishing; 2017. p. 87–104.
17. Chen LW, McShane PJ, Karkowsky W, Gray SE, Adegunsoye A, Stock W, Artz A, White SR, Montner SM, Strek ME. De novo development of bronchiectasis in patients with hematologic malignancy. Chest. 2017;152(3):683–5.
18. Birch J, Victorelli S, Rahmatika D, Anderson RK, Jiwa K, Moisey E, Ward C, Fisher AJ, De Soyza A, Passos JF. Telomere dysfunction and senescence-associated pathways in bronchiectasis. Am J Respir Crit Care Med. 2016;193(8):929–32.
19. Lehmann D, Baarsma HA, Konigshoff M. WNT Signaling in Lung Aging and Disease. Ann Am Thorac Soc. 2016;13(Supplement_5):S411–6.
20. Rojas M, Mora AL, Kapetanaki M, Weathington N, Gladwin M, Eickelberg O. Aging and lung disease. Clinical impact and cellular and molecular pathways. Ann Am Thorac Soc. 2015;12(12):S222–7.

21. Volkova M, Zhang Y, Shaw AC, Lee PJ. The role of toll-like receptors in age-associated lung diseases. J Gerontol A Biol Sci Med Sci. 2012;67(3):247–53.
22. King PT. The pathophysiology of bronchiectasis. Int J Chron Obstruct Pulmon Dis. 2009;4:411–9.
23. Brower KS, Del Vecchio MT, Aronoff SC. The etiologies of non-CF bronchiectasis in childhood: a systematic review of 989 subjects. BMC Pediatr. 2014;14:4.
24. Goyal V, Grimwood K, Marchant J, Masters IB, Chang AB. Pediatric bronchiectasis: no longer an orphan disease. Pediatr Pulmonol. 2016;51(5): 450–69.
25. Wurzel DF, Chang AB. An update on pediatric bronchiectasis. Expert Rev Respir Med. 2017;11(7):517–32.
26. Boyton RJ, Altmann DM. Bronchiectasis: current concepts in pathogenesis, immunology, and microbiology. Annu Rev Pathol. 2016;11:523–54.
27. McDonnell MJ, Aliberti S, Goeminne PC, Restrepo MI, Finch S, Pesci A, Dupont LJ, Fardon TC, Wilson R, Loebinger MR, et al. Comorbidities and the risk of mortality in patients with bronchiectasis: an international multicentre cohort study. Lancet Respir Med. 2016;4(12):969–79.
28. Anwar GA, McDonnell MJ, Worthy SA, Bourke SC, Afolabi G, Lordan J, Corris PA, DeSoyza A, Middleton P, Ward C, et al. Phenotyping adults with non-cystic fibrosis bronchiectasis: a prospective observational cohort study. Respir Med. 2013;107(7):1001–7.
29. Buscot M, Pottier H, Marquette CH, Leroy S. Phenotyping adults with non-cystic fibrosis bronchiectasis: a 10-year cohort study in a French regional university hospital center. Respiration. 2016;92(1):1–8.
30. Martinez-Garcia MA, Vendrell M, Giron R, Maiz-Carro L, de la Rosa CD, de Gracia J, Olveira C. The multiple faces of non-cystic fibrosis bronchiectasis: a cluster analysis approach. Ann Am Thorac Soc. 2016;
31. Shoemark A, Ozerovitch L, Wilson R. Aetiology in adult patients with bronchiectasis. Respir Med. 2007;101(6):1163–70.
32. Pasteur MC, Helliwell SM, Houghton SJ, Webb SC, Foweraker JE, Coulden RA, Flower CD, Bilton D, Keogan MT. An investigation into causative factors in patients with bronchiectasis. Am J Respir Crit Care Med. 2000;162(4 Pt 1): 1277–84.
33. McShane PJ, Naureckas ET, Strek ME. Bronchiectasis in a diverse US population: effects of ethnicity on etiology and sputum culture. Chest. 2012; 142(1):159–67.
34. Das L, Kovesi TA. Bronchiectasis in children from Qikiqtani (Baffin) region, Nunavut, Canada. Ann Am Thorac Soc. 2015;12(1):96–100.
35. Kovesi T. Respiratory disease in Canadian first nations and Inuit children. Paediatr Child Health. 2012;17(7):376–80.
36. Marostica PJ, Fischer GB. Non-cystic-fibrosis bronchiectasis: a perspective from South America. Paediatr Respir Rev. 2006;7(4):275–80.
37. Kadowaki T, Yano S, Wakabayashi K, Kobayashi K, Ishikawa S, Kimura M, Ikeda T. An analysis of etiology, causal pathogens, imaging patterns, and treatment of Japanese patients with bronchiectasis. Respir Investig. 2015; 53(1):37–44.
38. Singleton R, Morris A, Redding G, Poll J, Holck P, Martinez P, Kruse D, Bulkow LR, Petersen KM, Lewis C. Bronchiectasis in Alaska native children: causes and clinical courses. Pediatr Pulmonol. 2000;29(3):182–7.
39. Singleton RJ, Valery PC, Morris P, Byrnes CA, Grimwood K, Redding G, Torzillo PJ, McCallum G, Chikoyak L, Mobberly C, et al. Indigenous children from three countries with non-cystic fibrosis chronic suppurative lung disease/bronchiectasis. Pediatr Pulmonol. 2014;49(2):189–200.
40. Fleshman JK, Wilson JF, Cohen JJ. Bronchiectasis in Alaska native children. Arch Environ Health. 1968;17(4):517–23.
41. Twiss J, Metcalfe R, Edwards E, Byrnes C. New Zealand national incidence of bronchiectasis "too high" for a developed country. Arch Dis Child. 2005; 90(7):737–40.
42. Munro KA, Reed PW, Joyce H, Perry D, Twiss J, Byrnes CA, Edwards EA. Do New Zealand children with non-cystic fibrosis bronchiectasis show disease progression? Pediatr Pulmonol. 2011;46(2):131–8.
43. Bibby S, Milne R, Beasley R. Hospital admissions for non-cystic fibrosis bronchiectasis in New Zealand. N Z Med J. 2015;128(1421):30–8.
44. Chang AB, Grimwood K, Mulholland EK, Torzillo PJ. Bronchiectasis in indigenous children in remote Australian communities. Med J Aust. 2002; 177(4):200–4.
45. Dimakou K, Triantafillidou C, Toumbis M, Tsikritsaki K, Malagari K, Bakakos P. Non CF-bronchiectasis: Aetiologic approach, clinical, radiological, microbiological and functional profile in 277 patients. Respir Med. 2016; 116:1–7.
46. Ringshausen FC, de Roux A, Diel R, Hohmann D, Welte T, Rademacher J. Bronchiectasis in Germany: a population-based estimation of disease prevalence. Eur Respir J. 2015;46(6):1805–7.
47. Ringshausen FC, de Roux A, Pletz MW, Hamalainen N, Welte T, Rademacher J. Bronchiectasis-associated hospitalizations in Germany, 2005-2011: a population-based study of disease burden and trends. PLoS One. 2013;8(8): e71109.
48. Monteagudo M, Rodriguez-Blanco T, Barrecheguren M, Simonet P, Miravitlles M. Prevalence and incidence of bronchiectasis in Catalonia, Spain: a population-based study. Respir Med. 2016;121:26–31.
49. Sanchez-Munoz G, Lopez de Andres A, Jimenez-Garcia R, Carrasco-Garrido P, Hernandez-Barrera V, Pedraza-Serrano F, Puente-Maestu L, de Miguel-Diez J. Time trends in hospital admissions for bronchiectasis: analysis of the Spanish National Hospital Discharge Data (2004 to 2013). PLoS One. 2016; 11(9):e0162282.
50. Saynajakangas O, Keistinen T, Tuuponen T, Kivela SL. Bronchiectasis in Finland: trends in hospital treatment. Respir Med. 1997;91(7):395–8.
51. Saynajakangas O, Keistinen T, Tuuponen T, Kivela SL. Evaluation of the incidence and age distribution of bronchiectasis from the Finnish hospital discharge register. Cent Eur J Public Health. 1998;6(3):235–7.
52. Seitz AE, Olivier KN, Adjemian J, Holland SM, Prevots DR. Trends in bronchiectasis among medicare beneficiaries in the United States, 2000 to 2007. Chest. 2012;142(2):432–9.
53. Weycker D, Hansen GL, Seifer FD. Prevalence and incidence of noncystic fibrosis bronchiectasis among US adults in 2013. Chron Respir Dis. 2017; 14(4):377–84.
54. Leung JM, Olivier KN. Bronchiectasis and connective tissue diseases. Curr Pulm Rep. 2016;5(4):169–76.
55. Aksamit TR, O'Donnell AE, Barker A, Olivier KN, Winthrop KL, Daniels MLA, Johnson M, Eden E, Griffith D, Knowles M, et al. Adult patients with bronchiectasis: a first look at the US bronchiectasis research registry. Chest. 2017;151(5):982–92.
56. Dhar R, Mohan M, D'Souza G, Rajagopalan S, Singh V, Jindal A, Archana B, Ghewade B, Joshi G, Sahasrabuddhe T, et al. Phenotype characterization of non cystic fibrosis bronchiectasis in India: baseline data from an Indian bronchiectasis registry. In: ATS 2017, vol. 195. Washington D.C; 2017. p. A4726.
57. Guan WJ, Gao YH, Xu G, Lin ZY, Tang Y, Li HM, Lin ZM, Zheng JP, Chen RC, Zhong NS. Aetiology of bronchiectasis in Guangzhou, southern China. Respirology (Carlton, Vic). 2015;20(5):739–48.
58. Qi Q, Wang W, Li T, Zhang Y, Li Y. Aetiology and clinical characteristics of patients with bronchiectasis in a Chinese Han population: a prospective study. Respirology (Carlton, Vic). 2015;20(6):917–24.
59. Chan-Yeung M, Lai CK, Chan KS, Cheung AH, Yao TJ, Ho AS, Ko FW, Yam LY, Wong PC, Tsang KW, et al. The burden of lung disease in Hong Kong: a report from the Hong Kong thoracic society. Respirology (Carlton, Vic). 2008; 13(Suppl 4):S133–65.
60. Tsang KW, Tipoe GL. Bronchiectasis: not an orphan disease in the east. Int J Tuberc Lung Dis. 2004;8(6):691–702.
61. Palwatwichai A, Chaoprasong C, Vattanathum A, Wongsa A, Jatakanon A. Clinical, laboratory findings and microbiologic characterization of bronchiectasis in Thai patients. Respirology (Carlton, Vic). 2002;7(1):63–6.
62. Kumar A, Lodha R, Kumar P, Kabra SK. Non-cystic fibrosis bronchiectasis in children: clinical profile, etiology and outcome. Indian Pediatr. 2015;52(1):35–7.
63. Kwak HJ, Moon JY, Choi YW, Kim TH, Sohn JW, Yoon HJ, Shin DH, Park SS, Kim SH. High prevalence of bronchiectasis in adults: analysis of CT findings in a health screening program. Tohoku J Exp Med. 2010;222(4):237–42.
64. Borekci S, Halis AN, Aygun G, Musellim B. Bacterial colonization and associated factors in patients with bronchiectasis. Ann Thorac Med. 2016; 11(1):55–9.
65. Duff RM, Simmonds NJ, Davies JC, Wilson R, Alton EW, Pantelidis P, Cox MJ, Cookson WO, Bilton D, Moffatt MF. A molecular comparison of microbial communities in bronchiectasis and cystic fibrosis. Eur Respir J. 2013;41(4): 991–3.
66. Rogers GB, van der Gast CJ, Cuthbertson L, Thomson SK, Bruce KD, Martin ML, Serisier DJ. Clinical measures of disease in adult non-CF bronchiectasis correlate with airway microbiota composition. Thorax. 2013;68(8):731–7.
67. Cox MJ, Turek EM, Hennessy C, Mirza GK, James PL, Coleman M, Jones A, Wilson R, Bilton D, Cookson WO, et al. Longitudinal assessment of sputum microbiome by sequencing of the 16S rRNA gene in non-cystic fibrosis bronchiectasis patients. PLoS One. 2017;12(2):e0170622.

68. Evans SA, Turner SM, Bosch BJ, Hardy CC, Woodhead MA. Lung function in bronchiectasis: the influence of Pseudomonas aeruginosa. Eur Respir J. 1996;9(8):1601–4.
69. King PT, Holdsworth SR, Freezer NJ, Villanueva E, Holmes PW. Microbiologic follow-up study in adult bronchiectasis. Respir Med. 2007;101(8):1633–8.
70. McDonnell MJ, Jary HR, Perry A, MacFarlane JG, Hester KL, Small T, Molyneux C, Perry JD, Walton KE, De Soyza A. Non cystic fibrosis bronchiectasis: a longitudinal retrospective observational cohort study of pseudomonas persistence and resistance. Respir Med. 2015;109(6):716–26.
71. Purcell P, Jary H, Perry A, Perry JD, Stewart CJ, Nelson A, Lanyon C, Smith DL, Cummings SP, De Soyza A. Polymicrobial airway bacterial communities in adult bronchiectasis patients. BMC Microbiol. 2014;14:130.
72. Davies G, Wells AU, Doffman S, Watanabe S, Wilson R. The effect of Pseudomonas aeruginosa on pulmonary function in patients with bronchiectasis. Eur Respir J. 2006;28(5):974–9.
73. Guan WJ, Gao YH, Xu G, Lin ZY, Tang Y, Li HM, Lin ZM, Zheng JP, Chen RC, Zhong NS. Sputum bacteriology in steady-state bronchiectasis in Guangzhou, China. Int J Tuberc Lung Dis. 2015;19(5):610–9.
74. Ho PL, Chan KN, Ip MS, Lam WK, Ho CS, Yuen KY, Tsang KW. The effect of Pseudomonas aeruginosa infection on clinical parameters in steady-state bronchiectasis. Chest. 1998;114(6):1594–8.
75. Finch S, McDonnell MJ, Abo-Leyah H, Aliberti S, Chalmers JD. A comprehensive analysis of the impact of Pseudomonas aeruginosa colonization on prognosis in adult bronchiectasis. Ann Am Thorac Soc. 2015;12(11):1602–11.
76. Wilson CB, Jones PW, O'Leary CJ, Hansell DM, Cole PJ, Wilson R. Effect of sputum bacteriology on the quality of life of patients with bronchiectasis. Eur Respir J. 1997;10(8):1754–60.
77. Loebinger MR, Wells AU, Hansell DM, Chinyanganya N, Devaraj A, Meister M, Wilson R. Mortality in bronchiectasis: a long-term study assessing the factors influencing survival. Eur Respir J. 2009;34(4):843–9.
78. Goeminne PC, Nawrot TS, Ruttens D, Seys S, Dupont LJ. Mortality in non-cystic fibrosis bronchiectasis: a prospective cohort analysis. Respir Med. 2014;108(2):287–96.
79. Aksamit TR, Philley JV, Griffith DE. Nontuberculous mycobacterial (NTM) lung disease: the top ten essentials. Respir Med. 2014;108(3):417–25.
80. Bonaiti G, Pesci A, Marruchella A, Lapadula G, Gori A, Aliberti S. Nontuberculous mycobacteria in noncystic fibrosis bronchiectasis. Biomed Res Int. 2015;2015:197950.
81. Faverio P, Stainer A, Bonaiti G, Zucchetti SC, Simonetta E, Lapadula G, Marruchella A, Gori A, Blasi F, Codecasa L, et al. Characterizing non-tuberculous mycobacteria infection in bronchiectasis. Int J Mol Sci. 2016;17(11).
82. Maiz L, Vendrell M, Olveira C, Giron R, Nieto R, Martinez-Garcia MA. Prevalence and factors associated with isolation of aspergillus and Candida from sputum in patients with non-cystic fibrosis bronchiectasis. Respiration. 2015;89(5):396–403.
83. Mirsaeidi M, Sadikot RT. Gender susceptibility to mycobacterial infections in patients with non-CF bronchiectasis. Int J Mycobacteriol. 2015;4(2):92–6.
84. Mirsaeidi M, Hadid W, Ericsoussi B, Rodgers D, Sadikot RT. Non-tuberculous mycobacterial disease is common in patients with non-cystic fibrosis bronchiectasis. Int J Infect Dis. 2013;17(11):e1000–4.
85. Edwards EA, Asher MI, Byrnes CA. Paediatric bronchiectasis in the twenty-first century: experience of a tertiary children's hospital in New Zealand. J Paediatr Child Health. 2003;39(2):111–7.
86. Wickremasinghe M, Ozerovitch LJ, Davies G, Wodehouse T, Chadwick MV, Abdallah S, Shah P, Wilson R. Non-tuberculous mycobacteria in patients with bronchiectasis. Thorax. 2005;60(12):1045–51.
87. Hare KM, Grimwood K, Leach AJ, Smith-Vaughan H, Torzillo PJ, Morris PS, Chang AB. Respiratory bacterial pathogens in the nasopharynx and lower airways of Australian indigenous children with bronchiectasis. J Pediatr. 2010;157(6):1001–5.
88. Kapur N, Grimwood K, Masters IB, Morris PS, Chang AB. Lower airway microbiology and cellularity in children with newly diagnosed non-CF bronchiectasis. Pediatr Pulmonol. 2012;47(3):300–7.
89. Zaid AA, Elnazir B, Greally P. A decade of non-cystic fibrosis bronchiectasis 1996-2006. Ir Med J. 2010;103(3):77–9.
90. Li AM, Sonnappa S, Lex C, Wong E, Zacharasiewicz A, Bush A, Jaffe A. Non-CF bronchiectasis: does knowing the aetiology lead to changes in management? Eur Respir J. 2005;26(1):8–14.
91. Eastham KM, Fall AJ, Mitchell L, Spencer DA. The need to redefine non-cystic fibrosis bronchiectasis in childhood. Thorax. 2004;59(4):324–7.
92. Sibila O, Suarez-Cuartin G, Rodrigo-Troyano A, Fardon TC, Finch S, Mateus EF, Garcia-Bellmunt L, Castillo D, Vidal S, Sanchez-Reus F, et al. Secreted mucins and airway bacterial colonization in non-CF bronchiectasis. Respirology (Carlton, Vic). 2015;20(7):1082–8.
93. Goeminne PC, Scheers H, Decraene A, Seys S, Dupont LJ. Risk factors for morbidity and death in non-cystic fibrosis bronchiectasis: a retrospective cross-sectional analysis of CT diagnosed bronchiectatic patients. Respir Res. 2012;13:21.
94. Tunney MM, Einarsson GG, Wei L, Drain M, Klem ER, Cardwell C, Ennis M, Boucher RC, Wolfgang MC, Elborn JS. Lung microbiota and bacterial abundance in patients with bronchiectasis when clinically stable and during exacerbation. Am J Respir Crit Care Med. 2013;187(10):1118–26.
95. Rogers GB, Bruce KD, Martin ML, Burr LD, Serisier DJ. The effect of long-term macrolide treatment on respiratory microbiota composition in non-cystic fibrosis bronchiectasis: an analysis from the randomised, double-blind, placebo-controlled BLESS trial. Lancet Respir Med. 2014;2(12):988–96.
96. Fowler SJ, French J, Screaton NJ, Foweraker J, Condliffe A, Haworth CS, Exley AR, Bilton D. Nontuberculous mycobacteria in bronchiectasis: prevalence and patient characteristics. Eur Respir J. 2006;28(6):1204–10.
97. Park J, Kim S, Lee YJ, Park JS, Cho YJ, Yoon HI, Lee KW, Lee CT, Lee JH. Factors associated with radiologic progression of non-cystic fibrosis bronchiectasis during long-term follow-up. Respirology (Carlton, Vic). 2016;21(6):1049–54.
98. Steinfort DP, Brady S, Weisinger HS, Einsiedel L. Bronchiectasis in Central Australia: a young face to an old disease. Respir Med. 2008;102(4):574–8.
99. King PT, Holdsworth SR, Freezer NJ, Villanueva E, Holmes PW. Characterisation of the onset and presenting clinical features of adult bronchiectasis. Respir Med. 2006;100(12):2183–9.
100. Rogers GB, Zain NM, Bruce KD, Burr LD, Chen AC, Rivett DW, McGuckin MA, Serisier DJ. A novel microbiota stratification system predicts future exacerbations in bronchiectasis. Ann Am Thorac Soc. 2014;11(4):496–503.
101. Rogers GB, van der Gast CJ, Serisier DJ. Predominant pathogen competition and core microbiota divergence in chronic airway infection. ISME J. 2015;9(1):217–25.
102. Rogers GB, Daniels TW, Tuck A, Carroll MP, Connett GJ, David GJ, Bruce KD. Studying bacteria in respiratory specimens by using conventional and molecular microbiological approaches. BMC Pulm Med. 2009;9:14.
103. Nguyen LD, Viscogliosi E, Delhaes L. The lung mycobiome: an emerging field of the human respiratory microbiome. Front Microbiol. 2015;6:89.
104. Krause R, Moissl-Eichinger C, Halwachs B, Gorkiewicz G, Berg G, Valentin T, Prattes J, Hogenauer C, Zollner-Schwetz I. Mycobiome in the lower respiratory tract - a clinical perspective. Front Microbiol. 2016;7:2169.
105. Bateman ED, Hayashi S, Kuwano K, Wilke TA, Hogg JC. Latent adenoviral infection in follicular bronchiectasis. Am J Respir Crit Care Med. 1995;151(1):170–6.
106. Rytel MW, Conner GH, Welch CC, Kraybill WH, Edwards EA, Rosenbaum MJ, Frank PF, Miller LF. Infectious agents associated with cylindrical bronchiectasis. Dis Chest. 1964;46:23–8.
107. Gao YH, Guan WJ, Xu G, Lin ZY, Tang Y, Lin ZM, Gao Y, Li HM, Zhong NS, Zhang GJ, et al. The role of viral infection in pulmonary exacerbations of bronchiectasis in adults: a prospective study. Chest. 2015;147(6):1635–43.
108. Kapur N, Mackay IM, Sloots TP, Masters IB, Chang AB. Respiratory viruses in exacerbations of non-cystic fibrosis bronchiectasis in children. Arch Dis Child. 2014;99(8):749–53.
109. Einsiedel L, Cassar O, Goeman E, Spelman T, Au V, Hatami S, Joseph S, Gessain A. Higher human T-lymphotropic virus type 1 subtype C proviral loads are associated with bronchiectasis in indigenous australians: results of a case-control study. Open Forum Infect Dis. 2014;1(1):ofu023.
110. Honarbakhsh S, Taylor GP. High prevalence of bronchiectasis is linked to HTLV-1-associated inflammatory disease. BMC Infect Dis. 2015;15:258.
111. Becroft DM. Bronchiolitis obliterans, bronchiectasis, and other sequelae of adenovirus type 21 infection in young children. J Clin Pathol. 1971;24(1):72–82.
112. Chotirmall SH, Al-Alawi M, Mirkovic B, Lavelle G, Logan PM, Greene CM, McElvaney NG. Aspergillus-associated airway disease, inflammation, and the innate immune response. Biomed Res Int. 2013;2013:723129.
113. Chotirmall SH, Branagan P, Gunaratnam C, McElvaney NG. Aspergillus/allergic bronchopulmonary aspergillosis in an Irish cystic fibrosis population: a diagnostically challenging entity. Respir Care. 2008;53(8):1035–41.
114. Chotirmall SH, Martin-Gomez MT. Aspergillus species in bronchiectasis: challenges in the cystic fibrosis and non-cystic fibrosis airways. Mycopathologia. 2017;

115. Yii AC, Koh MS, Lapperre TS, Tan GL, Chotirmall SH. The emergence of aspergillus species in chronic respiratory disease. Front Biosci (Schol Ed). 2017;9:127–38.
116. Woolnough KF, Richardson M, Newby C, Craner M, Bourne M, Monteiro W, Siddiqui S, Bradding P, Pashley CH, Wardlaw AJ. The relationship between biomarkers of fungal allergy and lung damage in asthma. Clin Exp Allergy. 2017;47(1):48–56.
117. Menzies D, Holmes L, McCumesky G, Prys-Picard C, Niven R. Aspergillus sensitization is associated with airflow limitation and bronchiectasis in severe asthma. Allergy. 2011;66(5):679–85.
118. Fairs A, Agbetile J, Hargadon B, Bourne M, Monteiro WR, Brightling CE, Bradding P, Green RH, Mutalithas K, Desai D, et al. IgE sensitization to aspergillus fumigatus is associated with reduced lung function in asthma. Am J Respir Crit Care Med. 2010;182(11):1362–8.
119. Goh KJ, Yii ACA, Lapperre TS, Chan AK, Chew FT, Chotirmall SH, Koh MS. Sensitization to aspergillus species is associated with frequent exacerbations in severe asthma. J Asthma Allergy. 2017;10:131–40.
120. Ghannoum MA, Jurevic RJ, Mukherjee PK, Cui F, Sikaroodi M, Naqvi A, Gillevet PM. Characterization of the oral fungal microbiome (mycobiome) in healthy individuals. PLoS Pathog. 2010;6(1):e1000713.
121. Aliberti S, Masefield S, Polverino E, De Soyza A, Loebinger MR, Menendez R, Ringshausen FC, Vendrell M, Powell P, Chalmers JD. Research priorities in bronchiectasis: a consensus statement from the EMBARC clinical research collaboration. Eur Respir J. 2016;
122. Kunst H, Wickremasinghe M, Wells A, Wilson R. Nontuberculous mycobacterial disease and aspergillus-related lung disease in bronchiectasis. Eur Respir J. 2006;28(2):352–7.
123. Zoumot Z, Boutou AK, Gill SS, van Zeller M, Hansell DM, Wells AU, Wilson R, Loebinger MR. Mycobacterium avium complex infection in non-cystic fibrosis bronchiectasis. Respirology (Carlton, Vic). 2014;19(5):714–22.
124. Kim ST, Choi JH, Jeon HG, Cha HE, Hwang YJ, Chung YS. Comparison between polymerase chain reaction and fungal culture for the detection of fungi in patients with chronic sinusitis and normal controls. Acta Otolaryngol. 2005;125(1):72–5.
125. Tipton L, Ghedin E, Morris A. The lung mycobiome in the next-generation sequencing era. Virulence. 2016:1–8.
126. Aliberti S, Lonni S, Dore S, McDonnell MJ, Goeminne PC, Dimakou K, Fardon TC, Rutherford R, Pesci A, Restrepo MI, et al. Clinical phenotypes in adult patients with bronchiectasis. Eur Respir J. 2016;47(4):1113–22.
127. Guan WJ, Jiang M, Gao YH, Li HM, Xu G, Zheng JP, Chen RC, Zhong NS. Unsupervised learning technique identifies bronchiectasis phenotypes with distinct clinical characteristics. Int J Tuberc Lung Dis. 2016;20(3):402–10.
128. Nicotra MB, Rivera M, Dale AM, Shepherd R, Carter R. Clinical, pathophysiologic, and microbiologic characterization of bronchiectasis in an aging cohort. Chest. 1995;108(4):955–61.
129. Angrill J, Agusti C, de Celis R, Rano A, Gonzalez J, Sole T, Xaubet A, Rodriguez-Roisin R, Torres A. Bacterial colonisation in patients with bronchiectasis: microbiological pattern and risk factors. Thorax. 2002;57(1):15–9.

Global lung function initiative 2012 reference values for spirometry in Asian Americans

Jingzhou Zhang[1,2], Xiao Hu[1,3], Xinlun Tian[1] and Kai-Feng Xu[1*]

Abstract

Background: Spirometry reference values specifically designed for Asian Americans are currently unavailable. The performance of Global Lung Function Initiative 2012 (GLI-2012) equations on assessing spirometry in Asian Americans has not been evaluated. This study aimed to assess the fitness of relevant GLI-2012 equations for spirometry in Asian Americans.

Methods: Asian subjects who never smoked and had qualified spirometry data were extracted from the National Health and Nutrition Examination Survey (NHANES) 2011–2012. Z-scores of forced expiratory volume in 1 s (FEV_1), forced vital capacity (FVC), and FEV_1/FVC were separately constructed with GLI-2012 equations for North East (NE) Asians, South East (SE) Asians, and individuals of mixed ethnic origin (Mixed). In addition, Proportions of subjects with observed spirometry data below the lower limit of normal (LLN) were also evaluated on each GLI-2012 equation of interest.

Results: This study included 567 subjects (250 men and 317 women) aged 6–79 years. Spirometry z-scores (z-FEV_1, z-FVC, and z-FEV_1/FVC) based on GLI-2012 Mixed equations had mean values close to zero (− 0.278 to − 0.057) and standard deviations close to one (1.001 to 1.128); additionally, 6.0% (95% confidence interval (CI) 3.1–8.9%) and 6.4% (95% CI 3.7–9.1%) of subjects were with observed data below LLN for FEV_1/FVC in men and women, respectively. In contrast, for NE Asian equations, all mean values of z-FEV_1 and z-FVC were smaller than − 0.5; for SE Asian equations, mean values of z-FEV_1/FVC were significantly smaller than zero in men (− 0.333) and women (− 0.440).

Conclusions: GLI-2012 equations for individuals of mixed ethnic origin adequately fitted spirometry data in this sample of Asian Americans. Future studies with larger sample sizes are needed to confirm these findings.

Keywords: Asian Americans, Lung function, LLN, Spirometry, Z-score

Background

Accurate interpretation of pulmonary function test results, which requires valid spirometry reference values, is of material importance to respiratory medicine. In addition to gender, age, and height, race/ethnicity acts as another major determinant of lung function [1–3]. Therefore, it is recommended that spirometry reference values established with healthy people of similar race/ethnicity be applied to a certain population whenever possible. The European Respiratory Society (ERS)/American Thoracic Society (ATS) recommended spirometry reference values that were based on a sample from the third National Health and Nutrition Examination Survey (NHANES III) for population aged 8–80 years in US [4, 5]. Nonetheless, limited by race/ethnicity classification in NHANES III, spirometry reference values for Asian Americans were unable to be produced through Hankinson et al.'s study [5].

Previous studies showed that Asian Americans had clinically significantly lower forced expiratory volume in 1 s (FEV_1) and forced vital capacity (FVC) compared with Caucasian people in US [6–11]. Accordingly, a correction factor for FEV_1 and FVC has been developed and calibrated to be applied to NHANES III Caucasian equations when assessing spirometry in Asian Americans. Specifically, 0.94 and

---

* Correspondence: xukf@pumch.cn
[1]Department of Respiratory Medicine, Peking Union Medical College Hospital, Peking Union Medical College & Chinese Academy of Medical Sciences, Beijing 100730, China
Full list of author information is available at the end of the article

0.88 have been sequentially proposed as the correction factor for FEV_1 and FVC [4, 12, 13]. A recent systemic review suggested that a correction factor of 0.88 was more suitable than 0.94 to be applied to NHANES III Caucasian reference values for FEV_1 and FVC evaluation in Asian Americans [14].

In 2012, the Global Lung Function Initiative (GLI-2012) published all-age-covering spirometry predictive equations for multiple ethnicities, including North East (NE) Asian and South East (SE) Asian [15]. In addition, a set of GLI-2012 equations were designed for individuals of mixed ethnic origin (Mixed) [15]. Although with mixed results, GLI-2012 equations showed clinically acceptable generalisability to spirometry in several validation samples [16–21]. Therefore, relevant GLI-2012 equations are potentially useful for evaluating lung function of Asian Americans. Nonetheless, performance of GLI-2012 reference equations on assessing spirometry in Asian Americans has not been evaluated.

Asian people, including Asian alone and in combination with other races, account for more than 17.3 million (5.6%) of total American population in 2010 [22]. Of note, the total US Asian population increased by 5.4 million (45.6%) from 2000 to 2010, and is projected to grow to 48.6 million by 2060 [23, 24]. Owing to the remarkable quantity and rapid growth of Asian population in US, it is clinically important to assess spirometry reference values that have been recommended for or can be potentially used in that population. Herein, we conducted this study to assess the fitness of relevant GLI-2012 equations and NHANES III reference values for spirometry in Asian Americans.

Methods
Study design
Asian subjects from NHANES 2011–2012, where spirometry data were available, were included in this study. The NHANES utilized a complex, multistage, probability sampling design to collect health and nutrition data from a nationally representative sample of civilian, non-institutionalized people in US each year. Since the year of 2011, NHANES has started to oversample Asian population in US and code them as "non-Hispanic Asian" for race/ethnicity, which provided opportunity for investigating health conditions specifically on Asian Americans [25]. NHANES 2011–2012 finally released demographic, nutritional, and health data of 1282 non-Hispanic Asian participants, which served as the basis for this study. NHANES protocols were reviewed and approved by the Research Ethics Review Board of National Center for Health Statistics, and written informed consent was obtained from each NHANES participant.

This study's exclusion criteria were: 1) examinees who did not qualify for a baseline spirometry test; 2) current or past smokers (defined as those who had smoked at least 100 cigarettes in life); 3) participants who reported respiratory illnesses (cough, cold, phlegm, runny nose, or other respiratory illnesses) seven days prior to the examination; 4) baseline spirometry effort quality attribute of "B", "C" or "D", or baseline FEV_1 or FVC quality attribute of "D (questionable results, use with caution)" or "F (results not valid)" [26, 27]. A detailed study sample inclusion and exclusion process is shown in Fig. 1.

Spirometry measurements
Participants aged 6–79 years were eligible for spirometry tests in NHANES 2011–2012. Examinees who had breathing problem requiring oxygen/taking deep breath, current ear infection, eye/chest/abdominal surgery, or stroke/heart attack in the past three months, tuberculosis in the past year, or coughing up blood in the past month were excluded from a baseline spirometry. Technicians received formal training and used an Ohio 822/827 dry-rolling seal volume spirometer (Ohio Medical, Gurnee, IL, USA) for spirometry tests. Regular calibration of spirometry equipment and rigorous spirometry curves quality control were conducted by health technicians and were subsequently verified by supervisory staff [28].

Statistical analysis
The fitness of GLI-2012 reference equations designed for NE Asians, SE Asians, and individuals of mixed ethnic origin and Caucasians were evaluated for spirometry in this sample. GLI-2012 equations were designed using the "Generalized Additive Models for Location, Scale, and Shape (GAMLSS)" method, which permitted the fitness of mean (M), coefficient of variance (S), and skewness (L) of spirometry data [15, 29]. Z-scores of FEV_1 (z-FEV_1), FVC (z-FVC), and FEV_1/FVC (z-FEV_1/FVC) were calculated using the formula: z-score = ((observed value/M) ^ L - 1) / (L*S). The z-score is defined as how many standard deviations (SDs) a measured value is from predicted value (z-score = (observed - predicted)/SD). One may argue that the z-score is a more appropriate approach to reporting lung function data than using % predicted by considering lung function related variables (age, height, ethnicity, etc.) [30]. The proportion of subjects with observed spirometry data below lower limit of normal (LLN), which corresponds to the 5th percentile of predicted values, were also evaluated for FEV_1, FVC, and FEV_1/FVC on each GLI-2012 equation of interest. The cutoff z-score of LLN was calculated with the formula: LLN z-score = − 1.6445 * (SD of z-scores).

Student's t-tests were used to examine the difference between the mean of z-scores and zero. Bland-Altman plots of spirometry predictions based on NHANES III

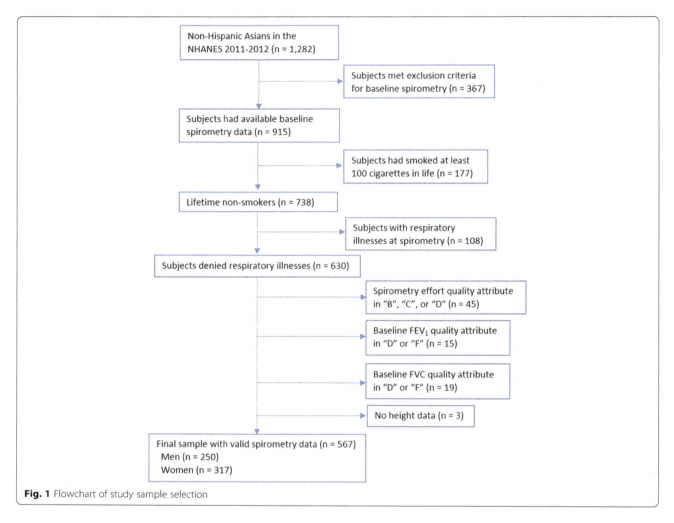

Fig. 1 Flowchart of study sample selection

Caucasian equations with 0.88 as the correction factor for FEV_1 and FVC against GLI-2012 Mixed equations were generated (difference = NHANES III prediction − GLI-2012 prediction). Bland-Altman plots are used to describe agreement between two quantitative methods of measurement by calculating the mean difference and 95% limits of agreement (1.96*SD of the difference) between the two measurements [31]. A two-sided $P < 0.05$ was considered statistically significant for all tests. Data analyses were performed with SAS 9.4 (SAS Institute, Cary, NC, USA) and R version 3.4.0 (R Foundation for Statistical Computing, Vienna, Austria).

Results

Sample characteristics (Table 1)

Five hundred and sixty-nine Asian participants (250 men and 317 women) were finally included in this analysis. The mean (SD) age were 28.4 (17.8) years for men and 34.3 (19.7) years for women; and the age range for men and women were 6 to 75 years and 6 to 79 years, respectively (Fig. 2). The mean (SD) height for men and women were 164.1 (15.6) cm and 154.2 (11.4) cm, respectively. In this sample, there were 17 (6.8%) men and 19 (6.0%) women who had a BMI ≥ 30 kg/m². Additionally, 38.4% of men and 31.6% of women were born in US. Among those who were not born in US, 31.6% of men and 37.3% of women had lived in US for more than 20 years, whereas 27.0% of men and 20.6% of women had been in US for less than 5 years.

Performance of GLI-2012 equations (Table 2)

For NE Asian equations, all mean (median) values of z-FEV_1 and z-FVC were smaller than − 0.5 in both men and women, with the lowest as − 0.743 (− 0.819) for z-FVC in women. For SE Asian equations, mean values of z-FEV_1/FVC were − 0.333 in men and − 0.440 in women, all significantly different from zero. In terms of the Mixed equations, all mean values of z-FEV_1, z-FVC, and z-FEV_1/FVC were not significantly different from zero in men; and in women, although statistically significantly different from zero, all absolute differences were within 0.3. SDs of z-scores based on GLI-2012 SE Asian

Table 1 Baseline characteristics of sample subjects by gender [a]

Characteristics	Gender	
	Men (n = 250)	Women (n = 317)
Age (year)	28.4 ± 17.8	34.3 ± 19.7
	23 (14, 41)	32 (16, 51)
Height (cm)	164.1 ± 15.6	154.2 ± 11.4
Weight (kg)	62.8 ± 19.4	53.9 ± 14.4
BMI (kg/m^2)	22.7 ± 4.7	22.3 ± 4.6
Born in the U.S.	96 (38.4%)	100 (31.6%)
Length of time in U.S. [b]		
Less than 5 years	41 (27.0%)	44 (20.6%)
5 to 10 years	28 (18.4%)	26 (12.2%)
10 to 20 years	35 (23.0%)	64 (29.9%)
More than 20 years	48 (31.6%)	80 (37.3%)
FEV$_1$ (L)	3.159 ± 0.904	2.344 ± 0.634
FVC (L) [c]	3.761 ± 1.052	2.785 ± 0.710
FEV$_1$/FVC [c]	0.84 ± 0.07	0.84 ± 0.08

BMI body mass index, *FEV$_1$* forced expiratory volume in 1 s, *FVC* forced vital capacity

[a]data were presented as mean ± standard deviation, median (interquartile range), or as number (percentage)

[b]for participants who were not born in the United States; 2 missing these data for men and 3 missing these data for women

[c]1 missing these data for men and 6 missing these data for women

equations and the Mixed equations ranged from 1.002 to 1.089 and 1.001 to 1.128, respectively, indicating that those equations adequately fitted variations of our spirometry data. In contrast, SDs of z-FEV$_1$ and z-FVC based on GLI-2012 NE Asian equations were 1.512 and 1.517, respectively. Distributions of z-scores based on GLI-2012 equations were showed in Fig. 3. For Caucasian equations, mean values of z-FEV$_1$ and z-FVC were substantially smaller than zero in both men and women (Additional file 1: Fig. S1). Also, plots of spirometry z-scores for GLI-2012 reference eqs. (NE, SE, and the Mixed) against age in men and women were showed in Additional file 2: Fig. S2 and Additional file 3: Fig. S3, respectively.

Regarding proportion of observed spirometry data below LLN (% < LLN), the Mixed equations showed a satisfactory overall performance. Specifically, 6.0% (95% confidence interval (CI): 3.1–8.9%) and 6.4% (95% CI: 3.7–9.1%) of z-FEV$_1$/FVC were below LLN for men and women, respectively. In contrast, according to SE Asian equations, 9.2% (95% CI: 5.6–12.8%) of z-FEV$_1$/FVC in men and 10.0% (95% CI: 6.7–13.3%) of z-FEV$_1$/FVC in women were below LLN; for NE Asian equations, all % < LLN for z-FEV$_1$ and z-FVC were significantly larger than 5% (11.2 to 16.2%).

In addition, we confirmed that the NHANES III Caucasian reference values with a correction factor of 0.88 for FEV$_1$ and FVC satisfactorily fitted the spirometry data (FEV$_1$ and FVC) of this sample (data not shown).

Agreement between NHANES III and GLI-2012 predictions

Overall, lung function predictions based on NHANES III Caucasian reference values with a correction factor of 0.88 for FEV$_1$ and FVC were smaller than those based on the GLI-2012 equations for FEV$_1$, FVC, and FEV$_1$/FVC (Fig. 4). The average differences in FEV$_1$ (L), FVC (L), and FEV$_1$/FVC (%) predictions were − 0.187, − 0.130, and − 2.46 for men, and − 0.131, − 0.095, and − 2.12 for women, respectively.

Discussion

In this population-based cross-sectional analysis of lung function, we were the first to assess the generalisability of relevant GLI-2012 reference equations to spirometry in Asian Americans. In addition, we evaluated the agreement of lung function predictions between the NHANES III Caucasian values with a correction factor of 0.88 for

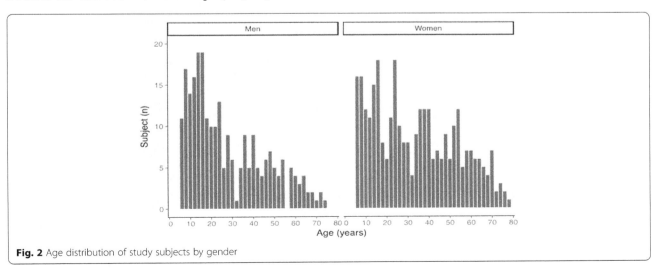

Fig. 2 Age distribution of study subjects by gender

Table 2 Spirometry z-scores of the present study population based on the GLI-2012 equations for North East Asians, South East Asians, and individuals of mixed ethnic origin

GLI-2012 equations	Statistics	z-FEV$_1$		z-FVC		z-FEV$_1$/FVC	
		Men	Women	Men	Women	Men	Women
North East Asians	Mean ± SD	−0.571 ± 1.512	−0.703 ± 1.029	−0.695 ± 1.517	−0.743 ± 1.223	0.021 ± 1.177	−0.135 ± 1.089
	95% CI of mean	(−0.759, −0.382) *	(−0.817, −0.589) *	(−0.884, −0.506) *	(−0.880, −0.607) *	(−0.124, 0.167)	(−0.257, −0.014) *
	Median	−0.558	−0.730	−0.619	−0.819	0.148	−0.152
	(5th, 95th percentile)	(−3.143, 1.855)	(−2.313, 0.799)	(−3.458, 1.909)	(−2.797, 1.099)	(−1.928, 1.798)	(−1.999, 1.716)
	N (%) < LLN	28 (11.2%)	51 (16.1%)	33 (13.3%)	42 (13.5%)	12 (4.8%)	20 (6.4%)
	95% CI of % < LLN	(7.3, 15.1%)	(12.1, 20.1%)	(9.1, 17.5%)	(9.7, 17.3%)	(2.1, 7.5%)	(3.7, 9.1%)
South East Asians	Mean ± SD	−0.037 ± 1.052	0.105 ± 1.080	0.177 ± 1.002	0.312 ± 1.089	−0.333 ± 1.055	−0.440 ± 1.010
	95% CI of mean	(−0.094, 0.168)	(−0.014, 0.225)	(0.051, 0.302) *	(0.190, 0.433) *	(−0.465, −0.201) *	(−0.552, −0.327) *
	Median	0.017	0.126	0.251	0.290	−0.203	−0.462
	(5th, 95th percentile)	(−1.736, 1.733)	(−1.619, 1.667)	(−1.610, 1.899)	(−1.502, 1.994)	(−2.073, 1.264)	(−2.154, 1.239)
	N (%) < LLN	13 (5.2%)	8 (2.5%)	12 (4.8%)	10 (3.2%)	23 (9.2%)	31 (10.0%)
	95% CI of % < LLN	(2.4, 8.0%)	(0.8, 4.2%)	(2.1, 7.5%)	(1.2, 5.2%)	(5.6, 12.8%)	(6.7, 13.3%)
Individuals of mixed ethnic origin	Mean ± SD	−0.101 ± 1.051	−0.278 ± 1.079	−0.112 ± 1.050	−0.212 ± 1.128	−0.057 ± 1.020	−0.152 ± 1.001
	95% CI of mean	(−0.232, 0.030)	(−0.397, −0.159) *	(−0.229, 0.033)	(−0.338, −0.086) *	(−0.185, 0.070)	(−0.264, −0.040) *
	Median	−0.111	−0.284	−0.051	−0.266	0.055	−0.167
	(5th, 95th percentile)	(−1.881, 1.591)	(−1.975, 1.282)	(−2.007, 1.702)	(−2.096, 1.508)	(−1.745, 1.484)	(−1.865, 1.547)
	N (%) < LLN	18 (7.2%)	20 (6.3%)	20 (8.0%)	25 (8.0%)	15 (6.0%)	20 (6.4%)
	95% CI of % < LLN	(4.0, 10.4%)	(3.6, 9.0%)	(4.6, 11.4%)	(5.0, 11.0%)	(3.1, 8.9%)	(3.7, 9.1%)

GLI Global Lung Function Initiative, *SD* standard deviation, *CI* confidence interval, *FEV$_1$* forced expiratory volume in 1 s, *FVC* forced vital capacity, *z-FEV$_1$* z-score, *z-FVC* FVC z-score, *z-FEV$_1$/FVC* FEV$_1$/FVC z-score, *LLN* lower limit of normal

*$P < 0.05$ for student's t-tests comparing mean values of z-scores and zero

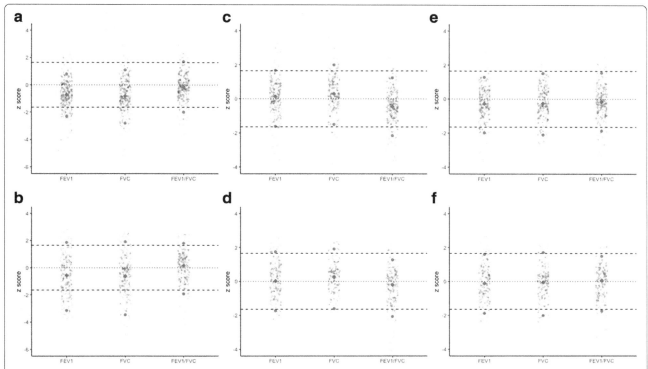

Fig. 3 Distributions of z-scores of FEV_1, FVC, and FEV_1/FVC based on GLI-2012 equations for North East Asians, South East Asians, and individuals of mixed ethnic origin. Panels A and B showed z-score distributions based on GLI-2012 equations for North East Asians in women and men, respectively; panels C and D showed z-score distributions based on GLI-2012 equations for South East Asians in women and men, respectively; and panels E and F showed z-score distributions based on GLI-2012 equations for individuals of mixed ethnic origin in women and men, respectively. In this graph, red dot denotes 5th and 95th percentiles of observed spirometry data; blue diamond denotes median of observed values; solid line represents a z-score of zero; and dotted line represents z-scores of ±1.96. *FEV_1: forced expiratory volume in 1 s; FVC: forced vital capacity; GLI: Global Lung Function Initiative*

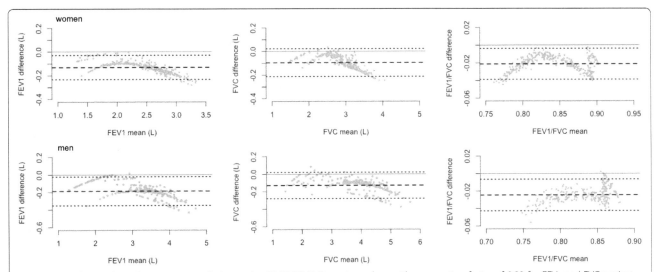

Fig. 4 Bland-Altman plots of spirometry predictions using NHANES III Caucasian values with a correction factor of 0.88 for FEV_1 and FVC against those with GLI-2012 equations for individuals of mixed ethnic origin (difference = NHANES III prediction − GLI-2012 prediction). In this graph, dashed line represents the mean difference; dotted line represents 95% confidence interval of the mean difference; solid line represents the value of zero. *NHANES III: The Third National Health and Nutrition Examination Survey; FEV_1: forced expiratory volume in 1 s; FVC: forced vital capacity; GLI: Global Lung Function Initiative*

FEV_1 and FVC and the GLI-2012 equations for individuals of mixed ethnic origin.

Our findings showed that GLI-2012 Mixed equations adequately fitted FEV_1, FVC, and FEV_1/FVC data of our sample for both gender. GLI-2012 Mixed equations were designed for people of mixed ethnic origin, which we believe current Asian Americans could be categorized into due to the following several reasons. First, in the year 2010, around 16% of Asian Americans were Asian in combination with one or more other races, among whom Asian in combination with White were the majority [22]. Second, US Asian population consists of more than twenty subgroups, with Chinese, Indian, Filipino, Vietnamese, Korean, and Japanese accounting for the most in quantity [22]. Third, due to diversities of birth country and years living in US, which is readily translated into difference in environmental exposures and socioeconomic status, Asian Americans may have quite different lung function development [32–37]. Therefore, Asian Americans are genetically, environmentally, and socioeconomically heterogeneous in nature, which may explain the satisfactory performance of GLI-2012 Mixed equations in fitting spirometry data in this sample.

GLI-2012 NE Asian equations were built based on two datasets, one collected from North China and the other from South Korea; whereas the GLI-2012 SE Asian equations were derived from a collated dataset consisting of five subsamples from South Asia and a subsample from US [15]. Quanjer et al. found that the two subsamples of NE Asians had significantly larger lung function than the six subsamples of SE Asians, and therefore they constructed spirometry predictive equations separately for NE Asians and SE Asians [15]. Not surprisingly, GLI-2012 NE Asian equations led to substantially larger FEV_1 and FVC predictions compared with observed data in our sample for both gender, strongly suggesting against the application of those equations to assessing spirometry in Asian Americans. GLI-2012 SE Asian equations, while performed satisfactorily in fitting FEV_1 and FVC, contributed to significantly larger FEV_1/FVC predictions compared with the observed data, which will potentially result in an overdiagnosis of chronic obstructive pulmonary disease in Asian Americans.

Generally, both the GLI-2012 Mixed equations and the NHANES III Caucasian reference values with a correction factor of 0.88 adequately fitted the lung function data in this sample. However, GLI-2012 equations possess several potential advantages over the NHANES III reference values. First, as all-age-covering spirometry reference values, GLI-2012 equations are valid for people aged 3 to 95 years old [38]; the NHANES III equations, in contrast, have a comparably narrower valid age range of 8 to 80 years. Of note, in this study we were not able to evaluate the fitness of GLI-2012 equations for spirometry in Asian Americans aged outside 6 to 79 years. Secondly, GLI-2012 equations were designed with a semiparametric predictive modelling method, which was able to fit variance and skewness of spirometry data in addition to the mean value [39]. Moreover, splines used in GLI-2012 equations modeled age-related variations for spirometry data. NHANES III equations were built based on quadratic function for FEV_1 and FVC and linear function for FEV_1/FVC. Thus, compared with GLI-2012 equations, NHANES III equations were less likely to reflect actual patterns of spirometry data due to their fixed function formats. Thirdly, NHANES III equations for FEV_1/FVC LLN and equations for FEV_1/FVC are same as each other except different intercepts. Therefore, according to NHANES III equations, LLN for FEV_1/FVC differs from FEV_1/FVC by a constant magnitude regardless of a subject's age. However, since LLN theoretically corresponds to the 5th percentile of spirometry data and lung function varies with age, it is conceptually insufficient to define LLN as a constant difference to the mean for the entire age range. GLI-2012 reference values address this issue by defining LLN with spirometry z-scores, a way comprehensively taking mean, variance, and skewness of spirometry data into consideration.

The GLI-2012 equations have been proposed to be adopted worldwide in order to standardise the interpretation of lung function [40]. Admittedly, the application of a correction factor to the NHANES III Caucasian reference values offers a practical solution to assessing spirometry in Asian Americans. However, the rationale behind the development of a correction factor, which is only for temporary use, is not conceptually and methodologically ideal. Based on the current findings and what has been discussed above, it is reasonable to regard GLI-2012 Mixed equations as superior to the NHANES III Caucasian reference values with a correction factor for evaluating spirometry in Asian Americans. In particular, the ready availability of spirometry z-scores and LLN from the GLI-2012 equations could possibly provide a convenient approach to the diagnosis and severity stratification of obstructive lung diseases. Therefore, with the rapid increase of Asian population in US, the application of GLI-2012 Mixed equations to Asian Americans is clinically important.

This study has several limitations. First, the sample size of this study is relatively small. However, we would argue that our sample sizes of men and women are both large enough for validating spirometry reference values, which requires at least 150 subjects for each gender [41]. Second, as shown in Fig. 2, the distributions of age are right skewed in both men and women. Especially for men, the proportion of adults and elderly people is relatively small, which may limit the power of this study in that population. This issue is clinically relevant in that obstructive lung diseases, where lung function references are widely used, are most prevalent in elderly people. As the accrual of NHANES data of Asian Americans, the fitness of GLI-2012 equations could be better evaluated in the near future.

Conclusions

In this cross-sectional analysis of lung function from a nationally representative sample of US Asian population, we showed that the GLI-2012 reference equations for individuals of mixed ethnic origin performed adequately on fitting spirometry data of this sample. Considering the strengths of GLI-2012 equations such as all-age-covering capacity and readily z-score calculation and LLN definition, the GLI-2012 equations for individuals of mixed ethnic origin are reasonably considered as a useful set of tools in evaluating spirometry in Asian Americans. Further studies with larger sample sizes covering wider age ranges, especially the most elderly (> 80 years) people, are warranted to confirm these findings.

Abbreviations
ATS: American Thoracic Society; ERS: European Respiratory Society; FEV_1: Forced Expiratory Volume in 1 s; FVC: Forced Vital Capacity; GLI: Global Lung Function Initiative; LLN: Lower Limit of Normal; NHANES: National Health and Nutrition Examination Survey; North East Asian: NE Asian; South East Asian: SE Asian

Acknowledgements
We thank all NHANES participants for their willingness to spare valuable time and contribute health data to this epidemiologic study.

Funding
This study was supported by the National Key Basic Research Program of China (973 Program) (Grant No. 2015CB553402).

Authors' contributions
JZ, XH, XT, and KFX designed this study. JZ and XH collected, analyzed data, and drafted the manuscript. All authors interpreted data, critically reviewed the paper, and approved the final version of manuscript for publication.

Competing interests
The authors declare that they have no competing interests.

Author details
[1]Department of Respiratory Medicine, Peking Union Medical College Hospital, Peking Union Medical College & Chinese Academy of Medical Sciences, Beijing 100730, China. [2]Department of Epidemiology, Mailman School of Public Health, Columbia University, New York, NY, USA. [3]Yale School of Public Health, Yale University, New Haven, CT, USA.

References
1. Yang TS, Peat J, Keena V, Donnelly P, Unger W, Woolcock A. A review of the racial differences in the lung function of normal Caucasian, Chinese and Indian subjects. Eur Respir J. 1991;4(7):872–80.
2. Braun L, Wolfgang M, Dickersin K. Defining race/ethnicity and explaining difference in research studies on lung function. Eur Respir J. 2013;41(6):1362–70.
3. Strippoli MP, Kuehni CE, Dogaru CM, Spycher BD, McNally T, Silverman M, et al. Etiology of ethnic differences in childhood spirometry. Pediatrics. 2013;131(6):e1842–9.
4. Pellegrino R, Viegi G, Brusasco V, Crapo RO, Burgos F, Casaburi R, et al. Interpretative strategies for lung function tests. Eur Respir J. 2005;26(5):948–68.
5. Hankinson JL, Odencrantz JR, Fedan KB. Spirometric reference values from a sample of the general US population. Am J Respir Crit Care Med. 1999;159(1):179–87.
6. Fulambarker A, Copur AS, Javeri A, Jere S, Cohen ME. Reference values for pulmonary function in Asian Indians living in the United States. Chest. 2004;126(4):1225–33.
7. Korotzer B, Ong S, Hansen JE. Ethnic differences in pulmonary function in healthy nonsmoking Asian-Americans and European-Americans. Am J Respir Crit Care Med. 2000;161(4 Pt 1):1101–8.
8. Lin FL, Kelso JM. Pulmonary function studies in healthy Filipino adults residing in the United States. J Allergy Clin Immunol. 1999;104(2 Pt 1):338–40.
9. Marcus EB, MacLean CJ, Curb JD, Johnson LR, Vollmer WM, Buist AS. Reference values for FEV1 in Japanese-American men from 45 to 68 years of age. Am Rev Respir Dis. 1988;138(6):1393–7.
10. Sharp DS, Enright PL, Chiu D, Burchfiel CM, Rodriguez BL, Curb JD. Reference values for pulmonary function tests of Japanese-American men aged 71 to 90 years. Am J Respir Crit Care Med. 1996;153(2):805–11.
11. Massey DG, Fournier-Massey G. Japanese-American pulmonary reference values: influence of environment on anthropology and physiology. Environ Res. 1986;39(2):418–33.
12. Hankinson JL, Kawut SM, Shahar E, Smith LJ, Stukovsky KH, Barr RG. Performance of American Thoracic Society-recommended spirometry reference values in a multiethnic sample of adults: the multi-ethnic study of atherosclerosis (MESA) lung study. Chest. 2010;137(1):138–45.
13. Townsend MC. Occupational, environmental lung disorders C: spirometry in the occupational health setting–2011 update. J Occup Environ Med. 2011;53(5):569–84.
14. Redlich CA, Tarlo SM, Hankinson JL, Townsend MC, Eschenbacher WL, Von Essen SG, et al. American Thoracic Society Committee on spirometry in the occupational S: official American Thoracic Society technical standards: spirometry in the occupational setting. Am J Respir Crit Care Med. 2014;189(8):983–93.
15. Quanjer PH, Stanojevic S, Cole TJ, Baur X, Hall GL, Culver BH, et al. Multi-ethnic reference values for spirometry for the 3-95-yr age range: the global lung function 2012 equations. Eur Respir J. 2012;40(6):1324–43.
16. Arigliani M, Canciani MC, Mottini G, Altomare M, Magnolato A, Loa Clemente SV, et al. Evaluation of the global lung initiative 2012 reference values for spirometry in African children. Am J Respir Crit Care Med. 2017;195(2):229–36.
17. Langhammer A, Johannessen A, Holmen TL, Melbye H, Stanojevic S, Lund MB, et al. Global lung function initiative 2012 reference equations for spirometry in the Norwegian population. Eur Respir J. 2016;48(6):1602–11.
18. Hall GL, Thompson BR, Stanojevic S, Abramson MJ, Beasley R, Coates A, et al. The global lung initiative 2012 reference values reflect contemporary Australasian spirometry. Respirology. 2012;17(7):1150–1.
19. Bonner R, Lum S, Stocks J, Kirkby J, Wade A, Sonnappa S. Applicability of the global lung function spirometry equations in contemporary multiethnic children. Am J Respir Crit Care Med. 2013;188(4):515–6.
20. Zhang J, Hu X, Shan G. Spirometry reference values for population aged 7-80 years in China. Respirology. 2017;22(8):1630–6.
21. Backman H, Lindberg A, Sovijarvi A, Larsson K, Lundback B, Ronmark E. Evaluation of the global lung function initiative 2012 reference values for spirometry in a Swedish population sample. BMC Pulm Med. 2015;15:26.
22. The Asian Population: 2010 [https://www.census.gov/library/publications/2012/dec/c2010br-11.html].
23. The Asian Population: 2000 [https://www.census.gov/library/publications/2002/dec/c2kbr01-16.html].

24. US Census Bureau. 2014 National Population Projections Tables [https://www.census.gov/data/tables/2014/demo/popproj/2014-summary-tables.html].
25. Paulose-Ram R, Burt V, Broitman L, Ahluwalia N. Overview of Asian American data collection, release, and analysis: National Health and nutrition examination survey 2011-2018. Am J Public Health. 2017;107(6):916–21.
26. Johannessen A, Omenaas ER, Eide GE, Bakke PS, Gulsvik A. Feasible and simple exclusion criteria for pulmonary reference populations. Thorax. 2007;62(9):792–8.
27. Hankinson JL, Eschenbacher B, Townsend M, Stocks J, Quanjer PH. Use of forced vital capacity and forced expiratory volume in 1 second quality criteria for determining a valid test. Eur Respir J. 2015;45(5):1283–92.
28. NHANES 2011-2012 Respiratory Health Spirometry Procedures Manual 2011, https://wwwn.cdc.gov/nchs/data/nhanes/2011-2012/manuals/spirometry_procedures_manual.pdf.
29. Quanjer GLI-2012 Regression Equation and Lookup Tables [http://www.ers-education.org/guidelines/global-lung-function-initiative/tools/quanjer-gli-2012-regression-equations-and-lookup-tables.aspx].
30. Stanojevic S, Quanjer P, Miller MR, Stocks J. The global lung function initiative: dispelling some myths of lung function test interpretation. Breathe. 2013;9(6):462–74.
31. Myles PS, Cui J. Using the bland-Altman method to measure agreement with repeated measures. Br J Anaesth. 2007;99(3):309–11.
32. Gehring U, Gruzieva O, Agius RM, Beelen R, Custovic A, Cyrys J, et al. Air pollution exposure and lung function in children: the ESCAPE project. Environ Health Perspect. 2013;121(11-12):1357–64.
33. Raju PS, Prasad KV, Ramana YV, Balakrishna N, Murthy KJ. Influence of socioeconomic status on lung function and prediction equations in Indian children. Pediatr Pulmonol. 2005;39(6):528–36.
34. Fulambarker A, Copur AS, Cohen ME, Patel M, Gill S, Schultz ST, et al. Comparison of pulmonary function in immigrant vs US-born Asian Indians. Chest. 2010;137(6):1398–404.
35. Gauderman WJ, Urman R, Avol E, Berhane K, McConnell R, Rappaport E, et al. Association of improved air quality with lung development in children. N Engl J Med. 2015;372(10):905–13.
36. Gauderman WJ, Avol E, Gilliland F, Vora H, Thomas D, Berhane K, et al. The effect of air pollution on lung development from 10 to 18 years of age. N Engl J Med. 2004;351(11):1057–67.
37. Hegewald M, Crapo RO. Socioeconomic status and lung function. Chest. 2007;132(5):1608–14.
38. Stanojevic S, Wade A, Stocks J, Hankinson J, Coates AL, Pan H, et al. Reference ranges for spirometry across all ages - a new approach. Am J Respir Crit Care Med. 2008;177(3):253–60.
39. Rigby RA, Stasinopoulos DM. Generalized additive models for location, scale and shape. Journal of the Royal Statistical Society Series C-Applied Statistics. 2005;54:507–44.
40. Swanney MP, Miller MR. Adopting universal lung function reference equations. Eur Respir J. 2013;42(4):901–3.
41. Quanjer PH, Stocks J, Cole TJ, Hall GL, Stanojevic S, Global Lungs I. Influence of secular trends and sample size on reference equations for lung function tests. Eur Respir J. 2011;37(3):658–64.

Asthma exacerbations in a subtropical area and the role of respiratory viruses

Lusmaia Damaceno Camargo Costa[1*], Paulo Augusto Moreira Camargos[2], Paul L. P. Brand[3], Fabíola Souza Fiaccadori[4], Menira Borges de Lima Dias e Souza[4], Divina das Dôres de Paula Cardoso[4], Ítalo de Araújo Castro[4], Ruth Minamisava[5] and Paulo Sérgio Sucasas da Costa[1]

Abstract

Background: Multiple factors are involved in asthma exacerbations, including environmental exposure and viral infections. We aimed to assess the association between severe asthma exacerbations, acute respiratory viral infections and other potential risk factors.

Methods: Asthmatic children aged 4–14 years were enrolled for a period of 12 months and divided into two groups: those with exacerbated asthma (group 1) and non-exacerbated asthma (group 2). Clinical data were obtained and nasopharyngeal samples were collected through nasopharyngeal aspirate or swab and analysed via indirect fluorescent immunoassays to detect influenza A and B viruses, parainfluenza 1–3, adenovirus and respiratory syncytial virus. Rhinovirus was detected via molecular assays. Potential risk factors for asthma exacerbation were identified in univariate and multivariate analyses.

Results: In 153 children (group 1: 92; group 2: 61), median age 7 and 8 years, respectively, the rate of virus detection was 87.7%. There was no difference between groups regarding the frequency of virus detection ($p = 0.68$); however, group 1 showed a lower frequency (19.2%) of inhaled corticosteroid use (91.4%, $p < 0.01$) and evidence of inadequate disease control. In the multivariate analysis, the occurrence of three or more visits to the emergency room in the past 12 months (IRR = 1.40; $p = 0.04$) and nonadherence to inhaled corticosteroid (IRR = 4.87; $p < 0.01$) were the only factors associated with exacerbation.

Conclusion: Our results suggest an association between asthma exacerbations, poor disease control and nonadherence to asthma medication, suggesting that viruses may not be the only culprits for asthma exacerbations in this population.

Keywords: Asthma, Exacerbations, Virus, Child

Background

Asthma exacerbations generate considerable morbidity, affecting various aspects of the patient's quality of life, and producing high costs for the health system [1]. The multifactorial origin of asthma exacerbations has been well described and includes allergen exposure, acute viral respiratory tract infections, pollutants, climate changes, exercise, amongst other factors [1–3]. Despite the existence of effective drugs, poor asthma control remains common in many children worldwide [4]. A key characteristic of poor asthma control is the occurrence of asthma exacerbations, and a history of recent emergency room visits for asthma is a strong and independent predictor of future asthma exacerbations [5]. Asthma tends to be poorly controlled in the socially disadvantaged population [6] and the reasons are multifactorial with complex interactions [7]. On the other hand, authors have identified specific genetic variants associated with susceptibility to viral respiratory infections, severity of infection and virus-induced exacerbations of asthma during childhood [8].

* Correspondence: lusmaiapneumoped@gmail.com
[1]Pediatric Pulmonology Unit, University Hospital, Federal University of Goiás, Primeira Avenida, S/N. Setor Leste Universitária, Goiânia CEP: 746050-20, Brazil
Full list of author information is available at the end of the article

Since the early 1970s, viral respiratory infections have been associated with the onset of asthma exacerbations. However, studies in children, who are particularly susceptible to viral infection due to their relative immunological immaturity, increased in the 1990s, when molecular techniques became more sensitive allowing for the identification of more respiratory viruses and facilitating a better understanding of this association [9–16]. Studies using *reverse transcription-polymerase chain reaction* (RT-PCR) detected respiratory viruses in more than 90% of asthma exacerbations [9].

Acute respiratory tract infections are responsible for high morbidity and mortality, accounting for around 20% of the estimated 9 million deaths of children worldwide in 2007, according to the World Health Organization. Viruses are responsible for most of these infections, causing generally mild and self-limited infections, though some may become very severe or complicate the clinical course of patients with underlying chronic lung diseases, including asthma [17]. Moreover, the association between viral infection and environmental exposure is described as a trigger for exacerbations and type 2 inflammation is associated with an increased risk of virus-induced exacerbations [18, 19]. Achieving asthma control remains a global challenge, especially in poor-resource populations. Although viral infection is an important trigger, few studies in this area have been conducted in tropical countries. To add more details about this possible association in Latin American children, we examined the viral detection rate in a group of Brazilian asthmatic children with and without exacerbation. We hypothesize that in a population of a low income country, living in a subtropical area, viruses may not be the main trigger of an asthmatic exacerbation.

Methods

Setting

This study was carried out in the city of Goiânia, capital of Goiás state, located in Central Brazil, a region with semi-humid tropical climate with an estimated population of 1,302,001 inhabitants. Public health care is provided free of charge by the Brazilian Unified Health System, and an estimated 70% of the population use the public health system [20].

Study population

From June 2012 through August 2013, asthmatic children were screened for respiratory viruses if they met the following inclusion criteria: 4–14 year olds, admitted to emergency rooms of three hospitals, which attend children from public and private health insurance due to asthma exacerbation (group 1). We only included in the study patients who had at least three previous episodes of bronchospasm and fulfill the GINA criteria for asthma definition [1]. We did not include children under 4 years old because of the difficulty in differentiation of asthma from wheezing episodes of other origin in very young children. Exacerbations were defined as increased symptoms that required a change in medication as judged by the attending physician according to ATS/ERS statement [21]. Exacerbations requiring a course of oral corticosteroids or admission to hospital were considered severe.

Asthmatic children without exacerbation (group 2), were invited to participate in this study during their appointment in the major respiratory outpatient clinic of the city, which attend children from public health insurance (Brazilian Unified Health System). They were only eligible for inclusion when they reported not having symptoms of upper respiratory tract infection, such as rhinorrhoea, fever and nasal congestion in the 4 weeks prior to the clinic visit. All patients had similar access to primary care and maintenance medications. Exclusion criteria for both groups were premature birth and the presence of cardiorespiratory chronic diseases, neurologic and metabolic disorders and immunosuppression.

The study protocol was approved by the Clinical Research Ethics Committee (HC/UFG Protocol 175/2011). Written informed consent was obtained from parents, and written assent was obtained from older children (over 8 years old).

Data and sample collection

For each child, data on sociodemographic data, asthma related symptoms, hospitalisations in the last 12 months and environmental exposure to aeroallergens and secondhand tobacco was collected by two researchers (LDCC and PSSC). A nasopharyngeal aspirate was obtained from each patient upon admission to the emergency ward (Group 1) or during the interview (Group 2). The nasopharyngeal swab specimens were obtained from the nostril from a depth of 2 to 3 cm by using a sterile ray swab that was then inserted into a vial containing 2.5 ml of viral transport medium (MEM). For the nasopharyngeal aspirate, a disposable catheter connected to a mucus extractor was inserted into the nostril to a depth of 5 to 7 cm and drawn back while applying gentle suction with an electric suction device [22]. Nasopharyngeal flocked swab (Chemicon-Millipore Corporation, Billerica, MA, USA) was obtained in cases of absence of sufficient sample by nasopharyngeal aspirate.

Samples were transported at 4 °C to the Human Virology Laboratory, Federal University of Goias, Tropical Medicine and Public Health Institute and processed immediately. The supernatant was stored at −70 °C for molecular study, and the pellet was used in the immunofluorescence assay.

Viral detection

Each sample was analysed using a Respiratory Panel I Viral Screening and Identification IFA Reagent immunofluorescence kit (Chemicon-Millipore Corporation, Billerica, MA, USA) consisting of a panel of monoclonal antibodies specific to influenza virus A (FLUVA), influenza virus B (FLUVB), human respiratory syncytial virus (hRSV), human adenovirus (hADV), and human parainfluenza viruses (hPIV) 1, 2, and 3 following the manufacturer's instructions.

For molecular identification of rhinovirus, all samples were submitted to ribonucleic acid (RNA) extraction using a QIAamp® cador® Pathogen Mini Kit (Qiagen, Germany), and conventional RT-PCR was conducted using primers described previously [23]. Briefly, 20 μL of viral RNA was extracted using random hexamers (Random Primer – Invitrogen® life technologies, USA) in a final volume of 50 μL. The reaction was incubated at 25 °C for 5 min, 42 °C for 10 min, 50 °C for 20 min, and 85 °C for 5 min, all in a single cycle. For the polymerase chain reaction (PCR) reaction, the commercial kit Platinum PCR SuperMix HF (Invitrogen® life technologies, USA), 0.4 mM of each primer (P1–1 e P3–1), and 2.5 μL of cDNA were mixed and submitted to amplification in a thermocycler (Mastercycler Personal/Eppendorf) with the following cycling parameters: 94 °C for 2 min, followed by 35 cycles of 94 °C for 20 s, 53 °C for 30 s, 72 °C for 40 s, and a final extension of 72 °C for 10 min. The products were submitted to 1.5% agarose gel electrophoresis and visualised using a UV transilluminator. The samples were compared to a molecular marker (100 bp ladder), and the expected amplicon size for Rhinovirus was 390 bp. In all reactions, positive (previously sequenced Rhinovirus samples) and negative (MilliQ water) controls were used.

Statistical analysis

Kruskal-Wallis, Chi-square and Fisher's exact tests were used to compare medians and proportions between groups. Poisson multivariate regression analysis was performed to identify the variables associated with the outcome (asthma exacerbation), including the independent variables significantly or near-significantly ($p \leq 0.1$) in bivariate analysis. Results are presented as the incidence risk ratio (IRR) with the 95% confidence interval (95% CI). All analyses were performed using STATA v 12.0 (Stata Corp, College Station, TX, USA).

Results

During the study period, respiratory secretion samples were collected from 158 children. Five patients (3.2%) were excluded from analysis (three from group 1 and two from group 2) due to an insufficient amount of material for the examinations. Of the 153 samples analysed, 92 (60.1%) belonged to group 1 and 61 (39.9%) to group 2. The median age was 7.0 years (IQR =5.0–8.7) in group 1 and 8.0 years (6.0–11.0) in group 2. Table 1 shows clinical and socio-demographic characteristics of the patients in the study.

In 134 children (87.6%), the nasal sample was obtained by nasopharyngeal aspirate and in 19 children (12.4%) by nasal swab. Most patients (72.0%) were recruited between April and June (autumn in the southern hemisphere); the highest detection rate of viruses (63.2%) also occurs during this time period.

Of the 153 samples tested, 136 were positive (88.9%; 95% CI 83.1–93.2) for at least one virus, and the detection rate of viruses was similar in both groups ($p = 0.7$). More than one viral agent was identified in 27.9% (36) of the samples, with no difference between groups ($p = 0.1$). The most common virus was hRV (82.4, 95% CI 75.77–87.8), followed by FLUVA (15.0%), hADV (6.5%), hPIV2 (4.6%), hRSV (3.9%), FLUVB (2.6%) and hPIV1 (2.6%). None of the samples were positive for hPIV3. FLUVB and hPIV1 were only found with other viruses (Table 2).

We performed an analysis of the severity of exacerbations and did not find statistically significant differences between the groups with and without virus infection regarding severity, such as hospitalization ($p = 0.4$), oxygen use ($p = 0.8$), and systemic use of corticosteroids ($p = 0.5$).

There were no differences in the viral rates between children with and without exacerbation. The results of univariate analysis evidenced that some variables were associated with asthma exacerbation: at least one hospitalisation for asthma in the past 12 months, at least three emergency room visits in the past 12 months, white ethnicity, monthly family income below 200 US$, cough or dyspnoea on exertion, nocturnal cough, exposure to mould and poor medication adherence (Table 1). After multivariate analysis, at least three visits to hospital for asthma in the last 12 months and nonadherence in inhaled corticosteroids (ICS) remained associated with the outcome (Table 3).

Discussion

In this study, we assessed asthmatic children in emergency room and in an outpatient clinic from a tropical region in Brazil and the results were consistent with those observed by several authors around the world, with high viral detection rates [9–11], with rhinovirus being the most frequent agent similar with others studies [9, 12, 15, 16, 23–25]. However the presence of respiratory viruses was similar in children with and without asthma exacerbation (regardless of severity) and although most studies have shown a higher prevalence of viruses in patients with acute asthma than controls, others studies found a similar detection rate of viruses between children with and without exacerbation [26–29].

The high detection rate of viruses among patients without asthma exacerbation may reflect the increased

Table 1 Clinical and social demographic features of patients with and without exacerbation

	G1 (92) N (%)	G2 (61) N (%)	P
Male gender	56 (60.9)	42 (68.9)	0.20
White ethnicity	62 (67.4)	28 (45.9)	< 0.01
Monthly family income ≤200 US$	41 (44.6)	39 (63.9)	0.01
Maternal schooling level ≤ 8 years	47 (51.1)	25 (41.0)	0.14
≥ 3 emergency room visits in the past 12 months	73 (76.0)	23 (24.0)	< 0.01
1 or more hospitalisations for asthma in the past 12 months	58 (80.6)	14 (19.4)	< 0.01
Cough or dyspnoea on exertion (yes)	66 (75.0)	22 (25.0)	< 0.01
Nocturnal cough, in-between exacerbations (yes)	70 (80.5)	17 (19.5)	< 0.01
Use of ICS (yes)	6 (19.2)	84 (91.4)	< 0.01
Exposure to furry animals (yes)	58 (65.9)	30 (34.1)	0.09
Exposure to mould (yes)	44 (71.0)	18 (29.0)	0.02
Exposure to house dust mite (yes)	66 (59.5)	45 (40.5)	0.80
Exposure to second hand tobacco smoking (yes)	33 (56.9)	25 (43.1)	0.61

G1 group 1(exacerbated asthmatics), *G2* group 2 (non-exacerbated asthmatics), *ICS* inhaled corticosteroids

sensitivity of PCR, which detects nucleic acid from current or previous infections, especially in the case of rhinovirus, which may be present up to 5 to 6 weeks after the beginning of symptomatic infection [30]. Regarding obtaining the sample, previous studies have shown that diagnostic yields of nasopharyngeal swab are comparable to the results obtained with nasopharyngeal aspirate specimens for all of the viruses identified by PCR methods [31–33]. In the present study the rates of virus detection was as high as in previous studies and rhinovirus was the most prevalent, in both group, independent of the sample colletion method.

Although it has been shown that viruses are associated with asthma exacerbations, several studies suggest that other factors, like allergen exposure, in combination with viral infection may increase the risk. In the subjects of this study, according to the results of bivariate analysis some variables were associated with asthma exacerbation: at least one hospitalization for asthma in the past 12 months, at least three emergency room visits in the past 12 months, white ethnicity, monthly family income below 200 US$, cough or dyspnea on exertion, nocturnal cough, exposure to mold and poor medication adherence. After multivariate analysis, the variables that remained associated with a higher risk of exacerbation were at least three emergency visits due to exacerbation in the last 12 months and nonadherence to asthma treatment.

It is known that exposure to allergens in combination with viral infection may increase the likelihood of an exacerbation, and in this population, allergic exposure was more prevalent in the exacerbated group, although without statistical significance. Exposure to mold was associated with exacerbation in the univariate analysis, but this association was not maintained in a multivariate analysis. We know that asthma prevalence in tropical areas is high and it may be linked to exposure to dust mites, parasitic infestation and other unknown aspects [34]. Exposure to molds is associated with allergic diseases, however, it prevalence vary widely probably because of environmental differences, and wide range of diagnostic tests used [2]. We assessed aeroallergen exposure through a questionnaire, not with objective measures, however, the results was similar to data obtained by Brazilian studies, with sensitization prevalence between 46.8% [35] and 54% [36] to at least one aeroallergen in asthmatic children evaluated by skin prick test or standard allergen extracts panel.

In the present study, nonadherence to inhaled corticosteroid was an important risk factor for asthma exacerbation, which indicates that the likelihood of viruses triggering an exacerbation of asthma can be minimized

Table 2 Rates of virus detection and co-detection between groups

Virus	G1 N (%)	G2 N (%)	Total N (%)	P
hRV	74 (80.4)	52 (85.2)	126 (82.4)	0.19
FLUVA	17 (18.5)	6 (9.8)	23 (15.0)	0.17
hAdV	5 (5.4)	5 (8.2)	10 (6.5)	0.30
HPIV2	6 (6.5)	1 (1.6)	7 (4.6)	0.20
hRSV	5 (5.4)	1 (1.6)	6 (3.9)	0.30
FLUV B	3 (3.3)	1 (1.6)	4 (2.6)	0.50
HPIV1	4 (4.3)	0 (0.0)	4 (2.6)	0.16
Any detected virus	81 (88.0)	55 (90.2)	136 (88.9)	0.70
Co-detection	27 (20.9)	9 (7.0)	36 (27.9)	0.10

G1 group 1, *G2* group 2, *hRV* human rhinovirus, *FLUVA* influenza virus A, *hAdV* human adenovirus, *FLUVB* influenza virus B, *hRSV* human respiratory syncytial virus, *HPIV2* human parainfluenza virus type 2, *HPIV1* parainfluenza virus type 1

Table 3 Variables associated with asthma exacerbation, multivariate analysis final model

Variables	IRR	95% CI	p-value
≥ 3 visits for asthma, 12 months	1·40	1·01–1·95	0·04
Nonadherence to inhaled corticosteroids	4·87	2·43–9·76	< 0·01

by daily ICS controller therapy. Our results are in accordance with a study in the United Kingdom, in which the regular use of daily ICS controller therapy protected from virus-related asthma exacerbations and hospital admissions [37].

Experimental studies have demonstrated that ICS inhibit respiratory tract viral replication and reduce cytokines in bronchial epithelial cells [38]. These effects of reducing virus-induced inflammation may help to explain the findings observed among patients using ICS in the present study who, despite presence of viral genetic material, showed no clinical evidence of viral disease. This association may have previously gone unnoticed because most of the studies in this area have been performed in countries in which most if not all children with asthma in the studies were on ICS maintenance treatment [7, 10, 14]. In contrast, the present study was conducted in a different setting with a lower rate of ICS use.

This is one of a few studies on viruses related to asthma exacerbations in a low-middle income country and using a control comparison group, which enhances the relevance of the results. This study not only downplays the importance of viruses as the sole culprit in asthma exacerbations, but also highlights the need of a comparison group in similar investigations. Moreover, it is possible that different populations can behave differently in terms of triggering exacerbations and genetic mechanisms may be involved in the association [8, 34]. Thus, larger studies are necessary to provide more insights into the pathogenesis of viral respiratory infections and virus-induced exacerbations of asthma in different populations.

In conclusion, while there is no doubt that viruses are associated with asthma exacerbations, the results of the present study suggest that viral infections per se are insufficient to cause an exacerbation. The proportion of acute respiratory viral infections among children with current asthma exacerbation was similar to that observed among children without exacerbation. The only significant risk factors for acute asthma exacerbations were previous emergency room visits for uncontrolled asthma and nonadherence in asthma treatment. The present study suggests that the occurrence of virus-induced exacerbations in children can be attenuated by the proper use of inhaled corticosteroids.

Abbreviations
95% CI: 95% confidence interval; ATS/ERS: American Thoracic Society/European Thoracic Society; FLUVA: Influenza virus A; FLUVB: Influenza virus B; hADV: Human adenovirus; hPIV: Human parainfluenza viruses; hRSV: Human respiratory syncytial virus; ICS: Inhaled corticosteroids; IRR: Incidence risk ratio; PCR: Polymerase chain reaction; RT-PCR: Reverse transcription-polymerase chain reaction

Acknowledgements
We thank Sarah de Faria and Arielli Evangelista for the collection of samples. We also thank the Clinical Research Unit of Federal University of Goiás and FAPEGO.

Funding
The study was sponsored by the State of Goias Research Foundation (FAPEG), wich had no participation in the study design, data analysis or interpretation and in the writing of the manuscript.

Authors' contributions
LDCC carried out the study design, collected the clinical data, analysed and interpreted the patient data and was a major contributor in writing the manuscript. PAMC carried out the study design, analysed and interpreted the patient data and was a major contributor in writing the manuscript. PLPB analysed and interpreted the patient data and was a major contributor in writing the manuscript. FSF and DDPC performed the laboratorial analysis and interpreted the data and contributed in writing the manuscript. MBLDS performed the laboratorial analysis and interpreted the data. IAC performed the laboratorial analysis and interpreted the data. RM performed the statistical analysis and interpreted the data and contributed in writing the manuscript. PSSC carried out the study design, collected the clinical data, analysed and interpreted the patient data and was a major contributor in writing the manuscript. All authors read and approved the final manuscript.

Competing interests
The authors declare that they have no competing interests.

Author details
[1]Pediatric Pulmonology Unit, University Hospital, Federal University of Goiás, Primeira Avenida, S/N. Setor Leste Universitária, Goiânia CEP: 746050-20, Brazil. [2]Pediatric Pulmonology Unit, University Hospital, Federal University of Minas Gerais, Belo Horizonte, Brazil. [3]Princess Amalia Children's Centre, Isala Hospital, Zwolle, and UMCG Postgraduate School of Medicine, University Medical Centre and University of Groningen, Groningen, the Netherlands. [4]Human Virology Department, Public Health and Tropical Pathology Institute, Federal University of Goiás, Goiânia, Brazil. [5]Faculty of Nursing, Universidade Federal de Goiás, Goiânia, GO, Brazil.

References
1. Global Initiative for Asthma. Global strategy for asthma management and prevention: Updated 2016. http//ginasthma.org. Accessed 15 Feb 2017.
2. Dick S, Doust E, Cowie H, Ayres JG, Turner S. Associations between environmental exposures and asthma control and exacerbations in young children: a systematic review. BMJ Open. 2014;4(2):e003827.
3. Fuchs O, Mutios E. Prenatal and childhood infections: implications for the development and treatment of childhood asthma. Lancet Respir Med. 2013;1:743–54.
4. Miller MK, Lee JH, Miller DP, Wenzel SE. Recent asthma exacerbations: a key predictor of future exacerbations. Respir Med. 2007;101(3):481–9.
5. Lai CKW, Beasley R, Crane J, Foliaki S, Shah J, Weiland S. The ISAAC phase three study group. Global variation in the prevalence and severity of asthma symptoms: phase three of the international study of asthma and allergies in childhood (ISAAC). Thorax. 2009;64(6):476–83.
6. Kopel LS, Phipatanakul W, Gaffin JM. Social disadvantage and asthma control in children. Paediatr Respir Rev. 2014;15(3):256–63.
7. Brand PLP. Inhaled corticosteroids should be the first line of treatment for children with asthma. Paediatr Respir Rev. 2011;12:245–9.

8. Loisel DA, Du G, Ahluwalia TS, Tisler CJ, Evans MD, Myers RA, Gangnon RE, Kreiner-Moller E, Bonnelykke K, Bisgaard H, et al. Genetic associations with viral respiratory illnesses and asthma control in children. Clin Exp Allergy. 2016;46:112–24.
9. Bizzintino J, Lee WM, Laing IA, Vang F, Pappas T, Zhang G, Martin AC, Khoo SK, Cox DW, Geelhoed GC, et al. Association between human rhinovirus C and severity of acute asthma in children. Eur Respir J. 2011;37(5):1037–42.
10. Maffey AF, Barrero PR, Venialgo C, Fernandez F, Fuse VA, Saia M, Villalba A, Fermepin MR, Teper AM, Mistchenko AS. Viruses and atypical bacteria associated with asthma exacerbations in hospitalized children. Pediatr Pulmonol. 2010;45:619–25.
11. Fujitsuka A, Tsukagoshi H, Arakawa M, Goto-Sugai K, Ryo A, Okayama Y, Mizuta K, Nishina A, Yoshizumi M, Kaburagi Y, et al. A molecular epidemiological study of respiratory viruses detected in Japanese children with acute wheezing illness. BMC Infect Dis. 2011;11:168.
12. Kato M, Tsukagoshi H, Yoshizumi M, Saitoh M, Kunihisa K, Yamada Y, Maruyama K, Yasuhie H, Kimura H. Different cytokine profile and eosinophil activation are involved in rhinovirus and RS virus-induced acute exacerbation of childhood wheezing. Pediatr Allergy and Immunol. 2011;22:e87–94.
13. Khetsuriani N, Kazerouni NN, Erdman DD, Lu X, Redd SC, Anderson LJ, Teague WG. Prevalence of viral respiratory tract infections in children with asthma. J Allergy Clin Immunol. 2007;119(2):314–21.
14. Mandelcwajg A, Moulin F, Menager C, Rozenberg F, Lebon P, Gendrel D. Underestimation of influenza viral infection in childhood asthma exacerbations. J Pediatr. 2010;157(3):505–6.
15. Rawlinson WD, Waliuzzaman Z, Carter IW, Belessis YC, Gilbert KM, Morton JR. Asthma exacerbations in children associated with rhinovirus but not human metapneumovirus infection. J Infect Dis. 2003;187(8):1314–8.
16. Ozcan C, Toyran M, Civelek E, Erkocoglu M, Altas AB, Albayrak N, Korukluoglu G, Kocabas CN. Evaluation of respiratory viral pathogens in acute asthma exacerbations during childhood. J Asthma. 2011;48(9):888–93.
17. Child Health Epidemiology Reference Group of WHO and UNICEF. Global, regional and national causes of child mortality: an updated systematic analysis for 2010 time trends since 2000. Lancet. 2012;379:2151–61.
18. Murray CS, Poletti G, Kebadze T, Morris J, Woodcock A, Johnston SL, Custovic A. Study of modifiable risk factors for asthma exacerbations: virus infection and allergen exposure increase the risk of asthma hospital admissions in children. Thorax. 2006;61(5):376–82.
19. Bjerregaard A, Laing IA, Backer V, Sverrild A, Khoo SK, Chidlow G, Sikazwe C, Smith DW, Souëf PL, Porsbjerg C. High fractional exhaled nitric oxide and sputum eosinophils are associated with an increased risk of future virus-induced exacerbation- a prospective cohort study. Clin Exp Allergy. 2017; https://doi.org/10.1111/cea12935.
20. Instituto Brasileiro de Geografia e Estatística (IBGE). Pesquisa nacional de saúde 2013: percepção do estado de saúde, estilos de vida e doenças crônicas - Brasil, grandes regiões e unidades da federação. Rio de Janeiro, 2014.
21. Reddel HK, Taylor DR, Bateman ED, Boulet LP, Boushey HC, Busse WW, et al. An official American Thoracic Society/European Respiratory Society statement: asthma control and exacerbations: standardizing endpoints for clinical asthma trials and clinical practice. Am J Respir Crit Care Med. 2009;180(1):59–99.
22. Brazilian Ministry of Health. Manual of norms and procedures for the laboratory diagnosis of Influenza. In: Brazilian plan of preparation for an influenza pandemic. Brasília; 2006. p. 164–72.
23. Lee WM, Kiesner C, Pappas T, Lee I, Grindle K, Jartti T, Jakiela B, Lemanske RF, Shult PA, Gern JE. A diverse group of previously unrecognized human rhinoviruses are common causes of respiratory illnesses in infants. PLoS One. 2007;2(10):e966.
24. Litwin CM, Bosley JG. Seasonality and prevalence of respiratory pathogens detected by multiplex PCR at a tertiary care medical center. Arch Virol. 2014;159(1):65–72.
25. Arden KE, Chang AB, Lambert SB, Nissen MD, Sloots TP, Mackay IM. Newly identified respiratory viruses in children with asthma exacerbation not requiring admission to hospital. J Med Virol. 2010;82(8):1458–61.
26. Camara AA, Silva JM, Ferriani VPL, Tobias KRC, Macedo IS, Padovani MA, Harsi CM, Cardoso MRA, Chapman MD, Arruda E. Risk factors for wheezing in a subtropical environment: Role of respiratory viruses and allergen sensitization. J Allergy Clin Immunol. 2004;113(3):551–7.
27. Kloepfer KM, et al. Increased H1N1 infection rate in children with asthma. Am J Resp Crit Care Med. 2012;185(12):1275–9.
28. Advani S, Sengupt AA, Forman M, Valsamakis A, Milstone AM. Detecting respiratory viruses in asymptomatic children. Pediatr Infect Dis J. 2012;31(12):122.
29. Ohrmalm L, Malinovsch A, Levinson WP, Janson C, Broliden K, Alving K. Presence of rhinovirus in the respiratory tract of adolescents and young adults with asthma without symptoms of infection. Respir Med. 2016;115:1–6.
30. Jartti T, Lehtinen P, Vuorinen T, Koskenvuo MK, Ruuskanen O. Persistence of rhinovirus and enterovirus RNA after acute respiratory illness in children. J Med Virol. 2004;72(4):695–9.
31. Sung RYT, Chan PKS, Choi KC, Yeung ACM, Li AM, Tang JW, et al. Comparative study of nasopharyngeal aspirate and nasal swab specimens for diagnosis of acute viral respiratory infection. J Clin Microbiol. 2008;46(9):3073. https://doi.org/10.1128/JCM.01209-08.
32. Blaschke J, Allison MA, Meyers L, Rogatcheva M, et al. Non-invasive sample collection for respiratory vírus testing by multiplex PCR. JClin Virol. 2011;52(3):210–4.
33. Tunsjo HS, Berg AS, Inchley CS, Roberg IK, Leegaard TM. Comparison of nasopharyngeal aspirate with flocked swab for PCR-detection of respiratory viruses in children. APMIS. 2015;123(6):473–7.
34. Caraballo L, Zakzuk J, Lee BW, Acevedo N, Soh JY, Sánchez-Borges M, Hossny E, Garci E, Rosario N, Ansotegui I, et al. Particularities of allergy in the tropics. World All Org J. 2016;9(1):20.
35. Pastorino AC, Kuschnir FC, Arruda LK, Casagrande RR, de Souza RG, Dias GA, et al. Sensitisation to aeroallergens in Brazilian adolescents living at the periphery of large subtropical urban centres. Allergol Immun(Madr). 2008;36(1):9–16.
36. Sarinho EC, Mariano J, Sarinho SW, Medeiros D, Rizzo JÁ, Almerinda RS, et al. Sensitisation to aeroallergens among asthmatic and non-asthmatic adolescents living in a poor region in the northeast of Brazil. Allergol Immun(Madr). 2009;37(5):239–43.
37. Prazma CM, Kral KM, Nadeem G, Yancey SW, Stempel DA. Controller medications and their effects on asthma exacerbations temporally associated with upper respiratory infections. Respir Med. 2010;104:780–7.
38. Bochkov YA, Busse WW, Brockman-Schneider RA, Evans MDE, Jarjour NN, McCrae C, Miller-Larsson A, Gern JE. Budesonide and formoterol effects on rhinovirus replication and epithelial cell cytokine responses. Respir Res. 2013;14(1):98.

The lung microbiome in children with HIV-bronchiectasis

Refiloe Masekela[1,2]*, Solize Vosloo[3], Stephanus N. Venter[3], Wilhelm Z. de Beer[3] and Robin J. Green[1]

Abstract

Background: Data on the lung microbiome in HIV-infected children is limited. The current study sought to determine the lung microbiome in HIV-associated bronchiectasis and to assess its association with pulmonary exacerbations.

Methods: A cross-sectional pilot study of 22 children (68% male; mean age 10.8 years) with HIV-associated bronchiectasis and a control group of 5 children with cystic fibrosis (CF). Thirty-one samples were collected, with 11 during exacerbations. Sputum samples were processed with 16S rRNA pyrosequencing.

Results: The average number of operational taxonomy units (OTUs) was 298 ± 67 vs. 434 ± 90, for HIV-bronchiectasis and CF, respectively. The relative abundance of *Proteobacteria* was higher in HIV-bronchiectasis (72.3%), with only 22.2% *Firmicutes*. There was no correlation between lung functions (FEV_1% and $FEF_{25/75}$%) and bacterial community ($r = 0.154$; $p = 0.470$ and $r = 0.178$; $p = 0.403$), respectively. Bacterial assemblage of exacerbation and non-exacerbation samples in HIV-bronchiectasis was not significantly different (ANOSIM, $R_{HIV-bronchiectasis} = 0.08$; $p = 0.14$ and $R_{CF} = 0.08$, $p = 0.50$). Higher within-community heterogeneity and lower evenness was associated with CF (Shannon-Weiner (H') = 5.39 ± 0.38 and Pielou's evenness (J) 0.79 ± 0.10 vs. HIV-bronchiectasis (Shannon-Weiner (H') = 4.45 ± 0.49 and Pielou's (J) 0.89 ± 0.03.

Conclusion: The microbiome in children with HIV-associated bronchiectasis seems to be less rich, diverse and heterogeneous with predominance of *Proteobacteria* when compared to cystic fibrosis.

Keywords: Paediatrics, Microbiology, HIV-associated bronchiectasis, Bacterial diversity, Lung microbiome

Background

Bronchiectasis is a chronic inflammatory lung disease that, in high-income countries, has been declining outside of the context of cystic fibrosis (CF) in children, as compared to adults where the incidence and prevalence is on the rise [1]. However, this is not so in low-middle income countries and some economically disadvantaged groups in high-income countries [2–4]. The burden of disease is linked to inequity in access to quality health care, lack of essential medicines, high tuberculosis (TB) rates, indoor pollution and secondary immunodeficiency states such as human immunodeficiency virus (HIV) infection [5].

Bronchiectasis is characterized by interspersed episodes of quiescence and pulmonary exacerbations (PEs). The consequence of PEs is chronic respiratory disability and poor quality of life. A key factor in the initiation of PEs are airway microbes, which are thought to establish recurrent respiratory tract infections and therefore maintain an inflammatory milieu in the airway [6]. Traditionally, microorganisms are obtained from respiratory samples via microscopy and culture and this is then utilized to guide anti-microbial therapy. Recently, there has been a renewed interest in research on the microbial community in the lung of individuals in both diseased and in healthy lungs; this research is based on culture-independent phylogenetic profiling approaches based on genetic biomarkers such as 16S rRNA sequencing [7, 8].

Microbial communities isolated in the upper airways have been found to closely resemble those present in the lung compartment [9]. In the context of both CF

* Correspondence: masekelar@ukzn.ac.za
[1]Department of Paediatrics and Child Health, Faculty of Health Sciences, University of Pretoria, Pretoria, South Africa
[2]Department of Maternal and Child Health, Nelson R Mandela School of Medicine, College of Health Sciences, University of KwaZulu-Natal, 719 Umbilo Road, Congella, Durban 4013, South Africa
Full list of author information is available at the end of the article

and non-CF bronchiectasis, there is evidence that bacterial diversity is critical in the maintenance of "homeostasis" and that this prevents PEs and is associated with better lung function [10, 11]. The contribution of microbes to the specific community of individuals' lungs may either suppress (resilience microbiota) or precipitate (risk microbiota) pulmonary exacerbations [8, 10]. In the context of HIV infection, which is known to affect both innate and adaptive immune pulmonary responses, recent data suggests that there is a change in the lung microbiome of HIV-infected individuals which is attributed to the immunosuppressive state; however these studies have been in adult cohorts [12, 13].

To our knowledge, there is currently no published data on the airway microbiome in children with HIV-associated bronchiectasis on antiretroviral therapy and the changes in the microbiome during or between exacerbations episodes. The primary aim of this pilot study was to evaluate the microbiome in HIV-infected children with established chronic lung disease, to assess the diversity of the microbiome, and to assess for any changes that may occur during exacerbation episodes. We also sampled a small group of children with bronchiectasis secondary to cystic fibrosis to evaluate any differences between these children and those with HIV-bronchiectasis in the same environment.

Methods
Setting
Children were recruited during routine or unscheduled visits at the Steve Biko Academic Hospital, Chest Clinic, Pretoria, South Africa during a 17-month period between May 2013 and October 2014. This clinic serves as a referral centre for children from Tshwane Metropolitan region in Gauteng with over 2.5 million children living in a peri-urban setting, where 27.0% of the people live in informal settlements with a high HIV prevalence rate at 11.2% in 2015. The clinic also serves the adjoining Mpumalanga province with a largely rural population. All the children in the study were from communities in Tshwane (urban/pre-urban) and Mpumalanga province (rural). For the HIV-bronchiectasis group, HIV status was based on a positive enzyme-linked immunosorbent assay (ELISA). All subjects had to have been on antiretroviral therapy for a minimum of 6 months prior to enrolment. All children at the clinic are screened routinely every 3 months for TB and none of the subjects had positive TB cultures. Subjects with cystic fibrosis (CF) confirmed by genetics and/or two positive sweat tests were invited to participate to serve as controls in a 3:1 design.

Exacerbations were defined according to the following criteria: a change in the nature of cough or increasing shortness of breath; development of new constitutional symptoms (fever, malaise) or changes in sputum characteristics (e.g. sputum colour and/or increase in sputum quality and/or increase in sputum volume). The sputum quality was assessed using the Barlett score which is based on the average number of neutrophils per low power field, average number of epithelial cells per low power field and presence of mucus/saliva in the specimen [14]. A value of < 0 indicates either either no inflammation or a poor quality specimen. Immune staging with HIV viral load and $CD4^+$ T cells was performed. Presence of bronchiectasis was confirmed for each child by a CT chest scan carried out by an independent radiologist and pulmonologist. Lung function testing was performed using Viasys SpiroPro Jaeger Spirometer (Hoechberg, Germany).

Sputum collection, processing and DNA extraction
All sputum samples were collected by sputum induction after nebulization with hypertonic saline and collected by mucus extractors after percussions by a physiotherapist. Prior to DNA extraction, the sputum samples were washed with two times the volume, 0.85% Phosphate Buffered Saline (PBS) (8.00 g/L NaCl, 0.2 g/L KCl, 1.44 g/L Na_2HPO_4, 0.24 g/L KH_2PO_4, pH 7.4). Excess PBS was removed and the remaining sputum was incubated with equal volume Sputasol (Thermo Scientific), a mucolytic agent, at 37 °C. The liquefied suspension was centrifuged at 11000 x g for 5 min. The supernatant was removed and the pellet was washed with 750 μl PBS and centrifuged at 10000 x g for 5 min. The wash step was repeated two more times. DNA was extracted from the processed sputum samples using the Zymo Research Genomic DNA™ Tissue MiniPrep kit (Zymo Research, South Africa), in accordance with the manufacturer's protocol. The protocol includes a pre-treatment step with Proteinase K to improve lysis of Gram-positive bacteria. DNA concentration and purity (OD260/280 and OD 230/260) were determined using the Nanodrop ND-1000™ Spectrophotometer. All genomic DNA was stored at − 20 °C until further analysis.

16S rRNA gene amplification and pyrosequencing
Full length 16S rRNA libraries were constructed using primers: 27F (5′AGAGTTTGATCCTGGCTCAG-3′) and 1492R (5′-GGTTACCTTGTTACGACT-3′) adapted from Edward et al. [15]. In order to increase sequencing depth, five 16S rRNA amplicon libraries were constructed for each sample. The five generated amplicon libraries of corresponding samples were pulled and sent to Inqaba Biotec (Pretoria, South Africa) for variable region, V1-V3 amplicon library construction and

pyrosequencing, using the GS Junior System (Roche Applied Science, Basel). Bacterial 16S rRNA amplicons obtained were subjected to variable region V1 – V3 bacterial community profiling, using the 454-pyrosequencing platform. Polymerase chain reaction (PCR) was carried out using the BIO-RAD T100™ Thermal Cycler. The polymerase chain reaction (PCR) mixtures (25 μl) consisted of 1 x reaction buffer, 1.5 mM $MgCl_2$, 250 μM of each nucleotide (dATP, dCTP, dGTP, dTTP), 10 pmol of each primer (forward and reverse), 1.5 U Taq DNA polymerase, 16.85 μl nuclease free water (Qiagen) and 0.5 μl genomic DNA. The cycling conditions for the 16S rRNA amplicons consisted of an initial denaturation step at 92 °C for 10 min, followed by 30 cycles of denaturation at 92 °C for 1 min, annealing at 58 °C for 1 min, extension at 75 °C for 1 min, and a final extension at 75 °C for 5 min. At the end of the 30 cycles, the reaction was kept at 4 °C. Each DNA amplification step within the 16S profiling process included standard negative controls using nuclease-free water instead of the sample DNA. Samples were not processed to the next step unless the negative controls were confirmed to be negative. During the study, all negative controls showed no amplification. Standard negative controls were also included during the sequencing process. No extra measures typically required for low microbial biomass samples were performed, as all the DNA extractions yielded high concentrations of DNA (determined with nanodrop) and no more than 30 cycles were required for any of the PCR amplification steps [16]. Normal positive control samples (bacterial DNA) as well as the positive reactions obtained for all the samples indicated that the various steps in the analysis provided the expected results.

Sequence processing and data analysis
Sequence processing and data analysis were conducted using the MOTHUR software package (version 1.35.1) and processing pipeline as described on the MOTHUR website: www.mothur.org/wiki/454_SOP [17]. Briefly described, raw pyrosequencing reads were initially screened to remove all sequences that did not meet the required quality criteria. Processed sequences following initial screening included sequences with a minimum quality score of 35, minimum sequence length of 150 nucleotides, maximum sequence length of 600 nucleotides, maximum of six ambiguous nucleotides and absence of mismatches in barcodes and primers. Following quality filtering the processed sequences were aligned to a reference alignment, which was generated from the SILVA seed ribosomal RNA database (Release 119) [18]. After alignment, the sequence data set were screened to cull all sequences that did not align to the alignment region, variable region V1 – V3 of the 16S rRNA gene. The ends of the aligned sequences were subsequently trimmed to ensure that the sequences all started and ended at the same alignment coordinates.

The aligned sequences were screened for chimeras using UCHIME [19]. Taxonomic affiliation was assigned to each processed and chimeric-free sequence using the GreenGenes reference taxonomy database at a pseudo-bootstrap confidence score of 80%. Unwanted lineages were culled by removing sequences that could not be classified to kingdom level, or that classified as *Eukaryota*, chloroplast, or mitochondria. The remaining high quality reads were clustered into operational taxonomic units (OTUs) at a 97% similarity threshold. Representative sequences for each OTU were obtained and classified against the GreenGenes dataset (August 2013 of gg_13_8) as described above.

Sample diversity comparisons and statistics
In order to ensure that all samples were compared at the same sequence depth, a computation of alpha and beta diversity indices was performed. This was performed after sub-sampling of the entire sequence dataset 1000 times to a defined number of sequences. The sub-sampling threshold was determined following rarefaction analysis. The rarefaction curves of the samples reached completed saturation at about 1200 sequences per sample. In light of this, the sequence database were subsampled to a threshold of 1200 sequences per sample. Alpha and beta diversity indexes were calculated using functions provided in the MOTHUR software package (version 1.35.1) [17]. Three alpha diversity indexes, e.g. Chao1, Shannon-Weiner index (H′) and Pielou's evenness index (J) were calculated. Chao1 was used as a measure of within community species richness, whereas H′ and J were used as measures of within community heterogeneity and evenness, respectively.

For OTU-based beta diversity analysis, variability in the bacterial species assemblage between samples was analysed using two ecological coefficients of compositional dissimilarity, namely, Jaccard and Bray-Curtis [20, 21]. Jaccard coefficients were used to address community structure, as calculated pair-wise dissimilarity among selected samples is based on incidence-data (presence/absence), whereas Bray-Curtis coefficients were used to address community membership, as pair-wise dissimilarity between selected samples is calculated on the basis of incidence and abundance data. In addition, comparative analysis of compositional variability within the community assemblage of individual samples was visualized by performing non-metric multi-dimensional scaling (NMDS) on the Bray-Curtis distances using the vegan package (metaMDS function) in R [22]. This was followed by the analysis of similarities (ANOSIM) to statistically explain the compositional variability observed among samples categorized according to defined groupings [23].

Analysis included descriptive statistics for age, gender and lung functions. Associations between bacterial communities, disease, exacerbations and lung function parameters i.e. FEV_1% predicted and FEF_{25-75}% were investigated using Pearson correlation coefficients utilizing STATA 13.0 (StataCorp LP. 2013 Stata: Release 13, College Station, TX, USA). For all statistical analyses, the null hypothesis was rejected at a probability of $p < 0.05$. Written informed consent was provided by parents or guardians for all children under the age of 18 years and assent for all children over the age of 7 years. Ethical approval for the study was granted by the Research Ethics Committee of the Faculty of Health Sciences of the University of Pretoria (HREC No 315/2013).

Results
Clinical data
The demographics and baseline data of the 27 subjects recruited for the study are reflected in Table 1. The 22 HIV-bronchiectasis subjects (72% male) included had a mean age of 10.8 years. For the CF controls, six patients were enrolled; of these, one patient was excluded from analysis due to poor sputum quality. The final analysis therefore included only 5 subjects (60% males) with a mean age of 8.4 years.

In total, 31 sputum samples were collected. Twenty-one sputum samples (HIV-bronchiectasis = 18 and CF = 3) were collected from clinically stable subjects (non-exacerbation samples); the remaining ten samples were collected prior to the initiation of antibiotics for an exacerbation (HIV-bronchiectasis = 8 and CF = 2).

The HIV-bronchiectasis subjects had been on highly active antiretroviral therapy (HAART) for a mean duration of 4 years, and WHO stage 4 with evidence of moderate immune suppression and inadequate HIV viral suppression. Of these children, 4 had HIV-viral loads greater than 100,000 copies/ml, despite being on HAART for more than 6 months reflecting treatment failure. The respiratory morbidity in the HIV-bronchiectasis group was severe with a lower mean FEV_1% predicted and significant lower airway obstruction. For the CF group, the children were younger with more preserved lung function when compared to the HIV-bronchiectasis group.

Pyrosequencing data analysis
The total number of raw 16S rRNA variable region, V1 – V3 pyrosequencing reads were 223,458, with a Mean $\pm SD$ of $6983 \pm 12,146$ per sample. The average number V1 – V3 pyrosequencing reads of processed sequences obtained within HIV-bronchiectasis and CF samples were (mean $\pm$ SD) 3762 ± 2568 and 1409 ± 283, respectively. Subsequent classification of the processed sequences into operational taxonomic units (OTUs) at a 97% similarity threshold identified 4779 OTUs. The average number of OTUs detected among HIV-bronchiectasis samples were (mean $\pm$ SD) 298 ± 67, whereas those for CF samples were 434 ± 90.

Bacterial diversity analysis
The visual display of the rarefaction curves infers a continued emergence of new observed species as the sequence output increases (Fig. 1). The rarefaction curves of the samples reached completed saturation at about 1200 sequences per sample. In light of this, the sequence database was subsampled to a threshold of 1200 sequences per sample. Following computation Chao1, Shannon-Weiner (H′) and Pielou's evenness indices (J), there were no significant differences in Chao1 [$F(1, 29) = 0.69$, $p = 4.12E-01$); however, there was significant differences in

Table 1 Demographic, immunological and lung function data of children with HIV-associated bronchiectasis and CF-bronchiectasis

Variable	HIV associated bronchiectasis		CF-bronchiectasis [δ]	
	Mean	95% CI	Mean	95% CI
Age (years)	10.8	9.4–12.3	8.4	6.9–9.7
Gender (M/F)*	16/6 (72/28)		3/2 (60/40)	
Height z score **	−2.3	−2.9 – −1.46	−1.0	−4.3 – 2.2
BMI z-scores**	−1.9	−2.9 – −0.6	−0.9	−3.5 – 1.6
CD4% count	22.9	19.3–25.5		
HIV-viral load (copies/ml)	11,455	1768–74,199		
Duration HAART (months)	48.0	34.5–62.6		
FEV_1% predicted	52.5	45.6–59.4	84.8	45.5–124.0
$FEF_{25/75}$% predicted	47.8	36.6–59.1	72.7	63.2–82.3
Bartlett score [§]	1.6	1.4–1.9	1.75	0.9–2.5
Mutation (%)			p.F508del (67)	3120 (33)

*numbers expressed in parentheses percentage of males and females; **: height and body mass index expressed as z-scores (SD) as per WHO criteria with normal between 0 and 2 z-scores; [§] Bartlett score from reference 14; [¶]p.508.del p F508del./p.F508.del; 3120: 3120 = 1G > A/3120 + 1G > A; [δ] results for 5 children

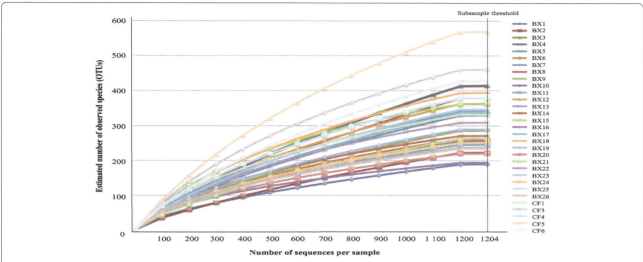

Fig. 1 Rarefaction analysis displaying estimated number of observed species (OTUs at 97% similarity) detected at different sequence intervals. The subsampling threshold limit was set at 1204 sequences per sample (dotted black line). BX: bronchiectasis and CF: cystic fibrosis

Shannon-Weiner (H) [$F(1, 29) = 16.22$, $p = 3.72E-04$] and Pielou's (J) [$F(1, 29) = 5.26$, $p = 3.00E-02$]. Specifically, the community of the CF samples was significantly more diverse (H', mean ± SD = 5.39 ± 0.38) and uneven (J, mean ± SD = 0.79 ± 0.10) when compared with the HIV-bronchiectasis samples (mean ± SD for Shannon-Weiner = 4.45 ± 0.49 and Pielou's 0.89 ± 0.03, respectively) (Figs. 2 and 3).

Jaccard (D_J) and Bray-Curtis (D_{BC}) were used to compare the bacterial community structure and membership between samples. Within the HIV-bronchiectasis group, the average dissimilarity in the community membership was about 92% (D_J, mean ± SD = 0.92 ± 0.08), whereas the average dissimilarity in the community structure was about 95% (D_{BC}, mean ± SD = 0.95 ± 0.07). Similarly, within the CF group the average dissimilarity in the community membership was about 80% (D_J, mean ± SD = 0.80 ± 0.10), whereas the average dissimilarity in the community structure was about 88% (D_{BC}, mean ± SD = 0.88 ± 0.05). To depict the degree of compositional variability amongst the HIV-bronchiectasis and CF samples, all the samples were ordinated in a two-dimensional non-metric multidimensional scaling (NMDS) plot (based on Bray-Curtis dissimilarity measures) (Fig. 4). To test for localized bacterial community assemblage confined to HIV-bronchiectasis and CF groups, analysis of similarity test (ANOSIM) test was performed using on Bray-Curtis distances. Following ANOSIM tests there was a significant difference in the community structures of the HIV-bronchiectasis and CF samples (ANOSIM, $R = 0.21$, $p = 0.04$). In contrast, there was no significant difference in the community structures between the exacerbation and non-exacerbation samples for either disease groups (ANOSIM, $R_{HIV\text{-}bronchiectasis} = 0.08$, $p = 0.14$; $R_{CF} = 0.08$, $p = 0.50$).

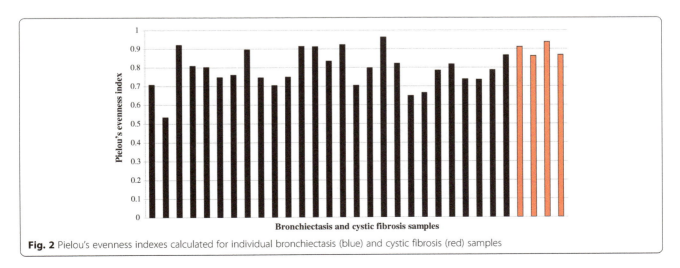

Fig. 2 Pielou's evenness indexes calculated for individual bronchiectasis (blue) and cystic fibrosis (red) samples

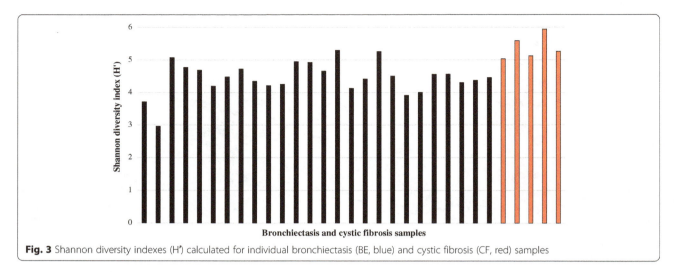

Fig. 3 Shannon diversity indexes (H') calculated for individual bronchiectasis (BE, blue) and cystic fibrosis (CF, red) samples

Bacterial community profiling

For bacterial community profiles, eight bacterial phyla – *Actinobacteria*, *Bacteroidetes*, *Firmicutes*, *Fusobacteria*, *Proteobacteria*, *Spirochetes*, *Tenericutes* and *Candidatus Saccharibacteria* were recovered from all samples. Three phyla – *Spirochetes*, *Tenericutes* and *Candidatus Saccharibacteria* were encountered only within the bronchiectasis group, where they were infrequently detected at relative abundances < 1%. *Proteobacteria* and *Firmicutes* were the two dominating phyla detected within the HIV-bronchiectasis and CF groups with combined average relative abundances of these two phyla reaching 94.0 and 89.0%, respectively. The average relative abundance of *Proteobacteria* was higher in the HIV-bronchiectasis group than in CF 72.3% vs. 40.1%, respectively. In contrast, the average relative abundance of *Firmicutes* was higher within the CF group (49.0% vs. 22.2%). The remaining three phyla in decreasing order had an average relative abundance of: *Fusobacteria*, 2.4%; *Bacteroidetes*, 1.9% and *Actinobacteria*, 0.5% within the HIV-bronchiectasis group. For the CF groups *Bacteroidetes* 8.4%, *Fusobacteria* 1.0% and *Actinobacteria* 0.7% were the other predominant phyla. In addition, several samples were dominated by other phyla that contributed towards a significant proportion of the phyla assemblage. *Fusobacteria* was detected in HIV-bronchiectasis (BE) samples: BE6 (36.8%), BE12 (9.3%) and BE18 (6.7%), whereas *Bacteroidetes* were detected in BE15 (16.1%), BE18 (9.4%) and BE22 (12.9%). Five genera *Moryella*, *Parvimonas*, *Peptostreptococcus*, *Pseudomonas* and *Sneathia* were confined to HIV-bronchiectasis samples.

As with the HIV-bronchiectasis samples, the fluctuating dominance of *Proteobacteria* and *Firmicutes* was also observed within CF samples. *Proteobacteria* dominated two CF samples - CF1 and CF6 [69.7%, range 64.8 - 74.7%)],

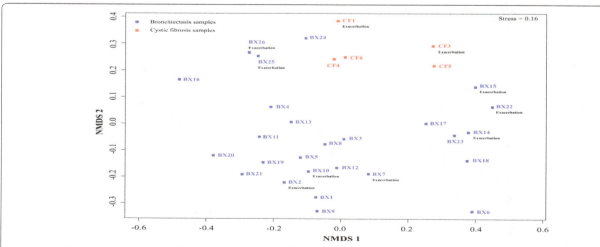

Fig. 4 Two-dimensional nonmetric multidimensional scaling (NMDS) plot displaying the spatial ordination of 31 sputum samples collected from 22 bronchiectasis subjects (BX, blue) and 5 cystic fibrosis subjects (CF, red)

whereas *Firmicutes* dominated the remaining 4 CF samples [59.9%, range (47.1- 70.1%)]. In addition, *Bacteroidetes* were present at high relative abundances (range 4.0 - 20.8%) with the exception of sample CF1 in which the phylum was not detected. *Staphylococcus* was detected only within CF samples. Exacerbations had no impact on the microbial community composition.

Taxonomic affiliation at a genus level was used to explain the bacterial community profiles. *Haemophilus* had a higher prevalence in the HIV-bronchiectasis group (64.7%) than the CF group (28.0%). In contrast, *Streptococcus* was more prevalent in the CF group (41.4% vs. 15.2%) than in the HIV-bronchiectasis group. The genera assemblage harboured by each sample was structurally diverse. *Haemophilus* (*Proteobacteria* phylum) and *Streptococcus* (*Firmicutes* phylum) were the dominant genera within HIV-bronchiectasis and CF samples with combined average abundances of these two genera reaching 79.9 and 69.4% within each group, respectively.

Compositional similarity within the genera assemblage of individual samples was displayed in the heat map, which was constructed following UPGMA hierarchical cluster analysis (Fig. 5). The samples were categorized into three distinct groupings that were distinguishable from one another based on their bacterial genera assemblage composition. The groups were designated as: Group A, *Haemophilus*-dominating with *Streptococcus*; Group B, *Streptococcus*-dominating with *Haemophilus* and Group C, *Pseudomonas*-dominating with *Prevotella*.

The majority of the HIV-bronchiectasis samples and one CF samples (CF6) clustered within Group A, with relative abundances of *Haemophilus* 85.7% (range: 62.6 – 99.3%) and *Streptococcus* 27.3% (range: 0.1 – 34.6%). Group B included the CF samples, with the exception of CF6, as wells as 4 bronchiectasis samples (BE14, BE17, BE18, and BE23). This group was dominated by Streptococcus 53.8% (range: 32.8 – 79.2%), and *Haemophilus* 11.4% (range: 0.30- 35.4%). Group C contained only two samples (BE22 and BE15), which had high relative abundances of *Pseudomonas* (BE15 = 57.0% and BE22 = 35.0%) and *Prevotella* (BE15 = 14.8% and BE22 = 12.7%). For lung function parameters there was no correlation between FEV_1% nor $FEF_{25/75}$% and the predominance of *Proteobacteria* ($r = 0.154$; $p = 0.4706$ and $r = 0.178$; $p = 0.4034$), respectively.

Discussion

In this study of the microbiome of children with HIV-associated bronchiectasis there was higher relative abundance of *Proteobacteria* when compared to a limited number of CF-bronchiectasis subjects, where *Furmicutes* predominated. *Pseudomonas* and *Prevotella* were also identified, but in less than 1% of the samples. There was no correlation between relative abundance of specific taxa and lung function parameters, although these children had significant morbidity with low lung functions. The community richness within the bronchiectasis subjects had relatively fewer OTUs and less sample heterogeneity when compared to the limited CF

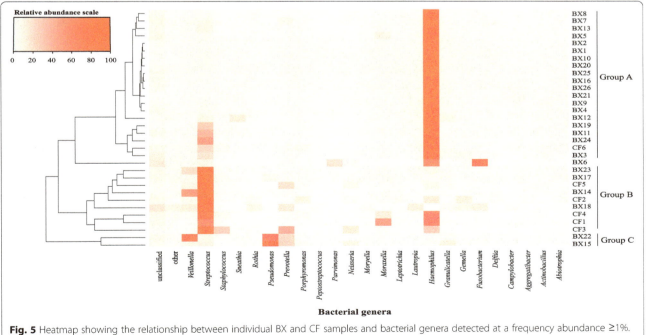

Fig. 5 Heatmap showing the relationship between individual BX and CF samples and bacterial genera detected at a frequency abundance ≥1%. The UPGMA tree shown on the left side of the figure depicts hierarchical clustering of 26 BX and 5 CF samples based on Bray-Curtis dissimilarity coefficient

samples. Bacterial assemblage was not affected by the presence or absence of pulmonary exacerbations in the HIV-bronchiectasis group.

There is conflicting data in the literature with regards to the level of immunosuppression and its impact on the lung microbiome. In one study in HIV-positive adults with acute pneumonia in two cohorts in Uganda and San Francisco, the Ugandan subjects revealed a richer and more diverse microbiome and higher prevalence of *P. aeruginosa* despite having more advanced HIV-disease staging [24]. A more recent study has shown that HIV-infected subjects with advanced disease demonstrated decreased alpha diversity (richness and diversity) when compared to HIV-uninfected individuals and that this difference persisted up to 3 years after initiation of HAART [12]. These studies suggest that HIV may impact the interaction between host and environment via perturbation in the bacterial diversity in the respiratory tract. The question of the impact of innate immunity and HIV also requires further study; so far there is one study in HIV-positive children that demonstrated lower saliva bacterial species in the study group, despite comparable levels of secretory IgA to an uninfected cohort [25]. In HIV-positive individuals, the use of antimicrobials, antifungals and antiretroviral therapy may be contributing to the changing microbiome. The impact of polypharmacy and its role on dysbiosis in HIV still requires further elucidation. In the current study, we found lower bacterial diversity in the HIV-infected group when compared to an admittedly small control group of CF children.

Severity of lung disease has also been shown to impact the microbiome. In chronic obstructive pulmonary disease (COPD), more advance staging of disease with global initiative of chronic obstructive lung disease (GOLD) stage 4, was found to be associated with reduced bacterial diversity when compared to healthy individuals and COPD sufferers with milder disease [26, 27]. In the current study, the CF group had more preserved lung function than the HIV-bronchiectasis group and we postulate that the differences in severity of lung impairment may account for the differences in the microbiome in the two groups although the numbers were small. *Pseudomonas aeruginosa* was identified only in the HIV-bronchiectasis group, and this pathogen has been previously been associated with lung inflammation and reduced lung function [11, 28]. In the current study the subjects with CF were younger and the sample size small, possibly explaining the lack of *P. aeruginosa* in this group.

Currently utilised tools for assessment of *P. aeruginosa* are crude, with bacterial densities, bacterial counts and bacterial numbers being unreliable to predict exacerbations [29–31]. Studies using the microbiome to guide therapeutic interventions have also yielded disappointing results. The use of antibiotics during exacerbation has been shown in both animal and human studies to have minimal impact on the microbial community composition, and the bacterial load with qPCR testing with the exception of *Pseudomonadales* [11, 29, 32]. The relative abundance of *Pseudomonas* as a target for assessment of treatment response is an attractive option, particularly in CF, bronchiectasis and COPD where *P. aeruginosa* colonization influences pulmonary outcomes and exacerbations. Further studies are needed in this area, particularly on the role of the microbial community and its change pre- and post-exacerbations; as well as for treatment response assessment.

The strength of the current study is that it provides pilot data on the microbiome in bronchiectasis in the context of HIV-infected children where little data exists. The differences shown reflects results found by other authors on the impact of HIV on the lung microbiome, showing reduced diversity and reduced richness [12, 24, 32]. There seems to be a signal of less diversity in HIV-bronchiectasis when compared to CF, although this should be interpreted with caution due to the small numbers in the CF group.

The study is limited by the small sample size and lack of an HIV-positive group without chronic lung disease, which could have provided insight to the effect of HIV-infection alone on the microbiome. Without the HIV "control" group, conclusions on the microbiome may not be based on lung disease severity but rather on the infection with HIV. A previous study by the Lung HIV Microbiome Project showed similarities in the microbiome of lower airway broncho-alveolar lavage samples of HIV-negative, HIV-positive HAART "naïve" and HIV-positive on HAART in adults [33]. In the current study, there was no comparison of the microbiome data with conventional sputum microscopy and sensitivity results. The number of CF 'controls' is also small and any conclusions should be interpreted with caution. We also collected induced samples and not broncho-alveolar protected brush samples, as previous studies in children have shown induced samples to provide adequate samples similar to those of the upper airway [34]. The numbers of patients with exacerbations are also small, limiting their interpretation and generalization.

The current findings, showing that *Haemophilus* and *Streptococcus* dominated the microbiome of both groups of patients were supported by previous culture based studies [6, 35]. Although the impact of reagent contamination on the microbiome was not addressed specifically, the possibility that these dominant groups could be directly linked to reagent contamination was small. *Haemophilus* was not identified as a typical contaminant previously and due to the high level of microbial biomass in all samples, high concentrations of DNA could be extracted [16, 36]. Comparison of the relative abundance data (Fig. 5) also did not provided any indication of issues with contamination of DNA in the reagents.

Conclusion
The microbiome in children with HIV-associated bronchiectasis seems to be less rich, diverse and heterogeneous than in children with CF-bronchiectasis, with predominance of *Proteobacteria*.

Funding
This study was funded with a grant for RM from the University of Pretoria Institutional Research –Genomics 2013. The University had no role in the design of the study, data collection, analysis, and interpretation of data and in writing the manuscript.

Authors' contributions
RM, SV and SNV contributed to the study concept, data collection, data analysis and the writing up of the manuscript. RJG contributed to the study concept, data analysis and writing of the manuscript. WZdB contributed to the study concept, data collection and data analysis of the manuscript. All authors read and approved the final manuscript.

Competing interests
The authors declare that they have no competing interests.

Author details
[1]Department of Paediatrics and Child Health, Faculty of Health Sciences, University of Pretoria, Pretoria, South Africa. [2]Department of Maternal and Child Health, Nelson R Mandela School of Medicine, College of Health Sciences, University of KwaZulu-Natal, 719 Umbilo Road, Congella, Durban 4013, South Africa. [3]Department of Microbiology and Plant Pathology, University of Pretoria, Pretoria, South Africa.

References
1. Quint JK, Millett ERC, Joshi M, Navaratnam V, Thomas SL, Hurst JR, Smeeth L, et al. Change in the incidence, prevalence and mortality of bronchiectasis in the UK from 2004 to 2013: a population-based cohort study. Eur Respir J. 2016;47(1):186–93.
2. Singleton RJ, Valery PC, Morris P, Brynes CA, Grimwood K, Reddding G, et al. Indigenous children from three countries with non-cystic fibrosis chronic suppurative lung disease/bronchiectasis. Pediatr Pulmonol. 2014;49(2):189–200.
3. Karadag B, Karakoc F, Ersu R, Kut A, Bakac S, Dagli E. Non-cystic-fibrosis bronchiectasis in children: a persisting problem in developing countries. Respiration. 2005;72:233–8.
4. Kapur N, Karadag B. Differences and similarities in non-cystic fibrosis bronchiectasis between developing and affluent countries. Paediatr Respir Rev. 2011;12(2):91–6.
5. Masekela R, Anderson R, Moodley T, Kitchin OP, Risenga SM, Becker PJ, et al. HIV-related bronchiectasis in children: an emerging spectre in high tuberculosis burden areas. Int J Tuberc Lung Dis. 2011;15(12):1702–7.
6. Cole PJ. Inflammation: a two-edged sword-the model of bronchiectasis. Eur J Respir Dis Suppl. 1986;147:6–15.
7. Marsland BJ, Yadava K, Nicod LP. The airway microbiome and disease. Chest. 2013;14(2):63–637.
8. Segal LN, Rom W, Widen MD. Lung microbiome for clinicians. New discoveries about bugs in healthy and diseased lungs. Ann Am Thorac Soc. 2014;11(1):108–16.
9. Bassis CM, Erb-Downward JR, Dickson RP, Freeman CM, Schmidt TM, Young VB, et al. Analysis of the upper respiratory tract microbiotas as the source of the lung and gastric microbiotas in healthy individuals. MBio. 2015;6(2): e00037. https://doi.org/10.11128/mBio.0003715.
10. Rogers GB, van der Gast CJ, Cuthberson L, Thomson SK, Bruce KD, Martin LM, et al. Clinical measures of disease in adult non-CF bronchiectasis correlate with airway microbiota composition. Thorax. 2013;68:731–137.
11. Zemanick ET, Harris KJ, Wagner BD, Robertson CE, Sagel SD, Stevens MJ, et al. Inflammation and airway microbiota during cystic fibrosis pulmonary exacerbations. PLoS One. 2013;8(4):e62917. https://doi.org/10.1371/journal.pone.0062917. Print 2013
12. Twigg HL 3rd, Knox KS, Zhou J, Crothers KA, Nelson DE, Toh E, Day RB, et al. Effect of advanced HIV infection on the respiratory microbiome. Am J Respir Crit Care Med. 2016; https://doi.org/10.1164/rccm.201509-1875OC. [Epub ahead of print]
13. Twigg HL 3rd, Weinstock GM, Knox KS. Lung microbiome in human immunodeficiency virus infection. Transl Res. 2017;179:97–107.
14. Bartlett RC. Medical microbiology: quality cost and clinical relevance. New York: Wiley; 1974.
15. Edward U, Rogall T, Blöckerl H, Emde M, Böttger EC. Isolation and direct complete nucleotide determination of entire genes. Characterization of a gene coding for 16S ribosomal RNA. Nucleic Acids Res. 1989;17:7843–53.
16. Kim D, Hofstaedter CE, Zhao C, Mattei L, Tanes C, Clarke E, et al. Optimizing methods and dodging pitfalls in microbiome research. Microbiome. 2017;5(1):52.
17. Schloss P, Westcott S, Ryabin T, Hall J, Hartmann M, Hollister E, et al. Introducing MOTHUR: open source, platform-independent, community-supported software for describing and comparing microbial communities. Appl Environ Microbiol. 2009;75(23):7537–41.
18. Pruesse E, Quast C, Knittel K, Fuchs BM, Ludwig W, Peplies J, et al. A comprehensive online resource for quality checked and aligned ribosomal RNA sequence data compatible with ARB. Nucleic Acids Res. 2007;35:7188–96.
19. Edgar RC, Haas BJ, Clemente JC, Quince C, Knight R. UCHIME improves sensitivity and speed of chimera detection. Bioinform. 2011;27:2194–200.
20. Jaccard P. Contributing au problem de l'immigration post-glaciare de la flore alpine. Bull Soc Vaudoise Science Nat. 1990;36:87–130.
21. Bray JR, Curtis JT. An ordination of the upland forest communities of southern Wisconsin. Ecol Monogr. 1957;27:325–49.
22. Oksanen J. Multivariate analysis of ecological communities in R: vegan tutorial; 2015. p. 1–43.
23. Clarke KR. Non-parametric multivariate analysis of changes in community structure. Austr J Ecol. 1993;18:117–43.
24. Iwai S, Huang D, Fonc S, Jarlsberg LG, Worodria W, Yoo S, Cattamanchi A, et al. The lung microbiome of Ugandan HIV-infected pneumonia patients is compositionally and functionally distinct from that of a san Fransciscan patients. PLoS One. 2014;9(4):e95726. https://doi.org/10.1371/journal.pone.0095726.
25. Silva-Boghossian C, Castro GF, Teles RP, De Souza IP, Colombo AP. Salivary microbiota in HIV-positive children and its correlation with HIV status, oral disease, and total secretory IgA. Int J Paediatr Dent. 2008;18:205–16.
26. Galiana A, Aguirre E, Rodriguez JC, Mira A, Santivanez M, Candela I, et al. Sputum microbiota in moderate versus severe patients with COPD. Eur Respir J. 2014;43:1787–90.
27. Garcia-Nuñez M, Millares L, Pomares X, Ferrari R, Pérez-Brocal V, Gallego M, et al. Severity-related changes of bronchial microbiome in chronic obstructive pulmonary disease. J Clin Microbiol. 2014;52(12):4217–23.
28. Rogers GB, Zain NM, Bruce KD, Burr LD, Chen AC, Rivett DW, et al. A novel microbiota stratification system predicts future exacerbations in bronchiectasis. Ann AM Thorac Soc. 2014;1194:496–503.
29. Collie D, Glendinning L, Govan J, Wright S, Thornton E, Tennant P, et al. Lung microbiota changes associated with chronic pseudomonas aeruginosa lung infection and the impact of intravenous colistimethate sodium. PLoS One. 2015;10(11):e0142097. https://doi.org/10.1371/journal.pone.0142097. eCollection 2015
30. Burkett A, Vandemheen KL, Giesbrecht-lewis T, Ramotar K, Ferris W, Chan F, et al. Persistency of pseudomonas aeruginosa in sputum cultures and clinical outcome in adult patients with cystic fibrosis. Eur J Clin Microbiol Infect Dis. 2012;31(7):1603–10.

31. Stressmann FA, Rogers GB, Marsh P, Lilley AK, Daniels TW, Carroll MP, et al. Does bacterial density in cystic fibrosis sputum increase prior to pulmonary exacerbation? J Cyst Fibros. 2011;10(5):357–65.
32. Tunney MM, Einarsson GG, Wei L, Drain M, Klem ET, Cardwell C, et al. Lung microbiota and bacterial abundance in patients with bronchiectasis when clinically stable and during exacerbation. Am J Respir Crit Care Med. 2013;187(10) 1118–26.
33. Beck JM, Schloss PD, Venkataraman A, Twigg H. Iii, Jablonski KA, bushman FD, et al. multicenter comparison of lung and oral microbiomes of HIV-infected and HIV-uninfected individuals. Am J Respir Crit Care Med. 2015; 192(11):1335–44.
34. Boutin S, Graeber SY, Weitnauer M, Panitz J, Stahl M, Clausznitzer D, et al. Comparison of microbiomes from different niches of upper and lower airways in children and adolescents with cystic fibrosis. PLoS One. 2015;10(1):eC116029. https://doi.org/10.1371/journal.pone.0116.
35. Verwey C, Velaphi S, Khan R. Bacteria isolated from airways of paediatric patients with bronchiectasis according to HIV status. S Afr Med J. 2017;107(5):435–9.
36. Salter SJ, Cox MJ, Turek EM, Calus ST, Cookson WO, et al. Reagent and laboratory contamination can critically impact sequence-based microbiome analyses. BMC Biol. 2014;12:87.

Latent class analysis to define radiological subgroups in pulmonary nontuberculous mycobacterial disease

Steven A. Cowman[1,2]*, Joseph Jacob[1,3], Sayed Obaidee[4], R. Andres Floto[4,5], Robert Wilson[1,2], Charles S. Haworth[4,5] and Michael R. Loebinger[1,2]

Abstract

Background: Nontuberculous mycobacterial (NTM) pulmonary disease has conventionally been classified on the basis of radiology into fibrocavitary and nodular-bronchiectatic disease. Whilst being of great clinical utility, this may not capture the full spectrum of radiological appearances present. The aim of this study was to use latent class analysis (LCA) as an unbiased method of grouping subjects with NTM-pulmonary disease based on their CT features and to compare the clinical characteristics of these groups.

Methods: Individuals with NTM-pulmonary disease were recruited and a contemporaneous CT scan obtained. This was scored using an NTM-specific scoring system. LCA was used to identify groups with common radiological characteristics. The analysis was then repeated in an independent cohort.

Results: Three classes were identified in the initial cohort of 85 subjects. Group 1 was characterised by severe bronchiectasis, cavitation and aspergillomas, Group 2 by relatively minor radiological changes, and Group 3 by predominantly bronchiectasis only. These findings were reproduced in an independent cohort of 62 subjects. Subjects in Group 1 had a lower BMI and serum albumin, higher serum CRP, and a higher mortality.

Conclusions: These findings suggest that NTM-pulmonary may be divided into three radiological subgroups, and that important clinical and survival differences exist between these groups.

Keywords: Nontuberculous mycobacteria, Latent class analysis, High resolution computed tomography

Background

Pulmonary non-tuberculous mycobacterial disease is a challenging infection which is associated with a high mortality [1–3]. Treatment is frequently poorly tolerated, expensive, and in many cases response rates are poor [4]. Radiology is essential for the diagnosis of disease and has important implications in guiding treatment. NTM-pulmonary disease has been observed to commonly fall into two clinico-radiological patterns of disease, fibrocavitary and nodular-bronchiectatic disease, and this classification forms the basis of treatment recommendations in guidelines [5] and has important prognostic implications [6–8]. Whilst being of great clinical utility this division may not capture the spectrum of radiological appearances, some of which may not fit clearly into either group [3, 9–11].

The aim of this study was to characterise the radiological features of NTM-pulmonary disease using an NTM-specific scoring system, to use latent class analysis (LCA) as an unbiased method to identify subgroups sharing common patterns of radiological features, and to examine the clinical characteristics associated with any such patterns.

Methods

Individuals with NTM-pulmonary disease were recruited prospectively from the outpatient department of the Royal Brompton Hospital and Chelsea and Westminster Hospital between September 2012 and November 2013.

---

* Correspondence: s.cowman12@imperial.ac.uk
[1]National Heart and Lung Institute, Imperial College London, London, UK
[2]Host Defence Unit, Royal Brompton Hospital, London, UK
Full list of author information is available at the end of the article

All met American Thoracic Society 2007 disease criteria [5]. Subjects were excluded if they had a diagnosis of cystic fibrosis, HIV infection or other primary or secondary immunodeficiency or if they were receiving any immunosuppressant medication other than oral prednisolone. A HRCT scan of the thorax was performed in subjects who had not undergone such a scan in the previous 6 months. In those who declined additional imaging as part of the study their most recent clinical HRCT was obtained. Subjects also underwent a full clinical assessment, blood and sputum sampling, St George's Respiratory Questionnaire (SGRQ) and lung function testing. Written consent was gained from all participants and the study was approved by the local Research Ethics Committee (reference 12/LO/1034). Further details are provided in the supplementary materials.

CT scoring was performed as previously described [12] by a specialist radiologist with 5 years of experience in thoracic imaging, blinded to clinical details. For bronchiectasis extent, bronchiectasis severity, tree-in-bud opacification, nodules and consolidation, tertiles of the maximum possible score for each feature were used to categorise the features as low, medium or high. Cavitating nodules, severe cavitation and aspergilloma scores were dichotomised as present or absent. As a measure of the overall severity of an individual's radiological disease burden, composite CT scores were calculated for each participant by expressing the individual scores for bronchiectasis extent, bronchiectasis severity, tree-in-bud opacification, nodules, consolidation, cavitating nodules, severe cavitation and aspergilloma as a percentage of the maximum possible score for that feature, then summing the scores together. The scoring proforma is detailed in Additional file 1: Table S1 of the supplementary material.

Statistical analysis was performed in the R environment version 3.4.0 [13]. Latent class analysis (LCA) was performed on the matrix of CT scores using the fpc and flexmix packages [14, 15]. LCA is a statistical method which takes a set of multivariate data and uses this to identify groups of related subjects ('latent classes') within the data which share similar characteristics. The Aikake information criteria (AIC) was used to identify the optimum number of classes in the model as the number giving the lowest value of AIC [16]. Composite CT scores were compared between groups using analysis of variance (ANOVA). Clinical characteristics were compared between groups using ANOVA, Tukey's Honestly Significant Difference test and Fisher's exact test. Survival curves were generated using the survival package [17] and compared using the Log-rank test. Correction for multiple testing was performed using the Benjamini-Hochberg method.

To examine the reproducibility of the groups identified by LCA and their radiological characteristics, the analysis was repeated on an independent cohort from another tertiary centre. Subjects with NTM-pulmonary disease at Papworth Hospital who underwent CT scanning at as part of their clinical care were identified retrospectively, their anonymised imaging and clinical data were retrieved and data analysed using the exact methodology used for the original cohort.

Results

A total of 85 subjects were recruited, their clinical and radiological characteristics are shown in Additional file 1: Tables S2 and S3 of the supplementary material. Twelve subjects declined further imaging but had undergone HRCT for clinical purposes which were obtained for analysis. The median interval between imaging and recruitment was 23 days. In 80 (94%) subjects a HRCT was obtained within twelve months of recruitment.

Identification of latent classes

Three latent classes were identified using the AIC (see Additional file 1: Figure S1). There were 14 subjects (16.4%) in class 1, 38 (44.7%) in class 2 and 33 (38.8%) in class 3. The individual CT features of each of the latent classes are shown in Fig. 1 and the total composite CT scores in each class are shown in Fig. 2a.

The first class, referred to as "Cavitary" disease, was characterised by the universal presence of severe cavitation with medium or highly extensive bronchiectasis. There was a high incidence of aspergilloma in this group, seen in almost half, whereas they were almost absent from the other groups. The second class, referred to as "Nodular" disease had the lowest composite CT scores and a relative lack of radiological changes, with the exception of nodules (medium levels in 13.5%) and cavitating nodules which were present in 22.5%. The third class, referred to as "Bronchiectatic" disease had the most extensive bronchiectasis (high in 71.2%) which was of high severity in the majority (56%), and the highest frequency of tree-in-bud changes (medium or high levels in 28%), although cavitation and nodules were uncommon.

The composite CT score (Fig. 2a) was highest in Cavitary disease (mean 2.62), intermediate in Bronchiectatic disease (mean 1.96) and lowest in Nodular disease (0.95). All differences were significant at $P < 0.001$.

Clinical differences

The clinical characteristics of the latent classes are shown in Table 1. Subjects from the Cavitary group were significantly older than those in other classes ($P = 0.003$ vs Nodular, $P = 0.079$ vs Bronchiectatic groups). They had a higher prevalence of semi-invasive aspergillosis, were more likely to have received treatment for NTM and over one-third were receiving systemic corticosteroids, although these

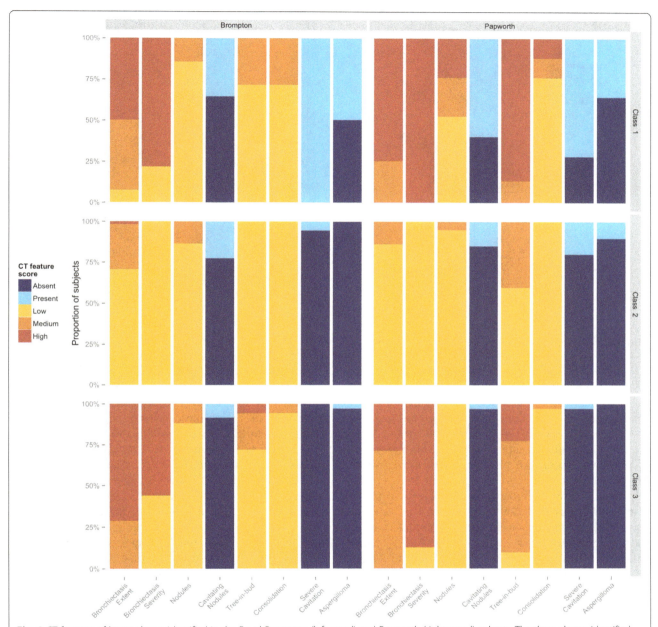

Fig. 1 CT features of latent classes identified in the Royal Brompton (left panel) and Papworth (right panel) cohorts. The three classes identified by latent class analysis in each cohort are shown in the top, middle and bottom panels. The individual CT features used in the NTM scoring system are shown on the x-axes and the proportion of subjects on the y-axes. Colours represent the severity (low, medium or high), or the presence or absence of the CT feature

differences were not significant. The mean C-reactive protein level was higher than both other classes ($P < 0.001$ vs Nodular, $P = 0.002$ vs Bronchiectatic groups), body mass index was lower ($P = 0.003$ vs Nodular, $P = 0.008$ vs Bronchiectatic groups) and serum albumin was lower than in the Nodular ($P = 0.007$) but not the Bronchiectatic ($P = 0.246$) group. The mean corrected carbon monoxide transfer factor (TLCOc) was the lowest of the three groups, but this did not reach significance. Dyspnoea and quality of life scores were not significantly worse than the other two classes.

Compared to the other groups, the Nodular group had a more even mix of underlying respiratory pathology and 21% had no underlying disease. Lung function indices were the highest of the three groups. This group had the shortest mean duration of NTM disease prior to enrolment ($P = 0.307$ vs Cavitary, $P = 0.008$ vs Bronchiectatic groups).

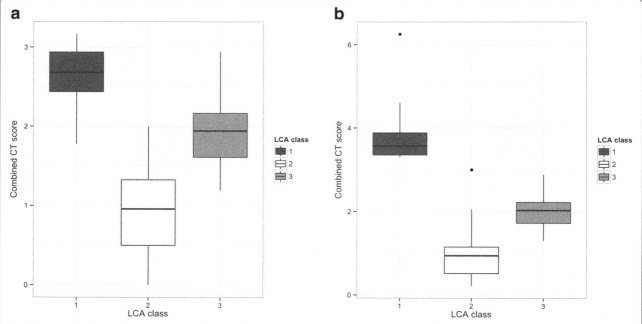

Fig. 2 Composite CT scores between latent classes in the a) Royal Brompton and b) Papworth cohorts. The three classes identified by latent class analysis in each cohort are shown on the x-axes, the composite CT score for each class are shown on the y-axis

Significantly more subjects (75.8%) in the Bronchiectatic group had previously diagnosed underlying bronchiectasis and 21.2% were chronically infected with Pseudomonas, which was uncommon in the other groups. The Bronchiectatic group had the highest rates of antibiotic prophylaxis and the lowest rate of current NTM treatment.

Survival data were available for 78 subjects with a median follow-up time of 126 weeks. There were significant differences in survival seen between groups, with the Cavitary group showing the highest mortality of 42.9% compared with the bronchietatic (9.1%) and Nodular (16.1%) groups (logrank test $P = 0.011$, Fig. 3).

Replication cohort

CT scans from 62 patients were available from Papworth Hospital. Demographic details of the cohort are given in Additional file 1: Table S4 of the supplementary material. LCA identified three groups using the AIC (see Additional file 1: Figure S1). Class 1 comprised 8 (12.9%) subjects, class 2 comprised 19 (30.6%) subjects and class 3 comprised 35 (56.5%) subjects. The CT features of each class showed high similarity to the Brompton cohort (Fig. 1).

Class 1 corresponded to the Cavitary group with universally severe bronchiectasis which was highly extensive in 74.6%. Aspergillomas were present in 35.7% and the majority had severe cavitation (71.9%) although this was less than the universal presence seen in the Brompton cohort. Another point of difference was the high level of severe tree-in-bud change, seen in 87% but not seen in the Brompton cohort. Class 2 corresponded to the Nodular group, with generally mild changes except cavitating nodules which were present in 14.9% and severe cavitation in 20%. In contrast to the Brompton cohort, aspergillomas were present in 10% and a medium level of tree-in-bud changes in 40.2%. Class 3 corresponded to the Bronchiectatic group with all subjects having high severity bronchiectasis and 87.3% having highly extensive bronchiectasis. In contrast to the Brompton cohort the majority (90.5%) had a medium or high degree of tree-in-bud changes and no subjects had medium or high nodule scores compared with 12% in the Brompton cohort. Similarly, the vast majority had no cavitating nodules or severe cavitation, and aspergillomas were not seen. As with the Brompton cohort, class 1 showed the highest composite CT scores (mean 3.95), class 2 the lowest (mean 0.97) and class 3 intermediate values (mean 1.99). All differences were significant with $P < 0.001$ (Fig. 2b).

The mean age was youngest in class 2 and highest in the class 1, although this difference was not significant. There was significantly more underlying bronchiectasis in class 3. There was significantly more MAC (87.5%) in class 1 compared to other classes, whereas in the corresponding Cavitary group from the Brompton cohort this species accounted for only 50% of subjects.

Subgroup analysis of subjects with bronchiectasis

A subgroup analysis was performed restricted to subjects with an underlying diagnosis of bronchiectasis. In the

Table 1 Clinical characteristics of latent classes in the Royal Brompton cohort

	Class			P value	Adjusted P value
	1 N = 14	2 N = 38	3 N = 33		
Female Sex	9 (64.3%)	22 (57.9%)	23 (69.7%)	0.571	0.670
Age (years)	72.4 (±10.0)	61.5 (±11.1)	66.8 (±9.1)	**0.003**	**0.037**
Smoking				0.411	0.575
Never smoker	6 (42.9%)	18 (47.4%)	17 (51.5%)		
Ex-smoker	5 (35.7%)	16 (42.1%)	15 (45.5%)		
Current smoker	3 (21.4%)	4 (10.5%)	1 (3.0%)		
White - British Ethnicity	12 (85.7%)	30 (78.9%)	28 (84.8%)	0.747	0.747
Diagnosis				**0.006**	**0.039**
Bronchiectasis	5 (35.7%)	13 (34.2%)	25 (75.8%)		
COPD	5 (35.7%)	11 (28.9%)	4 (12.1%)		
Other	0 (0.0%)	6 (15.8%)	2 (6.1%)		
No underlying disease	4 (28.6%)	8 (21.1%)	2 (6.1%)		
Systemic corticosteroids	4 (28.6%)	7 (18.4%)	5 (15.2%)	0.574	0.670
Oral antibiotic prophylaxis	2 (14.3%)	9 (23.7%)	11 (33.3%)	0.404	0.575
Nebulised antibiotic prophylaxis	1 (7.1%)	2 (5.3%)	4 (12.1%)	0.677	0.702
Chronic *Pseudomonas* infection	0 (0.0%)	3 (7.9%)	7 (21.2%)	0.088	0.176
Semi-invasive Aspergillosis	2 (14.3%)	1 (2.6%)	0	0.069	0.155
NTM species				0.612	0.685
M. abscessus	4 (28.6%)	4 (10.5%)	6 (18.2%)		
M. avium complex	7 (50.0%)	18 (47.4%)	19 (57.6%)		
M. kansasii	1 (7.1%)	4 (10.5%)	4 (12.1%)		
M. xenopi	1 (7.1%)	8 (21.1%)	2 (6.1%)		
Other species	1 (7.1%)	4 (10.5%)	2 (6.1%)		
Sputum smear positive	1 (7.1%)	3 (7.9%)	5 (15.2%)	0.639	0.688
Currently receiving NTM treatment	6 (42.9%)	8 (21.1%)	4 (12.1%)	0.072	0.155
Ever received NTM treatment	11 (78.6%)	15 (39.5%)	11 (33.3%)	**0.015**	0.060
Duration of NTM disease (years)	3.4 (±3.2)	1.6 (±2.6)	4.3 (±4.7)	**0.01**	**0.047**
Age at diagnosis (years)	69.6 (±9.9)	60.0 (±11.5)	62.5 (±10.6)	**0.035**	0.098
BMI (kg/m^2)	18.3 (±3.2)	22.6 (±4.3)	22.3 (±3.4)	**0.004**	**0.037**
SGRQ total score	51.3 (±24.6)	42.1 (±26.1)	48.1 (±21.6)	0.443	0.591
MRC dyspnoea score	2.9 (±1.4)	2.4 (±1.5)	2.6 (±1.1)	0.513	0.653
FEV1 (% predicted)	58.7 (±13.3)	69.5 (±27.6)	53.9 (±20.1)	**0.024**	0.081
FVC (% predicted)	83.1 (±27.0)	97.7 (±20.8)	85.8 (±16.8)	**0.026**	0.081
TLCOc (% predicted)	47.9 (±24.1)	62.2 (±26.0)	59.2 (±18.2)	0.25	0.389
Haemoglobin (g/dL)	12.7 (±1.7)	13.7 (±1.6)	13.7 (±1.1)	**0.049**	0.125
Neutrophil count (× 10^9/L)	7.0 (±2.9)	5.3 (±3.0)	6.1 (±3.1)	0.186	0.326
Lymphocyte count (× 10^9/L)	1.4 (±0.5)	1.6 (±0.6)	1.8 (±0.7)	0.242	0.389
Serum albumin (g/L)	36.0 (±6.3)	40.2 (±3.7)	38.2 (±3.9)	**0.007**	**0.039**
CRP (mg/L)	37.2 (±51.1)	7.1 (±13.7)	10.0 (±13.5)	**< 0.001**	**0.017**
Platelet count (× 10^9/L)	298 (±126)	244 (±62)	255 (±86)	0.126	0.235

Continuous variables are given as mean ± standard deviation and compared using ANOVA, categorical values are given as number and percentage and compared using Fisher's exact test

COPD chronic obstructive pulmonary disease, *BMI* body mass index, *SGRQ* St George's Respiratory Questionnaire, *MRC* Medical Research Council dyspnoea scale, *FEV1* forced expiratory volume in 1 s, *FVC* forced vital capacity, *TLCOc* corrected transfer factor for carbon monoxide, *CRP* C-reactive protein

Values shown in bold indicate $P < 0.05$

Brompton cohort ($N = 43$), two classes were identified by LCA representing 58 and 42% of the group (Additional file 1: Fig. S2). The first class was characterised by bronchiectasis of predominantly low severity and an absence of consolidation, severe cavitation or aspergillomas. It contained all 13 subjects in the Nodular subgroup of the full analysis, none from the Cavitary subgroup, and 12 subjects from the Bronchiectatic subgroup (see Additional file 1: Table S5 of the supplementary material). The second class was characterised by extensive and severe bronchiectasis, with severe cavitation in 30% and aspergillomas in 24%. This class contained all 5 subjects from the Cavitary subgroup of the full analysis, no subjects from the Nodular subgroup and 13 subjects from the Bronchiectatic subgroup.

In the Papworth cohort ($N = 45$) three classes were identified representing 62, 21 and 16% of the group. The features of these groups (Additional file 1: Fig. S3) closely resembled those found in the larger cohort (Fig. 1), corresponding to the 'Bronchiectatic', 'Nodular' and 'Cavitary' subgroups respectively. When compared with the original classification, 96% of subjects remained in the same subgroup (see Additional file 1: Table S5 of the supplementary material).

Discussion

In this study, LCA identified three groups with distinct radiological characteristics in two independent cohorts of subjects with NTM-pulmonary disease. The finding of compatible radiological changes is a cornerstone of the diagnosis of NTM-pulmonary disease [5]. Historically the radiological pattern associated with NTM-pulmonary disease was one of cavitation similar to tuberculosis, typically seen in older males with underlying lung disease such as emphysema [18]. In the later twentieth century the first reports were published of a pattern of disease characterised by nodules and bronchiectasis which in contrast occurred in those with no underlying lung disease and was more common in women [19, 20]. The differentiation between the former 'fibrocavitary' disease and latter 'nodular-bronchiectatic' disease is of major clinical importance, as several studies have consistently demonstrated an association between fibrocavitary disease and mortality [6–8], disease progression [7] and treatment failure [21, 22]. This has been reflected in successive guidelines which recommend more aggressive treatment of fibrocavitary disease [5]. Other patterns of disease have been reported, in particular consolidation and infiltrative patterns have been associated with poor outcomes [9–11] however with no agreed consensus regarding definitions for these patterns, the findings remain unique to the individual studies. Even when an additional 'consolidative' category was used, one study found that 27% of subjects still did not clearly fit any category [3] and another was still unable to classify the radiological appearances of 229/481 subjects [9].

Our current study used a predefined scoring system to reduce subjectivity in assessing NTM related radiological changes, and latent class analysis as an unbiased method to identify groups sharing radiological characteristic without presupposing the existence of any specific patterns of disease.

The findings support the existence of fibrocavitary disease as a distinct pattern, identifying a group characterised by severe cavitation associated with markers of disease severity and a high mortality. There was a

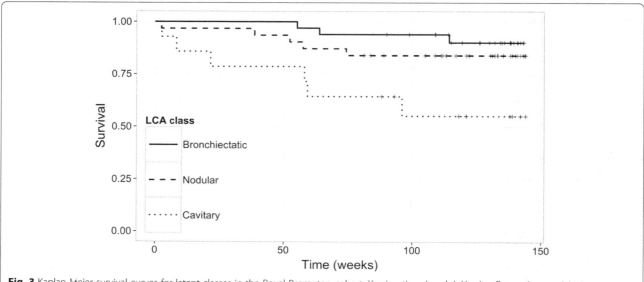

Fig. 3 Kaplan-Meier survival curves for latent classes in the Royal Brompton cohort. X-axis = time (weeks), Y-axis = Proportion surviving, lines = latent classes

high prevalence of aspergilloma within this group, which has been associated with increased mortality in NTM-pulmonary disease [12].

Within the remaining majority of subjects, LCA identified two distinct subgroups, split evenly into those with very few radiological changes apart from nodules, and those with marked bronchiectasis. As may be expected, significantly more subjects in the latter Bronchiectatic group has pre-existing bronchiectasis, although this was also the case in over a third of those with 'nodular' disease. Interestingly despite having the best-preserved lung function and lowest symptom scores, there was no significant difference in mortality between the nodular and bronchiectatic groups. The duration of disease was significantly shorter in the nodular group, raising the possibility that this represents early disease which may progress to Cavitary or Bronchiectatic forms. A pattern of nodules and bronchiectasis have been associated with *M. avium* complex infection in a single study [23] however there were no differences in species prevalence between groups.

The validation cohort confirms the presence of three subgroups whose radiological characteristics shared many similarities with the Brompton cohort. There was a smaller group characterised by high composite CT scores with severe cavitation, the common presence of aspergillomas and severe and extensive bronchiectasis, corresponding to the Cavitary group. The other subjects were divided into those dominated by severe and extensive bronchiectasis without nodules, cavitation or aspergilloma (corresponding to the Bronchiectatic group) and those with low composite CT scores and low scores for most CT features (corresponding to the Nodular group). A higher proportion of subjects fell into the Bronchiectatic group, likely due to the higher overall prevalence of underlying bronchiectasis in this cohort.

The only major difference to the Brompton cohort was the higher prevalence of tree-in-bud changes, which were moderate or severe in 76% compared with 17%. The prevalence was higher in all three disease subgroups and does not appear to be due to the increased prevalence of underlying bronchiectasis. As the scoring of the validation cohort was performed separately to the Brompton cohort observer bias may be responsible for this difference, although this was performed by the same individual, alternatively it may be that differences in treatment, coinfection, or other clinical factors between centres is responsible. There was also more severe cavitation and aspergilloma in the nodular Papworth group compared with the Brompton, however only four subjects accounted for this difference.

In contrast to other studies mentioned previously, the presence of a separate consolidative pattern of NTM-pulmonary disease was not seen in this study.

The vast majority of subjects in both cohorts had only mild consolidation, although this feature was slightly more prominent in the Cavitary group. Only one subject had consolidation and no other feature of NTM disease. Our findings may in part be explained by the absence of immunocompromised or critically ill subjects from our cohorts. When the analysis was restricted to subjects with known underlying bronchiectasis only two subgroups were identified, with the Bronchiectatic group being split in half dividing the cohort into groups more consistent with the conventional 'fibrocavitary' and 'nodular-bronchiectatic' patterns. However, in the validation cohort the three subgroups were still clearly identified.

The principle limitation of the study is the heterogeneous nature of the cohort, comprising subjects with differing underlying respiratory diseases, NTM species, antibiotic treatments and infecting co-pathogens. Nevertheless the findings were replicable in an independent cohort suggesting they are not merely related to the specific case mix at a single centre. Furthermore, such a mix of subjects is representative of real-life clinical practice, although as both cohorts come from tertiary centres the proportion of subjects with severe bronchiectasis and aspergillomas may be higher than the wider population of individuals with NTM-pulmonary disease. A number of subjects had previously undergone HRCT and declined further imaging, therefore in some subjects the collected clinical data may not reflect the point in time when the HRCT was performed and in 10% of cases more than a year had elapsed from imaging to study enrolment. A single radiologist was responsible for performing CT scoring and despite the use of an objective scoring system this remains a potential source of bias, although the scoring system was based on the Bhalla score [24] which has been shown to have low interobserver variability [25].

Conclusions

This study provides validation of the existence of cavitary disease as a distinct phenotype of NTM-pulmonary disease associated with a poor prognosis. In addition they suggest that 'nodular-bronchiectatic' disease is formed of two separate groups with important radiological and clinical differences, which may possibly reflect differences in underlying lung disease or duration of infection. These data underline that fact that NTM-pulmonary disease is a heterogeneous condition and more precise phenotyping will be valuable in clinical decision making and stratification in clinical trials.

Abbreviations
AIC: Aikake information criteria; ANOVA: Analysis of variance; BMI: Body mass index; COPD: Chronic obstructive pulmonary disease; CRP: C-reactive protein; CT: Computed tomography; FEV_1: Forced expiratory volume in 1 s;

FVC: Forced vital capacity; HIV: Human immunodeficiency virus; HRCT: High resolution computed tomography; LCA: Latent class analysis; MRC: Medical Research Council dyspnoea scale; NTM: Nontuberculous mycobacteria; SGRQ: St George's Respiratory Questionnaire; TLCOc: Corrected transfer factor for carbon monoxide

Funding
S.A.C. and M.R.L. were funded by a grant from the Welton Foundation. The Welton Foundation played no role in the conception or conduct of this study, nor the preparation of the manuscript.

Authors' contributions
MRL and SAC conceived and designed the study. SAC performed the data analysis and prepared the manuscript. JJ performed the scoring of CT scans. SO, RAF, RW, CSH and RW were responsible for the clinical care of the subjects and provided CT scans and clinical data. All authors contributed substantially to the interpretation of data and preparation of the final manuscript. MRL had full access to the data of the study and takes responsibility for the integrity of the data and the accuracy of the data analysis. All authors read and approved the final manuscript.

Competing interests
S.A.C., S.O., R.A.F. and R.W. have no conflicts of interest to declare. J.J. reports personal fees from Boehringer Ingelheim, outside of the submitted work. C.S.H reports grants and personal fees from Insmed, outside of the submitted work. M.R.L. reports personal fees from Insmed, outside of the submitted work.

Author details
[1]National Heart and Lung Institute, Imperial College London, London, UK. [2]Host Defence Unit, Royal Brompton Hospital, London, UK. [3]Department of Radiology, Royal Brompton Hospital, London, UK. [4]Cambridge Centre for Lung Infection, Papworth Hospital, Cambridge, UK. [5]Department of Medicine, University of Cambridge, Cambridge, UK.

References
1. Fleshner M, Olivier KN, Shaw PA, Adjemian J, Strollo S, Claypool RJ, et al. Mortality among patients with pulmonary non-tuberculous mycobacteria disease. Int J Tuberc Lung Dis. 2016;20:582–7.
2. Novosad SA, Henkle E, Schafer S, Hedberg K, Ku J, Siegel SAR, et al. Mortality after respiratory isolation of nontuberculous mycobacteria. A comparison of patients who did and did not meet disease criteria. Ann Am Thorac Soc American Thoracic Society. 2017;14:1112–9.
3. Gommans EPAT, Even P, Linssen CFM, van Dessel H, van Haren E, de Vries GJ, et al. Risk factors for mortality in patients with pulmonary infections with non-tuberculous mycobacteria: a retrospective cohort study. Respir Med. 2015;109:137–45.
4. Stout JE, Koh W-J, Yew WW. Update on pulmonary disease due to non-tuberculous mycobacteria. Int J Infect Dis Elsevier. 2016;45:123–34.
5. Griffith DE, Aksamit T, Brown-Elliott BA, Catanzaro A, Daley C, Gordin F, et al. An official ATS/IDSA statement: diagnosis, treatment, and prevention of nontuberculous mycobacterial diseases. Am J Respir Crit Care Med. 2007; 175:367–416.
6. Hayashi M, Takayanagi N, Kanauchi T, Miyahara Y, Yanagisawa T, Sugita Y. Prognostic factors of 634 HIV-negative patients with Mycobacterium avium complex lung disease. Am J Respir Crit Care Med. 2012;185:575–83.
7. Gochi M, Takayanagi N, Kanauchi T, Ishiguro T, Yanagisawa T, Sugita Y. Retrospective study of the predictors of mortality and radiographic deterioration in 782 patients with nodular/bronchiectatic Mycobacterium avium complex lung disease. BMJ Open. 2015;5:e008058.
8. Okumura M, Iwai K, Ogata H, Ueyama M, Kubota M, Aoki M, et al. Clinical factors on Cavitary and nodular Bronchiectatic types in pulmonary Mycobacterium avium complex disease. Intern Med. 2008;47:1465–72.
9. Shu C-C, Lee C-H, Hsu C-L, Wang J-T, Wang J-Y, Yu C-J, et al. Clinical characteristics and prognosis of nontuberculous mycobacterial lung disease with different radiographic patterns. Lung. 2011;189:467–74.
10. Shu C-C, Lee C-H, Wang J-Y, Jerng J-S, Yu C-J, Hsueh P-R, et al. Nontuberculous mycobacteria pulmonary infection in medical intensive care unit: the incidence, patient characteristics, and clinical significance. Intensive care med. Springer-Verlag. 2008;34:2194–201.
11. Andréjak C, Lescure F-X, Pukenyte E, Douadi Y, Yazdanpanah Y, Laurans G, et al. Mycobacterium xenopi pulmonary infections: a multicentric retrospective study of 136 cases in north-East France. Thorax. 2009;64:291–6.
12. Zoumot Z, Boutou AK, Gill SS, van Zeller M, Hansell DM, Wells AU, et al. Mycobacterium avium complex infection in non-cystic fibrosis bronchiectasis. Respirology. 2014;19:714–22.
13. Core TRR. A language and environment for statistical computing. Vienna, Austria: R Foundation for Statistical Computing; 2014.
14. Hennig C. Fpc: flexible procedures for clustering. R package version. 2014;2:1–9.
15. Leisch F. FlexMix: a general framework for finite mixture models and latent class regression in R. J Stat Softw. 2004;11:1-18.
16. Akaike H. A new look at the statistical model identification. IEEE Trans Autom Control. 1974;19:716–23.
17. Therneau TM, Grambsch PM. Modeling survival data: extending the cox model. New York: Springer; 2000.
18. LEWIS AG, DUNBAR FP, LASCHE EM, BOND JO, LERNER EN, WHARTON DJ, et al. Chronic pulmonary disease due to atypical mycobacterial infections. Am Rev Respir Dis. 1959;80:188–99.
19. Prince DS, Peterson DD, Steiner RM, Gottlieb JE, Scott R, Israel HL, et al. Infection with Mycobacterium avium complex in patients without predisposing conditions. N Engl J Med. 1989;321:863–8.
20. Reich JM. Mycobacterium avium complex pulmonary disease presenting as an isolated lingular or middle lobe pattern. The Lady Windermere syndrome Chest. 1992;101:1605.
21. Rosenzweig DY. Pulmonary mycobacterial infections due to Mycobacterium intracellulare-avium complex. Clinical features and course in 100 consecutive cases. Chest. 1979;75:115–9.
22. Lam PK, Griffith DE, Aksamit TR, Ruoss SJ, Garay SM, Daley CL. Factors related to response to intermittent treatment of Mycobacterium avium complex lung disease. Am J Respir Crit Care Med. 2006;173:1283–9.
23. Hollings NP, Wells AU, Wilson R, Hansell DM. Comparative appearances of non-tuberculous mycobacteria species: a CT study. Eur Radiol. 2002;12:2211–7.
24. Bhalla M, Turcios N, Aponte V, Jenkins M, Leitman BS, McCauley DI, et al. Cystic fibrosis: scoring system with thin-section CT. Radiology. 1991;179:783–8.
25. Reiff DB, Wells AU, Carr DH, Cole PJ, Hansell DM. CT findings in bronchiectasis: limited value in distinguishing between idiopathic and specific types. AJR Am J Roentgenol. 1995;165:261–7.

Pulmonary arterial hypertension in Latin America: epidemiological data from local studies

Ana Beatriz Valverde[1], Juliana M. Soares[1], Karynna P. Viana[1], Bruna Gomes[1], Claudia Soares[1] and Rogerio Souza[2*]

Abstract

Background: Pulmonary arterial hypertension is a rare, progressive disease with poor prognosis. However, there is limited information available on the characteristics of PAH patients outside of North America and Europe. This is particularly important as researchers have described that there are potential geographical and regional differences which are vital to consider in the design of clinical trials as well as PAH treatment. The aim of this study was to describe the epidemiology of PAH (PH group 1) in Latin America.

Methods: A search of electronic databases for studies published in English, Spanish or Portuguese was conducted specifying publication dates from the 1st of January 1987 until 10th October 2016. Two authors independently assessed papers for inclusion and extracted data. A narrative synthesis of the findings was conducted.

Results: The search revealed 22 conference abstracts and articles, and on application of the inclusion criteria, six conference abstracts and articles were included in the final review. Studies/registries were based in Argentina, Brazil and Chile. In contrast to the available literature from developed countries, in Latin America, most patients were diagnosed at younger age; nevertheless, the higher prevalence of idiopathic PAH (IPAH) and the advanced stage of the disease at diagnosis were comparable to the existing literature, as the long term survival, despite the lower availability of targeted therapies.

Conclusion: This study highlights the regional characteristics in the epidemiology of group 1 PH. The recognition of these differences should be considered when developing clinical guidelines and extrapolating diagnostic and treatment algorithms. Equitable access to health care and therapies are also issues that need to be addressed in Latin America. Information coming from a large prospective registry representing the different populations in Latin America is of critical importance to increase disease awareness in the region and improve diagnosis and management.

Keywords: Pulmonary arterial hypertension, Epidemiology, Prognosis, Latin America

Background

Pulmonary arterial hypertension (PAH), a clinical classification of group 1 pulmonary hypertension (PH), is a rare, progressive disease with poor prognosis. It has a worldwide estimated prevalence ranging from 10 to 16 cases per million inhabitants per year and an incidence between 2.0 to 3.2 cases per million inhabitants [1, 2]. In the last two decades, knowledge of the basic pathobiology of PAH, its natural history, prognostic indicators, and therapeutic options have improved. National registries have provided a better understanding of the epidemiology and clinical evolution of the disease [3] as well as valuable information on disease characteristics, demographics and outcomes of patients with PAH [4], allowing the development of risk stratification tools [5]. Two recent reviews [2, 6] have identified 11 PAH registries based in the United States (US), China, France, Scotland, United Kingdom (UK), Spain and a European Union consortium. However, limited information is available on the characteristics of PAH patients outside of North America and

* Correspondence: souza.rogerio@me.com
[2]Pulmonary Hypertension Unit, Pulmonary Department – Heart Institute, University of Sao Paulo Medical School, Av. Dr. Eneas de Carvalho Aguiar, 44, Sao Paulo 05403-000, Brazil
Full list of author information is available at the end of the article

Europe. Moreover, no Latin American studies were included in these reviews. This is particularly important as researchers have described that there are potential geographical and regional differences which are vital to consider in the design of clinical trials as well as PAH treatment [2, 6, 7]. The aim of this study was to describe the epidemiology of PAH (group 1) in Latin America.

Methods

To identify relevant studies, a search was conducted using Medline, PubMed, LILACS, EMBASE, SciElo, PAHO, BVS, Cochrane, Latindex, CAPES and Searchlight (a GlaxoSmithKline database that includes conference abstracts) specifying publication dates from the 1st of January 1987 until 10th October 2016. The search terms included "pulmonary arterial hypertension", combined with "registry", "cohort study" and "observational study". A web-based search, using the Internet search engine 'Google Scholar', was also conducted.

Studies were included if they were based in Latin America (Central and South America) and the Caribbean [8], examined PAH (PH group 1) adult patients aged between 18 and 65 years old and were available in English, Spanish and/or Portuguese. Studies were required to report on at least one of the following topics: clinical characteristics (etiology, time from onset of symptoms to diagnosis, hemodynamic parameters and severity of the disease based on the World Health Organization – WHO – classification); demographic characteristics (age and gender); treatment pattern or survival rates in a cohort of PAH patients. Publications were excluded if they focused on a subgroup of PAH patients and not a cohort of all PAH or all IPAH patients, for example articles that investigated PAH only in pregnant women or pediatric patients, and/or PAH patients treated with a particular treatment. Additionally, studies that focused on patients with a specific etiology associated with group 1 PH such as schistosomiasis, HIV, lupus or coronary heart disease were also excluded. Due to the paucity of data, the decision was made to include conference abstracts if they have any publication describing the study design to assure the correct understanding of the data collection, patient inclusion, study results and methodology.

The following items were extracted from each article: inclusion and exclusion criteria; sample size; country where the study was conducted; study design; study population, period of enrollment and follow up; incidence and prevalence; diagnosis criteria; PAH patient's demographic characteristics (age and gender); co-morbidities; time from onset of symptoms until the diagnosis; PAH etiologies; PAH survival and PAH treatment. Two reviewers independently extracted data using a standardized data extraction form.

Results

A total of 22 publications including articles and conference abstracts were retrieved by the literature search. Fourteen conference abstracts were screened. From these, twelve were excluded. The Mexican registry [9], two abstracts that reported data from the Colombian registry [10, 11] and a study from Puerto Rico [12] were excluded as they did not report data separately for group 1 PH patients. The Paraguayan registry [13] was excluded as data was reported according to the treatment received by each patient's group (for example, group A: patients only treated with Sildenafil). Five conference abstracts were excluded as they reported on the same results from the **HI**pertensió**N PUL**monar y **AS**ociaciones en la **AR**gentina (HINPULSAR) registry [14–18]. Also, one publication from the **R**egistro **Co**laborativo de **Hi**pertensión **P**ulmonar en Argentina (RECOPILAR) registry [19] was excluded because it reported duplicate data. Additionally, one registry from Uruguay [20] was excluded as they did not provide another publication detailing the study design.

Two conference abstracts, one from the HINPULSAR registry [21] and one from RECOPILAR registry [22], both based in Argentina were included in the final analysis. The data from the abstracts was complemented with methodological information from the study protocols [23, 24].

Eight full text articles were found of which four were excluded from the analysis. One study conducted in Brazil [25] was excluded because unlike the other studies, PH diagnosis was made based only on echocardiography results and did not consider hemodynamic parameters. The other study from Chile [26] was excluded as the study included group 1 and 4 PH patients but did not report data separately for group 1 PH. The other two excluded publications were conducted in Argentina and described only the study protocol and methodology of the HINPULSAR [23] and the RECOPILAR registries [24] but did not report results. Four articles were included in the final analysis: two Chilean [27, 28] one Argentinean [29] and one Brazilian [7]. The characteristics of the PAH registries are provided in Table 1. In total, six publications (two conference abstracts and four full articles) were qualified for inclusion according to the eligibility criteria (see Fig. 1). The publications excluded are described in Additional file 1.

All studies were conducted in South America, mainly in Argentina, Brazil and Chile. The number of patients with group 1 PH varied from 17 in Chile [28] to 178 in Brazil [7]. The number of centres involved in the registries/studies varied from 1 to 31 [21]. The studies found did not report on or calculate the incidence and prevalence of PAH in Latin America (see Table 1).

The mean age of PAH patients in Latin America varied from 34 [29] to 51 years [22]. All the studies included just adult patients, except the Argentinean by Talavera et al., [29] that included 16 patients (12.8%) younger than

Table 1 Characteristics of PAH registries/studies included in the review

Characteristic	Argentina [29]	Brazil [7]	Chile [28]	HINPULSAR [21]	RECOPILAR [22]	Chile [27]
Study design and time period	Prospective January 2004–March 2012	Prospective January 2008–December 2013	1999–2005	Prospective January 2010–December 2011	Prospective July 2014–May 2015	Prospective June 2003–March 2005
Number of centres	1	1	2	31	Multicenter[a]	1
Study cohort	Group 1 PH	Group 1 PH	Group 1 PH	Group 1 PH	Group 1 PH	Group 1 PH and Group 4 PH
Percentage of patients with group 1 PH (number of PAH patients)	100% (125)	100% (178)	100% (17)	100% (124)	100% (170)	93% (27)
% IPAH patients	49	29	80	52	52	41
% CTD-PAH	14	26	13	15	15	26
% CHD-PAH	28	8	–	27	27	33
% Sch-PAH	–	20	–	–	–	–
% Others[b]	9	18	7	6	6	–
% female	79	77	60	78	79	86
Mean age (years-old)	34 ± 16	46 ± 15	45	45 ± 17	51	41 ± 14
% FC III/IV	58	46	47	62	70	85
6MWD (m)	360	383 ± 152	348 ± 98	–	373	378 ± 113
RAP (mm Hg)	8	10 ± 5	12 ± 8	–	10	8 ± 7
mPAP (mm Hg)	54	52 ± 18	57 ± 15	55 ± 20	–	59 ± 12
PVR (woods units)	12	10 ± 6	–	–	–	–
CI (L/min/m^2)	2	3 ± 1	2 ± 1	–	3	3 ± 1
Time from onset of symptoms until diagnosis (years)	1.4	–	–	–	–	2.9

CTD connective tissue disease, *CHD* congenital heart disease, *Sch* schistosomiasis-associated, *FC* functional class, *6MWD* 6-minute walking distance, *RAP* right atrial pressure, *mPAP* mean pulmonary artery pressure, *PVR* pulmonary vascular resistance, *CI* cardiac index
[a]The number of centres was not provided
[b]Others: PAH associated to drugs and toxins, associated to HIV and portal hypertension

18 years. All studies reported greater frequency of PAH in female patients ranging from 60% [28] up to 86% [27], both values found in small cohorts in Chile.

The most commonly reported subtype among PAH patients was IPAH. One of the Chilean studies [28] showed the highest percentage of IPAH patients (80%) and the Brazilian registry [7] had the lowest with 29%. However, the Brazilian registry [7] mentioned schistosomiasis as one of the most common subtypes of PAH (Sch-PAH in 20% of total patients). As can be seen in Fig. 2, the percentage of IPAH patients is higher in Latin America compared to European studies and the REVEAL registry from the United States (US).

All the studies defined PAH as the presence of mean pulmonary arterial pressure (mPAP) greater than 25 mmHg at rest and a pulmonary artery wedge pressure (PCWP) less than 15 mmHg after right heart catheterization (RHC) [30]. Only one of the Argentinean studies [29] and one of the Chilean studies [27] reported the time from onset of symptoms to diagnosis (1.4 and 2.9 years, respectively).

The Brazilian registry [7] reported the lowest proportion of patients in the New York Heart Association (NYHA)/WHO functional class III or IV (46%). The Argentinean registries reported similar proportion of patients with functional class III or IV (ranging from 58 to 70%) [21, 22, 29]. One Chilean study [27] with 27 group 1 PH patients showed the highest proportion of patients with severe functional class (85%). Despite the differences, these values are considered high and demonstrate that most of the patients were in an advanced stage of the disease. Regarding the 6-min walk distance (6MWD), in general, the studies exhibited the same pattern for exercise capacity, ranging from 348 m in Chile [28] up to 383 m in Brazil [7].

The hemodynamic parameters exhibited the same pattern in all studies. Mean right atrial pressure (RAP) ranged from 8 in the Chilean [27] and Argentinean [29] registries up to 12 ± 8 mmHg in the Chilean study [28]. The mean pulmonary artery pressure (mPAP) ranged from 52 ± 18 mmHg in the Brazilian study [7] up to 59 ± 12 mmHg in Chile [27]. Regarding the pulmonary vascular resistance (PVR), only the Brazilian [7] and the Argentinean [29] registries reported this parameter and it was similar (10 ± 6 and 12 woods units, respectively). The studies also exhibited the same pattern for cardiac index (CI) (See Table 1).

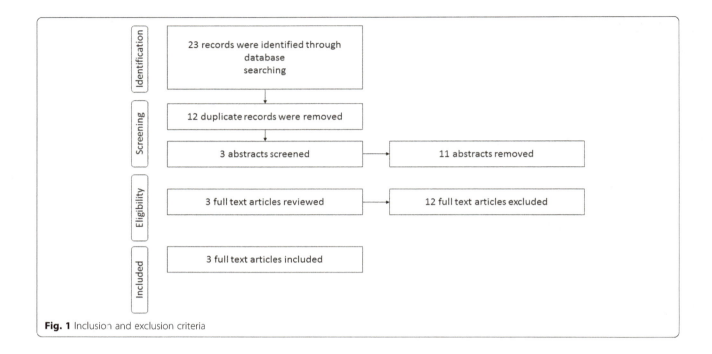

Fig. 1 Inclusion and exclusion criteria

Three studies reported the survival rates at 1, 2 and 3 years after diagnosis. The Brazilian registry [7] described survival only for incident patients and the Argentine study [29] showed survival for incident and prevalent patients. The Chilean study [28] did not specify if they included incident and/or prevalent patients. Comparing the Brazilian [7] and Argentinean [29] registries in the first year, the survival was similar (92.7 and 94% respectively), but in the second (79.6% vs 90%) and third year (73.9% vs 83%), the survival of the Argentinean cohort was higher. The Chilean study by Enríquez et al. [28] with a small sample size ($N = 17$) showed at first year a 88% of survival and the same survival rate at years 2 and 3 (82%). Figure 3 shows the survival rates in these Latin American studies compared to other international registries.

Most of the studies described the treatment received by patients [7, 16, 28, 29]. The Argentinean [29] and the Brazilian [7] studies reported that nearly 30% of patients were treated with Bosentan. It is important to note that the Brazilian registry only included incident patients [7] and hence only first-line treatment. On the other hand, the HINPULSAR and the Chilean registries reported that only 12% of the patients were treated with Bosentan. Sildenafil was considered as first line treatment in Argentina and Brazil [7]. The highest percentage of Sildenafil use was in Argentina [29] (83%) and lowest in Chile [28] (24%). However, the Chilean registry [28] reported the highest percentage of patients receiving treatment with Ambrisentan (82%). Inhaled Iloprost use was mentioned in HINPULSAR [21] (11%), in the Argentinean registry [29] (32%) and also

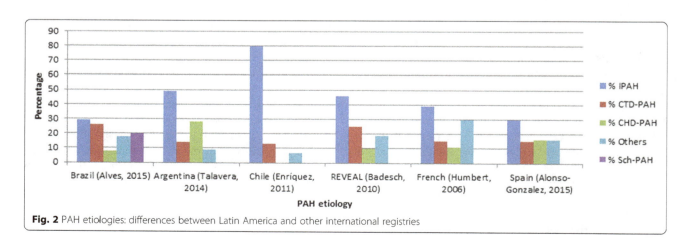

Fig. 2 PAH etiologies: differences between Latin America and other international registries

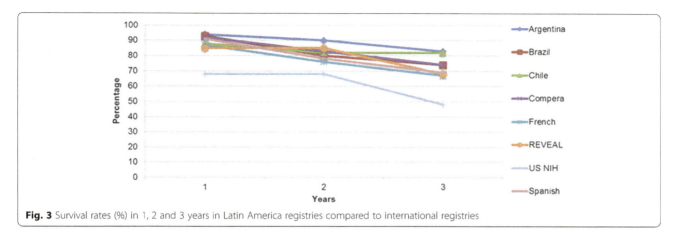

Fig. 3 Survival rates (%) in 1, 2 and 3 years in Latin America registries compared to international registries

in Chile [28] (29%). This is despite the fact that in Chile the use of inhaled Iloprost was approved in 2005, when the study was finished and Ambrisentan was first approved in 2014, several years after the recruitment period of this study.

Discussion

To our knowledge, this is the first article to describe the epidemiology of PAH (group 1 PH) in Latin America. As previously described, there is limited data from Latin America making it difficult to understand the disease and patient's characteristics in the region as a whole. While registries are an instrumental source of information regarding the epidemiology and outcomes, they can be influenced by external factors related to local circumstances such as access to health care, disease awareness and living conditions [5, 31].

While there was variation in the average age among the Latin American countries, most patients diagnosed were young and of working age. As previously mentioned, the Argentinean study by Talavera et al. [29] had a lower mean age due to the fact that 16 patients aged under 18 years old were included in the registry. This is in contrast with results from developed countries where patients were older at diagnosis. The mean age of patients in the Giessen Pulmonary Hypertension Registry [30], the French registry [32], the US Registry to Evaluate Early and Long-Term PAH disease management (REVEAL) [33] and the Comparative, Prospective Registry of Newly Initiated Therapies for Pulmonary Hypertension (COMPERA) [34] was higher (≥ 50 years). Hoeper et al. [5], noticed that differences between countries may be explained by population age distribution (older population in Europe and US) and health care systems. However, other factors may play a role such as: referral patterns, PAH awareness, increase patient access to information and widespread use of non-invasive screening tools [6]. As noted by McGoon et al. [6], phenotypes may be related to the healthcare environment rather than to different expressions of the disease.

Similar to the results of international registries, the prevalence of PAH in female patients was higher [2, 6].

The studies reviewed described differences in the prevalence of IPAH. For example, in Brazil the percentage of IPAH was lower but this could be explained by a high percentage of other etiologies such as the Sch-PAH. According to WHO, schistosomiasis affects more than 200 million people worldwide [7]. Estimates indicate that 8 to 12 million people are infected by schistosomiasis in Brazil [31], suggesting that schistosomiasis could be one of the main causes of PAH in the country. It is noteworthy that the proportion of PAH patients with congenital heart disease (CHD-PAH) reported in Argentina [29] (28%) was higher than what was described in Europe [32, 35] and North America [33] (below 15%). A recent review [35] emphasized the remarkable differences that might exist in specific areas of the world, as schistosomiasis in Brazil, or HIV in Africa, that should not be neglected when developing health policies for the appropriate diagnosis and management of PAH.

Functional class is a powerful predictor of outcomes in patients with PAH [36]. The majority of patients in the studies were in NYHA/WHO functional class III or IV. Patients in the Brazilian registry of incident cases [7] had lower proportion NYHA/WHO III/IV (46%), compared to most international (> 50%) [2, 6] and other Latin America studies [21, 22, 27]. It appears NYHA/WHO III/IV is higher in the US and Europe [2, 6] compared to Latin America (See Table 1). This is still the case when studies consider only incident or both prevalent and incident cases. However, even lower than in US and Europe, the percentage of patients in advanced functional class is still very high in Latin America, evidencing that patients are still diagnosed at late stages suggesting a lack of disease awareness and limited access to health care.

Hemodynamic parameters such as RAP, mPAP and PVR were similar to those reported in other international registries [2, 6]. The mean 6MWD in the Latin American studies (See Table 1) was higher compared to

US and European registries [2, 6]. However, it is important to consider that the mean age of patients was lower in Latin America, which could contribute to a better 6MWD. Compared to older patients, younger patients (< 50 years) have a shorter duration of symptoms, fewer comorbidities associated, better exercise capacity, and despite more severe hemodynamic impairment, better survival [2]. As previously noted, the percentage of patients in advanced functional class III/IV in Latin America was lower than in other regions, which may also contribute to a better exercise capacity. Alves et al. [7], have hypothesized that intrinsic characteristic of the patients or perhaps environmental factors associated with the socioeconomic conditions may also influence the level of daily activity of these patients. For example, patients may need to walk and/or travel more to reach the treating hospital.

Three studies reported survival rates. The Argentine registry had the highest 3-year survival rate [29]. The Brazilian study with only incident patients showed a high survival rate in the first year but in the second and third years the survival rate decreased [7]. As noted by McGoon et al. [6] and demonstrated by different studies, as the French and the Giessen registries [30, 31], compared to incident cases, prevalent ones had a better prognosis which could explain the differences between these studies. In general, Latin American patients had similar survival rates as patients in developed countries. The French [32] and REVEAL [33] studies exhibited a survival rate lower than the Argentinean [29] and Brazilian studies [7], despite the lower availability of targeted therapies in Latin America. A recent analysis of the COMPERA registry divided the PAH group into typical and atypical PAH, according to the presence of 3 or more risk factor for the existence of left heart disease, characterizing the atypical subgroup [37]. Patients with typical PAH were younger, without any remarkable difference in the hemodynamics profile. Although with similar overall survival, the response to treatment was higher in the subgroup with typical PAH. The study suggests that the presence of comorbidities might significantly influence the spectrum of PAH disease by adding different pathophysiological mechanisms to the more isolated vascular disease seen in the typical PAH. The lower mean age evidenced in Latin American patients suggests a lower prevalence of comorbidities which could contribute to a better survival rate in the region. Nevertheless, the lack of appropriate description of the comorbidities in the selected studies prevented a proper evaluation of the role of typical and atypical PAH prevalences in the overall survival.

Despite the fact that data on PAH treatment in Latin America is limited, oral drugs appear to be the main form of first line therapy with Sildenafil being the most commonly used drug for PAH treatment within the region. The lack of data on combination therapy may be due to the fact that it is not approved in most Latin American countries. It is also important to point out that some treatments that were reported in the studies have not been approved for PAH use in the countries where data was collected. This highlights the fact that entering a clinical trial may be one way of providing PAH patients an opportunity to receive specific treatment [31]. Timely and improved access to medicines may still be limited in the region. Efforts should be made to improve early diagnosis and the availability of new treatments which in turn may increase survival rates of PAH patients in Latin America.

Our study has limitations that need to be acknowledged. There is a clear paucity of available data regarding PAH in the region. Most of the PAH data in Latin America is available only in conference abstracts, making it difficult to evaluate the profile of PAH patients among the region. Research from non-English speaking countries is underrepresented in high-impact medical journals and indexation problems for journals in Spanish and Portuguese hinder the screening of studies.

While national registries are currently being implemented in different Latin American countries, accurate epidemiologic information on PAH is still limited. However, a new international multicenter registry "Registro Latinoamericano de Hipertensión Pulmonar (RELAHP)" was launched in 2014. This registry has been designed to collect medical history, diagnostic methods and treatment of patients suffering from pulmonary hypertension (PH) under optimal medical care in an effort to better fill the existing gap on the knowledge about the broader distribution of PAH in the region. Although there are some local registries in progress, more efforts and investments are still needed to ensure the dissemination of PAH data in Latin America.

Conclusion

This study highlights the regional differences in the epidemiology of PAH. In contrast to Europe and North America, there is a clear heterogeneity in the distribution of the PAH forms in Latin America and the profile of patients described in the regional registries seems to be different from international ones. The recognition of these differences should be considered when developing clinical guidelines and extrapolating diagnostic and treatment algorithms. Specific health policies should address these differences while taking into account the limited health care access in some regions within Latin America. Equitable access to health care and therapies are issues that need to be addressed in Latin America. Information coming from a large prospective registry representing the different populations in Latin America is of critical importance to increase disease awareness in the region and improve diagnosis and management.

Abbreviations

6MWD: 6-minute walking distance; CHD: Congenital heart disease; CI: Cardiac index; COMPERA: Comparative, prospective registry of newly initiated therapies for pulmonary hypertension; CTD: Connective tissue disease; FC: Functional class; HINPULSAR: HIpertensión Pulmonar y Asociaciones en la Argentina; IPAH: Idiopathic pulmonary arterial hypertension; mPAP: Mean pulmonary artery pressure; NYHA: New York heart association; PAH: Pulmonary arterial hypertension; PCWP: Pulmonary artery wedge pressure; PH: Pulmonary hypertension; PVR: Pulmonary vascular resistance; RAP: Right atrial pressure; RECOPILAR: Registro Colaborativo de Hipertensión Pulmonar en Argentina; RELAHP: Registro Latinoamericano de Hipertensión Pulmonar; REVEAL: Registry to evaluate early and long-term PAH disease management; Sch: Schistosomiasis; UK: United Kingdom; US: United States of America; WHO: World Health Organization

Funding

This study (GSK study number LS2579) was funded and supported by GlaxoSmithKline (GSK). Dr. Rogerio Souza received no funding from GSK to work on this study. RANDOM Foundation (Colombia) provided medical writing services funded by GSK.

Authors' contributions

JMS and BG collected and analysed the data. CS and KV analysed the data and assisted on the writing process. ABV and RS designed the study, analysed the data and assisted on the writing process. All authors had full access to the data, participated on the study reviews and gave final approval to submit for publication.

Competing interests

ABV, CS, JMS, KV and BG are employees of GSK. ABV and CS hold GSK shares. RS received no funding from GSK to perform this work; however, he received lecture and consultancy fees from GSK, Actelion, Bayer and Pfizer.

Author details

[1]Latin America Medical Department – GlaxoSmithKline, Estrada dos Bandeirantes, Rio de Janeiro 8464, Brazil. [2]Pulmonary Hypertension Unit, Pulmonary Department – Heart Institute, University of Sao Paulo Medical School, Av. Dr. Eneas de Carvalho Aguiar, 44, Sao Paulo 05403-000, Brazil.

References

1. Frost AE, Badesch DB, Barst RJ, Benza RL, Elliott CG, Farber HW, et al. The changing picture of patients with pulmonary arterial hypertension in the United States: how REVEAL differs from historic and non-US contemporary registries. Chest. 2011;139(1):128–37. https://doi.org/10.1378/chest.10-0075. PubMed PMID: 20558556
2. Jiang X, Jing ZC. Epidemiology of pulmonary arterial hypertension. Curr Hypertens Rep. 2013;15(6):638–49. https://doi.org/10.1007/s11906-013-0397-5. PubMed PMID: 24114080
3. Humbert M, Khaltaev N, Bousquet J, Souza R. Pulmonary hypertension - from an orphan disease to a public health problem. Chest. 2007;132(2):365–7. https://doi.org/10.1378/chest.07-0903. PubMed PMID: WOS:000248779700002
4. McLaughlin W, Shah SJ, Souza R, Humbert M. Management of Pulmonary Arterial Hypertension. J Am Coll Cardiol. 2015;65(18):1976–97. https://doi.org/10.1016/j.jacc.2015.03.540
5. Hoeper MM, Simon RGJ. The changing landscape of pulmonary arterial hypertension and implications for patient care. Eur Respir Rev. 2014;23(134):450–7. https://doi.org/10.1183/09059180.00007814. PubMed PMID: 25445943
6. McGoon MD, Benza RL, Escribano-Subias P, Jiang X, Miller DP, Peacock AJ, et al. Pulmonary arterial hypertension: Epidemiology and Registries. J Am Coll Cardiol. 2013;62(25, Supplement):D51–D9. https://doi.org/10.1016/j.jacc.2013.10.023
7. Alves JL Jr, Gavilanes F, Jardim C, Fernandes CJCDS, Morinaga LTK, Dias B, et al. Pulmonary arterial hypertension in the southern hemisphere: results from a registry of incident brazilian cases. Chest. 2015;147(2):495–501. https://doi.org/10.1378/chest.14-1036
8. United Nations. Standard country or area codes for statistical use (M49) - Methodology Geographic Regions Latin America and the Caribbean New York: The United Nations Statistics Division; 2017. Available from: https://unstats.un.org/unsd/methodology/m49/. Cited 16 2017 June
9. Ramirez-Rivera A, Sanchez CJ, Garcia Badillo EV, Medellin B, Rivera SR, Palacios JM, et al. Northeast mexican registry on pulmonary arterial hypertension (RENEHAP). Chest. 2010;138:372a. https://doi.org/10.1378/chest.9942.
10. Conde R, Villaquiran C, Duenas R, Torres A. Diagnosis and Treatment of Pulmonary Arterial Hypertension and Chronic Thromboembolic Pulmonary Hypertension in Five Reference Centers In Bogota-Colombia, at 2.640 Meters Above Sea Level. Am J Respir Crit Care Med. 2015;191:A4847.
11. Villaquiran C, Duenas R, Conde R, Torres A. Description of the Clinical, Functional and Hemodynamic Characteristics of Patients with Pulmonary Arterial Hypertension in Five Reference Centers in Bogota - Colombia, at 2.640 Meters Above Sea Level. Am J Respir Crit Care Med. 2015. 191; 2015:A3842
12. Aranda A, Martin E, Fernandez R, Nieves J, Basora J, Torrellas P. Puerto Rico pulmonary artery hypertension registry scheme. Chest. 2014;145:517A. https://doi.org/10.1378/chest.1824935.
13. Chamorro F, Medina D, Melgarejo G. Clinical management of pulmonary arterial hypertension. Eur J Heart Fail. 2015;17(Suppl 1):114–5.
14. Perna ER, Coronel ML, Echazarreta D, Cursack G, Marquez LL, Alvarez S, et al. The epidemiology of pulmonary arterial hypertension in HINPULSAR Registry showed areas for intervention in Argentina: promote early identification, improve the diagnostic strategy and treatment. Eur Heart J. 2012;33:419. PubMed PMID: WOS:000308012403295
15. Coronel M, Perna E, Echazarreta D, Lema L, Zini GP, Aristimuno G, et al. Treatment of pulmonary arterial hypertension according with functional class in the Argentinean HINPULSAR registry. Eur J Heart Fail. 2012;11(SUPPL 1):S55–S6. PubMed PMID: WOS:000307009200139
16. Coronel M, Perna E, Echazarreta D, Lema L, Zini GP, Aristimuno G, et al. Pulmonary arterial hypertension in Argentina: insights from HINPULSAR registry. Circulation. 2012;125(19):E696. PubMed PMID: WOS:000307009200139
17. Echazarreta D, Coronel ML, Perna ER, Colque R, Cursack G, Nunez C, et al. Characterization of pulmonary hypertension and associations in Argentina: results of HINPULSAR registry. Eur J Heart Fail. 2012;11(S1):S108.
18. Coronel ML, Perna ER, Nunez C, Cursack G, Fleitas M, Botta C, et al. Severe right ventricular dysfunction in pulmonary arterial hypertension: prevalence, clinical markers and treatment in Argentinean HINPULSAR registry. Eur J Heart Fail. 2014;16:293–4. PubMed PMID: WOS:000335966801086
19. Perna ER, Coronel ML, Diez M, Atamanuk N, Nitsche A, Caneva J, et al. First collaborative registry of pulmonary hypertension in Argentina (RECOPILAR registry): a clinical snapshot from a developing country. Eur J Heart Fail. 2016;18:267. PubMed PMID: WOS:000377107502205
20. Gruss Al, Pascal G, Salisbury JP, Trujillo P, Grignola JC, Curbelo P. Uruguayan National reference center in pulmonary hypertension: a population descriptive study. American Thoracic Society 2014 International Conference; San Diego: Am J Respir Crit Care Med. 2016. p. A4705.
21. Perna ER, Coronel ML, Echazarreta D, Cursack G, Marquez LL, Alvarez S, et al. Epidemiological profile of pulmonary arterial hypertension in Argentina: insights from HINPULSAR registry. Eur J Heart Fail. 2012;SUPPL 1: S55.
22. Lescano A, Talavera L, Mazzei J, Barimboim E, Saurit V, Varela B, et al. The advanced functional class and the variables of poor prognosis in pulmonary hypertension. Eur J Heart Fail. 2016;18:122. PubMed PMID: WOS: 000377107501048.
23. Federacion Argentina de Cardiologia - Comité de Insuficiencia Cardíaca e Hipertensión Pulmonar. Diseño del Registro HINPULSAR: HIpertensióN PULmonar y aSociaciones en la ARgentina. Insuficiencia cardíaca. 2010;5:126–31.
24. Echazarreta D, Perna E, Coronel MI. Registro Colaborativo de Hipertensión Pulmonar en Argentina (RECOPILAR). Rev Fed Arg Cardiol. 2014;43:146–9.
25. Lapa MS, Ferreira EVM, Jardim C, Martins BCS, Arakaki JSO, Souza R. Características clínicas dos pacientes com hipertensão pulmonar em dois centros de referência em São Paulo. Revista da Associação Médica Brasileira. 2006;52:139–43.
26. Herrera S, Gabrielli L, Paredes A, Saavedra R, Ocaranza MP, Sepúlveda P, et al. Sobrevida a mediano plazo en los pacientes con hipertensión arterial pulmonar en la era de terapias vasodilatadoras específicas del territorio vascular pulmonar. Rev Med Chil. 2016;144:829–36.
27. Zagolin BM, Wainstein GE, Uriarte G de CP, Parra RC. [Clinical, functional and hemodynamic features of patients with pulmonary arterial hypertension]. Caracterizacion clinica, funcional y hemodinamica de la poblacion con

hipertension pulmonar arterial evaluada en el Instituto Nacional del Torax. Rev Med Chi. 2006;134(5):589–95. PubMed PMID: Medline:16802051

28. Enriquez A, Castro P, Sepulveda P, Verdejo H, Greig D, Gabrielli L, et al. Changes long term prognosis of 17 patients with pulmonary artery hypertension. Rev Med Chil. 2011;139(3):327–33. doi: /S0034-98872011000300007. PubMed PMID: 21879164

29. Talavera ML, Cáneva JO, Favaloro LE, Klein F, Boughen RP, Bozovich GE, et al. Hipertensión arterial pulmonar: Registro de un centro de referencia en Argentina. Rev Am Med Respir. 2014;14:144–52.

30. Costa E, Jardim C, Bogossian H, Amato M, Roberto C, Carvalho R, et al. Acute vasodilator test in pulmonary arterial hypertension: evaluation of two response criteria. Vasc Pharmacol. 2005;43(3):143–7. https://doi.org/10.1016/j.vph.2005.05.004. PubMed PMID: WOS:000231711300001

31. Lopes AA, Bandeira AP, Flores PC, Santana MV. Pulmonary hypertension in Latin America: pulmonary vascular disease: the global perspective. Chest. 2010;137(6 Suppl):78S–84S. https://doi.org/10.1378/chest.09-2960. PubMed PMID: 20522583

32. Humbert M, Sitbon O, Chaouat A, Bertocchi M, Habib G, Gressin V, et al. Pulmonary arterial hypertension in France: results from a national registry. Am J Respir Crit Care Med. 2006;173(9):1023–30. https://doi.org/10.1164/rccm.200510-1668OC. PubMed PMID: 16456139

33. Badesch DB, Raskob GE, Elliott CG, Krichman AM, Farber HW, Frost AE, et al. Pulmonary arterial hypertension: baseline characteristics from the REVEAL registry. Chest. 2010;137(2):376–87. https://doi.org/10.1378/chest.09-1140. PubMed PMID: 19837821

34. Hoeper MM, Huscher D, Ghofrani HA, Delcroix M, Distler O, Schweiger C, et al. Elderly patients diagnosed with idiopathic pulmonary arterial hypertension: results from the COMPERA registry. Int J Cardiol. 2013;168(2):871–80. https://doi.org/10.1016/j.ijcard.2012.10.026.

35. Alonso-Gonzalez R, Lopez-Guarch CJ, Subirana-Domenech MT, Ruíz JMO, González IO, Cubero JS, et al. Pulmonary hypertension and congenital heart disease: an insight from the REHAP National Registry. Int J Cardiol. 2015;184:717–23. https://doi.org/10.1016/j.ijcard.2015.02.031.

36. Galiè N, Humbert M, Vachiery J-L, Gibbs S, Lang I, Torbicki A, et al. 2015 ESC/ERS Guidelines for the diagnosis and treatment of pulmonary hypertensionThe Joint Task Force for the Diagnosis and Treatment of Pulmonary Hypertension of the European Society of Cardiology (ESC) and the European Respiratory Society (ERS): Endorsed by: Association for European Paediatric and Congenital Cardiology (AEPC), International Society for Heart and Lung Transplantation (ISHLT). Eur Heart J. 2016;37(1):67–119. https://doi.org/10.1093/eurheartj/ehv317.

Comorbidities and COPD severity in a clinic-based cohort

Chantal Raherison[1,2,10*], El-Hassane Ouaalaya[1], Alain Bernady[3], Julien Casteigt[4], Cecilia Nocent-Eijnani[5], Laurent Falque[6], Frédéric Le Guillou[7], Laurent Nguyen[8], Annaig Ozier[8] and Mathieu Molimard[9]

Abstract

Background: Chronic obstructive pulmonary disease (COPD) is an important cause of morbidity and mortality around the world. The aim of our study was to determine the association between specific comorbidities and COPD severity.

Methods: Pulmonologists included patients with COPD using a web-site questionnaire. Diagnosis of COPD was made using spirometry post-bronchodilator FEV1/FVC < 70%. The questionnaire included the following domains: demographic criteria, clinical symptoms, functional tests, comorbidities and therapeutic management. COPD severity was classified according to GOLD 2011. First we performed a principal component analysis and a non-hierarchical cluster analysis to describe the cluster of comorbidities.

Results: One thousand, five hundred and eighty-four patients were included in the cohort during the first 2 years. The distribution of COPD severity was: 27.4% in group A, 24.7% in group B, 11.2% in group C, and 36.6% in group D. The mean age was 66.5 (sd: 11), with 35% of women. Management of COPD differed according to the comorbidities, with the same level of severity. Only 28.4% of patients had no comorbidities associated with COPD. The proportion of patients with two comorbidities was significantly higher ($p < 0.001$) in GOLD B (50.4%) and D patients (53.1%) than in GOLD A (35.4%) and GOLD C ones (34.3%). The cluster analysis showed five phenotypes of comorbidities: cluster 1 included cardiac profile; cluster 2 included less comorbidities; cluster 3 included metabolic syndrome, apnea and anxiety-depression; cluster 4 included denutrition and osteoporosis and cluster 5 included bronchiectasis. The clusters were mostly significantly associated with symptomatic patients i.e. GOLD B and GOLD D.

Conclusions: This study in a large real-life cohort shows that multimorbidity is common in patients with COPD.

Keywords: COPD, Comorbidities, Cluster analysis, Management

Background

COPD has emerged as the most important respiratory disease worldwide. The epidemiology of COPD had changed in recent years, with more women affected [1], fewer old subjects and more medications available for health providers.

To improve the management of COPD and take into account the heterogeneity of the disease, the Global Obstructive Lung Disease Initiatives [2] proposed a new classification in 2011 that takes into account respiratory symptoms, the burden of exacerbations and lung function.

Comorbidities in COPD have received considerable attention as COPD patients frequently suffer from comorbidities such as cardiovascular and cerebrovascular disease, lung cancer and diabetes, with a significant impact on mortality that was termed by Divo et al. known as the "comorbidome" [3]. They constructed a comorbidity index (COTE index) based on 12 comorbidities that seem to negatively influence survival. However, the use of indexes like the COTE and the BODE [4] in clinical practice needs to be clarified. The validity of the COTE has been questioned since patients with GOLD B

* Correspondence: Chantal.raherison@chu-bordeaux.fr
[1]Univ. Bordeaux, Inserm, Bordeaux Population Health Research Center, team EPICENE, UMR 1219, F-33000 Bordeaux, France
[2]Pole cardiothoracique, Respiratory Diseases Department, CHU de Bordeaux, F-33000 Bordeaux, France
Full list of author information is available at the end of the article

seem to have worse survival than patients with GOLD C, because of the particular heart disease found in a very large population study in Copenhagen area [5]. Some authors suggest that the presence of comorbidities should influence the relationship between the GOLD score and lung function measurements, the former perhaps being more representative of morbidity than of COPD severity [6].

The distribution and the type of comorbidities seem to vary between studies, except for cardiovascular disease which seems to be stable across them [7]. The complexity of COPD was reported in the Eclipse cohort, suggesting that COPD includes several different phenotypes when taking into account clinical parameters, survival, hospitalization, comorbidities and systemic inflammation [8]. Recently, in a complex analysis using network analysis, Divo et al. showed that comorbidities in COPD do not occur by chance [9].

In 213 patients included in a rehabilitation center, Vanfleteren et al. identified 13 comorbidities and five comorbidity clusters: less comorbidity, cardiovascular, cachectic, metabolic and psychological [10]. However, little is known about the reproducibility of these comorbidity phenotypes in COPD patients in real life and their association with COPD severity. Recently, the ATS/ERS consensus statement recommended that studies be performed either to confirm or rule out an association between specific comorbidities and COPD [11]. In an ongoing prospective observational cohort of outpatients with COPD followed up by pulmonologists, the aim of our study was to determine the association between specific comorbidities and COPD severity.

Methods
Study design and population
The Palomb cohort is an ongoing, prospective, multicenter, observational study of subjects with COPD recruited in pulmonary clinics in South-West of France in a real-life setting since the first January 2014 and followed up for 3 years (Additional file 1).

The CNIL (National Data Protection and Privacy Commission) and the CCTIRS (Advisory Committee for Data Processing in Health Research) approved the study, and informed consent was obtained before enrollment. The authors had asked the local ethics committee for feedback regarding the need for ethical clearance for such a retrospective analysis, and were advised that this was not warranted.

Consent for publication statement is not applicable as no personal information is provided in this manuscript.

Between January 2014 and February 2016, $n = 1584$ patients were enrolled in the study by pulmonologist and followed up in everyday practice, the data was obtained using a web-site questionnaire fulfilled by the pulmonologist on a secure platform and with specific agreement obtained for the storage of health data.

The inclusion criterion was a diagnosis of COPD on the basis of a lung function test according to the ATS/ERS standards [12] and made using spirometry with post-bronchodilator FEV1/FVC < 70%. Patients were excluded if they didn't have the lung function criteria of COPD.

Measurements
The website questionnaire included the following domains: demographic criteria (age, gender), smoking habits, clinical symptoms (mMRC dyspnea, chronic cough, exacerbations during past 12 months), body mass index (BMI) [4], lung function, comorbidities and therapeutic management (vaccinations, pulmonary rehabilitation, smoking cessation and prescribed inhaler medication).

Comorbidities
Comorbidities ($n = 19$) were recorded systematically in a standardized manner by the pulmonologist. The diagnosis of comorbidity was assessed first by patient report then confirmed by either reviewing the patient's medication list or when complementary tests were available in medical records. Bronchiectasis was recorded by clinical and/or radiologic criteria, as usual in clinical practice.

COPD severity
Severity of COPD was classified as A,B,C or D according to GOLD 2011 [2]: 1) high/low symptoms using the mMRC dyspnea score < or ≥ 2; 2) the severity of airflow limitation [13]; and 3) the number of exacerbations per year. Despite the recent publication of GOLD 2017, GOLD 2011 was chosen because this classification was used by the pulmonologist in clinical practice during the study.

Statistical analysis
Analysis of variance was used for continuous variables and Chi-squared tests were used for categorical variables. We performed a univariate analysis between comorbidities and COPD severity (GOLD 2011). We decided to retain for further analysis only the comorbidities that were significantly more frequent in more severe COPD stages (B,C,D) than in the mild stage (A). Then we performed a principal component analysis and a non-hierarchical (K-means) cluster analysis to describe the cluster of comorbidities. To better define the number of appropriate clusters, we used three statistical methods: the scree plot method, the percentage of variance explained, and the Kaiser-Guttman method.

Lastly, we performed a cluster analysis (ward method) to ensure stability of the different clusters. All analyses were performed with SAS software version 9.4. All statistical tests were two sided, with $P < 0.05$ considered to indicate statistical significance.

Results

Patients' characteristics

A total of 1584 patients were included in the cohort during the first 2 years.

The GOLD 2011 distribution was as follows: 27.4% in group A, 24.7% in group B, 11.2% in group C, and 36.6% in group D, with no significant gender difference. The mean age was 66.5 (sd: 11), with 30% of women. Clinical symptoms, exacerbations, lung function and management according to COPD severity are presented in Table 1. 28.7% of the patients had had 2 or more exacerbations during the past year.

The onset of symptoms (i.e. cough, exacerbations or dyspnea) occurred between 25 and 49 years in 6% of the patients, 49–59 years in 20%, 59–69 years in 35%, 69–79 years in 25.3% and after 79 years in 13.26%.

16% had a BMI below 21 kg/m2, 34.8% between 21 and 26 kg/m2, 20% were overweight and 28.7% were obese (BMI > 29 kg/m2). BMI was significantly associated with severity of dyspnea and age (data not shown).

Prescription of pulmonary rehabilitation was rather infrequent in the whole population and was significantly more frequent in GOLD D patients (Table 1). By contrast, influenza vaccination was more frequent in GOLD B and D patients than pneumococcal vaccination, which increased with COPD severity (trend).

Frequency of comorbidities

Only 28.4% of patients had no comorbidities associated with COPD, whatever the severity of their COPD. The

Table 1 Description of 1584 subjects with COPD according to GOLD 2011 Classification (frequency of each variable by COPD severity)

	A N = 435	B N = 391	C N = 178	D N = 580	p
Males, %	68.5	62.6	62.9	64.6	0.3006
Age, yr (SD)	63.2(10.4)	69(10.8)	63.6(10.6)	68.2(11)	0.0006
BMI, (kg/m2), % < 21					0.0001
(underweight) [21–26[(normal)	12.4	13.3	21.3	19.6	
[26–29[(overweight)	37.7	30.2	33.2	36.4	
> 29 (obese)	21.8	21.2	22.5	17.6	
	28.3	35.3	23	26.4	
FEV1, % pred					0.0001
> 80%	109(25)	55(14)	26(14.6)	13(2.2)	
50–80%	326(75)	336(86)	62(34.9)	141(24.3)	
30–50%	–	–	85(47.8)	328(56.5)	
< 30%	–	–	5(2.8)	98(16.9)	
mMRC 0–1, n(%)	435(100)	0	178(100)	0	0.0001
mMRC > =2, n(%)	0	391(100)	0	580(100)	0.0001
Chronic cough, n(%)	190(43.6)	222(56.7)	96(53.9)	402(69.3)	< 0.0001
Current smokers, n(%)	170(39.8)	131(34.5)	68(39.5)	195(34.5)	0.2394
0–1 exacerbation previous year, n(%)	435(100)	391(100)	71(40)	231(39.8)	0.0001
> = 2 exacerbations, previous year, n(%)	0	0	107(60)	349(60.2)	0.0001
Pulmonary rehabilitation, n(%)	12(2.7)	23(5.8)	10(5.6)	97(16.7)	< 0.0001
Smoking cessation, n(%)	35(8.0)	23(5.8)	26(14.6)	58(10)	0.0053
SABA, %	28.7	44.2	37	47	< 0.0001
LABA, or LAMA, %	53.1	72.1	66.8	71.2	< 0.0001
ICS and LABA, %	18.1	24.8	24.2	39	< 0.0001
Annual influenza vaccination, n(%)	166(38.1)	230(58.8)	93(52.2)	410(70.6)	< 0.0001
Pneumococcal vaccination, n(%)	141(32.4)	204(52.1)	100(56.1)	379(65.3)	< 0.0001

Abbreviations: *SABA* short-acting bronchodilators *LABA* long-acting bronchodilators. *LAMA* long-acting muscarinic antagonist

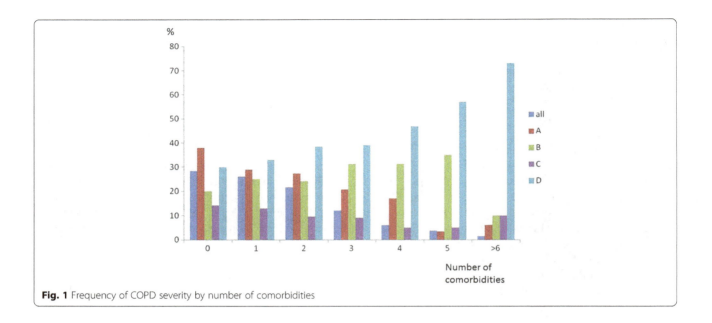

Fig. 1 Frequency of COPD severity by number of comorbidities

number of comorbidities by COPD severity is shown in Fig. 1, the number of comorbidities increased with severity of COPD. Cardiac comorbidities were more frequent in men whereas anxiety-depression and osteoporosis were more frequent in women.

Hypertension, ischemic cardiopathy, heart rhythm disorder and left cardiac insufficiency were significantly higher in overweight and obese subjects (p: 0.0001).

Prevalence of obstructive apnea syndrome (OAS) was higher in group A. Hypertension, OAS, dyslipidemia,

Table 2 Frequency of comorbidities in 1584 subjects with COPD according to GOLD 2011 Classification (frequency of each variable by COPD severity)

	A N = 435	B N = 391	C N = 178	D N = 580	p
Hypertension	139(31.9)	173(44.2)	52(29.2)	237(40.8)	0.0001
Obstructive apnea syndrome	118(27.1)	75(19.2)	23(12.9)	63(10.9)	0.0001
Dyslipidemia	97(22.3)	114(29.2)	37(20.8)	143(24.7)	0.072
Cancer, all causes	79(18.2)	70(17.9)	20(11.2)	90(11.5)	0.14
Ischemic cardiopathy	59(12.5)	99(25.3)	30(16.8)	127(21.9)	0.0001
Past asthma	47(10.8)	48(12.3)	19(10.7)	71(12.3)	0.84
Depression	43(9.9)	50(12.8)	15(8.4)	113(19.5)	0.0001
Anxiety	30(6.9)	70(17.9)	23(12.9)	154(26.5)	0.0001
Heart rhythm disorder	41(9.4)	65(16.6)	24(13.4)	86(14.8)	0.016
Diabetes	41(9.4)	51(13)	18(10.1)	88(15.2)	0.035
Undernutrition, BMI < 21 kg/m2	1(0.2)	3(0.7)	4(2.2)	25(4.3)	0.0001
Osteoporosis	2(0.4)	23(5.8)	1(0.5)	35(6.0)	0.0001
Atheroma	20(4.6)	27(6.9)	9(5.0)	51(8.8)	0.048
Left cardiac insufficiency	8(1.8)	21(5.3)	12(6.7)	50(8.6)	0.0001
Vascular Stroke	16(3.7)	22(5.6)	5(2.8)	20(3.5)	0.26
Pulmonary hypertension	3(0.7)	7(1.8)	1(0.6)	26(4.5)	0.0002
Metabolic syndrome	10(2.3)	16(4.1)	5(2.8)	27(4.7)	0.21
Rhinitis/rhinosinusitis	8(3.2)	14(7)	7(7.8)	19(7.4)	0.16
Bronchiectasis	7(3.9)	31(4.1)	34(9.2)	6(6.4)	0.004

Table 4 Comorbidities frequency (> = 2 vs 0–1) by COPD severity (statistical test to compare the distribution of comorbidity frequency in each severity stage)

Comorbidity frequency	GOLD 2011				p value
	A N = 435	B N = 391	C N = 178	D N = 580	
0–1864(54.55%)	281(32.5%)	194(22.4%)	117(13.5%)	272(31.4%)	< 0.0001
≥2720(45.45%)	154(21.3%)	197(27.3%)	61(8.4%)	308(42.7%)	

ischemic cardiopathy and heart rhythm disorder were more frequent in groups B and D than in groups A and C. The frequencies of all comorbidities for COPD stage are presented in Table 2.

We have identified 13 comorbidities which were more frequent in higher COPD stages (B,C,D) than in the mild stage (A). OAS was more frequent in mild stage (A) than in others.

Anxiety and depression was higher in groups D and B than in the other groups. Undernutrition was higher in group D. Osteoporosis was higher in groups B and D.

Number of comorbidities

In the group of patients with one comorbidity, 36.7% had hypertension, 11.8% had Obstructive Syndrome Apnea (OSA), 10.4% had depression and 10% had ischemic cardiopathy. The proportion of patients with two comorbidities was significantly higher ($p < 0.001$) in GOLD B (50.4%) and D patients (53.1%) than in GOLD A (35.4%) and C ones (34.3%). The median of comorbidities was 1.6 (box plot) in the whole sample.

The proportion of GOLD B and D patients, increased significantly with the number of comorbidities, particularly among those with more than two comorbidities (Fig. 1). The number of comorbidities was higher in GOLD B and D patients (Table 3). The number of patients with two comorbidities or more was significantly higher in patients GOLD B and D patients than in GOLD A and C ones (Table 4).

Management of COPD according to number of comorbidities

In GOLD A and B patients, prescription of treatment as needed and regular treatment did not differ according to the number of comorbidities (Table 5), unlike for GOLD C and D patients. In GOLD C patients, LABA were more frequently prescribed in those with comorbidities than in those without. In GOLD D patients, SABA was prescribed significantly more frequently in those with comorbidities. Pulmonary rehabilitation and vaccination were prescribed significantly more in GOLD B and D patients with comorbidities than in those with the same degree of severity but without comorbidities. Finally, smoking cessation was prescribed significantly more in GOLD C and D patients with comorbidities.

Comorbidity clusters

The cluster analysis showed five phenotypes of comorbidities: cluster 1 included cardiac profile; cluster 2 included less comorbidity; cluster 3 included metabolic syndrome, apnea and anxiety-depression; cluster 4 included cachectic and osteoporosis and cluster 5 included mainly bronchiectasis. The label of each cluster was given, comparing the prevalence of comorbidity in the whole population with prevalence of comorbidity in each cluster (Table 6).

The different clusters were distributed in the four stages of COPD severity, however cardiac cluster was more frequent in patients with GOLD B. Cluster with less comorbidity was more frequent in patient GOLD C and A. Metabolic syndrome was more frequent in GOLD C and D. Cachectic and osteoporotic profile were most frequent in GOLD B and D. Lastly, bronchiectasis profile was more frequent in patient GOLD D (Table 7).

Discussion

This study sought to determine whether comorbidities were associated with COPD severity in a clinic-based

Table 3 Number of comorbidities n (%) by COPD severity (frequency of Number of comorbidities in each COPD severity stage)

Number of comorbidities	A N = 435	B N = 391	C N = 178	D N = 580	p
0	160 (36.7)	90(23)	64(35.9)	136(23.4)	< 0.0001
1	121(27.8)	104(26.6)	53(29.8)	136(23.4)	< 0.0001
2	94(21.6)	83(21.2)	33(18.5)	132(22.7)	< 0.0001
3	40(9.2)	60(15.3)	17(9.5)	75(12.9)	< 0.0001
4	16(3.7)	30(7.7)	5(2.8)	45(7.8)	< 0.0001
5	2(0.4)	21(5.4)	3(1.7)	34(5.9)	< 0.0001
6 and more	2(0.4)	3(0.7)	3(1.7)	22(2.1)	< 0.0001

Table 5 COPD treatment by number of comorbidities and COPD severity (P value refers to compare each pharmacologic treatment according to number of comorbidities in each severity stage)

Number of comorbidities	A N = 435			B N = 391			C N = 178			D N = 580		
	0-1 N = 281	>=2 N = 154	p	0-1 N = 194	>=2 N = 197	p	0-1 N = 117	>=2 N = 61	p	0-1 N = 272	>=2 N = 308	p
SABA, n(%)	83(29.5)	42(27.2)	0.61	81(41.7)	92(46.7)	0.32	46(39.3)	20(32.8)	0.39	94(34.5)	179(58.2)	<0.0001
LABA or LAMA, n(%)	152(54.0)	79(51.3)	0.57	139(71.6)	143(72.6)	0.83	72(61.5)	47(77.0)	0.03	186(68.4)	227(73.7)	0.15
ICS and LABA, n(%)	53(18.9)	26(16.9)	0.60	55(28.3)	42(21.3)	0.10	31(26.5)	12(19.7)	0.31	102(37.5)	124(40.3)	0.49
LABA and LAMA, n(%)	30(10.7)	23(14.9)	0.02	26(13.4)	38(19.3)	0.01	18(15.4)	19(31.1)	0.02	45(16.5)	94(30.5)	0.01
LABA and LAMA and ICS, n(%)	1(0.35)	1(0.64)	0.35	2(1.03)	2(1.01)	0.35	2(1.7)	2(3.2)	0.35	8(2.9)	21(6.8)	0.02
Pulmonary Rehabilitation, n(%)	8(2.8)	4(2.6)	0.87	6(3.9)	17(8.6)	0.02	7(6)	3(5)	0.76	31(11.4)	66(21.4)	0.0012
Annual influenza vaccination, n(%)	105(37.4)	61(39.6)	0.64	95(49)	135(68.5)	<0.0001	60(51.3)	33(54.1)	0.72	167(61.4)	243(79)	<0.0001
Pneumococcal vaccination, n(%)	85(30.2)	56(36.3)	0.19	81(41.7)	123(62.4)	<0.0001	65(55.5)	35(57.3)	0.81	145(53.3)	234(76)	<0.0001
Smoking cessation, n(%)	24(8.5)	11(7.14)	0.60	13(6.7)	10(5.0)	0.49	13(11.1)	13(21.3)	0.06	17(6.2)	41(13.3)	0.0047

Table 6 Prevalence of comorbidities in the five clusters

comorbidities (% in the whole population)	Cluster1 N = 360	Cluster2 N = 430	Cluster3 N = 233	Cluster4 N = 327	Cluster5 N = 234
OSA (17.6)	69(24.7)	36(12.9)	74(26.5)	60(21.5)	40(14.3)
Bronchiectasis (5.1)	17(21)	6(7.4)	20(24.7)	17(21)	21(25.9)
Left cardiac insufficiency (5.7)	19(20.9)	17(18.7)	23(25.3)	16(17.6)	16(17.6)
Hypertension (37.9)	130 (21.6)	98(16.3)	164 (27.3)	136 (22.6)	73(12.1)
Heart rhythm disorder (13.64)	48(22.2)	31(14.4)	54(25)	51(23.6)	32(14.8)
Atheroma (6.76)	23(21.5)	12(11.2)	35(32.7)	18(16.8)	19(17.8)
Pulmonary hypertension (2.3)	15(40.5)	4(10.8)	8(21.6)	5(13.5)	5(13.5)
Diabetes (12.5)	47(23.7)	26(13.1)	56(28.3)	51(25.8)	18(9.1)
Depression (13.95)	46(20.8)	33(14.9)	66(29.9)	44(19.9)	32(14.5)
Anxiety (17.5)	62(22.4)	15(5.4)	87(31.4)	67(24.2)	46(16.6)
Undernutrition (2)	10(30.3)	1(3)	8(24.2)	10(30.3)	4(12.1)
Ischemic cardiopathy (19.9)	61(19.4)	46(14.6)	83(26.3)	72(22.9)	53(16.8)
Osteoporosis (3.8)	13(21.3)	3(4.9)	14(23)	21(34.4)	10(16.4)

cohort of COPD patients, mostly GOLD A and B, followed up by pulmonologists. Only 28.4% of patients had no associated comorbidities. Fourteen comorbidities were significantly different with COPD severity. In this large population of patients, the median number of comorbidities was two.

Hypertension, OSA, dyslipidemia, ischemic cardiopathy and heart rhythm disorder were more frequent in GOLD B and D patients than in the other groups, as were anxiety and depression. Undernutrition was the most frequent in GOLD D patients and osteoporosis was the most frequent in GOLD B and D subjects. The number of comorbidities was the highest in GOLD B and D patients. Even when the severity of symptoms was similar, the management of COPD seemed to be different according to whether patients had comorbidities or not. Finally, five clusters of comorbidities were established, the most frequent being the cluster with cardiovascular disease and obstructive apnea syndrome.

Our approach was to analyze the relationship between these comorbidities and COPD severity by using three different approaches: the impact of the number of comorbidities, the univariate association between the comorbidities and COPD severity and cluster analysis to determine the association between the comorbidities i.e. to establish the existence of different phenotypes. Our findings are consistent with previous publications reporting a high prevalence of comorbidity in COPD, particularly cardio-vascular disease. Chen et al. [7] in a large review reported that compared with the non-COPD population, patients with COPD were more likely to be diagnosed with cardiovascular disease (odds ratio [OR] 2.4; 95% CI 2.02–3.00; $p < 0.0001$), including a two- to five-fold higher risk of

Table 7 Distribution of comorbidities cluster by COPD severity

Clusters	GOLD 2011				p value
	A N = 435	B N = 391	C N = 178	D N = 580	
Cluster 1 Cardiac (22.7%)	107(24.6)	102(26)	33(18.5)	118(20)	< 0.0001
Cluster 2 less comorbidity (27%)	137(31.5)	96(24.5)	57(32)	140(24.1)	< 0.0001
Cluster 3 metabolic, apneic and anxiety-depression (14.7%)	56(12.8)	39(9.9)	41(23)	97(16)	< 0.0001
Cluster 4 Cachectic and osteoporosis (20.6%)	70(16)	101(25.8)	22(12.3)	134(23)	< 0.0001
Cluster 5 bronchiectasis (14.7%)	65(14.9)	53(13.5)	25(14)	91(15.6)	< 0.0001

ischemic heart disease, cardiac dysrhythmia, heart failure, diseases of the pulmonary circulation, and arterial disease. Additionally, patients with COPD reported hypertension more often (OR 1·3, 95% CI 1·1–1·5; $p = 0.0007$), diabetes (1·3, 1·2–1·5; $p < 0.0001$], and ever smoking (4·2, 3·2–5·6; $p < 0.0001$). Divo et al. found in their cohort that cardiovascular disease was highly associated with the risk of mortality, but that the highest risk of mortality was associated with anxiety [3]. However, we found a high prevalence of OAS, probably owing to the overlap syndrome as reported by Soler et al. [14]. By contrast, OAS was the most frequent comorbidity is GOLD A and B patients although it seemed to be associated with moderate-to-severe COPD. It is essential to diagnose OAS in patients with COPD as patients with overlap syndrome who are not treated with CPAP have a higher mortality [15].

In our cohort, 14 comorbidities were significantly associated with COPD severity. Hypertension, OSA, dyslipidemia, ischemic cardiopathy, and heart rhythm disorder were more frequent in GOLD B and D compared to GOLD A and C. Anxiety and depression was higher in GOLD D and B, compared to the other groups of severity. These results are in line with the analysis performed in the Copenhagen cohort showing that GOLD B patients had more severe dyspnea and significantly poorer survival than group C ones, in spite of a higher FEV1 level [5]. The same trend concerned the number of comorbidities, with a prevalence of comorbidities (more than two) in GOLD B and D patients. At an equal level of severity, management of COPD seems to be different in severe COPD patients with comorbidities, with more LABA and SABA in severe COPD, suggesting that comorbidities could increase respiratory symptoms. Moreover, prevention of exacerbations requires interventions beyond the lungs, including treatment of comorbidities such as gastro-esophageal reflux disease, reduction of cardiovascular risks, and management of dyspnea and anxiety [16].

LABA were prescribed the most in GOLD A patients, which is not in agreement with the guidelines GOLD 2011. This could be due to the high prevalence of symptoms like cough in this group, as symptoms included in the GOLD classification are based on dyspnea and exacerbations but not on cough. We cannot rule out that symptomatic GOLD A patients could represent a specific phenotype. Recently, Woodruff et col. described a subgroup of symptomatic patients with no criteria for COPD regarding lung function [17]. In addition, management of COPD differed according to the comorbidities that patients had, even if those with or without had the same level of severity. This was particularly the case for rehabilitation and vaccination which were more prescribed in symptomatic GOLD B and D patients who had comorbidities than in those without.

We expected to have a gradient in COPD severity, perhaps patients GOLD B should be called differently, as they seemed to be more severe than GOLD C.

The cluster analysis revealed five clusters: The cluster analysis showed five phenotypes of comorbidities: cluster 1 included cardiac profile; cluster 2 included less comorbidities; cluster 3 included metabolic syndrome, apnea and anxiety-depression; cluster 4 included undernutrition and osteoporosis and cluster 5 included bronchiectasis. Vanfleteren found 13 comorbidities in a sample of 213 COPD patients [10] with five comorbid phenotypes: less comorbidity, cardiovascular, cachectic, metabolic, and psychological. Four of our clusters are concordant, i.e. cardiovascular, cachectic, metabolic and less comorbidities. Nevertheless, all the clusters were more significantly associated with GOLD D and in less manner with GOLD B. This finding could explain the higher risk of mortality in GOLD B and D patients, as previously reported elsewhere [5]. In the same way, Divo et al. [9] also identified a number of modules in the comorbidity network, including a cardiovascular one, and a module characterized by mil-moderate airflow limitation and metabolic syndrome with high BMI, these two modules are concordant with our findings.

Our results show that while comorbidity in COPD is a complex issue, comorbidities contributed prominently to the clinical severity of our patients, and that management of their severe COPD differed according to whether they had comorbidities or not, at the same level of obstruction.

Our study has some limitations. First, comorbidities were recorded by pulmonologists; previous studies showed that comorbidities are underdiagnosed in real life. This could also be the case in our study for most comorbidity except for OSA, as OSA was diagnosed by a polysomnography performed by the same pulmonologist who diagnosed COPD. However, we think that this bias is limited in our study, as we found a significant correlation between the comorbidities declared and compliance with the treatment given for them (data not shown). Second, we cannot generalize these findings to patients with COPD in the general population, as our population was managed both by a general practitioner and a pulmonologist. Third, we performed a multivariable exploratory analysis in order to better describe the associations between the different comorbidities [18]. This type of analysis uses a statistical method that processes a large amount of information from heterogeneous variables in homogeneous groups. It is well known that various factors can influence the analysis and therefore the results: the choice of the methods, hierarchical or nonhierarchical, the determination of the number of clusters before the analysis, the choice of the variables included in the analysis, the correlation between the selected variables and the clinical judgment of the investigators. To limit the impact of the specific correlation between the variables, we first performed a principal component analysis. Then we used the scree plot of the eigenvalue, the Kaiser-Guttman criterion and the percentage of variance explained to determine the number of clusters.

Lastly, we cannot validate our clusters in terms of survival as the study was performed with inclusion criteria, or with systemic inflammation. Further analysis with survival data from these COPD patients would provide important information for validating these clusters of comorbidity.

Conclusions

This study in a large clinic-based cohort shows that multimorbidity is common in patients with COPD, and that five comorbidity clusters can be identified. Patients GOLD B have more comorbidities than GOLD C.

The presence of comorbidities should therefore be included in any assessment of COPD severity. Further analysis is needed to validate these clusters in a future cohort.

Abbreviations
ATS/ERS: American Thoracic Society/European Respiratory Society; BODE: Bmi Obstruction Dyspnea Exercise; COPD: Chronic obstructive pulmonary disease; COTE index: Comorbidity index; FEV1: Forced expiratory Volume; GOLD: Global Obstructive Lung Disease Initiatives; ICS: Inhaled corticosteroids; LABA: Long acting bronchodilatator; LAMA: Long acting muscarinic antagonist; OSA: Obstructive Syndrome Apnea; SABA: Short acting bronchodilatator

Acknowledgements
The authors dedicate this manuscript to the memory and the contribution of their dear co-author and friend François Pellet, MD, for his outstanding contribution to the Palomb project. They also thank R. Goin and C. Bousquet, A. Le-Leon (Bordeaux University Foundation) for their support, R. Cooke for copyediting the manuscript and E. Berteaud for data management.
Inclusion centers: C. Roy, J. Moinard, Y. Daoudi, JM Dupis, E. Blanchard, H. Jungmann E. Monge, A. Prudhomme, M. Sapene, M. Sabatini.

Funding
Funding (unrestricted grants): Bordeaux University Foundation, Novartis Pharma, Isis Medical, Boehringer Ingelheim, Glaxo-Smith Kline. The funding sources had no role in the design or conduct of the study, in the collection, management, analysis and interpretation of the data, or in the preparation, review or approval of the manuscript.

Authors' contributions
Study concept and design: CR, AB, JC, CN, LF, FLG, LN, MM. Acquisition of data: all authors. Statistical analysis: CR, EO. Data access and responsibility: CR and EO had full access to the data of the study and take responsibility for the integrity of the data and the accuracy of the data analysis. All authors read and approved the final manuscript.

Competing interests
Dr. Raherison reports grants from Bordeaux University Foundation, during the conduct of the study; personal fees from Astra Zeneca, personal fees from Chiesi, personal fees from ALK, personal fees from Boehringer Ingelheim, personal fees from Glaxo SmithKline, personal fees from MundiPharma, personal fees from Novartis, outside the submitted work; Dr. Nocent-Eijnani has nothing to disclose.
Dr. Molimard reports personal fee from the University of Bordeaux, during the conduct of the study, other from Novartis Pharma, GSK, MundiPharma outside the submitted work. Dr. Nguyen has nothing to disclose. Dr. Falque has nothing to disclose. Dr. Casteigt has nothing to disclose. Dr. Le Guillou has nothing to disclose. Dr. Ozier has nothing to disclose. Dr. Bernady has nothing to disclose. Mr. Ouaalaya has nothing to disclose.

Author details
[1]Univ. Bordeaux, Inserm, Bordeaux Population Health Research Center, team EPICENE, UMR 1219, F-33000 Bordeaux, France. [2]Pole cardiothoracique, Respiratory Diseases Department, CHU de Bordeaux, F-33000 Bordeaux, France. [3]Rehabiliation Center, Cambo-les-Bains, France. [4]Pneumology Clinic, St Medard en Jalles, France. [5]General Hospital, Bayonne, France. [6]Pneumology Clinic, Bordeaux, France. [7]Pneumology Clinic, La Rochelle, France. [8]Pneumology Clinic, St Augustin, Bordeaux, France. [9]U1219 Pharmaco-epidemiology, Bordeaux University, Bordeaux, France. [10]Univ. Bordeaux, Inserm, Bordeaux Population Health Research Center, team EPICENE, UMR 1219, 146 rue Leo Saignat, 33076 Cedex Bordeaux, France.

References
1. Thun MJ, et al. 50-year trends in smoking-related mortality in the United States. N Engl J Med. 2013;368(4):351–64.
2. National Heart, L., and Blood Institute. World Health Organization., Global Strategy for the Diagnosis, Management, and Prevention of Chronic Obstructive Pulmonary Disease. NHLBI/WHO Workshop Report 2011. Vestbo J: National Institutes of Health; 2014. Available from: https://goldcopd.org/gold-reports-2017/.
3. Divo M, et al. Comorbidities and risk of mortality in patients with chronic obstructive pulmonary disease. Am J Respir Crit Care Med. 2012;186(2):155–61.
4. Celli BR, et al. The body-mass index, airflow obstruction, dyspnea, and exercise capacity index in chronic obstructive pulmonary disease. N Engl J Med. 2004;350(10):1005–12.
5. Lange P, et al. Prediction of the clinical course of chronic obstructive pulmonary disease, using the new GOLD classification: a study of the general population. Am J Respir Crit Care Med. 2012;186(10):975–81.
6. Weinreich UM, et al. The effect of comorbidities on COPD assessment: a pilot study. Int J Chron Obstruct Pulmon Dis. 2015;10:429–38.
7. Chen W, et al. Risk of cardiovascular comorbidity in patients with chronic obstructive pulmonary disease: a systematic review and meta-analysis. Lancet Respir Med. 2015;3(8):631–9.
8. Rennard SI, et al. Identification of five chronic obstructive pulmonary disease subgroups with different prognoses in the ECLIPSE cohort using cluster analysis. Ann Am Thorac Soc. 2015;12(3):303–12.
9. Divo MJ, et al. COPD comorbidities network. Eur Respir J. 2015;46(3):640–50.
10. Vanfleteren LE, et al. Clusters of comorbidities based on validated objective measurements and systemic inflammation in patients with chronic obstructive pulmonary disease. Am J Respir Crit Care Med. 2013;187(7):728–35.
11. Celli BR, et al. An official American Thoracic Society/European Respiratory Society statement: research questions in COPD. Eur Respir J. 2015;45(4):879–905.
12. Celli BR, MacNee W, Force AET. Standards for the diagnosis and treatment of patients with COPD: a summary of the ATS/ERS position paper. Eur Respir J. 2004;23(6):932–46.
13. Gold PM. The 2007 GOLD guidelines: a comprehensive care framework. Respir Care. 2009;54(8):1040–9.
14. Soler X, et al. High prevalence of obstructive sleep apnea in patients with moderate to severe chronic obstructive pulmonary disease. Ann Am Thorac Soc. 2015;12(8):1219–25.
15. Marin JM, et al. Outcomes in patients with chronic obstructive pulmonary disease and obstructive sleep apnea: the overlap syndrome. Am J Respir Crit Care Med. 2010;182(3):325–31.
16. Vanfleteren LE, et al. Management of chronic obstructive pulmonary disease beyond the lungs. Lancet Respir Med. 2016;4(11):911–24

Delayed isolation of smear-positive pulmonary tuberculosis patients in a Japanese acute care hospital

Sho Nishiguchi[1,4,5*], Shusaku Tomiyama[2], Izumi Kitagawa[1] and Yasuharu Tokuda[3]

Abstract

Background: Active pulmonary tuberculosis (TB) is associated with intra-hospital spread of the disease. Expeditious diagnosis and isolation are critical for infection control. However, factors that lead to delayed isolation of smear-positive pulmonary TB patients, especially among the elderly, have not been reported. The purpose of this study is to investigate factors associated with delay in the isolation of smear-positive TB patients.

Methods: All patients with smear-positive pulmonary TB admitted between January 2008 and December 2016 were included. The setting was a Japanese acute care teaching hospital. Following univariate analysis, significant factors in the model were analyzed using the multivariate Cox proportional hazard model.

Results: Sixty-nine patients with mean age of 81 years were included. The median day to the isolation of pulmonary TB was 1 day with interquartile range, 1–4 days. On univariate analysis, the time to isolation was significantly delayed in male patients ($p = 0.009$), in patient who had prior treatment with newer quinolone antibiotics ($p = 0.027$), in patients who did not have chronic cough ($p = 0.023$), in patients who did not have appetite loss ($p = 0.037$), and in patients with non-cavitary lesion ($p = 0.005$), lesion located other than in the upper zone ($p = 0.015$), and non-disseminated lesion on the chest radiograph ($p = 0.028$). On multivariate analysis, the time to isolation was significantly delayed in male patients (hazard ratio [HR], 0.47; 95% confidence interval [CI], 0.25 to 0.89; $P = 0.02$), in patients who did not have chronic chough (HR, 0.52; 95% CI, 0.28 to 0.95; $P = 0.033$), and in patients with non-cavitary lesion on the chest radiograph (HR, 0.46; 95% CI, 0.23 to 0.92; $P = 0.028$).

Conclusions: In acute care hospitals of an aging society, prompt diagnosis and isolation of TB patients are important for the protection of other patients and healthcare providers. Delay in isolation is associated with male gender, absence of chronic cough, and presence of non-cavitary lesions on the chest radiograph.

Keywords: Pulmonary tuberculosis, Delay, Isolation, Diagnosis, Smear-positive

Background

Tuberculosis (TB) control is of worldwide interest, especially among patients with active pulmonary TB who are smear-positive for acid-fast bacilli [1]. TB control requires early diagnosis and immediate initiation of treatment [2]. Delay in diagnosis adversely affects clinical outcome; besides, it increases transmission within the community and leads to higher transmission rates in an epidemic [3, 4].

Although the prevalence of TB had reduced to 16.7 per 100,000 among Japanese population in 2012, this figure remains 3–4 times higher than in Europe and North America [5, 6]. One reason for the relatively high prevalence of TB in Japan is an aging population with previous TB infection [7]. In the World Health Organization 2017 global report, Japanese patients with smear-positive pulmonary TB were older and had a higher mortality than in other countries [8, 9]. Given the high rates of hospital admission among elderly patients in developed countries, any delay in diagnosis and isolation of pulmonary TB can cause spread of infection [10]. Therefore, in aging societies

---

* Correspondence: sanazen@hotmail.co.jp
[1]Department of General Internal Medicine, Shonan Kamakura General Hospital, 1370-1 Okamoto, Kamakura, Kanagawa, Japan
[4]Department of Internal Medicine, Hayama Heart Center, Hayama, Kanagawa, Japan
Full list of author information is available at the end of the article

including Japan, it is important to seek reasons for delay in the isolation of pulmonary TB patients.

In previous studies, factors leading to delayed diagnosis of pulmonary TB have been well reported worldwide [2, 11–14]. These reports focused on 'patient delay' and 'health care system delay' [14–16]. Delayed diagnosis has been associated with human immunodeficiency virus infection, chronic cough, and presence of incidental lung disease [2]. Geographical and socio-psychological barriers include rural residence and poor access to healthcare [2, 11, 12]. Other factors that may delay diagnosis include old age, female gender, alcoholism and substance abuse, initial visitation at a low-level government healthcare facility, private practitioner, or traditional healer [2, 11, 12, 14]. History of immigration, poor education status, low awareness of TB, irrational beliefs, self-treatment, the associated stigma, consultation at a public hospital, and prior treatment with fluoroquinolones may also delay the diagnosis of active pulmonary TB [2, 11–14].

To the best of our knowledge, factors associated with delay in isolation of pulmonary TB patients have not been reported. In the clinical setting, any delay in isolation is critical to control of infection within hospitals. Therefore, we conducted this study to clarify factors associated with delayed isolation of active pulmonary TB patients.

Methods
Patients and setting
We conducted a retrospective study on patients who were diagnosed with smear-positive pulmonary TB in an urban teaching hospital between January 2008 and December 2016. The hospital provides primary through tertiary care in Kanagawa Prefecture, Japan, with a population of about nine million people. The hospital has no specific wards for patients with treatment of active pulmonary TB. Those who are suspected to have active pulmonary TB disease are immediately isolated in single rooms with negative air pressure for definite sputum smear diagnosis, particularly with three consecutive sputum or gastric aspiration analysis. After the diagnosis of smear-positive pulmonary TB is established, the patients are then transferred to another hospital that has special wards for the treatment of smear-positive pulmonary TB. Therefore, a delay in isolation on admission may spread the TB infection in-hospital. We studied 69 consecutive patients who were diagnosed with smear-positive pulmonary TB by examination of the sputum or gastric specimen.

Data collection
Data collection for each patient, collectively referred to as "patient-related factors": age, gender, history of smoking or alcoholism, welfare recipient or not, activities of daily living, past history of TB, contact with TB patients, diabetes mellitus, other lung disease, surgical history of gastric resection, human immunodeficiency virus infection, preceding treatment with newer quinolone antibiotics, steroid use, chronic cough, loss of appetite, body mass index, body temperature on arrival, systolic blood pressure, oxygen requirement, hemoglobin level, serum albumin level, C-reactive protein level, presence of a cavitary, upper zone or disseminated lesion on the chest radiograph, and the raw score. The raw score is a validated prognostic score for patients with smear-positive pulmonary TB [8].

We also collected data on the following "facility and physician-related factors": year of hospital visit, time of arrival (day or night), weekday or weekend arrival, the attending ER physician, medical care provided by the resident on arrival, medical care provided by male physician on arrival, and whether transferred to the hospital by ambulance.

Statistical analysis
We aimed to evaluate factors associated with delayed isolation of smear-positive pulmonary TB patients. The primary outcome measure was the duration day from hospital visit to the isolation of the patient with TB. Day-to-isolation analysis, based on the Cox proportional hazard model, was used to analyze factors associated with delay to the isolation of pulmonary TB patients. In a univariate model, the "patient-related factors" and "medical facility and physician-related factors" were evaluated as possible reasons for the delayed isolation of active pulmonary TB, based on log-rank test or univariate Cox hazard test, as appropriate. Significant factors in the univariate model were analyzed using the multivariate Cox proportional hazard model. A two-tailed p-value < 0.05 was considered statistically significant. All data analyses were undertaken using the SPSS Statistics version 21 J (IBM, Tokyo, Japan). This study was approved by the Institutional Review Board of the hospital (No. TGE00667-024).

Results
Sixty-nine patients with smear-positive pulmonary TB were enrolled. Base-line characteristics and univariate analysis were included in Table 1. The mean age of patients was 81 years, with 18 (26.1%) female patients. All patients were hospitalized and isolated for infection control. Two patients were discharged home, 55 were transferred to other hospitals for the treatment of TB, and 12 died in our hospital. The median length of hospital stay was 7 days with interquartile range (IQR), 5–18 days.

The median day to the isolation of pulmonary TB patients was 1 day with IQR, 1–4 days. Figure 1 showed that over 60% patients isolated within 1 day. However, approximately 10% patients isolated over 10 days (Fig. 1). On univariate analysis, male gender (p = 0.009), prior

Table 1 Clinical characteristics and day-to-isolation univariate analysis ($N = 69$)

Characteristic	No.(%) or mean ± SD	Day-to-isolation (95% CI)	p-value
Patient factor			
Age (years)	81.1 ± 10.0		0.827
Male gender-no.(%)	51 (73.9)	8.2 (3.90–12.41)	0.009*
Female gender-no.(%)	18 (26.1)	1.8 (0.70–2.86)	
Smoking-no.(%)	40 (58.0)	6.6 (3.16–10.09)	0.585
Non-smoking-no.(%)	29 (42.0)	6.3 (0.24–12.38)	
Alcoholism-no.(%)	4 (5.8)	1.5 (0.52–2.48)	0.217
Non-alcoholism-no.(%)	65 (94.2)	6.8 (3.40–10.21)	
Welfare recipient-no.(%)	4 (5.8)	1.3 (0.76–1.74)	0.172
Non-welfare recipient-no.(%)	65 (94.2)	6.8 (3.41–10.22)	
Dependent ADL-no.(%)	12 (17.4)	11.5 (2.67–20.33)	0.129
Partially dependent ADL-no.(%)	20 (29.0)	8.7 (0.08–17.22)	
Independent ADL-no.(%)	37 (53.6)	3.7 (1.28–6.13)	
Past history of tuberculosis-no.(%)	28 (40.6)	3.0 (1.44–4.49)	0.073
Non-past history of tuberculosis-no.(%)	41 (59.4)	8.9 (3.69–14.12)	
Contact with tuberculosis patients-no.(%)	7 (10.1)	3.3 (0.01–6.56)	0.519
Non-contact with tuberculosis patients-no.(%)	62 (89.9)	6.9 (3.30–10.41)	
Diabetes mellitus-no.(%)	25 (37.3)	3.8 (1.19–6.49)	0.248
Non-diabetes mellitus-no.(%)	42 (60.9)	8.3 (3.31–13.31)	
Other lung disease-no.(%)	18 (26.1)	5.3 (0.73–9.83)	0.864
Non-other lung disease-no.(%)	51 (73.9)	6.9 (2.86–10.99)	
Gastric resection-no.(%)	8 (11.6)	4.8 (0.00–11.02)	0.593
Non-gastric resection-no.(%)	61 (88.4)	6.7 (3.16–10.28)	
Human immunodificiency virus infection -no.(%)	1 (1.4)	1.0 (1.00–1.00)	0.366
Non-human immunodificiency virus infection-no.(%)	68 (98.6)	6.6 (3.31–9.84)	
Preceding newer quinolone antibiotics-no.(%)	6 (8.7)	23.0 (0.00–51.14)	0.027*
Non-preceding newer quinolone antibiotics-no.(%)	63 (91.3)	4.9 (2.77–7.07)	
Steroid use-no.(%)	15 (21.7)	6.5 (0.38–12.55)	0.923
Non-steriod use-no.(%)	54 (78.3)	6.5 (2.72–10.28)	
Chronic cough-no.(%)	19 (27.5)	2.3 (0.81–3.82)	0.023*
Absence of chronic cough-no.(%)	50 (72.5)	8.1 (3.74–12.42)	
Appetite loss-no.(%)	48 (70.6)	8.5 (3.96–13.00)	0.037*
Absence of appetite loss-no.(%)	20 (29.0)	2.0 (1.36–2.64)	
BMI (kg/m^2)	19.0 ± 3.3		0.213
BT on arrival (°C)	37.2 ± 1.8		0.335
sBP on arrical (mmHg)	123.5 ± 30.3		0.768
Oxygen requirement-no.(%)	25 (36.2)	8.2 (0.89–15.51)	0.555
Non-oxygen requirement-no.(%)	44 (63.8)	5.5 (2.60–8.44)	
Haemoglobin level (g/dL)	11.9 ± 1.9		0.783
Serum albumin level (g/dL)	2.9 ± 0.6		0.348
CRP level (mg/dL)	9.3 ± 5.6		0.748
Cavitary lesion on the chest radiograph-no.(%)	15 (21.7)	1.3 (1.04–1.50)	0.005*

Table 1 Clinical characteristics and day-to-isolation univariate analysis (N = 69) *(Continued)*

Characteristic	No.(%) or mean ± SD	Day-to-isolation (95% CI)	p-value
Non-cavitary lesion on the chest radiograph-no.(%)	54 (78.3)	7.9 (3.91–11.98)	
Upper zone lesion on the chest radiograph-no.(%)	36 (52.2)	3.3 (1.33–5.17)	0.015*
Lesion located other than in the upper zone on the chest radiograph-no.(%)	33 (47.8)	10.0 (3.80–16.26)	
Disseminated lesion on the chest radiograph-no.(%)	32 (46.4)	3.3 (0.72–5.91)	0.028*
Non-disseminated lesion on the chest radiograph-no.(%)	37 (53.6)	9.2 (3.79–14.70)	
Raw score (from −30 points to 60 points)	29.2 ± 18.0		0.973
Medical facility and doctor factor			
Year of hospital visit (from 2008 to 2016)	2012.4 ± 2.6		0.151
Night-time arrival-no.(%)	27 (39.1)	8.7 (1.87–15.47)	0.248
Day-time arrival-no.(%)	42 (60.9)	5.1 (2.11–8.08)	
Weekend arrival-no.(%)	13 (18.8)	3.8 (1.06–6.48)	0.517
Weekday arrival-no.(%)	56 (81.2)	7.1 (3.22–11.03)	
Medical care provided by resident-no.(%)	27 (39.1)	7.1 (0.72–13.58)	0.844
Medical care provided by non-resident-no.(%)	42 (60.9)	6.1 (2.71–9.44)	
Medical care provided by male doctor-no.(%)	60 (87.0)	5.9 (2.64–9.20)	0.407
Medical care provided by female doctor-no.(%)	9 (13.0)	10.3 (0.00–22.07)	
Transferred to the hospital by ambulance-no.(%)	39 (56.5)	7.9 (2.74–13.16)	0.523
Transferred to the hospital by non-ambulance-no.(%)	30 (43.5)	4.6 (1.63–7.57)	
Attending ER physician-no.(%)	55 (79.7)	6.3 (2.53–10.05)	0.580
Attending non-ER physician-no.(%)	14 (20.3)	7.3 (1.27–13.30)	

Raw score is tuberculosis prognostic score, which is calculated as follows:
age(years) + (oxygen requirement, 10 points) − 20 × albumin (g/dl) + (ADL: independent, 0 point; semi-dependent, 5 points; totally dependent, 10 points)
Resident indicate physician who was graduated within two years
Based on logrank test or cox hazard crude model, where appropriate, *$p < 0.05$
CI confidence interval, *SD* = standard deviation, *ADL* activities of daily living, *BMI* body mass index, *BT* body temperature, *sBP* systolic blood pressure, *CRP* C-reactive protein, *ER* emergency room

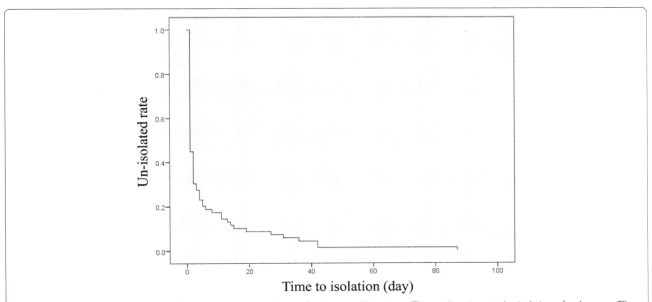

Fig. 1 Kaplan-Meier curve of the time from admission to isolation of pulmonary TB patients. The median time to the isolation of pulmonary TB patients was 1 day with interquartile range, 1–4 days

treatment with newer quinolone antibiotics ($p = 0.027$), absence of chronic cough ($p = 0.023$), appetite loss ($p = 0.037$), non-cavitary lesion on the chest radiograph ($p = 0.005$), lesion located other than in the upper zone on the chest radiograph ($p = 0.015$), and non-disseminated lesion on the chest radiograph ($p = 0.028$) were significant factors associated with a delayed isolation of pulmonary TB patients (Table 1).

On multivariate analysis using Cox hazard model, male gender (hazard ratio [HR], 0.47; 95% confidence interval [CI], 0.25 to 0.89; $P = 0.02$), absence of chronic cough (HR, 0.52; 95% CI, 0.28 to 0.95; $P = 0.033$), and non-cavitary lesion on the chest radiograph (HR, 0.46; 95% CI, 0.23 to 0.92; $P = 0.028$) were significantly associated with delayed isolation of TB patients (Table 2).

Figure 2 showed intergroup comparisons of day-to-isolation among significant factors associated with delayed isolation of pulmonary TB patients in the multivariate analysis.

Discussion

Our study revealed that male gender, absence of chronic cough, and non-cavitary lesion on the chest radiograph were associated with delayed isolation of active pulmonary TB patients.

A non-cavitary lesion on the chest radiograph and absence of chronic cough are factors consistent with previous reports of diagnostic delay in cases of pulmonary TB; our findings of association of male gender with diagnostic delay is contrary to the findings of previous studies. Chronic cough is an important symptom for the clinician to consider the diagnosis of pulmonary TB from the clinical history. Moreover, a previous report of in-hospital diagnostic delay from Southern Taiwan revealed non-cavitary lesion on the chest radiograph as an independent risk factor [14], similar to our finding. A chest radiograph is commonly employed and easy to perform; presence of a cavitary lesion is critical in the early detection of pulmonary TB. In previous systematic reviews and meta-analyses, female gender has been shown to be a risk factor for delayed diagnosis of pulmonary TB [11, 12]; there are no previous reports of male gender being associated with delay in isolation of pulmonary TB patients.

We speculate that the delay in isolation associated with male gender, absence of chronic cough and non-cavitary lesion on the chest radiograph, may be related to the advanced age of our patients (mean age: 81.1 years). Younger patients with smear-positive TB were referred to other hospitals with special wards, resulting in an increase in elderly patients with TB in our hospital. Elderly patients with TB can manifest with unusual features that may be confused with aspiration pneumonia [17], commonly observed in this population [18]. The typical symptoms of aspiration pneumonia are fever, cough with sputum, and dyspnea; however, non-specific symptoms including loss of consciousness and appetite loss are also important. Thus, the symptoms of pulmonary TB and aspiration pneumonia are similar. Moreover, aspiration pneumonia, a common disease in an aging society, can co-exist in patients with active pulmonary TB and has drawn increasing attention recently [19]. Although the incidence of active pulmonary TB has decreased, the number of elderly patients has increased in Japan [20]. There may be a lack of widespread awareness among healthcare workers, including physicians, of this development. This may have led to failure to consider pulmonary TB in elderly patients. Besides, the symptoms of pulmonary TB can mimic aspiration pneumonia in the elderly.

Although previous studies have described factors associated with delayed diagnosis of pulmonary TB [11–13, 15, 21–27], we focused on factors that delayed isolation, especially among elderly patients admitted to hospital. To the best of our knowledge, ours is the first study that deals with delayed isolation of pulmonary TB patients in an aging society [28, 29]. According to nation-wide Japanese data, the number of patients over 70 years with smear-positive pulmonary TB has increased by 2.5 times from 1980 to 2000 [20, 30]. In an aging society, the

Table 2 Associated factors with delayed isolation among patients with smear positive tuberculosis

Variable	Adjusted HR	95% CI for HR	P value
Male gender	0.47	(0.249 to 0.888)	0.020*
Appetite loss	0.63	(0.351 to 1.133)	0.123
Absence of chronic cough	0.52	(0.279 to 0.948)	0.033*
Preceding newer quinolone antibiotics	0.50	(0.190 to 1.290)	0.150
Non-cavitary lesion on the chest radiograph	0.46	(0.233 to 0.922)	0.028*
Non-upper zone lesion on the chest radiograph	0.64	(0.367 to 1.124)	0.120
Non-disseminated lesion on the chest radiograph	0.82	(0.479 to 1.404)	0.470

Multivariable Cox proportional hazards model including all factors $p < 0.05$ in univariate analysis
HR hazard ratio, CI confidence interval, CRP C-reactive protein
*$p < 0.05$

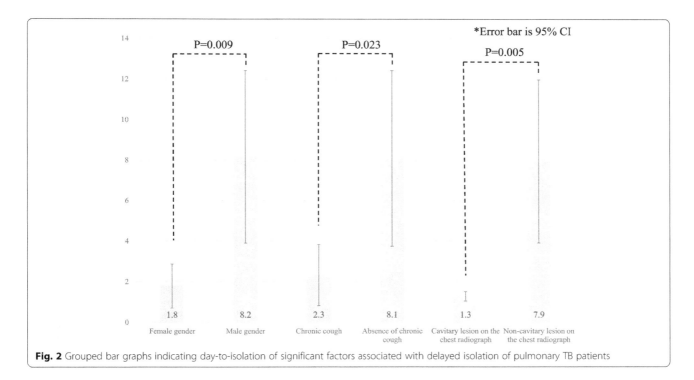

Fig. 2 Grouped bar graphs indicating day-to-isolation of significant factors associated with delayed isolation of pulmonary TB patients

number of older patients with smear-positive pulmonary TB may have increased in community-based acute care hospitals. However, there are few reports of elderly patients with pulmonary TB. Thus, our results may be of relevance in an aging society.

There are several limitations to our study. First, ours was based on a single center cohort study with a small sample size. The clinical ability of our residents was variable, depending on their level of training and experience, which may have led to bias. In our study model, a $p < 0.05$ was used as the cutoff level. This strict criteria though can prematurely exclude relevant variables, which may lead to selection bias. Second, we are unable to establish a causal relationship in this retrospective observational study. Further prospective studies are required to confirm such an association. Third, as it was a hospital-based study, we could not analyze factors involving delay from symptoms onset to hospital visit, reported as "patient delay" in a previous study [16]. Fourth, the present study may not include all in-hospital patients with smear-positive pulmonary TB, because there can be presence of the patients who discharged or died before the investigation of sputum or gastric smear.

Future research needs to be directed to understanding factors associated with a delayed diagnosis of active pulmonary TB; this information may help with earlier isolation of TB patients, improve infection control, and reduce adverse outcomes. Therefore, multi-center, prospective studies are required, across different population groups, in countries with aging populations, to corroborate our results.

Conclusion

Isolation of active pulmonary TB patients was delayed in male patients, patients without chronic cough, and patients with non-cavitary lesions on the chest radiograph. Elderly TB patients can present with atypical manifestations that mimic other diseases. Thus, physicians need to have a heightened awareness of active pulmonary TB, especially among elderly patients; this may prevent spread of infection within the hospital.

Abbreviations
CI: Confidence interval; ER: Emergency room; HR: Hazard ratio; IQR: Interquartile range; TB: Tuberculosis

Authors' contributions
NS and TS conceived the idea of the work and collected data. NS performed the analysis. NS and TY interpreted the results, KI supervised throughout the project. All authors read and approved the final manuscript.

Competing interests
The authors declare that they have no competing interests.

Author details
[1]Department of General Internal Medicine, Shonan Kamakura General Hospital, 1370-1 Okamoto, Kamakura, Kanagawa, Japan. [2]Department of General Medicine, Iizuka Hospital, Fukuoka, Japan. [3]Muribushi Okinawa Project for Teaching Hospitals, Okinawa, Okinawa Prefecture, Japan. [4]Department of Internal Medicine, Hayama Heart Center, Hayama, Kanagawa, Japan. [5]Unit of Public Health and Preventive Medicine, School of Medicine, Yokohama City University, Yokohama, Kanagawa, Japan.

References

1. Centers for Disease Control and Prevention. Guidelines for preventing the transmission of Mycobacterium tuberculosis in health-care settings. 2005. https://www.cdc.gov/mmwr/pdf/rr/rr5417.pdf. Accessed 21 May 2018.
2. Storla DG, Yimer S, Bjune GA. A systematic review of delay in the diagnosis and treatment of tuberculosis. BMC Public Health. 2008;8:15.
3. Dye C, Scheele S, Dolin P, Pathania V, Raviglione MC. Consensus statement. Global burden of tuberculosis: estimated incidence, prevalence, and mortality by country. WHO global surveillance and monitoring project. JAMA. 1999;232(7):677–86.
4. Bjune G. Tuberculosis in the 21st century: an emerging pandemic? Norsk Epidemiol. 2005;15(2):133–9.
5. Tuberculosis surveillance center. Tuberculosis Annual Report 2012. (1). Summary of tuberculosis notification statistics and foreign-born tuberculosis patients. Kekkaku. 2014;89(6):619–25.
6. Nakao M, Sone K, Kagawa Y, et al. Diagnostic delay of pulmonary tuberculosis in patients with acute respiratory distress syndrome associated with aspiration pneumonia: two case reports and a mini-review from Japan. Exp Ther Med. 2016;12(2):835–9.
7. Fukushima Y, Shiobara K, Shiobara T, et al. Patients in whom active tuberculosis was diagnosed after admission to a Japanese university hospital from 2005 through 2007. J Infect Chemother. 2011;17(5):652–7.
8. Horita N, Miyazawa N, Yoshiyama T, et al. Development and validation of a tuberculosis prognostic score for smear-positive in-patients in Japan. Int J Tuberc Lung Dis. 2013;17(1):54–60.
9. World Health Organization. Global tuberculosis report 2017: World Health Organization; 2017. http://www.who.int/tb/publications/global_report/gtbr2017_main_text.pdf. Accessed 21 May 2018.
10. Golub JE, Bur S, Cronin WA, et al. Delayed tuberculosis diagnosis and tuberculosis transmission. Int J Tuberc Lung Dis. 2006;10(1):24–30.
11. Cai J, Wang X, Ma A, Wang Q, Han X, Li Y. Factors associated with patient and provider delays for tuberculosis diagnosis and treatment in Asia: a systematic review and meta-analysis. PLoS One. 2015;10(3):e0120088.
12. Li Y, Ehiri J, Tang S, et al. Factors associated with patient, and diagnostic delays in Chinese TB patients: a systematic review and meta-analysis. BMC Med. 2013;11:156.
13. Chen TC, Lu PL, Lin CY, Lin WR, Chen YH. Fluoroquinolones are associated with delayed treatment and resistance in tuberculosis: a systematic review and meta-analysis. Int J Infect Dis. 2011;15(3):e211–6.
14. Lin CY, Lin WR, Chen TC, et al. Why is in-hospital diagnosis of pulmonary tuberculosis delayed in southern Taiwan? J Formos Med Assoc. 2010;109(4):269–77.
15. Yimer S, Bjune G, Alene G. Diagnostic and treatment delay among pulmonary tuberculosis patients in Ethiopia: a cross sectional study. BMC Infect Dis. 2005;5:112.
16. Chiang CY, Chang CT, Chang RE, Li CT, Huang RM. Patient and health system delays in the diagnosis and treatment of tuberculosis in southern Taiwan. Int J Tuberc Lung Dis. 2005;9(9):1006–12.
17. Yoshikawa TT. Tuberculosis in aging adults. J Am Geriatr Soc. 1992;40(2):178–87.
18. Teramoto S, Fukuchi Y, Sasaki H, Sato K, Sekizawa K, Matsuse T. High incidence of aspiration pneumonia in community- and hospital-acquired pneumonia in hospitalized patients: a multicenter, prospective study in Japan. J Am Geriatr Soc. 2008;56(3):577–9.
19. Ubukata S, Jingu D, Yajima T, Shoji M, Takahashi H. Occurrence and clinical characteristics of tuberculosis among home medical care patients. Kekkaku. 2014;89(7):649–54.
20. Ohmori M, Ishikawa N, Yoshiyama T, Uchimura K, Aoki M, Mori T. Current epidemiological trend of tuberculosis in Japan. Int J Tuberc Lung Dis. 2002;6(5):415–23.
21. Basnet R, Hinderaker SG, Enarson D, Malla P, Morkve O. Delay in the diagnosis of tuberculosis in Nepal. BMC Public Health. 2009;9:236.
22. Meyssonnier V, Li X, Shen X, et al. Factors associated with delayed tuberculosis diagnosis in China. Eur J Pub Health. 2013;23(2):253–7.
23. Gagliotti C, Resi D, Moro ML. Delay in the treatment of pulmonary TB in a changing demographic scenario. Int J Tuberc Lung Dis. 2006;10(3):305–9.
24. Liam CK, Tang BG. Delay in the diagnosis and treatment of pulmonary tuberculosis in patients attending a university teaching hospital. Int J Tuberc Lung Dis. 1997;1(4):326–32.
25. Rajeswari R, Chandrasekaran V, Suhadev M, Sivasubramaniam S, Sudha G, Renu G. Factors associated with patient and health system delays in the diagnosis of tuberculosis in South India. Int J Tuberc Lung Dis. 2002;6(9):789–95.
26. Sreeramareddy CT, Qin ZZ, Satyanarayana S, Subbaraman R, Pai M. Delays in diagnosis and treatment of pulmonary tuberculosis in India: a systematic review. Int J Tuberc Lung Dis. 2014;18(3):255–66.
27. Xu B, Jiang QW, Xiu Y, Diwan VK. Diagnostic delays in access to tuberculosis care in counties with or without the National Tuberculosis Control Programme in rural China. Int J Tuberc Lung Dis. 2005;9(7):784–90.
28. Severin J, Ruhe-van der Werff S, Bakker M, Vos MC. Risk factors for delayed isolation of tuberculosis patients in a tertiary care hospital in a low-incidence country. Antimicrob Resist Infect Control. 2015;4(Suppl 1):93.
29. Hsieh MJ, Liang HW, Chiang PC, et al. Delayed suspicion, treatment and isolation of tuberculosis patients in pulmonology/infectious diseases and non-pulmonology/infectious diseases wards. J Formos Med Assoc. 2009;108(3):202–9.
30. Japan Anti-Tuberculosis Association. Statistics of tuberculosis 2001. Tokyo: JATA; 2001.

"The missing ingredient": the patient perspective of health related quality of life in bronchiectasis

Emily K. Dudgeon[1], Megan Crichton[2] and James D. Chalmers[2*]

Abstract

Background: Bronchiectasis is a heterogeneous disease which affects quality of life. Measuring symptoms and quality of life has proved challenging and research is limited by extrapolation of questionnaires and treatments from other diseases. The objective of this study was to identify the major contributors to quality of life in bronchiectasis and to evaluate existing health related quality of life questionnaires in bronchiectasis.

Methods: Eight adults with bronchiectasis participated in one to one semi-structured interviews. These were recorded and transcribed verbatim. Thematic analysis was used to identify core themes relevant to disease burden and impact. Participant views on current health related quality of life questionnaires were also surveyed.

Results: Bronchiectasis symptoms are highly individual. Core themes identified were symptom burden, symptom variation, personal measurement, quality of life and control of symptoms. Themes contributing to quality of life were: social embarrassment, sleep disturbance, anxiety and modification of daily and future activities. Evaluation of 4 existing questionnaires established their individual strengths and weaknesses. A synthesis of the participants' perspective identified desirable characteristics to guide future tool development.

Conclusions: This qualitative study has identified core themes associated with symptoms and quality of life in bronchiectasis. Current treatments and quality of life tools do not fully address or capture the burden of disease in bronchiectasis from the patients' perspective.

Keywords: Bronchiectasis, Symptoms, Endpoints, Questionnaires, Qualitative

Background

Bronchiectasis is a chronic respiratory disease characterised by cough, sputum production and frequent chest infections [1, 2]. These symptoms impact health related quality of life (HRQL). HRQL questionnaires have become a useful tool for measuring the impact of disease on patients' lives and are essential to assess new treatments in clinical trials [3–5]. HRQL questionnaires have been developed for respiratory conditions such as COPD, asthma and chronic cough [6–9]. There is some overlap between symptoms of bronchiectasis and those of COPD and asthma, and two of these HRQL questionnaires (St George's Respiratory Questionnaire and Leicester Cough Questionnaire) have been validated for use in bronchiectasis. [3, 7]. However it was not until 2014 that a HRQL questionnaire designed specifically for bronchiectasis was published [10]. There are no large comparative studies to determine which is the best HRQL questionnaire for bronchiectasis.

The quality of life bronchiectasis questionnaire (QoL-B) was developed in the context of a clinical trial of an inhaled antibiotic and has not been tested widely in broad populations of patients with bronchiectasis [11].

In recent years, there has been a shift away from a traditional model of research where doctors or those working in the pharmaceutical industry decide on the best outcome measure when assessing new treatments. The patient led model of research recognises the value in patient involvement at every stage of clinical research, and best practices have now been identified [12]. There have been a series of unsuccessful trials in bronchiectasis. Treatments that are widely used in clinical

* Correspondence: jchalmers@dundee.ac.uk
[2]Division of Molecular and Clinical Medicine, University of Dundee, Dundee DD1 9SY, UK
Full list of author information is available at the end of the article

practice, and believed to be effective by clinicians and patients, may give only small changes in questionnaires, perhaps because we are unable to effectively measure what matters to patients with bronchiectasis [13–16].

A major limitation affecting all bronchiectasis research is that tools, approaches, questionnaires and treatments have generally been extrapolated from other diseases. There have been few studies specifically addressing the opinions, experiences and needs of patients with bronchiectasis.

Bronchiectasis is a distinct, heterogeneous condition in its own right [17]. Quality of life in particular is deeply personal and specific to an individual. Patients' quality of life may be determined by more than simply the number and frequency of physical symptoms but also by social, psychological and other personal factors [4–9].

In view of the importance of health related quality of life questionnaires for understanding bronchiectasis disease burden and as an outcome in clinical trials, we conducted a qualitative study to determine what contributes to quality of life in bronchiectasis patients and to gather patient views and opinions on how existing questionnaires reflect their quality of life. Finally we present a synthesis of bronchiectasis patients' evaluation of existing health related quality of life questionnaires, including the identification of desirable characteristics, with the aim of guiding development of more patient focussed, responsive and meaningful HRQL tools in future.

Methods

We performed a qualitative study of patients with bronchiectasis attending a regional specialist clinic at Ninewells Hospital in Dundee, UK.

The *inclusion criteria* were: A clinical diagnosis of bronchiectasis confirmed by CT scanning, an ability to communicate in English, respiratoy symptoms that are caused by the primary diagnosis of bronchiectasis. Key *exclusion criteria* were: Inability to give informed consent; diagnosis of cystic fibrosis, severe COPD or severe asthma. The study was approved by the North West Ethics Committee- approval number 16-NW-0100. All patients provided written informed consent for participate.

Study interviews

The study consisted of a single in depth semi-structured interview approximately one hour in length. Interviews explored the nature, variation and impact of symptoms, and the value of existing questionnaires as outlined below. Interviews were audio-recorded and transcribed verbatim. The interviewer was not involved in the clinical care of the participants, and was trained in qualitative methodology but did not have experience in bronchiectasis. This was desirable to avoid conscious or unconscious biases determined by prior experience with bronchiectasis patients.

Analysis

Transcripts were analysed by the researchers and common themes were identified by thematic analysis. Following Strauss and Corbin (1998) text was analysed line by line [18].

Responses were initially coded and grouped according to the research objectives [19]. Common themes and responses were identified. The researchers modified their coding and groups according to participant responses. Interviews were participant driven, with the researcher attending to understanding participants' perspectives from their point of view and using terminology common to participants identified through the interviews. Sample size was determined empirically, and was terminated at participant 8 after reaching data saturation, in which no new themes were identified.

The primary outcome of the study was to understand the symptom burden of bronchiectasis and the key determinants of quality of life. Secondary objectives were to evaluate those symptoms that change most frequently with exacerbations. Finally the study aimed to evaluate how well existing questionnaires captured participants' symptoms and quality of life, and the accessibility and ease of use of questionnaires from a patient perspective. The interview schedule which addresses each of these objectives is shown in Table 1.

Questionnaires

Participants were presented with the questionnaires at least 24 h before the interview in order to have time to become familiar with and to complete the questionnaires.

The questionnaires selected for use in this study were based on those identified in a systematic review of the literature as being used in bronchiectasis studies to evaluate symptoms or quality of life. These were

St. Georges Respiratory Questionnaire [3]
Quality of life bronchiectasis questionnaire version 3.1 [4]
Leicester Cough Questionnaire [7]
COPD assessment test [20]

Table 1 Interview outline

Symptom burden
   What daily symptoms of bronchiectasis do you experience?
   How do symptoms vary from day to day?
   Is there a way to quantify changes- how do participants express differences in how you are feeling (to doctors and to other patients)?
Exacerbations
   What changes when you have an exacerbation?
   What are the key symptoms that lead you to seek medical help?
Existing questionnaires
   How well do these reflect your symptoms and the changes in your symptoms?
   Do you find the questionnaires easy to understand and answer?
   How could you improve them?

The St George's Respiratory Questionnaire is a 50 item tool with 2–5 responses per item (mean 2.5), 5 A4 pages in length, giving a score of 0–100 points where 0 is no impairment of quality of life and 100 is maximum impairment. We note that there are 3 versions each with a different recall time (1 month, 3 months and 1 year), and the 3 month version was used in this study.

Quality of Life Bronchiectasis questionnaire is a 37 item tool with 2–6 responses per item (mean 4.1), 3 A4 pages in length, giving a score from 0 to 100 in each of 8 domains (respiratory symptoms, physical, role, emotional and social, vitality, health perceptions, treatment burden) and overall, where 0 is maximum impairment of quality of life and 100 is no impairment. It has a recall time of 1 week.

Leicester Cough Questionnaire is a 19 item tool with 7 responses per item on one A4 page, giving a score of 1–7 for each of 3 domains- physical, psychological and social and a total score of 3–21 with a higher score indicating minimal impairment on quality of life. It has a 24 h recall time.

COPD Assessment Test is an 8 item tool with 6 numerical responses per item, on one A4 page, giving a score out of 40. A higher score suggests a greater impact on quality of life. It has no specified recall time.

People living with bronchiectasis are referred to as patients and those who were interviewed for this study will be referred to as participants.

Results

Eleven consecutive patients were invited to participate and 8 interviews were carried out (5 female, 3 male). The mean age was 72 (63–80). 4 had idiopathic bronchiectasis, 2 had post-infective bronchiectasis. 1 participant had co-existing COPD and 1 participant had co-existing mild asthma (Table 2).

Thematic analysis of the interviews identified 5 key determinants of symptom burden and quality of life. Although our pre-specified analysis had intended to consider exacerbation impact separately from stable disease burden, our interviews revealed that participants regarded exacerbations as an integral part of daily disease impact. Participants did not regard exacerbations as a separate state from stable disease, but rather a continuum where daily symptoms become more severe or persistent. Participants defined an exacerbation as a worsening of symptoms, and recognised that this means they need to seek medical help, however, sometimes patients do not seek medical help and try to self-manage. In addition, all participants reported that exacerbations impacted on daily quality of life even when "well" because of anxiety around exacerbations and the modifying of activity and future plans due to risk of exacerbations (Fig. 1).

Table 2 Participant characteristics

Characteristics	N (%) or median (IQR)
N	8
Age- mean-range	72 (range 63–80)
Gender	5/8 (62.5%) female
Smoking history	6/8 (75%) never smokers
FEV1% predicted (mean-sd)	71.6% (24.4)
Bronchiectasis severity index (mean-sd)	8.6 (4.4)
Cause of bronchiectasis	
Idiopathic	4 (50%)
Post-infective	2 (25%)
Sjogrens syndrome	1 (12.5%)
Ulcerative colitis	1 (12.5%)
Exacerbations per year (mean-sd)	1.8 (1.3)
Pseudomonas aeruginosa infection	3 (38%)
Long term macrolide use	4 (50%)

Therefore exacerbations have been included in the following analysis as part of symptom burden. Table 3 shows an example of the analysis whereby individual responses were coded and then grouped into common themes.

The themes included were symptom burden, symptom variation, personal measurement of symptoms, quality of life and control. Symptom burden, symptom variation, and quality of life were pre-specified terms while personal measurement of symptoms and control were added based on consistent reporting by participants.

Theme 1: Symptom burden

A combination of cough, breathlessness and sputum production was present in all participants although the relative importance of each of these symptoms was highly variable when describing the impact on their quality of life.

Participant 4 "So, yeah, that, bronchiectasis, its, the biggest thing is breathlessness."

Participant 5 "The main one is that I, I cough a lot, and I cough a lot of phlegm up, erm I'm also very, I feel very short of breath sometimes."

5/8 described chest tightness as a prominent symptom in addition to breathlessness, cough and sputum production.

Participant 7 "I have like a film forms across my chest."

Additional symptoms that were reported were decreased energy levels (7/8), swallowing difficulties (3/8) and hoarse voice (2/8).

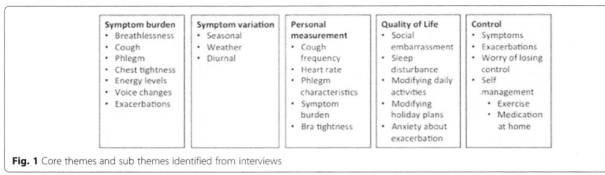

Fig. 1 Core themes and sub themes identified from interviews

Exacerbations were commonly (7/8) described as an increase in symptom burden accompanied by a feeling of being generally unwell.

Participant 1 "Erm, just general feeling not good, you know, and tired, and erm breathless, erm a lot more phlegm, using my inhaler a lot more"

Another participant described their exacerbations much more in terms of change in character of cough and increased sputum purulence, without necessarily feeling generally unwell.

Increased sputum purulence is regarded by guidelines as a core symptom of exacerbation. In this cohort, change in sputum colour was mentioned as a key symptom of exacerbation in only 4/8 participants. Participants described changes in sputum in many different ways using taste, volume, viscosity and colour with each giving different weight to each character.

Participant 7 "The mucus gets really tacky and it doesnae (does not) clear"

Theme 2: Symptom variation

Participants (5/8) commonly experienced diurnal variation in their symptoms. For some participants symptoms were worse in the morning, while for others they were worse in the afternoon or evening.

Participant 6 "I don't seem to have a problem until about 4 o clock in the afternoon… Yeah I do tend to avoid, meeting people you know, between four [pm] and six [pm]."

Environmental factors such as the weather, smoke, dust and paint also affected participants' symptoms.

Participant 7 "I like, like going to watch the football, but if it, if it's a damp rainy cold night then I'm no going. I'll just say nah because I'll feel really horrendous the next day."

There was no characteristic pattern to participants' symptoms with the diurnal variation being highly individual.

Theme 3: Personal measurement of symptoms

During the interviews it became clear that participants monitor their symptoms in different ways. Participants often expressed this in terms of the difference between a good day and a bad day. Most participants (6/8) had their own individual way of measuring how they are on any given day.

Interviewer: is there anything else that you can measure how bad you're feeling on one specific day?
Participant 1: "It's a strange one. My bra gets tight. [laughs]".

Participant 3 "I know I'm getting an infection if it [phlegm] goes through a colour change and my pulse rate goes up. My pulse rate is normally about 58/60 and that goes 70/75."

Some participants (4/8) know when an exacerbation is coming on because of symptoms that consistently occur at the onset.

Table 3 Example of the coding and grouping approaches for analysis

Participant information	Coding	Common theme
"I have like a film forming across my chest"	Chest tightness	Symptom burden
"Coughing usually starts about twelve O'Clock and it doesn't have any rhyme or reason"	Diurnal variation	Symptom variation
"Right, if somebody comes round to your house, you get a visitor who goes 'I'm not feeling well' then I just say 'well go away, just go, stay away from me'."	Social anxiety	Quality of life
"how do you define moderate difficulty and a little difficulty"	Questionnaire answers	Questionnaires

Participant 2 "When I have an exacerbation, yes, I tend first of all to start getting hot and cold flushes, …I then start to become dizzy. I start to cough a lot more."

The other participants had more heterogeneous, unpredictable events without characteristic symptoms at onset.

Theme 4: Quality of life
All of the participants agreed that the disease had a major impact on their quality of life. Impacts on quality life were diverse, taking in social embarrassment associated with cough and sputum, sleep disturbance, modification of activities and holiday plans, and anxiety or concern about developing exacerbations.

Participants feel embarrassed about sputum production in public.

Participant 5 "I'm worried about that [coughing when talking to someone] because 1) I don't like to do it 2) they might think its unhygienic and erm 3) I do think its unhygienic myself."

Participants feel they have to explain their symptoms.

Participant 4 "I have come out of church a couple of times and it upsets people because they think is she going to die out there or whatever."

Participant 5 "whoever it is will think you're giving them the bug of death or something you know."

Symptoms also cause participants to avoid certain situations.

Participant 7 "I wouldnae (would not) want to go to the pictures or a theatre… It would spoil other people's enjoyment."

Symptoms during the night can cause significant sleep disturbance, with several participants sleeping in separate rooms to their partner so as not to disturb them.

Participant 2 "I do cough a lot…especially at night time trying to get to sleep. That, erm, is a concern for me, not to unduly disturb my wife."

Symptom burden and seasonal and diurnal symptom variation has forced many participants to modify their daily activities.

Participant 7 "as I say you can't go in the winter months you cannae go out the walking that you do so you're confined to the house a wee bitty more, so you get a wee bitty fed up so you munch a wee bitty more and you put on a bit more weight that you've just took off."

The unpredictability of an exacerbation causes significant anxiety for participants and their families, particularly around planning travel and family events. For example, the word anxiety was mentioned 21 times by a single participant.

Theme 5: Control
Lack of control over symptoms was consistently reported (5/8) as a key impact of the disease. Control was frequently (7/8) mentioned in interviews and only one participant felt they were always in control of their condition. One participant cited control as the one thing they would change about the condition if they could.

Participant 4 " I don't have control over my cough…I mean you can grab the bottle of water and hope it shuts up for a minute or two but it's not, you know, I don't feel I control it all."

Regular exercise (4/8) and having antibiotics at home to self-manage exacerbations made participants feel that they had more control over their condition.

Participant 1 (regarding self-management with antibiotics at home) "And you feel as if you've got control. You know, that you can do something. Cos if the doctor's surgery is closed over the weekend, what do you do?"

Exacerbations can take away the feeling of having control which can cause anxiety.

Participant 2 "Well I feel very dependent on others. And that to some extent is debilitating. It's almost humiliating at times."

Evaluation of questionnaires
Evaluation of existing questionnaires identified desirable and undesirable characteristics (Fig. 2) for HRQL questionnaires used in bronchiectasis. Participants commented on the extent to which questions were understandable and reflective of their experience, the extent to which answer options gave them scope to express how they felt and the layout of questions in terms of ease of use and time taken for completion. Participants varied in their knowledge of medical terms. For example, commonly used terms like wheeze were considered jargon and poorly understood by many participants.

Figure 2 shows the aspects of questionnaires that participants did and did not value.

Desirable characteristics	Undesirable characteristics
Questions	
Cover full symptom burden and effect on quality of life	Cover only symptoms or quality of life or only elements of either
Appropriate for those with limited mobility/co morbidities	Inappropriate for immobility/co morbidities
Appropriate for those who retired before or because of condition	Questions asking about effect on work with no option for retirees
Recall time 1-4 weeks	Recall time <1 or >4 weeks
Clarity of question	Use of jargon
Answers	
3-7 answers	True/false
Use of numbers and phrases	Use of only numbers or phrases
Comparison to patient's baseline	No comparison to patient's baseline
N/A option	No N/A option
Opportunity to explain factors affecting symptom variation	No opportunity to explain factors affecting symptom variation
Layout	
Visual scale for answers	Answers as text
Clear text size	Too small
Length- 2 pages, 20 questions max	Length- more than 2 pages or 20 questions

Fig. 2 Participants' perspective on different health related quality of life and symptom questionnaires in bronchiectasis

Referring to specific questionnaires:
SGRQ- Participants reported that true and false answering method was very clear but gave too limited scope for answering questions, and suggested the use of a baseline. The questionnaire requires a recall time of 3 months which concerned some participants.

Participant 5 "again, the true and false, is just, it's not, you're not giving enough information to people.".

Participant 4 "Over the past 3 months, in an average week how many good days? Its, it's a long time to remember"

QolB- This was the most commonly preferred questionnaire (6/8 participants). The number of multiple choice answers were viewed favourably when compared to the true and false of the SGRQ and the seven choices of the LCQ, but participants felt the questions were sometimes ambiguous. While some participants felt that seven choices were too many, others viewed the increased number of options as favourable.

Participant 7 "During the past week indicate how often you have felt well. Again relative to what? What's your baseline? The word "well", is meaningless. It is its meaningless. No I'm no as well as I should be but am I as bad as I could be? No so what's well?"

CAT- The layout was praised for its simplicity and ease of reading but there was disagreement as to whether the visual scale from 0 to 5 was easy or difficult to answer.

Participant 2 "I like the layout... It's very visual."

Participant 4 "I found it very difficult to judge erm, which one, sort of, represented it"

LCQ- The layout was criticised but compared with the other questionnaires, the LCQ's answers have numbers and phrases which was considered favourable.

Participant 6 "Well it gave you more choices, there was, there was seven choices but it gave you much more, you could more accurately describe what your symptoms were."

Overall, the strengths and weaknesses of the different questionnaires from the bronchiectasis patient's perspective is summarised in Fig. 3.

Discussion

This qualitative study of symptom burden and quality of life in bronchiectasis has identified a disconnect between the classic symptoms of bronchiectasis (such as sputum production, purulence and exacerbations) and the impact on patients' quality of life. Our analysis suggests

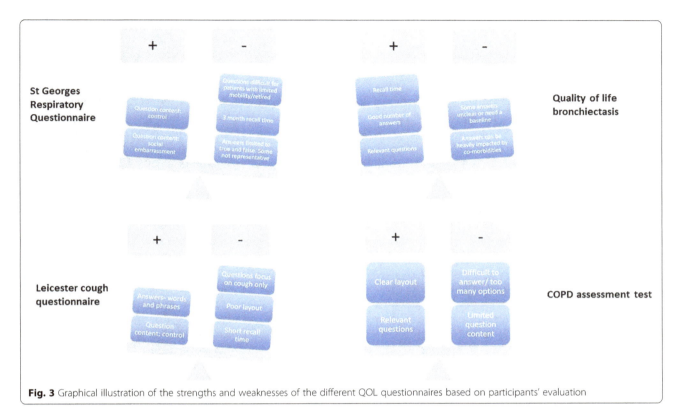

Fig. 3 Graphical illustration of the strengths and weaknesses of the different QOL questionnaires based on participants' evaluation

that what most strongly affects a patient's quality of life is highly personal to the individual, but includes an ability to feel in control of their symptoms, to achieve normal sleep and take part in social activities without embarrassment. Anxiety and fear of exacerbations had a major impact on quality of life.

These findings are important for clinical care, because many of these are aspects that are not frequently explored in a doctor-patient consultation. They are important for the development of new therapies because treatments aiming to improve quality of life need to be capable of addressing the major determinants of quality of life [21, 22].

Quality of life tools are used in clinical practice and in clinical trials to measure disease impact and response to therapy. We conducted what to the best of our knowledge is the only comparative "preference" study relating to quality of life tools in bronchiectasis. This analysis found that each of the questionnaires have different strengths and weaknesses. Discussion of these has allowed us to develop a framework for the "perfect" quality of life tool from a bronchiectasis patient's perspective. We identified that the quality of life bronchiectasis questionnaire was the most frequently preferred questionnaire from a patient perspective. It should be noted that the clinical value of a questionnaire includes its repeatability, responsiveness and clinical utility and that patient preference and ease of use is only one aspect of the evaluating a questionnaire [3, 4].

An interesting finding was disparity between how patients describe symptoms and how they are evaluated in questionnaires. A question may try to quantify exercise limitation in terms of mild or moderate difficulty, whereas patients do not think about symptoms in this way. Patients were consistently more focussed on "change from baseline" or differences between what they can achieve and what they want to achieve, which is highly individual. It is intuitively correct, and was expressed by the majority of patients, that you cannot accurately quantify something without a frame of reference. Patients find it much more straightforward to say they are "worse than usual" than to say they have "moderate difficulty" carrying out a task, without a frame of reference for how much difficulty a person without bronchiectasis might experience.

It is not surprising that bronchiectasis symptoms and quality of life determinants are heterogeneous because the disease itself is heterogeneous. It is caused by a range of underlying disorders, affecting all age groups and having a highly variable clinical course [23–26]. This emphasises one of the key findings of this research- it may be impossible to fully capture disease impact with categorical scales that do not account for patient's highly variable baseline symptoms, expectations and co-morbidities [22, 26]. As mentioned above, patients reported that anchoring questions within patients own baseline function could provide a solution to this heterogeneity. An example of an anchored question would be:

How is your breathlessness at the moment?

- My breathless is much better than normal
- My breathless is better than normal
- My breathless is normal for me
- My breathlessness is worse than normal for me
- My breathlessness is much worse than normal

compared to an unanchored question such as:
Walking up a flight of stairs makes me feel breathless.

- True
- False

Our study suggested the "perfect" questionnaire would use both anchored and unanchored questions to establish the patients baseline with a second question or set of questions to establish change from baseline.

There are similarities between our findings and those of qualitative studies in COPD and asthma in terms of symptom burden, anxiety, the benefit of exercise, control and self monitoring [27, 28]. It is interesting to note that the worry of asthma attacks is similar to that of exacerbations in bronchiectasis in impacting quality of life even when patients are not experiencing symptoms. Although it was not identified as a major theme, control was discussed in both the COPD and asthma studies. Similar to the current study, it was mentioned in a number of contexts: for example in asthma patients not being able to control the external environment leading to exposure to triggers and in COPD patients trying to take control of their condition.

Self monitoring differed between asthma and bronchiectasis patients. Whereas asthma patients are able to use the objective measure of peak expiratory flow rate, bronchiectasis patients have no objective measurement of their symptoms. As a result, self monitoring tends to be more subjective, and more individualised in bronchiectasis.

The COPD study reported that objective measurement of severity does not correlate with patient experience. The authors hypothesise that this may be attributable to variations in coping strategies and self management, and that patients with poor quality of life scores may be most suitable for non pharmacological interventions. The use of data measuring patient reported impact on quality of life in guiding management is an interesting suggestion, particularly as medicine and clinical research transition from a traditional paternalistic style to a patient led model.

Another qualitative study compared 3 quality of life questionnaires used in asthma [29]. Participants identified missing and irrelevant content when assessing questionnaires as weaknesses. Similar to the current study, confusing questions were identified as a weakness in several questionnaires and the questionnaire preferred by participants was one that covered both medical and psychosocial impact of disease. This is in line with our findings on how bronchiectasis impacts quality of life.

Therefore our findings are consistent with work in other chronic respiratory conditions but with disease specific features because of the subtle differences in the combination of symptoms present in each disease.

Limitations of this study must be acknowledged. This is a qualitative study and as is typical of such studies the sample size is small. This study is single centre and it is known that bronchiectasis can be quite heterogeneous across different healthcare systems. Nevertheless our patient population is typical/representative in terms of demographics of European bronchiectasis cohorts. [26, 30, 31] A small number of patients had previously completed questionnaires such as the QOL-B as part of clinical research studies and so we acknowledge prior experience as a potential source of bias. The length of interview and timing of interviews during working hours may have skewed the population towards older, retired participants. Nevertheless, as the average age of bronchiectasis patients is 65–70 years, we do not regard this as major bias [31, 32].

Conclusions

This study has characterised bronchiectasis symptom burden and its impact on quality of life and identified scope for improving existing health related quality of life questionnaires. [32] The framework we have developed can be used to evaluate future HRQL questionnaires for bronchiectasis.

Acknowledgements
We acknowledge the European Lung Foundation and the EMBARC/ELF patient advisory group for providing input into study design, analysis and interpretation. We also acknowledge Professor Sara Marshall for assistance with study design and interpretation.

Funding
Supported by the European Respiratory Society Clinical Research Collaboration (EMBARC).

Author contributions
JDC conceived the study, supervised the study and wrote the manuscript. MLC contributed to study design, recruited participants, contributed to literature review and wrote the manuscript. EKD performed data collection, analysed the data and wrote the manuscript. All authors read and approved the final manuscript.

Competing interests

JDC reports grant support from AstraZeneca, Boehringer-Ingelheim, Bayer Healthcare, Grifols, Glaxosmithkline and Pfizer Ltd. outside the submitted work. MLC and EKD report no conflicts of interest.

Author details

[1]Scottish Centre for Respiratory Research, University of Dundee, Ninewells Hospital and Medical School, Ninewells Drive, Dundee DD1 9SY, Scotland. [2]Division of Molecular and Clinical Medicine, University of Dundee, Dundee DD1 9SY, UK.

References

1. Quint JK, Millett ERC, Joshi M, Navaratnam V, Thomas SL, Hurst JR, Smeeth L, Brown JS. Changes in the incidence, prevalence and mortality of bronchiectasis in the UK from 2004 to 2013: a population-based cohort study. Eur Respir J. 2016;47:186–93.
2. Chalmers JD, McHugh BJ, Doherty CJ, Govan JRW, Kilpatrick DC, Hill AT. Mannose binding lectin deficiency and disease severity in non-CF bronchiectasis: a prospective study. Lancet Respiratory Medicine. 2013;1(3): 175–274.
3. Wilson CB, Jones PW, O'Leary CJ, Cole PJ, Wilson R. Validation of the St. George's respiratory questionnaire in bronchiectasis. Am J Respir Crit Care Med. 1997;156:536–41.
4. Quittner AL, O'Donnell AE, Salathe MA, Lewis SA, Li X, Montgomery AB, O'Riordan TG, Barker AF. Quality of Life Questionnaire-Bronchiectasis: final psychometric analyses and determination of minimal important difference scores. Thorax [Internet]. 2015;70:12–20. Available from: https://doi.org/10.1136/
5. Wong C, Jayaram L, Karalus N, Eaton T, Tong C, Hockey H, Milne D, Fergusson W, Tuffery C, Sexton P, Storey L, Ashton T. Azithromycin for prevention of exacerbations in non-cystic fibrosis bronchiectasis (EMBRACE): a randomised, double-blind, placebo-controlled trial. Lancet. 2012;380:660–7.
6. Birring SS, Prudon B, Carr AJ, Singh SJ, Morgan MDL, Pavord D. Develpoment of a symptom specific health status measure for patietns with chronic cough: Leicester cough questionnaire (LCQ). Thorax. 2003;58:339–43.
7. Murray MP, Turnbull K, MacQuarrie S, Pentland JL, Hill AT. Validation of the Leicester cough questionnaire in non-cystic bronchiectasis. Eur Respir J. 2009;34:125–31.
8. Jones PW, Quirk FH, Baveystock CM. The St Georges Respiratory Questionnaire. Respir Med. 1991;85(suppl B):25–31.
9. Jones PW, Harding G, Berry P, Wiklund I, Chen WH, Kline LN. Development and first validation of the COPD assessment test. Eur Respir J. 2009;34(3): 648–54.
10. Quittner AL, Marciel KK, Salathe MA, O'Donnell AE, Gotfried MH, Ilowite JS, Metersky ML, Flume PA, Lewis SA, McKevitt M, Montgomery AB, O'Riordan TG, Barker AF. A preliminary quality of life questionnaire-bronchiectasis: a patient-reported outcome measure for bronchiectasis. Chest. 2014;146(2): 437–48.
11. Barker AF, O'Donnell AE, Flume P, Thompson PJ, Ruzi JD, De Gracia J, Boersma WG, De Soyza A, Shao L, Zhang J, Haas L, Lewis SA, Leitzinger S, Montgomery AB, McKevitt MT, Gossage D, Quittner AL, O'Riordan TG. Aztreonam for inhalation solution in patients with non-cystic fibrosis bronchiectasis (AIR-BX1 and AIR-BX2): two randomised double-blind, placebo-controlled phase 3 trials. Lancet Respir Med. 2014;2:738–49.
12. Supple D, Roberts A, Hudson V, Masefield S, Fitch N, Rahmen M, Flood B, de Boer W, Powell P, Wagers S. From tokenism to meaningful engagement: best practices in patient involvement in an EU project. Research Involvement and Engagment. 2015;1:5.
13. Bilton D, Tino G, Barker AF, Chambers DC, De Soyza A, Dupont LJ, O'Dochartaigh C, Van EHJ H, Vidal LO, Welte T, Fox HG, Wu J, Charlton B. Inhaled mannitol for non-cystic fibrosis bronchiectasis: a randomised, controlled trial. Thorax [Internet]. 2014;69:1073–9.
14. Haworth CS, Foweraker JE, Wilkinson P, Kenyon RF, Bilton D. Inhaled colistin in patients with bronchiectasis and chronic pseudomonas aeruginosa infection. Am J Respir Crit Care Med. 2014;189:975 82.
15. Altenburg J. Effect of Azithromycin Maintenance Treatment on Infectious Exacerbations Among Patients With Non – Cystic Fibrosis Bronchiectasis. Jama [Internet]. 2013;309:1251–9.
16. De Soyza A, Pavord I, Elborn JS, Smith D, Wray H, Puu M, Larsson B, Stockley R. A randomised, placebo-controlled study of the CXCR2 antagonist AZD5069 in bronchiectasis. Eur. Respir. J. 2015;46:1021–32.
17. Aliberti S, Lonni S, Dore S, McDonnell MJ, Goeminne PC, Dimakou K, Fardon TC, Rutherford R, Pesci A, Restrepo MI, Sotgiu G, Chalmers JD. Clinical phenotypes in adult patients with bronchiectasis. Eur Respir J. 2016;47:1113–22.
18. Strauss A, Corbin J. Basics of qualitative research: techniques and procedures for developing grounded theory. 2nd ed. London: Sage Publications; 1998.
19. Charmaz K. Constructing grounded theory: a practical guide through qualitative analysis. London: Sage Publications; 2006.
20. Brill SE, Patel AR, Singh R, Mackay AJ, Brown JS, Hurst JR. Lung function, symptoms and inflammation during exacerbations of non-cystic fibrosis bronchiectasis: a prospective observational cohort study. Respir Res. 2015;16: 16. https://doi.org/10.1186/s12931-015-0167-9.
21. Mandal P, Chalmers JD, Graham C, Harley C, Sidhu MK, Doherty C, Govan JW, Sethi T, Davison DJ, Rossi AG, Hill AT. Atorvastatin as a stable treatment in bronchiectasis: a randomised controlled trial. Lancet Respiratory Medicine. 2014;2(6):455–63.
22. McDonnell MJ, Aliberti S, Goeminne PC, Restrepo MI, Pesci A, Dupont LJ, Fardon TC, Wilson R, Loebinger MR, Skrbic D, Obradovic D, De Soyza A, Ward C, Laffey JG, Rutherford R, Chalmers JD. Co-morbidities and the risk of mortality in patients with bronchiectasis. An international cohort study. Lancet Respiratory Medicine. 2016;4(12):969–79.
23. Lonni S, Chalmers JD, Goeminne PC, McDonnell MJ, Dimakou K, De Soyza A, Polverino E, Van De Kerkhove C, Rutherford R, Davison J, Rosales E, Pesci A, Restrepo MI, Torres A, Aliberti S. Etiology of non-cystic fibrosis bronchiectasis in adults and its correlation to disease severity. Ann Am Thorac Soc. 2015;12:1764–70.
24. Chalmers JD, Moffitt KL, Suarez-Cuartin G, Sibila O, Finch S, Furrie E, Dicker A, Wrobel K, Elborn JS, Walker B, Martin SL, Marshall SE, Huang JT-J, Fardon TC. Neutrophil Elastase Activity is Associated with Exacerbations and Lung Function Decline in Bronchiectasis. Am. J. Respir. Crit. Care Med. [Internet] 2016.
25. Chalmers JD, Goeminne P, Aliberti S, McDonnell MJ, Lonni S, Davidson J, Poppelwell L, Salih W, Pesci A, Dupont LJ, Fardon TC, De Soyza A, Hill AT. The bronchiectasis severity index an international derivation and validation study. Am J Respir Crit Care Med. 2014;189:576–85.
26. McDonnell MJ, Aliberti S, Goeminne PC, Dimakou K, Zucchetti SC, Davidson J, Ward C, Laffey JG, Finch S, Pesci A, Dupont LJ, Fardon TC, Skrbic D, Obradovic D, Cowman S, Loebinger MR, Rutherford RM, De Soyza A, Chalmers JD. Multidimensional severity assessment in bronchiectasis-analysis of 7 European Cohorts. Thorax. 2016; in press
27. O'Conor R, Martynenko M, Gagnon M, Hauser D, Young E, Lurio J, Wisnivesky JP, Wolf MS, Federman AD, SAMBA investigators. A qualitative investigation of the impact of asthma and self- management strategies among older adults. J Asthma. 2017;54(1):39–45.
28. Brien SB, Lewith GT, Thomas M. Patient Coping Strategies in COPD Across Disease Severity and Quality of Life: a Qualitative Study. NPJ Primary Care Respiratory Medicine. 2016;26:16051.
29. Apfelbacher CJ, Jones CJ, Frew A, et al. Validity of three asthma- specific quality of life questionnaires: the patients' perspective. BMJ Open. 2016;6: e011793.
30. Chalmers JD, Aliberti S, Polverino E, Vendrell M, Crichton M, Loebinger M, Dimakou K, Clifton I, van der Eerden M, Rohde G, Murris-Espin M, Masefield S, Gerada E, Shteinberg M, Ringshausen F, Haworth C, Boersma W, Rademacher J, Hill AT, Aksamit T, O'Donnell A, Morgan L, Milenkovic B, Tramma L, Neves J, Menendez R, Paggiaro P, Botnaru V, Skrgat S, Wilson R, et al. The EMBARC European Bronchiectasis Registry: protocol for an international observational study. ERJ Open Res. [Internet]. 2016;2 81-2015-81–2015.
31. Finch S, McDonnell MJ, Abo-Leyah H, Aliberti S, Chalmers JD. A comprehensive analysis of the impact of Pseudomonas aeruginosa colonisation on prognosis in adult bronchiectasis. Ann Am Thorac Soc. 2015;12(11):1602–11.
32. Aliberti S, Masefield S, Polverino E, De Soyza A, Loebinger MR, Menendez R, Ringshausen FC, Vendrell M, Powell P, Chalmers JD. Research priorities in bronchiectasis: a consensus statement from the EMBARC clinical research collaboration. Eur Respir J. 2016;48(3):632–47.

Characterization, localization and comparison of c-Kit+ lung cells in never smokers and smokers with and without COPD

Alejandra López-Giraldo[1,2,3], Tamara Cruz[2,3], Laureano Molins[1,2], Ángela Guirao[1,2], Adela Saco[2,4], Sandra Cuerpo[1,2,3], Josep Ramirez[2,4], Álvar Agustí[1,2,3] and Rosa Faner[2,3,5]*

Abstract

Background: c-Kit + lung stem cells have been described in the human healthy lung. Their potential relation with smoking and/or chronic obstructive pulmonary disease (COPD) is unknown.

Methods: We characterized and compared c-Kit+ cells in lung tissue of 12 never smokers (NS), 15 smokers with normal spirometry (S) and 44 COPD patients who required lung resectional surgery. Flow cytometry (FACS) was used to characterize c-Kit+ cells in fresh lung tissue disaggregates, and immunofluorescence (IF) for further characterization and to determine their location in OCT- embedded lung tissue.

Results: We identified 4 c-Kit+ cell populations, with similar proportions in NS, S and COPD: (1) By FACS, c-Kit^{high}/CD45 + cells (4.03 ± 2.97% (NS), 3.96 ± 5.30% (S), and 5.20 ± 3.44% (COPD)). By IF, these cells were tryptase+ (hence, mast cells) and located around the airways; (2) By IF, c-Kit^{low}/CD45+/tryptase- (0.07 ± 0.06 (NS), 0.03 ± 0.02 (S), and 0.06 ± 0.07 (COPD) cells/field), which likely correspond to innate lymphoid cells; (3) By FACS, c-Kit^{low}/CD45-/CD34+ (0.95 ± 0.84% (NS), 1.14 ± 0.94% (S) and 0.95 ± 1.38% (COPD)). By IF these cells were c-Kit^{low}/CD45-/CD31+, suggesting an endothelial lineage, and were predominantly located in the alveolar wall; and, (4) by FACS, an infrequent c-Kit^{low}/CD45-/CD34- population (0.09 ± 0.14% (NS), 0.08 ± 0.09% (S) and 0.08 ± 0.11% (COPD)) compatible with a putative lung stem cell population. Yet, IF failed to detect them and we could not isolate or grow them, thus questioning the existence of c-Kit+ lung stem-cells.

Conclusions: The adult human lung contains a mixture of c-Kit+ cells, unlikely to be lung stem cells, which are independent of smoking status and/or presence of COPD.

Keywords: Bronchitis, Chronic obstructive pulmonary disease emphysema, Lung repair, Smoking, Lung stem cells

Background

The mechanisms of lung repair and regeneration are not fully understood [1, 2]. A population of putative lung stem cells characterized by the surface expression of the c-Kit receptor (c-Kit+, also known as CD117) and the absence of hematopoietic, mesenchymal or epithelial cell markers, capable to repair the lung parenchyma in a cryoinjured mouse model has been described [3]. These results, however, have not been reproduced by other investigators who argued that this population of c-Kit+ cells might not have been adequately phenotyped and may in fact represent a population of endothelial progenitor cells [4–6] or even, mast cells, which share the c-Kit marker [7, 8].

Chronic obstructive pulmonary disease (COPD) is an important cause of morbidity and mortality worldwide [9]. Tobacco smoking is the main environmental risk factor for COPD, but not all smokers develop the disease [10]. We hypothesized that c-Kit+ lung dependent repair

* Correspondence: rfaner@clinic.cat
[2]Institut d'Investigacions Biomèdiques August Pi i Sunyer (IDIBAPS), Barcelona, Spain
[3]CIBER Enfermedades Respiratorias(CIBERES), Instituto de Salud Carlos III, Madrid, Spain
Full list of author information is available at the end of the article

mechanisms may be deficient in smokers with COPD. To test this hypothesis we: (1) carefully characterized the phenotype of pulmonary cells expressing c-Kit; (2) located stem cells (c-Kit+CD45-) cells in the lung parenchyma; and (3) compared their number and location in never smokers and smokers with or without COPD.

Methods

Methods are detailed in the on-line supplement.

Study design and ethics

This observational, prospective and controlled study was approved by the Ethics Committee of our institution (ID 2012/7731). All participants signed their informed consent.

Participants

We included 12 non-smokers, 15 smokers (> 10 pack/year) with normal spirometry and 44 smokers with COPD according to the GOLD criteria [10]. All of them required lung resectional surgery for diagnostic and/or therapeutic purposes due to early stage lung cancer or pulmonary solitary nodule. No participant received chemotherapy or radiotherapy before surgery or suffered from any other known chronic inflammatory condition.

Lung function

Forced spirometry, static lung volumes and carbon monoxide diffusing capacity (DLCO) were determined in all participants (Medisoft, Surennes, Belgium). Reference values correspond to the Mediterranean population [11, 12]. The severity of airflow limitation was graded following GOLD recommendations [10].

Tissue sampling & processing

Lung tissue was processed in less than 30 min after surgical extraction. After examination by a pathologist, non-tumoral affected tissue was selected; part was digested for flow cytometry (as described in the supplement) and the rest fixed in paraformaldehyde, embedded in OCT, frozen at − 50 °C in an isopentane bath and stored at − 80 °C until analysis.

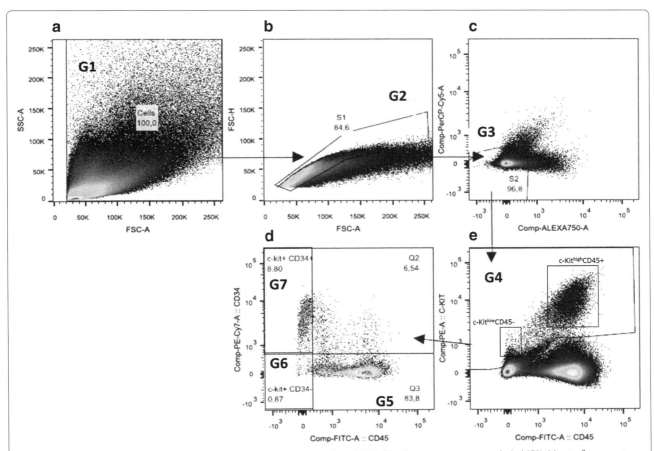

Fig. 1 Gating strategy of C-Kit+ cells in flow cytometry: (**a**) all events were selected (G1); (**b**) cells aggregates were excluded (G2); (**c**) auto fluorescent cells were excluded (G3); (**d**) the expression of CD45 and CD34 was assessed in C-Kit+ cells identifying C-Kit+CD45 + CD34- (G5) C-Kit+CD45-CD34- cells (G6) and C-Kit+CD45-CD34+ cells (G7); and, finally (**e**) the c-Kit cell population is selected (G4). For further explanations, see text

Flow cytometry
Cells were stained as follows: (1) c-Kit determination tube: anti CD45-FITC anti C-Kit-PE and anti CD34- PECy7; (2) a C-Kit isotype control tube: anti CD45-FITC, anti IL-17A and anti CD34- PECy7; and (3) a negative control. Acquisition was done in BD FACS-CANTO II (BD, US) and analysis in Flow-Jo X software (LLC, US) following the gating strategy shown in Fig. 1.

Immune-fluorescence
5 μm tissue slices were defrosted, rehydrated, subjected to antigen retrieval, permeabilised, washed and incubated overnight with primary antibodies: anti-CD117, anti-CD45, anti-tryptase, anti-CD31 (Additional file 1: Table S1). Specific staining was detected with secondary antibodies: Alexa Fluor 488/555 or 647 (Additional file 1: Table S1). Slices were mounted with prolong Gold with DAPI. Appropriate negative and cross reactivity controls were obtained (Additional file 1: Figure S1).

Imaging analysis
Images were acquired using a TCS-SP5 laser scanning spectral confocal microscope (Leica Microsystems, Germany). A mosaic composition of consecutive and adjacent images of 1024 × 1024 pixels in 5 laser channels each was processed with the Matrix Screening software (Leica microsystems) that allows to visualize a representative tissue area that covered in all cases small airways, pulmonary vessels and *alveolar septae* (Additional file 1: Figure S2). Analysis of the tissue mosaics images was done using a customized macro of Image J software [13].

Statistical analysis
Results are presented as n, proportion or mean ± SD, as appropriate. The Kruskal-Wallis test, followed by post-hoc Mann-Whitney contrast if needed, was used to compare continuous variables and Chi Square for discrete variables between groups. A p value < 0.05 was considered statistically significant.

Results
Table 1 summarizes the main characteristics of the population studied. Briefly, the proportion of females was higher in non-smokers. Age and body mass index (BMI) were similar across groups. Cumulative tobacco smoking (pack-yr) was higher in COPD patients who had moderate airflow limitation whereas spirometry was normal in the other two groups. Additional file 1: Table S2 shows that these characteristics were similar in the subsample of the study population used for immune-fluorescence analysis.

Characterization of c-kit+ cells by flow cytometry
As shown graphically in Fig. 1e and quantitatively in Table 2, the most abundant FACS population of c-Kit+ cells in fresh lung tissue disaggregates in the three groups studied were c-Kit+^{high}CD45+ cells. Differences between groups were not statistically significant (Additional file 1: Figure S3). Both mast cells and innate lymphoid cells (ILCs) co-express c-Kit and CD45 [14]. Additional file 1: Figure S4 shows that, by IF with tryptase co-staining the CD45 + c-Kit^{high} population represents mast cell, whereas ILCs are c-Kit^{low} CD45 + Triptase-.

Around 22% of the c-Kit+ population by flow cytometry (i.e., 1% of total gated cells) was not of hematopoietic lineage (CD45-, Fig. 1e); of note, c-Kit intensity of this CD45- lineage was lower than that of CD45+ cells (CD45-, Fig. 1e). Their proportions were not different in the three groups studied (Table 2). In c-Kit+ CD45- cells, we analyzed the co-expression of CD34 and observed two different cell populations: (1) C-Kit^{low}CD45-CD34+ cells (Fig. 1d. G6), which may represent a population of endothelial progenitor cells [15]; and, (2) C-Kit^{low}CD45-CD34- (Fig. 1d. G5), that can correspond to a putative resident stem cell population [3]. Of note, this latter cell population corresponds to less than 0.1% of the total live-gated cells, and they did not appear as a well-defined population in the flow cytometer plot (Fig. 1d. G5). Table 2 shows that the proportion of these cell populations was not different across groups.

Table 1 Characteristics (mean ± SD) of the individuals studied

	Non-smokers	Smokers	COPD	P value
	N = 12	N = 15	N = 44	
Age (years)	67.8 ± 9.3	61.4 ± 12.0	65.9 ± 7.6	0.18
Females/Males	10/2	5/10	9/35	0.0002
BMI (Kg/m^2)	28.5 ± 6.6	27.7 ± 4.6	25.7 ± 3.9	0.41
Current/Former smokers	0/0	9/6	27/17	0.99
Cumulative smoking exposure (packs-year)	0 ± 0	36.3 ± 24.8	49.9 ± 20.1	0.01
FEV1/FVC (%)	77.9 ± 4.0	77.3 ± 7.5	59.5.0 ± 7.3	< 0.001
FEV1 (% reference)	97.5 ± 8.1	95.3 ± 9.4	75.0 ± 15.6	< 0.001

BMI Body Mass Index, *FEV1* Forced expiratory volume in 1 s, *FVC* Forced vital capacity

Table 2 Percentage of C-Kit+ cells (in the population of live gated cells (G2)) determined by flow cytometry (mean ± SD)

% of gated cells	Non-smokers N = 12	Smokers N = 15	COPD N = 44	P value
C-Kit^{high}CD45+	4.03 ± 2.97	3.96 ± 5.30	5.20 ± 3.44	0.07
C-Kit^{low}CD45-	1.05 ± 0.92	1.22 ± 1.01	1.04 ± 1.41	0.44
C-Kit^{low}CD45-CD34+	0.95 ± 0.84	1.14 ± 0.94	0.95 ± 1.38	0.38
C-Kit^{low}CD45-CD34-	0.09 ± 0.14	0.08 ± 0.09	0.08 ± 0.11	0.94

Characterization of c-kit+ cell population by immunofluorescence (IF)

To localize the different lineages of c-Kit+ cells in lung tissue, we used triple IF staining containing c-Kit, CD45 and the mast cell marker tryptase, in a random subgroup of participants (Additional file 1: Table S2). In each of these patients we analyzed a mosaic composition of 169 consecutive images (× 40) covering a tissue area which included in all cases small airways, pulmonary vessels and alveolar *septae*. Additional file 1: Figure S2 is a representative image of the area studied per patient, and Additional file 1: Figure S4 an example of the staining of the three c-Kit different subpopulations identified.

As shown in Table 3, using IF the most abundant lung c-Kit+ cells were mast cells (c-Kit^{high}CD45 + tryptase+). We also observed a less abundant subpopulation of c-Kit^{low}CD45+ tryptase- cells (Table 3) that may represent ILCs [14]. Finally, less than 1% of c-Kit+ cells were negative for both mast cell markers (CD45 and tryptase), and their c-Kit staining intensity was lower than that of mast cells (c-Kit^{low}CD45-tryptase-). To rule out the potential endothelial lineage of this latter c-Kit^{low}CD45-tryptase- subpopulation, we evaluated if they also stained positive for CD31. We used this marker by IF instead of the CD34 used by FACS as in our hands the staining was able to better defined the cells. The c-Kit/CD31/CD45 was performed in a consecutive tissue sections to c-Kit/tryptase/CD45 and confocal images were obtained with additional 10 Z (axial) top to bottom slides. We found that all c-Kit^{low}CD45- tryptase- cells stained positive for CD31 (Additional file 1: Figure S5), suggesting their endothelial cell lineage [15]. Additionally, we did not find co-staining of the stem cell markers Oct-4, NANOG, and KLF4 with c-Kit+ cells (Additional file 1: Figure S6). Thus we were not able to identify by IF the lung tissue stem cells defined as c-Kit^{low}CD45-tryptase-CD31-. Finally, in agreement with FACS results, Table 3 shows that the number all the cell population identified by field was not different across groups.

Location of c-kit+ cells in the lung parenchyma

As expected, c-Kit^{high}CD45 + tryptase+ (mast cells) were mainly located around the peribronchial intestitium. On the other hand, we observed that 89.0% of the c-Kit^{low}CD45- tryptase- putative endothelial progenitor population was located in the alveolar wall, 8.9% in the bronchiolar epithelium, 1.6% in the vascular adventitia and 0.5% in the venous endothelium, without significant differences across groups (Fig. 2).

Relationship with smoking status and lung function

We did not observe any correlation between smoking status or the severity of airflow limitation or DLCO impairment with the number of the different c-Kit+ populations investigated here (data not shown).

Discussion

In 2011 Kajstura et al. reported the identification of a population of c-Kit+ putative stem cells in the human lung [3]. This publication generated both a great deal of interest and controversy [4–8]. To explore the role of c-Kit+ dependent repair mechanisms in COPD, we carefully characterized phenotypically all pulmonary cells expressing c-Kit, located them in the lung parenchyma and compared their number and location in never smokers and smokers with or without COPD. The two main and novel observations of our study were that, first, the human lung contains a heterogeneous mixture of, at least, four different c-Kit+ cell populations that likely include mast cells, innate lymphoid cells, endothelial progenitors and a putative but rare stem cell population; these observations clearly supports that c-Kit positivity cannot be used as "the" single stem cells marker [16]. And, second, that there were no significant differences in any c-Kit+

Table 3 Number of C-Kit+ cells per field (mean ± SD) by immunofluorescence

C-Kit+ cells /field	Non-smokers N = 5	Smokers N = 5	COPD N = 10	P value
C-Kit^{high}CD45 + Tryptase+	5.25 ± 3.28	2.89 ± 0.65	3.72 ± 1.36	0.19
C-Kit^{low}CD45-Tryptase-	0.07 ± 0.06	0.03 ± 0.02	0.06 ± 0.07	0.51
C-Kit^{high}CD45 + Tryptase-	0.79 ± 0.47	0.48 ± 0.51	0.50 ± 0.32	0.37

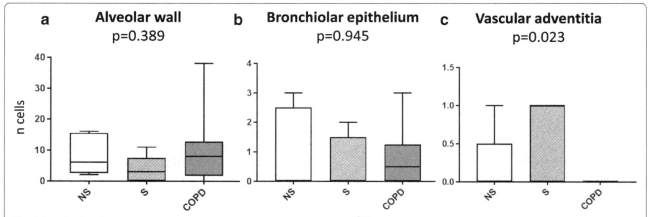

Fig. 2 Box plot (median, 5-95% IC and SD (bars)) comparing the number of c-Kit^{low}CD45-tryptase- cells (endothelial progenitors) in; panel (**a**) the alveolar wall, panel (**b**) bronchiolar epithelium, and panel (**c**) vascular adventitia in the three groups of subjects studied. Note the different Y range scales in the three different locations. For further explanations, see text

cell population studied here between never smokers and smokers with or without COPD, a hypothesis not previously tested to our knowledge.

Characterization and location of lung c-kit+ cells

In keeping with some similar previous studies in cardiac tissue [4, 5, 7, 8, 17], we found that the adult human lung contains a heterogeneous mixture of distinct c-Kit+ cell populations: (1) the majority of them (85% by IF) are mast cells, since c-Kit^{high}/CD45+ cells detected by FACS expressed the specific mast cell marker tryptase in IF [18], and were mainly located around the intestitium. The role of mast cells is well established in lung diseases associated with chronic inflammation [19] such as COPD [20] and asthma [21] and may contribute to their pathogenesis of bronchial remodeling [22]; (2) a smaller population (13% by IF) of c-Kit^{low}CD45+ were tryptase- and may represent ILC [23], a family of innate immune cells that participate in the regulation of the immune response and tissue inflammation [24]. ILC lack specific antigen receptors and can produce several cytokines according to which they are classified in three groups (ILC1, ICL2, ILC3). ILC3 are known to express c-Kit in lung tissue [23]. (3) An even smaller population (1.6% by IF) of c-Kit^{low}CD45- that express CD34+ and/or CD31+ likely represent endothelial cell progenitors, which have been already described in lung tissue [15, 25]. In our study, they mostly located in the alveolar walls (Fig. 2); and, (4) finally, we found (only by FACS) a very small population (< 0.1% of gated cells) of c-Kit^{low}CD45-CD34- cells that can potentially correspond to a potential putative lung stem cell population, as described by Kajstura et al.... [3] because they stained negative for cell linage markers. Yet, our IF analysis showed that c-Kit^{low} CD45-triptase- cells were positive for CD31, likely pinpointing towards an endothelial lineage. We were not able to identify a c-Kit^{low} lineage negative cells by IF.

In this context, some important differences between our study and that of Kajstura et al. [3] are worth mentioning. Firstly, they studied unused healthy young donor lungs whereas we obtained lung tissue samples from older patients requiring thoracic surgery for a variety of clinical reasons. Secondly, Kajstura et al reported high c-Kit staining intensity in lung stem cells [3] while in our study the bright c-Kit staining was only found in mast-cells, despite the fact we were used the c-Kit antibody from the same vendor. It is of note that, c-Kit is a receptor that is activated after binding its ligand, the stem cell factor (SCF). After binding SCF c-Kit receptors form homodimers that are internalized and degraded, so a low c-Kit expression (hence, intensity) is associated to an enhanced c-Kit consumption, thus cell activation [26]. Thirdly, Kajstura et al [3] reported that their c-Kit+ stem cells were mainly localized in the bronchioles whereas in this location we detected mast cells. Finally, our putative stem cell population (c-Kit^{low} CD45-CD34-) was detected by FACS only and we could not locate them in the lung parenchyma by IF. Unfortunately, we were not able to successfully sort and expand the c-Kit^{low}CD45-CD34- cell population observed by FACS. In our hands the < 3000 cells obtained after sorting did not expanded and were not enough to perform functional assays to assess their potential stem cell characteristics. Future studies will have to use alternatives methodologies, such as clonal derivation [16], to explore this possibility and eventually clarify if this c-Kit^{low}CD45-CD34- cells identified by FACS here really corresponds to a multipotent lung stem cell population.

Effects of smoking and COPD

To our knowledge, this is the first study that compares the quantity and localization of c-Kit+ cells in never smokers and smokers with and without COPD. We did not find differences between them. Likewise, we did not identify any significant relationship with physiological measures (severity of airflow limitation, DLCO) or smoking status. Hence, these results do not support our working hypothesis that c-Kit+ stem cells may be different in number and/or location in smokers with and without COPD. Yet, because we could not perform in vitro functional assays in this cell population, we cannot exclude that the function of these c-Kit+ cells may be different in these groups. In any case, these results contribute to delineate more precisely the quantity, type, localization and relationship with smoking and COPD of c-Kit+ cells in the adult human lung.

Strengths and limitations

Our study has a number of strengths and limitations. Among the former, the relative large number of participants included in the study, its controlled design, the use of combined FACS to characterize phenotypically these c-Kit+ cells and IF to locate them, as well as the comparison of smokers with and without COPD are strengths of our paper. Among the latter that, we acknowledge that the quantitation of putative stem cells in the context of very low cell numbers is very challenging so ours should be considered only as indicative data. Likewise, for this same reason, we could not isolate, expand in culture and perform functional assays in the putative stem cells population identified by FACS. Also, due to its low percentage, the failure to conform a well-defined population in forward side plots and the latter failure to detect them by IF we cannot exclude the possibility that these events are an artifact of the detection technique. In any case, however, our results cast serious doubts about the existence of c-Kit+ lung stem cells in humans.

Conclusions

This study shows that the adult human lung contains a heterogeneous population of c-Kit expressing cells, including mast cells, innate lymphoid cells and putative endothelial cell progenitors. Only using FACS we were able to identify < 0.1% cells meeting the cell-surface criterion of c-Kit+ stem cells, but we could not verify their presence by IF or functional analyses. All in all, these results question seriously the existence of c-Kit+ lung stem cells in humans. Finally, contrary to our original hypothesis, we failed to identify significant differences in c-Kit+ cells between smokers with and without COPD.

Abbreviations

COPD: Chronic obstructive pulmonary disease; DLCO: Carbon monoxide diffusing capacity; FACS: Flow cytometry; IF: Immunofluorescence; NS: Never smokers; S: Smokers with normal spirometry; SCF: Stem cell factor

Acknowledgments

Authors thank Maria Calvo, Anna Bosch and Elisenda Coll from the Advanced Optical Microscopy Unit (Campus Clinic) for their help and support with the confocal images acquisition and macro customization used in this study. We also thank Ms. Gemma Sunyer and Ms. Tamara García for their excellent technical support during the study.

Funding

Supported in part, by Fondo de Investigación Sanitaria, Instituto Carlos III (PI15/00799, SEPAR 192/2012), CIBERES and a PhD scholarship FI-DGR 2016. Cerca Program and Menarini. Rosa Faner is recipient of a Miguel Servet Research Program Contract (FEDER, CP16/00039). Funders had no roles in the design of the study and collection, analysis, and interpretation of data and in writing the manuscript.

Authors' contributions

Conception and design: ALG, AA, RF; Analysis and interpretation: ALG, TC, AA, RF; Recruitment, analysis and discussion of results: All. Drafting the manuscript for important intellectual content: All; Discussion and approval of the final manuscript: All.

Competing interests

The authors declare that they have no competing interests.

Author details

[1]Respiratory Institute, Hospital Clinic, University of Barcelona, Barcelona, Spain. [2]Institut d'investigacions Biomèdiques August Pi i Sunyer (IDIBAPS), Barcelona, Spain. [3]CIBER Enfermedades Respiratorias(CIBERES), Instituto de Salud Carlos III, Madrid, Spain. [4]Department of Pathology, Hospital Clinic, Barcelona, Spain. [5]Barcelona, Spain.

References

1. Kotton DN, Morrisey EE. Lung regeneration: mechanisms, applications and emerging stem cell populations. Nat Med. 2014;20:822–32.
2. Lau AN, Goodwin M, Kim CF, Weiss DJ. Stem cells and regenerative medicine in lung biology and diseases. Mol Ther. 2012;20:1116–30.
3. Kajstura J, Rota M, Hall SR, Hosoda T, D'Amario D, Sanada F, Zheng H, Ogorek B, Rondon-Clavo C, Ferreira-Martins J, et al: Evidence for human lung stem cells. N Engl J Med 2011, 364:1795–1806.
4. Sandstedt J, Jonsson M, Lindahl A, Jeppsson A, Asp J. C-kit+ CD45- cells found in the adult human heart represent a population of endothelial progenitor cells. Basic Res Cardiol. 2010;105:545–56.
5. Sultana N, Zhang L, Yan J, Chen J, Cai W, Razzaque S, Jeong D, Sheng W, Bu L, Xu M, et al. Resident c-kit(+) cells in the heart are not cardiac stem cells. Nat Commun. 2015;6:8701.
6. Sandstedt J, Jonsson M, Dellgren G, Lindahl A, Jeppsson A, Asp J. Human C-kit+CD45- cardiac stem cells are heterogeneous and display both cardiac and endothelial commitment by single-cell qPCR analysis. Biochem Biophys Res Commun. 2014;443:234–8.
7. Veinot JP, Prichett-Pejic W, Song J, Waghray G, Parks W, Mesana TG, Ruel M. CD117-positive cells and mast cells in adult human cardiac valves--observations and implications for the creation of bioengineered grafts. Cardiovasc Pathol. 2006;15:36–40.
8. Zhou Y, Pan P, Yao L, Su M, He P, Niu N, McNutt MA, Gu J. CD117-positive cells of the heart: progenitor cells or mast cells? J Histochem Cytochem. 2010;58:309–16.
9. Mannino DM, Buist AS. Global burden of COPD: risk factors, prevalence, and future trends. Lancet. 2007;370:765–73.
10. Alcorn JF, Crowe CR, Kolls JK. TH17 cells in asthma and COPD. Annu Rev Physiol. 2010;72:495–516.
11. Roca J, Sanchis J, Agusti-Vidal A, Segarra F, Navajas D, Rodriguez-Roisin R, Casan P, Sans S. Spirometric reference values from a Mediterranean population. Bull Eur Physiopathol Respir. 1986;22:217 24.

12. Roca J, Rodriguez-Roisin R, Cobo E, Burgos F, Perez J, Clausen JL. Single-breath carbon monoxide diffusing capacity prediction equations from a Mediterranean population. Am Rev Respir Dis. 1990;141:1026–32.
13. Schindelin J, Arganda-Carreras I, Frise E, Kaynig V, Longair M, Pietzsch T, Preibisch S, Rueden C, Saalfeld S, Schmid B, et al. Fiji: an open-source platform for biological-image analysis. Nat Methods. 2012;9:676–82.
14. Boyd A, Ribeiro JM, Nutman TB. Human CD117 (cKit)+ innate lymphoid cells have a discrete transcriptional profile at homeostasis and are expanded during filarial infection. PLoS One. 2014;9:e108649.
15. Suzuki T, Suzuki S, Fujino N, Ota C, Yamada M, Suzuki T, Yamaya M, Kondo T, Kubo H. C-kit immunoexpression delineates a putative endothelial progenitor cell population in developing human lungs. Am J Phys Lung Cell Mol Phys. 2014;306:L855–65.
16. Vicinanza C, Aquila I, Scalise M, Cristiano F, Marino F, Cianflone E, Mancuso T, Marotta P, Sacco W, Lewis FC, et al. Adult cardiac stem cells are multipotent and robustly myogenic: c-kit expression is necessary but not sufficient for their identification. Cell Death Differ. 2017;24:2101–16.
17. Bearzi C, Rota M, Hosoda T, Tillmanns J, Nascimbene A, De Angelis A, Yasuzawa-Amano S, Trofimova I, Siggins RW, Lecapitaine N, et al. Human cardiac stem cells. Proc Natl Acad Sci U S A. 2007;104:14068–73.
18. Schwartz LB, Kepley C. Development of markers for human basophils and mast cells. J Allergy Clin Immunol. 1994;94:1231–40.
19. Metz M, Grimbaldeston MA, Nakae S, Piliponsky AM, Tsai M, Galli SJ. Mast cells in the promotion and limitation of chronic inflammation. Immunol Rev. 2007;217:304–28.
20. Gosman MM, Postma DS, Vonk JM, Rutgers B, Lodewijk M, Smith M, Luinge MA, Ten Hacken NH, Timens W. Association of mast cells with lung function in chronic obstructive pulmonary disease. Respir Res. 2008;9:64.
21. Bradding P, Arthur G. Mast cells in asthma--state of the art. Clin Exp Allergy. 2016;46:194–263.
22. Okayama Y, Ra C, Saito H. Role of mast cells in airway remodeling. Curr Opin Immunol. 2007;19:687–93.
23. De Grove KC, Provoost S, Verhamme FM, Bracke KR, Joos GF, Maes T, Brusselle GG. Characterization and quantification of innate lymphoid cell subsets in human lung. PLoS One. 2016;11:e0145961.
24. Kumar V. Innate lymphoid cells: new paradigm in immunology of inflammation. Immunol Lett. 2014;157:23–37.
25. Montani D, Perros F, Gambaryan N, Girerd B, Dorfmuller P, Price LC, Huertas A, Hammad H, Lambrecht B, Simonneau G, et al. C-kit-positive cells accumulate in remodeled vessels of idiopathic pulmonary arterial hypertension. Am J Respir Crit Care Med. 2011;184:116–23.
26. Lennartsson J, Ronnstrand L. Stem cell factor receptor/c-kit: from basic science to clinical implications. Physiol Rev. 2012;92:1619–49.

Effectiveness of a standardized electronic admission order set for acute exacerbation of chronic obstructive pulmonary disease

Sachin R. Pendharkar[1,2,3,8*], Maria B. Ospina[4], Danielle A. Southern[3,5], Naushad Hirani[1], Jim Graham[4], Peter Faris[6], Mohit Bhutani[7], Richard Leigh[1], Christopher H. Mody[1,4] and Michael K. Stickland[7]

Abstract

Background: Variation in hospital management of patients with acute exacerbation of chronic obstructive pulmonary disease (AECOPD) may prolong length of stay, increasing the risk of hospital-acquired complications and worsening quality of life. We sought to determine whether an evidence-based computerized AECOPD admission order set could improve quality and reduce length of stay.

Methods: The order set was designed by a provincial COPD working group and implemented voluntarily among three physician groups in a Canadian tertiary-care teaching hospital. The primary outcome was length of stay for patients admitted during order set implementation period, compared to the previous 12 months. Secondary outcomes included length of stay of patients admitted with and without order set after implementation, all-cause readmissions, and emergency department visits.

Results: There were 556 admissions prior to and 857 admissions after order set implementation, for which the order set was used in 47%. There was no difference in overall length of stay after implementation (median 6.37 days (95% confidence interval 5.94, 6.81) pre-implementation vs. 6.02 days (95% confidence interval 5.59, 6.46) post-implementation, $p = 0.26$). In the post-implementation period, order set use was associated with a 1.15-day reduction in length of stay (95% confidence interval − 0.5, − 1.81, $p = 0.001$) compared to patients admitted without the order set. There was no difference in readmissions.

Conclusions: Use of a computerized guidelines-based admission order set for COPD exacerbations reduced hospital length of stay without increasing readmissions. Interventions to increase order set use could lead to greater improvements in length of stay and quality of care.

Keywords: Length of stay, Clinical decision support, Chronic obstructive pulmonary disease, Quality improvement

Background

Chronic obstructive pulmonary disease (COPD) is a common and progressive lung disease that is characterized by shortness of breath, activity limitation, and a predisposition to exacerbations. Acute exacerbations of COPD (AECOPD) adversely affect quality of life, [1] increase the risk of disease progression, [2] and reduce survival. [3] Hospitalizations for AECOPD cost approximately USD $3.8 billion [4] and account for 51% of overall expenditures for COPD. [5] Prolonged hospital length of stay (LOS) also have a negative impact on patient function and quality of life. [6]

Evidence-based management guidelines for AECOPD have been developed, [7, 8] and include recommendations regarding pharmacotherapy and post-exacerbation care. Despite these guidelines, hospital care of patients with AECOPD remains highly variable. [9] This variation may contribute to prolonged LOS [10] that, in turn, increases the risk of hospital-acquired complications and adversely impacts quality of life. [6, 11]

---

* Correspondence: sachin.pendharkar@ucalgary.ca
[1]Department of Medicine, Cumming School of Medicine, University of Calgary, Calgary, AB, Canada
[2]Department of Community Health Sciences, Cumming School of Medicine, University of Calgary, Calgary, AB, Canada
Full list of author information is available at the end of the article

Order sets are grouped medical orders intended to standardize evidence-based best practice. Computerized Physician Order Entry (CPOE) systems may improve workflow, promote appropriate testing and treatment, reduce errors and improve guideline adherence, [12–17] particularly when integrated into general order sets. [18] Standardized admission order sets have been used in other diseases with variable success at reducing hospital LOS. [14, 15]

Two observational studies have demonstrated that order sets likely improve the quality of hospital care for patients with AECOPD and reduce LOS. [13, 16] However, these studies used pre-post designs that could be influenced by secular trends in AECOPD management, and the studies did not account for the differential effects of the order set among physician groups.

The objective of this study was to determine whether the implementation of an evidence-based computerized admission order set would improve the quality of inpatient AECOPD care. A stepped wedge design was used to account for differential effects among physician groups and to minimize confounding related to the timing of order set implementation. Our hypothesis was that the implementation of a standardized order set would reduce hospital LOS of patients admitted for AECOPD without increasing emergency department (ED) or hospital readmissions. Preliminary study results have previously been reported in abstract form. [19]

Methods
Study design
This study is an analysis of administrative health data for a quality improvement project in which an electronic standardized admission order set for patients with AECOPD was implemented at a large, tertiary-care teaching hospital in Calgary, Alberta between March 1, 2013 and March 31, 2015. Since this was a quality improvement project, the University of Calgary Conjoint Health Research Ethics Board waived the requirement for formal ethics approval.

Study population
Patients were included if they were: older than 45 years of age; admitted to hospital between March 1, 2013 to March 31, 2015 with an International Classification of Diseases, Tenth Revision (ICD-10-CA) code indicative of AECOPD (J42 [unspecified chronic bronchitis], J43 [emphysema], or J44 [other chronic obstructive pulmonary disease]) in the primary diagnosis field of the hospital discharge abstract database; and admitted to the pulmonary, general internal medicine or hospitalist clinical services. Patients were excluded if they were admitted to the intensive care unit or any other clinical service. Historical controls from the 12 months prior to order set implementation in each group of ordering physicians were identified using similar criteria. Additional details on the methods are provided in an additional file (see Additional file 1).

Order set development
The AECOPD order set was based on published COPD guidelines, [7] and developed by a provincial COPD working group comprised of physicians, nurses, and respiratory therapists from a variety of clinical settings, in a series of face-to-face and teleconference meetings.

The order set contained recommended testing, medication (including suggested dosing and mode of delivery), consultations, and a priori discharge planning interventions specific to patients with AECOPD. Some interventions were pre-selected to encourage use (e.g., physiotherapy referral). The order set was built into the hospital's existing CPOE system, Sunrise Clinical Manager (Allscripts Solutions, Chicago IL). Screenshots are provided in an additional file (see Additional file 2).

Implementation
The order set was implemented using a stepped wedge design [20] among the three physician groups who admit patients with AECOPD: respirologists, general internists, and family physician hospitalists. It was implemented sequentially within physician groups with each group acting as its own control. Study outcome data were collected at baseline and at each implementation 'step'.

Implementation among respirologists, general internists and hospitalists occurred in March, May and August 2013, respectively. Prior to each implementation step, the research team met with physicians and allied health staff to introduce the order set. Order set use by each individual physician was voluntary. Monthly statistics on order set use were posted in clinical areas.

Analysis
Patient demographic, comorbidity and hospitalization data were obtained from provincial administrative data and linked to order set usage data from the CPOE system using the patient's provincial health number. [21]

The primary outcome was hospital LOS for patients admitted during the implementation period compared to those admitted during the previous 12 months (pre-post implementation analysis). Secondary outcomes included: hospital LOS of patients admitted with and without the order set after implementation (post-implementation analysis); all-cause readmissions at 7, 30 and 90 days after discharge; ED visits at 7 and 30 days; and in-hospital mortality.

Unadjusted and adjusted median regression models were constructed to assess the impact of the order set on LOS. [22–24] Covariates in adjusted models included age, sex, and five clinically relevant comorbidities (heart failure, dementia, liver disease, renal disease, and diabetes) that were strongly associated with the Charlson Comorbidity Index (Somers' D = 0.94). [25] Logistic regression was used to adjust 30-day readmission odds ratios for age, sex, comorbidity and admitting physician specialty.

All analyses were performed using SAS version 9.3 (Cary, NC) or R version 3.2.3; [26] $p < 0.05$ was considered statistically significant.

Results

Of 1435 AECOPD admissions to one of the three physician groups during the study period, 1413 with a LOS less than 90 days were included in the analysis (Fig. 1). There were 857 admissions after order set implementation, of which 406 patients (47%) were admitted using the order set.

Baseline characteristics of study participants are presented in Tables 1 and 2 for the pre-post and post-implementation analyses, respectively. The hospitalist service admitted most patients with AECOPD, but admitted fewer in the post-implementation period compared to the pre-implementation period (64.5% vs. 74.3%). Patients with co-existing heart failure and diabetes were more commonly admitted under general internists. Over 95% of patients were discharged home.

Order set uptake

In the post-implementation period, 57% of patients admitted to the hospitalist service were admitted using the order set, compared to 30% of patients admitted by general internists or respirologists. Time series analysis revealed that order set use increased gradually after implementation, mostly by general internists and hospitalists (Additional file 3: Figure S1).

Hospital LOS

Figure 2 shows the unadjusted and adjusted differences in median LOS for patients treated in the pre- and post-implementation periods. Median LOS was 6.37 days (95% confidence interval [CI] 5.94, 6.81; $n = 556$) for patients admitted before implementation and 6.02 days (95% CI 5.59, 6.46; $n = 857$) for patients admitted after implementation ($p = 0.26$).

Unadjusted and adjusted comparisons of median LOS in the post-implementation analysis are presented in Fig. 3. Order set use was associated with a 1.15-day (95% CI -0.50, − 1.81) shorter median LOS, due primarily to a 1.8-day (95% CI -0.95, − 2.61) decrease for the hospitalist group (Fig. 3). Median LOS for patients admitted by general internists or respirologists did not differ by order set use.

Readmissions

Neither order set implementation, nor order set use in the post-implementation period were associated with changes in readmissions or ED visits for all three physician groups (Tables 3 and 4 and Additional file 1 Table S1). Overall in-hospital mortality did not change with order set implementation, but was lower in the hospitalist group with order set use.

Discussion

This is the largest study to evaluate the impact of a standardized, guideline-based electronic order set for AECOPD on hospital LOS. We performed two analyses: a comparison of LOS before and after the order set was implemented, and a comparison of patients admitted with and without the order set after implementation. The results revealed that order set implementation did not result in an overall LOS reduction, perhaps because only 47% of admitting physicians used it. However, the post-implementation analysis revealed that when it was used, the order set was associated with a LOS reduction of 1.15 days. Use of the order set by hospitalists, who admitted 65% of AECOPD patients in the post-implementation cohort, resulted in the largest LOS reduction of 1.8 days. Importantly, there was

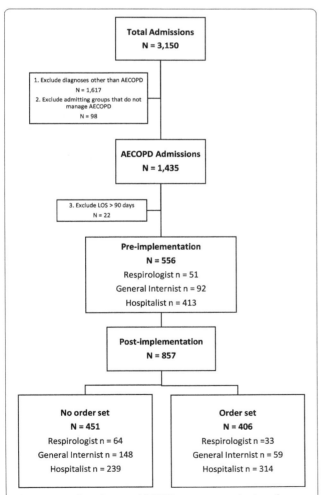

Fig. 1 Patient flow diagram. AECOPD – acute exacerbation of chronic obstructive pulmonary disease; LOS – length of stay

Table 1 Baseline characteristics for pre-post implementation analysis

Characteristics	Total	Pre-implementation	Post-implementation	p-value
Number of patients	1413	556	857	
Mean age, years (SD)	70 (12)	70 (12)	70 (12)	0.747
Age group, n (%)				
< 55	129 (9.1)	59 (10.6)	70 (8.2)	0.250
55–64	323 (22.9)	128 (23.0)	195 (22.8)	
65–74	428 (30.3)	157 (28.2)	271 (31.6)	
75–84	360 (25.5)	136 (24.5)	224 (26.1)	
85+	173 (12.2)	76 (13.7)	97 (11.3)	
Male sex, n (%)	727 (51.5)	279 (50.2)	448 (52.3)	0.441
Comorbidity, n (%)				
Heart failure	190 (13.5)	71 (12.8)	119 (13.9)	0.548
Dementia	45 (3.2)	24 (4.3)	21 (2.5)	0.051
Diabetes	318 (22.5)	131 (23.6)	187 (21.8)	0.444
Renal disease	36 (2.6)	13 (2.3)	23 (2.7)	0.687
Liver disease	13 (0.9)	6 (1.1)	7 (0.8)	0.614
Admitting specialty, n (%)				
Respirologist	148 (10.5)	51 (9.2)	97 (11.3)	0.0005
General internist	299 (21.2)	92 (16.6)	207 (24.2)	
Hospitalist	966 (68.4)	413 (74.3)	553 (64.5)	

SD = standard deviation

no increase in either ED or hospital readmissions, suggesting that earlier discharge resulting from order set use did not occur at the expense of harm to the patient.

Our findings extend observations from two recent studies examining the impact of order sets on AECOPD care. In a pre-post design of 243 patients hospitalized with AECOPD, Kitchlu et al. showed that implementation of an order set improved the quality of admission orders using pre-specified measures of guidelines-based care. [16] Using a similar design in a study of 275 patients, Brown et al. showed that physician prescribing practices for AECOPD could be

Table 2 Baseline characteristics for post-implementation analysis

Characteristics	Respirologist		General internist		Hospitalist	
	No order set (n = 64)	Order set (n = 33)	No order set (n = 148)	Order set (n = 59)	No order set (n = 239)	Order set (n = 314)
Mean age, years (SD)	63 (11)	64 (10)	69 (11)	71 (12)	72 (12)	71 (10)
Age group, n (%)						
< 55	8 (13)	6 (18)	12 (8)	8 (14)	15 (6)	21 (7)
55–64	27 (42)	10 (30)	37 (25)	14 (24)	39 (16)	68 (22)
65–74	20 (31)	9 (27)	50 (34)	14 (24)	72 (30)	106 (34)
75–84	9 (14)	8 (24)	36 (24)	18 (31)	65 (27)	88 (28)
85+	0	0	13 (9)	5 (9)	48 (20)	31 (10)
Male sex, n (%)	34 (53)	12 (36)	75 (51)	29 (49)	134 (56)	159 (51)
Comorbidity, n (%)						
Heart failure	4 (6)	2 (6)	39 (26)	11 (19)	37 (15)	26 (8)
Dementia	0	1 (3)	4 (3)	0	11 (5)	5 (2)
Diabetes	9 (14)	8 (24)	46 (31)	16 (27)	45 (19)	63 (20)
Renal disease	2 (3)	0	4 (3)	2 (3)	7 (3)	8 (3)
Liver disease	0	0	1 (1)	0	2 (1)	2 (1)

SD = standard deviation

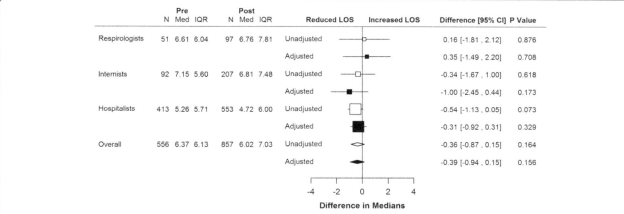

Fig. 2 Forest plot of implementation effects (pre-post implementation analysis). Adjusted model included age, sex, and five clinically relevant comorbidities selected from the Charlson Comorbidity Index (heart failure, dementia, mild or severe liver disease, renal disease, and diabetes. Pre – pre-implementation; Post – post-implementation; N – number of patients; Med – median length of stay; IQR – interquartile range; LOS – length of stay; CI – confidence interval

improved with an electronic order set. [13] Secondary analyses in both studies revealed LOS reductions without an increase in readmissions. The current study extends this work by demonstrating an improvement in hospital LOS in a larger study cohort. Unlike the previous studies, which reported on pre-post effects of order set implementation, we specifically examined the effect of actual use of the order set, demonstrating that it could reduce LOS compared to patients admitted without the order set. Furthermore, the stepped wedge design is robust to secular trends in care delivery and LOS of AECOPD patients, and allowed for subgroup analyses by different admitting physician groups. Both our study and the previous studies provide a strong rationale for the standardization of inpatient AECOPD care using computerized order sets.

A standardized order set is appealing due to high variability in inpatient AECOPD management. [9] Previous studies of order sets for AECOPD demonstrated more consistent use of systemic corticosteroids, appropriate antibiotics, and allied health providers such as physiotherapists, [13, 16] all of which have been shown to reduce hospital LOS. [27–29] The current order set similarly prompted admitting physicians to use these therapies, and pre-selection of some items (e.g., bronchodilator delivery, physiotherapy referral) provided additional clinical decision support around guidelines-based care.

The LOS reduction observed after order set implementation was driven by improvements for patients admitted by hospitalists, with no differences observed in the other physician groups; this was an interesting finding with many possible explanations. First, Sandhu et al. demonstrated high variability in AECOPD management

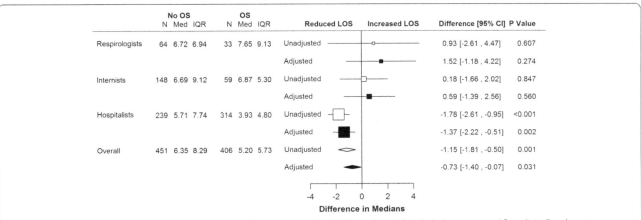

Fig. 3 Forest plot of the effects of the order set (post-implementation analysis). Adjusted model included age, sex, and five clinically relevant comorbidities selected from the Charlson Comorbidity Index (heart failure, dementia, mild or severe liver disease, renal disease, and diabetes. OS – order set; N – number of patients; Med – median length of stay; IQR – interquartile range; LOS – length of stay; CI – confidence interval; OS – order set

Table 3 Readmissions, emergency department visits and in-hospital mortality for pre-post implementation analysis

Results	Pre-implementation ($n = 556$)	Post-implementation ($n = 857$)	p-value
7-day readmission, n (%)	33 (5.9)	60 (7.0)	0.430
30-day readmission, n, (%)	91 (16.4)	166 (19.4)	0.153
90-day readmission, n, (%)	170 (30.6)	299 (34.9)	0.093
7-day ED visits, n (%)	42 (7.6)	55 (6.4)	0.409
30-day ED visits, n (%)	124 (22.3)	196 (22.9)	0.803
In-hospital mortality, n, (%)	19 (3.4)	31 (3.6)	0.842

ED = emergency department

among all specialties, with deviation from clinical guidelines occurring more often when care was provided by physicians other than respirologists. [9] This variability may be due to the diversity of medical problems managed by hospitalists, which could lead to a less uniform approach to inpatient AECOPD management. Thus, it is possible that the opportunity for standardization using an order set was greater for hospitalists than for other specialties. Second, heart failure and diabetes were more prevalent in patients admitted under general internists compared to hospitalist patients. These conditions have both been associated with longer LOS in patients with AECOPD, [30] and are unlikely to be impacted by order set use. Third, patients presenting with respiratory failure requiring noninvasive ventilation were only admitted by general internists or respirologists; these indicators of more severe AECOPD were not systematically captured, but could have reduced the effectiveness of the order set. [31] Although the order set's impact seemed to be isolated to only one admitting group, the 1.8-day reduction in median LOS is an important finding since hospitalists were responsible for providing almost two thirds of inpatient AECOPD care in our study, and this is likely to be similar in other large, tertiary-care urban hospitals in North America.

The order set was used by 47% of admitting physicians during the study period. This low uptake is a consistent finding for voluntary order sets [13, 16, 32, 33] and is a known limitation of their use. [34] Respirologists and general internists used the order set less frequently than hospitalists, for a number of possible reasons. First, the complexity of the patient's presentation (e.g., respiratory failure requiring noninvasive ventilation) may have made the order set less applicable at the time of admission. Second, respirologists may have greater perceived self-efficacy with AECOPD management, leading them to admit AECOPD patients without using an order set. Finally, whereas the AECOPD order set was the only respiratory order set embedded in the CPOE system, several admission order sets for medical problems typically admitted under hospitalists (e.g., pneumonia, heart failure) were already embedded. Thus, hospitalists may have more experience in order set use compared to other physicians. Importantly, end users were consulted to ensure the order set was intuitive and minimally disruptive to clinical workflow; these factors have been shown to increase uptake of clinical decision support systems such as standardized order sets. [14, 17, 18] The increase in order set use over time suggested that admitting physicians found it useful.

This study has a number of limitations. First, the non-randomized study design raises the possibility that improvements in LOS were due to other differences between groups admitted with and without the order set. However, when implementing complex healthcare interventions such as the AECOPD order set, traditional randomized controlled trials are impractical due to logistical constraints and the risk of contamination within clinical provider groups. The methodologically robust stepped wedge design minimized contamination

Table 4 Readmissions, emergency department visits and in-hospital mortality for post-implementation analysis

Results	Respirologist			General internist			Hospitalist		
	No order set ($n = 64$)	Order set ($n = 33$)	p value	No order set ($n = 148$)	Order set ($n = 59$)	p value	No order set ($n = 239$)	Order set ($n = 314$)	p value
7-day readmission, n (%)	4 (6.3)	2 (6.1)	0.971	18 (12.2)	4 (6.8)	0.257	13 (5.4)	19 (6.1)	0.760
30-day readmission, n (%)	19 (29.7)	5 (15.2)	0.116	29 (19.6)	14 (23.7)	0.508	41 (17.2)	58 (18.5)	0.689
90-day readmission, n (%)	30 (46.9)	13 (39.4)	0.482	59 (39.9)	19 (32.2)	0.305	75 (31.4)	103 (32.8)	0.723
7-day ED visits, n (%)	2 (3.1)	1 (3.0)	0.980	12 (8.1)	3 (5.1)	0.449	15 (6.3)	22 (7.0)	0.734
30-day ED visits, n (%)	18 (28.1)	5 (15.2)	0.155	28 (18.9)	14 (23.7)	0.437	54 (22.6)	77 (24.5)	0.597
In-hospital mortality, n (%)	0	1 (3.0)	0.162	8 (5.4)	5 (8.5)	0.411	12 (5)	5 (1.6)	0.021

ED = emergency department

by allowing implementation and evaluation of the order set in clusters [35] while still analyzing the effect of order sets within physician groups.

Second, the use of administrative data prevented analysis of patient characteristics that might have influenced a physician's decision to use the order set; it is thus possible that the reduced LOS in the post-implementation period is due to order set use in less complex cases. While our findings are consistent with studies performed in different geographic and clinical settings, [13, 16] we acknowledge the importance of future studies to examine whether COPD severity, presentation acuity, or use of specific interventions (e.g., noninvasive ventilation) impact order set use. Such an analysis would help to tailor strategies aimed at increasing order set uptake by specific physician groups.

The lack of clinical data on COPD severity (e.g., spirometry) or baseline performance status also precluded the determination of differential effects of the order set between COPD subgroups; it is also possible that these factors influenced LOS or readmission rates independently of the order set. However, this information is also often not available to clinicians at the time of admission. Thus, we chose to develop an order set that could be used for all patients admitted with AECOPD, consistent with actual clinical practice. Our statistical models did account for age, sex and clinically relevant comorbidities, indicating that our results were robust to these covariates. Future studies could further evaluate how patient characteristics impact order set use and outcomes from the order set.

Finally, we did not analyze individual components of the AECOPD order set, and thus do not know which orders were actually selected or executed (e.g., physiotherapy referral). We also cannot confirm whether there was concordance between pre-checked orders and actual orders selected by admitting physicians. These components may have differential impact on LOS and could help refine the order set. An understanding of how individual components were used may also help to identify areas for focused quality improvement. While the intent of this study was to evaluate the effectiveness of a comprehensive bundle of orders, the improvement in LOS provides compelling evidence to justify a secondary analysis of individual order set components.

Conclusion

In conclusion, this study found that when a standardized electronic order set was used to admit patients with AECOPD, LOS was reduced without increasing readmissions. Innovations such as order sets have the potential to lessen the burden of AECOPD hospitalizations on both patients and the healthcare system, and justify additional studies of clinical decision support tools for AECOPD.

Abbreviations
AECOPD: Acute exacerbation of chronic obstructive pulmonary disease; CI: Confidence interval; COPD: Chronic obstructive pulmonary disease; CPOE: Computerized physician order entry; ED: Emergency department; LOS: Length of stay

Acknowledgements
The authors acknowledge the members and staff of Alberta Health Services' Respiratory Health Strategic Clinical Network, who helped with design and implementation of the order set.

Funding
This project was supported by Alberta Health Services' Respiratory Health Strategic Clinical Network Seed Grant. Members of the Respiratory Health Strategic Clinical Network were involved in the design of the study and revision of the manuscript. However, the seed grant used to fund this project was obtained through an independent peer review process.

Authors' contributions
All authors have met the ICMJE guidelines for responsible authorship. The authors' substantial contributions to the study are listed below. All authors have critically revised previous versions of the manuscript, approve of the final version and agree to be accountable for all aspects of the work. Study conception and design: SRP, NH, JG, PF, MB, CHM, MKS, Project implementation: SRP, NH, JG, CHM, Data acquisition and analysis: SRP, MBO, DAS, PF, Manuscript preparation: SRP, MBO.

Competing interests
Dr. Leigh reports personal fees from AstraZeneca, grants from AstraZeneca, personal fees from Boehringer Ingelheim, grants from GlaxoSmithKline, grants from MedImmune, personal fees from Novartis, personal fees from TEVA Canada, outside the submitted work. The other authors have no disclosures.

Author details
[1]Department of Medicine, Cumming School of Medicine, University of Calgary, Calgary, AB, Canada. [2]Department of Community Health Sciences, Cumming School of Medicine, University of Calgary, Calgary, AB, Canada. [3]O'Brien Institute for Public Health, Cumming School of Medicine, University of Calgary, Calgary, AB, Canada. [4]Respiratory Health Strategic Clinical Network, Alberta Health Services, Edmonton, AB, Canada. [5]W21C Research and Innovation Centre, Cumming School of Medicine, University of Calgary, Calgary, AB, Canada. [6]Research Priorities and Implementation, Alberta Health Services, Calgary, AB, Canada. [7]Division of Pulmonary Medicine, Department of Medicine, Faculty of Medicine and Dentistry, University of Alberta, Edmonton, AB, Canada. [8]University of Calgary, TRW Building, Rm 3E23, 3280 Hospital Drive NW, Calgary, AB T2N 4Z6, Canada.

References
1. Seemungal TA, Donaldson GC, Paul EA, Bestall JC, Jeffries DJ, Wedzicha JA. Effect of exacerbation on quality of life in patients with chronic obstructive pulmonary disease. Am J Respir Crit Care Med. 1998;157(5):1418–22.
2. Kanner RE, Anthonisen NR, Connett JE. Lung health study research group. Lower respiratory illnesses promote FEV(1) decline in current smokers but not ex-smokers with mild chronic obstructive pulmonary disease: results from the lung health study. Am J Respir Crit Care Med. 2001;164(3):358–64.
3. Connors AF, Dawson NV, Thomas C, et al. Outcomes following acute exacerbation of severe chronic obstructive lung disease. The SUPPORT investigators (study to understand prognoses and preferences for outcomes and risks of treatments). Am J Respir Crit Care Med. 1996;154(4 Pt 1):959–67.

4. Wier LM, Elixhauser A, Pfuntner A, Au DH. Overview of hospitalizations among patients with COPD. Healthcare utilization project statistical brief #106. Rockville, MD: Agency for Healthcare Research and Quality; 2008. p. 2011.
5. Waye AE, Jacobs P, Ospina MB, Stickland MK, Mayers I. Economic surveillance for chronic obstructive pulmonary disease (COPD) in Alberta. Edmonton, AB: Institute for Health Economics; 2016.
6. Wang Q, Bourbeau J. Outcomes and health-related quality of life following hospitalization for an acute exacerbation of COPD. Respirol. 2005;10(3):334–40.
7. O'Donnell DE, Hernandez P, Kaplan A, et al. Canadian Thoracic Society recommendations for management of chronic obstructive pulmonary disease – 2008 update – highlights for primary care. Can Respir J. 2008;15(Suppl A):1A–8A.
8. Vestbo J, Hurd SS, Agustí AG, et al. Global strategy for the diagnosis, management, and prevention of chronic obstructive pulmonary disease: GOLD executive summary. Am J Respir Crit Care Med. 2013;187(4):347–65.
9. Sandhu SK, Chu J, Yurkovich M, Harriman D, Taraboanta C, Fitzgerald JM. Variations in the management of acute exacerbations of chronic obstructive pulmonary disease. Can Respir J. 2013;20:175–9.
10. Noon CE, Hankins CT, Cote MJ. Understanding the impact of variation in the delivery of healthcare services. J Healthc Manag. 2003;48(2):82–97.
11. Hoogerduijn JG, Schuurmans MJ, Duijnstee MS, de Rooij SE, Grypdonck MF. A systematic review of predictors and screening instruments to identify older hospitalized patients at risk for functional decline. J Clin Nurs. 2007;16(1):46–57.
12. Bates DW, Leape LL, Cullen DJ, et al. Effect of computerized physician order entry and a team intervention on prevention of serious medication errors. JAMA. 1998;280(15):1311–6.
13. Brown KE, Johnson KJ, Deronne BM, Parenti CM, Rice KL. Order set to improve the care of patients hospitalized for COPD exacerbations. Ann Am Thorac Soc. 2016;13:811–5.
14. Garg AX, Adhikari NK, McDonald H, et al. Effects of computerized clinical decision support systems on practitioner performance and patient outcomes: a systematic review. JAMA. 2005;293:1223–38.
15. Gillaizeau F, Chan E, Trinquart L, et al. Computerized advice on drug dosage to improve prescribing practice. Cochrane Database Syst Rev. 2013;11(11):CD002894.
16. Kitchlu A, Abdelshaheed T, Tullis E, Gupta S. Gaps in the inpatient management of chronic obstructive pulmonary disease exacerbation and impact of an evidence-based order set. Can Respir J. 2015;22:157–62.
17. Miller RA, Waitman LR, Chen S, Rosenbloom ST. The anatomy of decision support during inpatient care provider order entry (CPOE): empirical observations from a decade of CPOE experience at Vanderbilt. J Biomed Inform. 2005;38:469–85.
18. Munasinghe RL, Arsene C, Abraham TK, Zidan M, Siddique M. Improving the utilization of admission order sets in a computerized physician order entry system by integrating modular disease specific order subsets into a general medicine admission order set. J Am Med Inform Assoc. 2011;18(3):322–6.
19. Pendharkar S, Hirani N, Faris P, et al. Effectiveness of a standardized inpatient admission order set for acute exacerbation of COPD [abstract]. Am J Respir Crit Care Med. 2015;191:A6179.
20. Hemming K, Haines TP, Chilton PJ, Girling AJ, Lilford RJ. The stepped wedge cluster randomized trial: rationale, design, analysis, and reporting. Br Med J. 2015;350:h391.
21. Howe GR. Use of computerized record linkage in cohort studies. Epidemiol Rev. 1998;20:112–21.
22. Koenker R. Quantile Regression [computer program]. 2015. https://cran.r-project.org/web/packages/quantreg/index.html. Accessed 22 July 2016.
23. Koenker R, Bassett G Jr. Regression quantiles. Econometrica. J Econom Soc. 1978;46:33–50.
24. Portnoy S, Koenker R. The gaussian hare and the laplacian tortoise: computability of squared-error versus absolute-error estimators. Stat Sci. 1997;12(4):279–300.
25. Charlson ME, Pompei P, Ales KL, Mackenzie CR. A new method of classifying prognostic comorbidity in longitudinal studies: development and validation. J Chronic Dis. 1987;40:373–83.
26. R. A language and environment for statistical computing [computer program]. Vienna: R Foundation for Statistical Computing; 2015.
27. Niewoehner DE, Erbland ML, Deupree RH, et al. Effect of systemic glucocorticoids on exacerbations of chronic obstructive pulmonary disease. Department of Veterans Affairs cooperative study group. N Engl J Med. 1999;340:1941–7.
28. Quon BS, Gan WQ, Sin DD. Contemporary management of acute exacerbations of COPD: a systematic review and metaanalysis. Chest. 2008;133:756–66.
29. de Morton NA, Keating JL, Jeffs K. Exercise for acutely hospitalised older medical patients. Cochrane Database Syst Rev. 2007;1:CD005955.
30. Wang Y, Stavem K, Dahl FA, Humerfelt S, Haugen T. Factors associated with a prolonged length of stay after acute exacerbation of chronic obstructive pulmonary disease (AECOPD). Int J Chron Obstruct Pulmon Dis. 2014;9:99–105.
31. Matkovic Z, Huerta A, Soler N, et al. Predictors of adverse outcome in patients hospitalized for exacerbation of chronic obstructive pulmonary disease. Respiration. 2012;84:17–26.
32. Wright A, Feblowitz JC, Pang JE, et al. Use of order sets in inpatient computerized provider order entry systems: a comparative analysis of usage patterns at seven sites. Int J Med Inform. 2012;81(11):733–45.
33. Lennox L, Green S, Howe C, Musgrave H, Bell D, Elkin S. Identifying the challenges and facilitators of implementing a COPD care bundle. BMJ Open Respir Res. 2014;1:e000035.
34. Bobb AM, Payne TH, Gross PA. Viewpoint: controversies surrounding use of order sets for clinical decision support in computerized provider order entry. J Am Med Inform Assoc. 2007;14:41–7.
35. Portela MC, Pronovost PJ, Woodcock T, Carter P, Dixon-Woods M. How to study improvement interventions: a brief overview of possible study types. BMJ Qual Saf. 2015;24:325–36.

14

Patient information, education and self-management in bronchiectasis: facilitating improvements to optimise health outcomes

Katy L. M. Hester[1,2]*, Julia Newton[3], Tim Rapley[4] and Anthony De Soyza[1,2]

Abstract

Background: Bronchiectasis is an incurable lung disease characterised by irreversible airway dilatation. It causes symptoms including chronic productive cough, dyspnoea, and recurrent respiratory infections often requiring hospital admission. Fatigue and reductions in quality of life are also reported in bronchiectasis. Patients often require multi-modal treatments that can be burdensome, leading to issues with adherence. In this article we review the provision of, and requirement for, education and information in bronchiectasis.

Discussion: To date, little research has been undertaken to improve self-management in bronchiectasis in comparison to other chronic conditions, such as COPD, for which there has been a wealth of recent developments. Qualitative work has begun to establish that information deficit is one of the potential barriers to self-management, and that patients feel having credible information is fundamental when learning to live with and manage bronchiectasis. Emerging research offers some insights into ways of improving treatment adherence and approaches to self-management education; highlighting ways of addressing the specific unmet information needs of patients and their families who are living with bronchiectasis.

Conclusions: We propose non-pharmacological recommendations to optimise patient self-management and symptom recognition; with the aim of facilitating measurable improvements in health outcomes for patients with bronchiectasis.

Keywords: Bronchiectasis, Self-management, Information, Education, Qualitative, Adherence

Background

Bronchiectasis is a chronic lung condition that leads to a significant symptom and treatment burden for those affected, and significant costs to healthcare services such as the National Health Service. Worldwide prevalence is increasing [1–3], yet the evidence base for the management of bronchiectasis remains poor [4, 5]. Historically, there has been relatively little research conducted in this field and it is only recently that more attention has been paid to this previously somewhat neglected disease. Improvements in disease management interventions in bronchiectasis are required.

Interventions in bronchiectasis are likely to include better medical therapies, yet it is also apparent that bronchiectasis is a 'model' chronic disease in terms of its potential for improvements in self-management. If patients and their carers know how to recognise symptoms of deterioration or exacerbation, and know how and when to take action, this could facilitate improvements in self-management. This in turn has the potential to promote disease stability, reductions in unscheduled presentations to acute health care services and improvements in longer-term health.

Whilst clearly desirable, expecting patients to understand their condition, the treatments used and the implications of not using them appropriately, is potentially

* Correspondence: Katy.hester@ncl.ac.uk
[1]Institute of Cellular Medicine, Newcastle University, Newcastle upon Tyne NE2 4HH, UK
[2]Adult Bronchiectasis Service, Freeman Hospital, Newcastle upon Tyne NE7 7DN, UK
Full list of author information is available at the end of the article

challenging. Prior work has demonstrated that patients with bronchiectasis feel more confident with their treatments when they have received information about them in a specialist clinic [6]. Not every patient with bronchiectasis, however, has access to such information or specialist expertise. Despite recommendations for education and personalised management plans for patients with bronchiectasis [4, 7], there remains a lack of information material openly available to patients when compared to other chronic medical and respiratory conditions. For example, patients with chronic obstructive pulmonary disease (COPD) have a number of available resources [8–12]. In order to facilitate self-care, patients need to have accurate and accessible information about their condition, enabling them to recognise and respond to triggers appropriately and understand how their use of self-management could potentially alter their prognosis. Suitable education could lead to a level of self-management that results in clinically and biologically important endpoints in bronchiectasis. In this article we review the need for education and information in bronchiectasis and its current provision. We discuss options for future improvements in resource development to facilitate much needed improvements in health outcomes.

The burden of bronchiectasis: symptoms, prevalence and treatments

Bronchiectasis leads to symptoms of breathlessness, cough and a chronic infective syndrome and consequently, a poorer quality of life [13, 14] and clinically significant fatigue [15, 16]. Patients often have recurrent infective exacerbations, some of which result in costly hospital admissions. Patients with bronchiectasis are at an increased risk of anxiety and depression [17–19]. In cystic fibrosis, depression and anxiety rates are higher than in the general population, and therefore annual screening is recommended [20, 21]. Given the potential for such psychological distress to impact upon adherence and disease management, annual screening in bronchiectasis could also be of benefit. New data has additionally shown a greater risk of coronary heart disease and stroke in patients with bronchiectasis [22]. Multiple comorbidities are common in bronchiectasis [23]. The burden of disease for patients and carers is clearly significant.

The burden of bronchiectasis for healthcare services is also significant. Recently, UK data reported a prevalence of between 43.4/100,000 in those aged 18–30 and 1239.7/100,000 in those aged 70–79 [1]. There is further evidence that prevalence is increasing worldwide [2, 3]. Additionally, HRCT imaging studies report that up to 50% of patients with COPD have co-existent bronchiectasis [24, 25] and it has been proposed that COPD and bronchiectasis can co-exist as 'bronchiectasis COPD overlap syndrome' (BCOS) [26]. With approximately 1,000,000 patients with a diagnosis of COPD in the UK alone, [27] there is potential for the rise in prevalence of both bronchiectasis and BCOS to continue.

Bronchiectasis mortality rates have been reported in the UK as twice that of the general population [1], approximately 50% higher than that of uncomplicated COPD (calculated at 3% per annum) and are increasing [28, 29]. The presence of BCOS also leads to higher mortality rates [30–32]. Prognosis varies in bronchiectasis, with a study of 91 patients finding that the primary cause of death was usually respiratory, with survival rates of 91% at 4 years and 68.3% at 12.3 years [33]. The same study found factors such as chronic infection with *Pseudomonas aeruginosa* increase mortality. Two severity scores have been recently developed for use in bronchiectasis: the bronchiectasis severity index (BSI) [34] and the FACED score [35]. Although both predict mortality, the BSI is also predictive of severe exacerbations, hospital admissions and quality of life [36, 37]. Infective exacerbations lead to significant morbidity in bronchiectasis. The British Thoracic Society (BTS) national bronchiectasis audit reported that 38% of patients had three or more exacerbations per year [38]. Within cohorts of patients across Europe, reported average exacerbation rates have been from 1 to 4 per year [36, 39]. This is also consistent with American data on the increasing burden of bronchiectasis [40].

Earlier UK data also emphasised the burden of bronchiectasis, uncertainties in aetiology and lack of evidence for the treatments that are often used [41]. Although there are guidelines for investigation, diagnosis and management of bronchiectasis produced by the BTS, there is no cure for bronchiectasis and many therapies are empiric and not evidence based [4]. Bronchiectasis differs from some chronic diseases in both its periods of exacerbation and the role patients may play in managing these. In bronchiectasis, correct, timely recognition of exacerbation symptoms and prompt, appropriate management of infections could lead to increased disease stability. Failure to commence antibiotics promptly could result in a more severe exacerbation of bronchiectasis, potentially requiring hospital admission. This would lead to significant additional healthcare costs, and a much greater physical, psychological and social impact on patients and their families. Conversely, inappropriate and excessive antibiotic use can lead to antibiotic resistance. This could also have problematic repercussions in terms of response to future treatments and consequently longer-term health outcomes. Facilitating patients' understanding and ability to self-manage is therefore extremely important.

With some exceptions, treatments are broadly similar regardless of the aetiology of bronchiectasis, but specific treatment plans are tailored to the individual. These can range from no regular treatments at all, to daily use of nebulised therapies in conjunction with physiotherapy, inhalers and oral medications that collectively can be significantly complex and time-consuming for patients and their families. There is evidence that adhering to inhaled antibiotics decreases exacerbation rate and that poor adherence is associated with poorer outcomes [42, 43]. Understanding the importance of a variety of treatments can be problematic for patients and their families and suitable information and education is required to encourage adherence to mutually agreed treatment plans. Importantly, it is known that those with more frequent exacerbations suffer not only the physical effects, but also a reduction in quality of life [14]. Measuring how the psychological impacts and co-morbidities of bronchiectasis affect treatment adherence and self-management behaviours is a key challenge.

Current provision of information for patients with bronchiectasis

The education of patients with bronchiectasis is recommended; including explanations of the disease, recognition and importance of exacerbations, treatment approaches and a personal management plan [4, 7]. Although patients with bronchiectasis gain information through discussion with their clinician, there is relatively little additional information available to them in comparison to the number of resources available for other chronic conditions such as COPD or Cystic Fibrosis. When searching online for information about bronchiectasis, there are resources available. Some are produced by governmental bodies (e.g. the UK National Health Service (NHS) and the US National Institutes of Health), others by health information providers, and by hospitals and charitable organisations [44–48]. However, in addition to being limited in number when compared to other conditions, many are either very brief, with limited information provided, or are lengthy and potentially overwhelming. There are some resources run by patients which primarily serve as a patient's view or online forum rather than an information resource per se [49, 50]. To date there are no high quality trials nor systematic reviews of such information provision in bronchiectasis, as conducted in COPD [8–12, 51].

A tabulated summary (Table 1) shows examples of some of the bronchiectasis information resources that are available online. Determining credibility (affiliation with a well-known lung charity or a national healthcare provider, for example) is a necessary step in the selection process for patients seeking health information [52]. Despite the available information online, patients and carers with bronchiectasis have reported a lack of trustworthy and user-friendly information and felt they would benefit from credible, multi-format (text, images and video content) resources that they could continue to access outside of a clinic setting [53]. Further identification of the unmet information needs of affected individuals and preferred information formats would enable appropriate resource development. A key priority is to create an accessible, trustworthy resource containing information that users want, rather than information that providers have decided patients should have.

Provision of information for chronic conditions: General principles and its relationship to self-management

The importance of information provision for patients with long-term conditions and their carers is well recognised. There is longstanding evidence that patients want to access information [54] and that information can reduce anxiety [55] and improve patient outcomes [56, 57]. Self-management is increasingly recognised as an important part of chronic disease management and is recommended by the World Health Organisation (WHO) [58]. Information provision is key to facilitating self-care [59] and inadequacies in information provision are a potential reason for people managing their health poorly [60]. Information provision therefore plays an important role in supporting active participation in care and remains a priority area of health research for all chronic conditions.

Arguably, however, information alone does not always translate into behavioural change [61]. Providing patients with a simple factsheet about their condition is unlikely to result in any major tangible benefits. In a review of the role of education in asthma, it was recognised that information about asthma should not simply be factual but allow patients to acquire skills [62]. It is preferable to teach patients about their asthma treatments and inflammation rather than the structure and function of the lungs, for example [63]. Theoretical constructs and behavioural change techniques beyond information delivery are important to consider in development of any intervention that aims to produce changes in behaviour [64, 65]. Framing information, by establishing what is relevant to the patient group, and how it could be delivered in order to achieve the desired effects is therefore essential. For example, video demonstrations or instructions on how to perform certain tasks in bronchiectasis management such as chest clearance has been identified by patients as a priority [53]. This provision of instruction and demonstration of behaviours is in keeping with social-cognitive theory [66]. Information on behaviour-health links and consequences of actions or inactions, would be in keeping with an information-motivation-behavioural skills model [67]. Information is an intervention, the production of which

Table 1 A selection of available online bronchiectasis patient information resources (English language)

Resource	Provider	Description	User Co-production	Recognised healthcare service provider, academic organisation or charity?	Information in video format?
www.bronchiectasis.me	Produced by a multidisciplinary bronchiectasis team and patients and carers based at Newcastle University and Newcastle upon Tyne Hospitals NHS Foundation Trust	Content and format based upon findings of qualitative research with patients and carers. Comprehensive information in text (13,000 words. Sub-sectioned so small, relevant portions of information visible at a time) plus images and multiple videos. Option to download PDF. Updated and available open access June 2017	Yes. Co-produced with patients and carers and based upon prior research.	Yes	Yes
http://www.bronchiectasis.scot.nhs.uk/	NHS Lothian and input from patients with bronchiectasis	Online information with input from patients (Approximately 3000 words plus written patient stories). Option to download PDF brochure. Last updated Jan 2015.	Yes. User input during development.	Yes	No
https://www.blf.org.uk/support-for-you/bronchiectasis	British Lung Foundation (BLF)	Online and booklet version available. Previously quite brief information about bronchiectasis (900 words). Revised June 2017 to include more comprehensive information in keeping with the resources used in the BRIEF study [108].	User reviewers	Yes	No
http://www.nhs.uk/Conditions/Bronchiectasis/Pages/Diagnosis.aspx	U.K. National Health Service	Online information (3600 words). Lots of text on the page to scroll through plus extra items alongside. Last updated 2015	Not specified	Yes	No
http://patient.info/health/bronchiectasis-leaflet	Patient (patient and professional information provider)	Online text. Multiple adverts alongside. Includes discussion forum. Last Updated 2014	Not specified	No	No
http://www.bronchiectasishelp.org.uk/	Written by a patient with bronchiectasis	Patient's perspective with input from professionals. Not text-heavy. No Adverts.	Yes	No	No
https://www.nhlbi.nih.gov/health/health-topics/topics/brn	National Heart Lung and Blood Institute (USA)	Well organised sections. High volume of information and text (4500 words). No Adverts. Last updated 2014	Not specified	Yes	No
http://www.bronchiectasis.info/	Run by patients with bronchiectasis	Discussion forum and online community rather than an information resource.	Yes	No	No
https://en.wikipedia.org/wiki/Bronchiectasis	Wikipedia	Text and images. Last edited April 2017	Not specified	No	No
https://medlineplus.gov/ency/article/000144.htm	US National Library of Medicine	Concise information (570 words). Last updated April 2017.	Not specified	Yes	No
	British Medical Journal	Concise information (1200 words) no adverts. All text format, no pictorial content. Last updated October 2015.	Not specified	Yes	No
	BLF online presentation and question and answers with consultant and physiotherapist.	YouTube video of presentation slides and audio. Patient questions and answers. Published 2012.	Not specified	Yes	Yes
http://www.webmd.boots.com/a-to-z-guides/bronchiectasis	Boots, Pharmacy// WebMD. Last reviewed July 2015.	Online text information (1300 words). Lots of adverts on the page. Last updated July 2015.	Not specified	No (*)	No

(*) Provider notes: "subject to rigorous review and approval by doctors in the UK" is noted in the home page of the overall site but not noted on bronchiectasis specific pages

is a highly skilled process and ideally resources should be user tested, co-designed and co-produced where possible [68]. Such an approach should be taken to resource development for bronchiectasis [69].

Self-management and patient information provision are seemingly inextricably linked. In primary care, self-management has been referred to as 'patients with chronic disease making day to day decisions about their illnesses' [70] and 'the everyday tasks and activities that a person living with a chronic condition needs to carry out' [71]. The aim in supporting self-management is to allow patients to gain not only the knowledge but also the confidence and relevant skills to manage their condition; promoting patient 'activation' [72, 73]. An important concept embedded within this is self-efficacy: the confidence that one can carry out a behaviour necessary to achieve a desired goal [66]. Using self-efficacy as a measurable outcome, however, is not without flaws, as was shown when trialling the expert patient programme (EPP) [74–76]. The EPP was initially developed for patients with arthritis and designed to enhance disease specific information rather than replace it, as the programme is generic in nature. Although these studies found improvements in symptom control, pain and hospitalisations as well as gains in self-efficacy, there are some criticisms of the EPP. These include self-efficacy gains not leading to improvements in self-management and not necessarily reducing hospital presentations. Additionally, it has been suggested that participants in EPP studies were not representative of the general population and were possibly better at self-managing than most [77–79]. A UK study using a lay-led EPP ($n = 629$) showed an increase in participant self-efficacy and energy, yet no reduction in health care utilisation [80].

A number of self-management educational resources have been produced for chronic lung conditions other than bronchiectasis. For example, SPACE for COPD, a six week intervention [51]. At 6 months, there were gains in disease knowledge, anxiety and performance levels, yet the primary outcome measure of dyspnoea had not improved [9]. Living Well with COPD [10] is a website with information and videos requiring a password obtained by patients from their physician in order to access the full material. A two year randomised controlled trial conducted in primary care did not show long term benefits over usual care when using measures of self-efficacy and quality of life. The group with access to the living well programme, however, did seem more able to manage their exacerbations [81]. In asthma, a study using an educational programme based on repeated short interventions (face to face sessions at 3 month intervals over 1 year, a personalised action plan and inhaler technique training) saw improvements in asthma control in the intervention group, yet a degree of improvement within the control group was noted too [82]. Cost effectiveness was not examined and although the intervention was brief, it would involve staff time at considerable cost, and there was no provision for patient information needs at other time points.

Systematic reviews of such self-management education in chronic lung disease have also been conducted. A review of eight studies in COPD revealed inconclusive evidence of any benefits [12]. A more recent review and meta-synthesis, however, concluded that self-management education could reduce hospital admissions in COPD, and improve disease knowledge and quality of life. It did not lead to reductions in mortality or smoking rates, nor improve dyspnoea or lung function [11]. A recent systematic review and meta-analysis across different disease areas concluded that self-management interventions can be implemented without a detrimental effect on health outcomes and that they reduce service utilisation [57]. Although the effect sizes were small overall, it is of note that respiratory conditions were amongst the two groups that had the strongest evidence of benefit. In asthma, a Cochrane review reported that self-management education could improve health outcomes only when delivered in conjunction with medical reviews and a written action plan [83]. In cystic fibrosis, there were too few data to draw firm conclusions about recommendations for self-management [84]. In addition, a separate review of psychological interventions in cystic fibrosis highlighted that behavioural interventions had some effect in improving nutrition, and decision making tools regarding transplantation improved knowledge and expectations of transplant, yet there remained insufficient evidence overall [85]. A protocol for a systematic review of self-management in non-cystic fibrosis bronchiectasis has recently been published [86]. Conclusions are likely to be limited, however, reflecting the limited available literature on self-management in bronchiectasis.

Facilitating self-management in bronchiectasis: Use of information and considerations for resource development

An evidence-based intervention for use in bronchiectasis is still needed. In a study using focus groups, patients with bronchiectasis perceived lack of information and confidence as barriers to self-management and felt that disease specific information would be useful [87]. The use of an EPP as part of a self-management programme for patients with bronchiectasis has also been investigated [88]. The programme consisted of two group sessions of disease-specific information followed by a standard, generic EPP for six weeks. Improvement was found in six of ten domains of a self-efficacy scale, including managing symptoms and depression. The intervention group, however, also reported more symptoms and reduced quality of life post intervention. The educational sessions about bronchiectasis were not patient-driven in terms of content or format of delivery, and participants commented that the sessions should be condensed and be attended by physicians. Costs, staffing, time and patient commitment involved with such a course are considerable, making it potentially unfeasible to deliver at scale within a clinical setting. A successful intervention for bronchiectasis would need to meet patients' needs, be easily accessible and be feasibly deliverable on a long-term basis.

Another recent study has taken a different approach to aiding self-management in patients with bronchiectasis, using a novel tool, the Bronchiectasis Empowerment Tool [89]. The tool consisted of a one page action plan, within a pack containing information and optional notepads. The reported aim of the study was to work alongside existing care in order to improve self-management. At the time of writing the study is closed to recruitment but no published results are available.

In bronchiectasis, self-management includes making decisions surrounding adherence to treatments. Factors predicting adherence to treatments could include beliefs about treatments and burden of treatment [90]. Based on these findings, a theoretical approach is being used to work towards development of a behaviour change intervention to promote treatment adherence [91]. The need for information was again reported by patients during interviews. Participants thought that having knowledge about bronchiectasis and treatments improved adherence.

There is evidence, in COPD, that gaps in knowledge of health care professionals can impact upon patients' knowledge and understanding of their condition [92]. This finding may apply to other conditions. Patients who have bronchiectasis may not attend a specialist service, and general physicians may have less disease-specific knowledge than a specialist delivering a bronchiectasis service. In addition, they may not have sufficient exposure to have developed specific expertise in exchanging disease-specific information in a patient-focussed manner. Given this relative lack of exposure to patients who have bronchiectasis, further development of such skills in an area outside a healthcare providers' area of main expertise is likely to be problematic. In exploratory interviews with patients who had bronchiectasis, [52] participants referred to the fact that they had very little information until they started to attend a specialist bronchiectasis clinic. A trustworthy and patient-driven resource would enable both dissemination of good practice and equity of information access amongst the patient group.

Information seeking is another important aspect to consider in developing an understanding of patients' information needs and how such needs are fulfilled. Trust, particularly in relation to online resources, is a recognised issue [93, 94]. Reasons identified for avoiding seeking information in patients with bronchiectasis include not trusting sources, and fear of what they may find [52]. The potential for information to worsen rather than reduce anxiety has been proposed [95], and the concept of information avoidance is recognised [96]. Reviews of health information seeking behaviour have concluded that a better understanding of this concept will enable the provision of better information, and that information should meet patients' individual needs [95, 96]. Previous work exploring why patients with cancer may not want or seek information about their condition also identified that patients' attitudes and coping strategies can limit their seeking of information [97]. The importance of identifying the diversity of needs of the patient group in order to tailor resources to suit them rather than assume a 'one size fits all' approach will be effective was additionally highlighted. Having an in depth understanding of the information and education needs of both patients and their families, and how these could be met, in addition to an appreciation of how, why and when patients seek information would appear to be fundamental to the development and execution of novel interventions in bronchiectasis. Understanding these needs across a broad sample of potential users with differing backgrounds, ages and disease severities, for example, is also important. Those with bronchiectasis aetiologies that are associated with additional management challenges or poorer outcomes, for example, non-tuberculous mycobacterium infections, bronchiectasis-COPD overlap syndrome (BCOS) [26] and bronchiectasis rheumatoid arthritis syndrome (BROS) [98] may benefit from supplementary educational resources specific to their needs.

Patients use information to aid their decision making about various aspects of their management. Carers are often involved in shared decision-making in a variety of different ways and patients are rarely entirely autonomous in these processes [99, 100]. The role of family or carers in the adaptation of patients and coping with chronic illness is very important [101, 102]. Carers are just as likely to engage with information resources as patients. Therefore, any newly developed resource should accommodate the needs of carers and families of patients with bronchiectasis in addition to patients. A meta-synthesis of qualitative studies highlighted the importance of social networks (family, friends, communities) in the self-management of chronic illnesses [103]. A longitudinal study of patients with heart disease and diabetes also acknowledges this role of social networks in supporting self-management [104]. Participation in community organisations (including online communities and health education groups) has been associated with better physical and mental health within the self-management of diabetes [105, 106]. It is apparent that when considering educational and self-management support interventions they need to be tailored to users' approaches.

Work has begun in bronchiectasis, as yet published only in abstract form, to identify the unmet needs of patients and carers living with bronchiectasis, and co-develop a multi-format information resource [53, 107]. A feasibility study carried out using a resource developed with users, based on their needs and experiences, included user evaluations of the resource and web analytics [108]. A particular feature of this resource is the use of video in information delivery, from professionals, patients and carers. This use of video was based on the findings of prior qualitative interviews and was found to be a particularly engaging aspect of the resource [69, 109]. The website (www.bronchiectasis.me) had over 27,000 worldwide views during the study period of 16 months. By delivering interventions that have been designed in conjunction with patients, to complement their learning approaches, information resources can be tailored to meet needs and optimise uptake.

Conclusions

Patients and carers living with bronchiectasis have been relatively poorly provided for in terms of health information and self-management guidance, despite clear potential for such interventions to produce tangible benefits for patients and health care service providers. The prevalence of bronchiectasis is rising and makes this issue ever more pressing. This lack of provision should be addressed with a patient-centred approach, incorporating knowledge of information seeking and self-management in both other chronic diseases and bronchiectasis itself. In order to achieve development of patient-driven and user-friendly resources, the underlying needs and issues surrounding information and its uptake for patients with bronchiectasis must first be fully identified. The implementation of systematic annual screening for depression and anxiety could also identify patients with requirements for additional psychological support.

As with information delivered in a clinic setting, patients' needs vary. By ensuring the involvement of diverse groups during co-development processes, this range of views can be captured. By developing resources with clearly labelled and sub-sectioned subject areas, users can interact with the information they need, when they need it, and avoid what they may not need or want to know. Using healthcare experts across the multidisciplinary team, patients and carers to co-produce high quality information and education resources is an important step towards facilitating self-management advancements, improvements in adherence and consequent physical and psychological health improvements in bronchiectasis.

Funding
Katy Hester is funded by a National Institute for Health Research Doctoral Research Fellowship. This article presents independent work funded by the National Institute for Health Research (NIHR). The views expressed are those of the author(s) and not necessarily those of the NHS, the NIHR or the Department of Health.
ADS acknowledges funding to the BronchUK network from the UK Medical Research Council (grant MR/L011263/1) and a prior Higher Education Funding Council (HFCE senior lectureship).

Authors' contributions
KH is the main author of this review. TR, JN, ADS were contributors to the manuscript and all authors read and approved the final manuscript.

Competing interests
The authors declare that they have no competing interests.

Author details
[1]Institute of Cellular Medicine, Newcastle University, Newcastle upon Tyne NE2 4HH, UK. [2]Adult Bronchiectasis Service, Freeman Hospital, Newcastle upon Tyne NE7 7DN, UK. [3]Faculty of Medical Sciences, Newcastle University, Newcastle upon Tyne NE2 4HH, UK. [4]Department of Social Work, Education and Community Wellbeing, Northumbria University, Newcastle upon Tyne NE7 7XA, UK.

References
1. Quint JK, et al. Changes in the incidence, prevalence and mortality of bronchiectasis in the UK from 2004-2013: a population based cohort study. Eur Respir J. 2016;47(1):186–93.
2. Ringshausen FC, et al. Bronchiectasis in Germany: a population-based estimation of disease prevalence. Eur Respir J. 2015;46:1805–7.
3. Seitz AE, et al. Trends in bronchiectasis among medicare beneficiaries in the United States, 2000 to 2007. Chest. 2012;142:432–9.
4. Pasteur MC, Bilton D, Hill AT. British Thoracic Society guideline for non-CF bronchiectasis. Thorax. 2010;65(Suppl 1):i1–58.
5. Hester KLM, McDonnell MJ, De Soyza A. Bronchiectasis: what we don't know yet but should. BRN Rev. 2016;2(1):14–26.
6. Hester KLM, McAlinden P, De Soyza A. Education and information for patients with bronchiectasis: what do patients want? Eur Respir J. 2011; 38(supplement 35):P3622.
7. Bronchiectasis Quality Standards Working Group. Quality Standards for clinically significant bronchiectasis in adults. Br Thorac Soc Rep. 2012;4(1). ISSN 2040-2023.
8. Apps LD, et al. The development and pilot testing of the self-management programme of activity, coping and education for chronic obstructive pulmonary disease (SPACE for COPD). Int J ChronObstruct Pulmon Dis. 2013;8:317–27.
9. Mitchell KE, et al. A self-management programme for COPD: a randomised controlled trial. Eur Respir J. 2014;44(6):1538–47.
10. McGill University Health Centre and Quebec Asthma and COPD Network. Living well with COPD a plan of action for life. 2013 09042013]; Available from: http://www.livingwellwithcopd.com/.
11. Wang T, et al. Effectiveness of disease-specific self-management education on health outcomes in patients with chronic obstructive pulmonary disease: an updated systematic review and meta-analysis. Patient Educ Couns. 2017.
12. Monninkhof EEM, et al. Self-management education for patients with chronic obstructive pulmonary disease: a systematic review. Thorax. 2003;58:394–8.
13. O'Leary CJ, et al. Relationship between psychological well-being and lung health status in patients with bronchiectasis. Respir Med. 2002; 96(9):686–92.
14. Wilson CB, et al. Validation of the St George's respiratory questionnaire in bronchiectasis. Am J Respir Crit Care Mec. 1997;156(2 Pt 1):536–41.
15. Hester KLM, et al. Fatigue in bronchiectasis. Q J Med. 2012;105(3):235–40.

16. Macfarlane JG, et al. Fatigue in bronchiectasis: its relationship to pseudomonas colonisation, dyspnoea and airflow obstruction. Thorax. 2010;65:A60.
17. Ozgun Niksarlioglu EY, et al. Factors related to depression and anxiety in adults with bronchiectasis. Neuropsychiatr Dis Treat. 2016;12:3005–10.
18. Boussoffara L, et al. Anxiety-depressive disorders and bronchiectasis. Rev Mal Respir. 2014;31(3):230–6.
19. Olveira C, et al. Depression and anxiety symptoms in bronchiectasis: associations with health-related quality of life. Qual Life Res. 2013;22(3):597–605.
20. Quittner AL, et al. Prevalence of depression and anxiety in patients with cystic fibrosis and parent caregivers: results of the international depression epidemiological study across nine countries. Thorax. 2014;0:1–8.
21. Quittner AL, et al. International committee on mental health in cystic fibrosis: Cystic Fibrosis Foundation and European cystic fibrosis society consensus statements for screening and treating depression and anxiety. Thorax. 2016;71:26–34.
22. Navaratnam V, et al. Bronchiectasis and the risk of cardiovascular disease: a population-based study. Thorax. 2017;72:161–6.
23. McDonnell MJ, et al. Comorbidities and the risk of mortality in patients with bronchiectasis: an international multicentre cohort study. Lancet Respir Med. 2016;4(12):969–79.
24. Patel IS, et al. Bronchiectasis, exacerbation indices, and inflammation in chronic obstructive pulmonary disease. Am J Respir Critical Care Medicine. 2004;170(4):400–7.
25. O'Brien C, Guest PJ, Hill SL. Physiological and radiological characterisation of patients diagnosed with chronic obstructive pulmonary disease in primary care. Thorax. 2000;55:635–42.
26. Hurst JR, Elborn JS, De Soyza A. COPD-bronchiectasis overlap syndrome. Eur Respir J. 2015;45:310–3.
27. Shahab L, et al. Prevalence, diagnosis and relation to tobacco dependence of chronic obstructive pulmonary disease in a nationally representative population sample. Thorax. 2006;61(12):1043–7.
28. Roberts HJ, Hubbard R. Trends in bronchiectasis mortality in England and Wales. Respir Med. 2010;104(7):981–5.
29. Office for National Statistics, Mortality Statistics by cause. Series DH2. 2004, London: The Stationary Office.
30. Gatheral T, et al. COPD-related bronchiectasis; independent impact on disease course and outcomes. COPD. 2014;11:605–14.
31. Goeminne PC, et al. Mortality in non-cystic fibrosis bronchiectasis: a prospective cohort anlaysis. Respir Med. 2014;108:287–96.
32. De Soyza A, et al. Bronchiectasis rheumatoid overlap syndrome (BROS) is an independent risk factor for mortality in patients with bronchiectasis: a multicentre cohort study. Chest. 2017;151(6):1247-54.
33. Loebinger MR, et al. Mortality in bronchiectasis: a long-term study assessing the factors influencing survival. Eur Respir J. 2009;34(4):843–9.
34. Chalmers JD, et al. The bronchiectasis severity index an international derivation and validation study. Am J Respir Critic Care Med. 2014;189(5):576–85.
35. Martinez-Garcia MA, et al. Multidimensional approach to non-cystic fibrosis bronchiectasis: the FACED score. Eur Respir J. 2014;43:1357–67.
36. McDonnell MJ, et al. Multidimensional severity assessment in bronchiectasis: an analysis of seven European cohorts. Thorax. 2016;71:1110–8.
37. Ellis HC, et al. Predicting mortality in bronchiectasis using bronchiectasis severity index and FACED scores: a 19-year cohort study. Eur Respir J. 2016;47:482–9.
38. Hill AT, Routh C, Welham S. National BTS bronchiectasis audit 2012: is the quality standard being adhered to in adult secondary care? Thorax. 2013;0:1–3.
39. McDonnell MJ, et al. Non cystic fibrosis bronchiectasis: a longitudinal retrospective observational cohort study of Pseudomonas persistence and resistance. Respir Med. 2015;109(6):716–26.
40. Seitz AE, et al. Trends and burden of bronchiectasis-associated hospitalizations in the United States, 1993-2006. Chest. 2010;138(4):944–9.
41. Kelly MG, Murphy S, Elborn JS. Bronchiectasis in secondary care: a comprehensive profile of a neglected disease. Eur J Intern Med. 2003;14(8):488–92.
42. McCullough AR, et al. Treatment adherence and health outcomes in patients with bronchiectasis. BMC Pulmon Med. 2014;14:107.
43. Haworth CS, et al. Inhaled colistin in patients with bronchiectasis and chronic pseudomonas infection. Am J Respir Crit Care Med. 2014;189(8):975–82.
44. Newcastle upon Tyne Hospitals NHS Foundation Trust. Bronchiectasis Service. 2015 [cited 2016; Available from: http://www.newcastle-hospitals.org.uk/services/cardiothoracic_services_bronchiectasis.aspx.
45. Patient.co.uk. Bronchiectasis. 2016 [cited 2016; Available from: http://patient.info/health/bronchiectasis-leaflet
46. NHS Choices. Bronchiectasis. 2015 [cited 2016; Available from: http://www.nhs.uk/conditions/Bronchiectasis/Pages/Introduction.aspx.
47. National Heart Lung and Blood Institute. What is bronchiectasis? 2014; Available from: https://www.nhlbi.nih.gov/health/health-topics/topics/brn.
48. British Lung Foundation. Bronchiectasis. 2015 [cited 2016; Available from: https://www.blf.org.uk/support-for-you/bronchiectasis.
49. Angel. Bronchiectasis R Us. 2015 [cited 2015; Available from: http://www.bronchiectasis.info/.
50. Hunter, R. Bronchiectasis Help 2015 cited 2015; Available from: http://www.bronchiectasishelp.org.uk/.
51. Mitchell-Wagg K, et al. A self-management program of activity coping and exercise (SPACE) for COPD: results from a randomised controlled trial. Thorax. 2012;67 supplement II:A25.
52. Hester KLM, De Soyza A, Rapley T. Information and education needs of patients with bronchiectasis: a qualitative investigation. Thorax. 2012;67(supplement 2):A141.
53. Hester KLM, et al. Living your life with bronchiectasis: an exploration of patients and carers information needs informing development of a novel information resource. Thorax. 2015;70(Supplement 3):P201.
54. Bunker TD. An information leaflet for surgical patients. Ann R Coll Surg Engl. 1983;65(4):242–3.
55. George CF, Waters WE, Nicholas JA. Prescription information leaflets: a pilot study in general practice. Br Med J (Clin Res Ed). 1983;287(6400):1193–6.
56. Audit Commission, What seems to be the matter: communication between hospitals and patients. HMSO. 1993. ISBN 011886100X.
57. Panagioti M, et al. Self-management support interventions to reduce health care utilisation without compromising outcomes: a systematic review and meta-analysis. BMC Health Serv Res. 2014;14:356.
58. Epping-Jordan JE, et al. Improving the qaulity of health care for chronic conditions. Qual Saf Health Care. 2004;13:299–305.
59. Department of Health, Our health, our care, our say: a new direction for community services. 2006.
60. Wanless, D., Securing good health for the whole population, D.o. health, Editor. 2004, HMSO.
61. Becker MH. In: Shumaker SA, editor. Theoretical models of adherence and strategies for improving adherence, in the handbook of health behaviour change. New York: Springer Publishing Company; 1990. p. 5–43.
62. Partridge MR, Hill SR. Enhancing care for people with asthma: the role of communication, education, training and self-management. Eur Respir J. 2000;16(2):333–48.
63. Takakura S, Hasegawa T, Ishihara K. Assessment of patients' understanding of their asthmatic condition established in an outpatient clinic. Eur Respir J. 1998;12(supplement 29):24S.
64. Abraham C, Michie S. A taxonomy of behaviour change techniques used in interventions. Health Psychol. 2008;27(3):379–87.
65. Michie S, et al. Making psychological theory useful for implementing evidence based practice: a consensus approach on behalf on the "psychological theory" group. Qual Saf Health Care. 2005;14:26–33.
66. Bandura A. Self-efficacy: toward a unifying theory of behavioural change. Psychol Rev. 1977;84(2):191–215.
67. Fisher JD, Fisher WA. Changing AIDS risk behavior. Psychol Bull. 1992;111:455–74.
68. Patient Information Forum, Making the case for information. 2013.
69. Hester KLM, Newton J, Rapley T, et al. Information and education provision in bronchiectasis: co-development and evaluation of a novel patient-driven resource in a digital era. Eur Respir J. 2018;51:1702402. https://doi.org/10.1183/13993003.02402-2017.
70. Bodenheimer T, et al. Patient self-management of disease in primary care. JAMA. 2002;288(19):2469–75.
71. Eaton S, Roberts S, Turner B. Delivering person centred care in long term conditions. BMJ. 2015;350:h181.
72. Hibbard JH, Greene J. What the evidece shows about patient activation: better health outcomes and care experiences; fewer data on costs. Health Aff. 2013;32:207–14.
73. Eaton S. Delivering person-centred care in long-term conditions. Future Hospital Journal. 2016;3(2):128–31.
74. Lorig K, Holman H. Arthritis self-management studies: a twelve-year review. Health Educ Q. 1993;20(1):17–28.
75. Lorig K, et al. Outcomes of self-help education for patients with arthritis. Arthritis Rheum. 1985;28(6):680–5.

76. Lorig KR, et al. Chronic disease self-mangement program: 2-year health status and health care utilization outcomes. Med Care. 2001;39(11):1217–23.
77. Lindsay S, Vrijhoef HJM. A sociological focus on 'expert patients'. Health Sociol Rev. 2009;18(2):139–44.
78. Gately C, Rogers A, Sanders C. Re-thinking the relationship between long-term condition self-management education and the utilisation of health services. Soc Sci Med. 2007;65(5):934–45.
79. Taylor D, Bury M. Chronic illness, expert patients and care transition. Sociology of Health and Illness. 2007;29(1):27–45.
80. Kennedy A, et al. The effectiveness and cost effectiveness of a national lay led self care support programme for patients with long-term conditions: a pragmatic randomised controlled trial. J Epidemiol Community Health. 2007;61(3):254–61.
81. Bischoff E, et al. Comprehensive self-management and routine monitoring in chronic obstructive pulmonary disease patients in general practice: randomised controlled trial. BMJ. 2012;345:14.
82. Plaza V, et al. A repeated short educational intervention improves asthma control and quality of life. Eur Respir J. 2015;46(5):1298–307.
83. Gibson PG, et al. Self-management education and regular practitioner review for adults with asthma. Cochrane database of Sytematic Reviews. 2003;(1): CD001117.
84. Savage E, et al. Self-management education for cystic fibrosis (review). Cochrane Libr. 2011;7:CD007641.
85. Goldbeck L, et al. Psychological interventions for in dividuals with cystic fibrosis and their families. Cochrane database of Sytematic Reviews. 2014;6: CD003148
86. Kelly C, et al. Self-management for non-cystic fibrosis bronchiectasis. Cochrane Database of Sytematic Reviews. 2017;1:CD012528
87. Lavery K, et al. Self-management in bronchiectasis: the patients' perspective. Eur Respir J. 2007;29(3):541–7.
88. Lavery K, et al. Expert patient self-management program versus usual care in bronchiectasis: a randomized controlled trial. Arch Phys Med Rehabil. 2011;92:1194–201.
89. ISRCTN Registry. *Evaluation of Bronchiectasis Empowerment Tool (BET)*. 2015; Available from: http://www.isrctn.com/ISRCTN18400127.
90. McCullough AR, et al. Predictors of adherence to treatment in bronchiectasis. Respir Med. 2015;109(7):838–45.
91. McCullough AR, et al. Defining the content and delivery of an intervention to change adherence to treatment in bronchiectasis (CAN-BE): a qualitative approach incorporating the theoretical domains framework, behavioural change techniques and stakeholder expert panels. BMC Health Serv Res. 2015;15(1):342.
92. Edwards K, Singh S. The Bristol COPD knowledge questionnaire (BCKQ): assessing the knowledge of healthcare professionals involved in the delivery of COPD services. Thorax. 2012;67(Suppl 2):P235.
93. Henwood F, et al. 'Ignorance is bliss sometimes': constraints on the emergence of the 'informed patient' in the changing landscapes of health information. Sociology of Health and Illness. 2003;25(6):589–607.
94. Zulman D, et al. Trust in the internet as a health resource among older adults:analysis of data from a nationally representative survey. J Med Internet Res. 2011;13(1):e19.
95. Lambert SD, Loiselle CG. Health information–seeking behaviour. Qual Health Res. 2007;17:1006–19.
96. Case DO, et al. Avoiding versus seeking: the relationship of infromation seeking to avoidance, blunting, coping, dissonance and related concepts. Journal of the Medical Library Association. 2005;93(3):353–62.
97. Leydon GM, et al. Cancer patients' information needs and information seeking behaviour: in depth interview study. BMJ. 2000;320(7239):909–13.
98. De Soyza A, et al. Bronchiectasis rheumatoid overlap syndrome is an independent risk factor for mortality in patients with bronchiectasis: a multicenter cohort study. Chest. 2017;151(6):1247–54.
99. Ohlen J, et al. The influence of significant others in complementary and alternative medicine decisions by cancer patients. Soc Sci Med. 2006;63(6):1625–36.
100. Rapley T. Distributed decision making: the anatomy of decisions-in-action. Sociology of Health and Illness. 2008;30(3):429–44.
101. Anderson R, Bury M. Living the chronic illness: the experiences of patients and their families. London: Unwin Hyman; 1988.
102. Heijmans M, de Ridder D, Bensing J. Dissimilarity in patients' and spouses' representations of chronic illness: exploration of relations to patient adaptation. Psychol Health. 1999;14(3):451–66.
103. Vassilev I, et al. The influence of social networks on self-management support: a metasynthesis. BMC Public Health. 2014;14:719.
104. Reeves D, et al. The contribution of social networks to the health and management of patients with long-term conditions: a longitudinal study. PLoS One. 2014;9(6):e98340.
105. Koetsenruijter J, et al. Social support systems as determinants of self-management and quality of life of people with diabetes across Europe: study protocol for an observational study. Health Qual Life Outcomes. 2014;12:29.
106. Koetsenruijter J, et al. Social support and health in diabetes patients: an observational study in six European countries in an era of austerity. PLoS One. 2015;10(8):e0135079.
107. Hester KLM, et al. Living your life with bronchiectasis: an exploration of patients and carers information needs., in British sociological association medical sociology 47th annual conference. York: BSA; 2015. p. P106.
108. Hester KLM, et al. Evaluation of a novel information resource for patients with bronchiectasis: study protocol for a randomised controlled trial. Trials. 2016;17:210.
109. Hester KLM, et al. Evaluation of a novel intervention for patients with bronchiectasis: the bronchiectasis information and education feasibility (BRIEF) study. Thorax. 2016;71(Supplement 3):A265.

"Velcro-type" crackles predict specific radiologic features of fibrotic interstitial lung disease

Giacomo Sgalla[1,4*], Simon L. F. Walsh[2], Nicola Sverzellati[3], Sophie Fletcher[4], Stefania Cerri[5], Borislav Dimitrov[6^], Dragana Nikolic[7], Anna Barney[7], Fabrizio Pancaldi[8], Luca Larcher[8], Fabrizio Luppi[5], Mark G. Jones[4], Donna Davies[4] and Luca Richeldi[1,4]

Abstract

Background: "Velcro-type" crackles on chest auscultation are considered a typical acoustic finding of Fibrotic Interstitial Lung Disease (FILD), however whether they may have a role in the early detection of these disorders has been unknown. This study investigated how "Velcro-type" crackles correlate with the presence of distinct patterns of FILD and individual radiologic features of pulmonary fibrosis on High Resolution Computed Tomography (HRCT).

Methods: Lung sounds were digitally recorded from subjects immediately prior to undergoing clinically indicated chest HRCT. Audio files were independently assessed by two chest physicians and both full volume and single HRCT sections corresponding to the recording sites were extracted. The relationships between audible "Velcro-type" crackles and radiologic HRCT patterns and individual features of pulmonary fibrosis were investigated using multivariate regression models.

Results: 148 subjects were enrolled: bilateral "Velcro-type" crackles predicted the presence of FILD at HRCT (OR 13.46, 95% CI 5.85–30.96, $p < 0.001$) and most strongly the Usual Interstitial Pneumonia (UIP) pattern (OR 19.8, 95% CI 5.28–74.25, $p < 0.001$). Extent of isolated reticulation (OR 2.04, 95% CI 1.62–2.57, $p < 0.001$), honeycombing (OR 1.88, 95% CI 1.24–2.83, < 0.01), ground glass opacities (OR 1.74, 95% CI 1.29–2.32, $p < 0.001$) and traction bronchiectasis (OR 1.55, 95% CI 1.03–2.32, $p < 0.05$) were all independently associated with the presence of "Velcro-type" crackles.

Conclusions: "Velcro-type" crackles predict the presence of FILD and directly correlate with the extent of distinct radiologic features of pulmonary fibrosis. Such evidence provides grounds for further investigation of lung sounds as an early identification tool in FILD.

Keywords: Fibrotic interstitial lung disease, Idiopathic pulmonary fibrosis, Velcro crackles, Lung sounds, Breath sounds

Background

Fibrotic interstitial lung disease (FILD) represents a diverse and challenging group of disorders with varied treatment strategies and prognoses. Idiopathic pulmonary fibrosis (IPF) is the most frequent and deadly among FILD [1]. Recognition of signs and symptoms suggestive of FILD by healthcare practitioners represents a valuable point-of-care, low-cost opportunity for detection of early disease and timely diagnostic work up [2–4]. Chest auscultation remains an important clinical assessment in patients with respiratory disorders, providing immediate and reliable information to clinicians [5]. "Velcro-type" crackles are brief, discontinuous pathological lung sounds, explosive and transient in character, named after their similarity to the sound generated by Velcro strips separating [6]. Historically, "Velcro-type" crackles have been considered representative of established lung fibrosis [7], and quantitative analysis of crackles in ILD confirmed distinctive features as compared to those generated in other disorders such as

---

* Correspondence: giacomo.sgalla@guest.policlinicogemelli.it
^Deceased
[1]Division of Respiratory Medicine, University Hospital "A. Gemelli", Catholic University of Sacred Heart, Rome, Italy
[4]National Institute for Health Research Southampton Respiratory Biomedical Research Unit and Clinical and Experimental Sciences, University of Southampton, Southampton, UK
Full list of author information is available at the end of the article

chronic heart failure and pneumonia [8, 9]. While international consensus guidelines recommend that IPF is suspected in all patients with bibasilar inspiratory "Velcro-type" crackles [10], the direct association between "Velcro-type" crackles and specific radiologic features of pulmonary fibrosis has not been thoroughly clarified.

In this prospective case-control study, we systematically investigate the relationships between audible digitally recorded "Velcro-type" crackles and HRCT features and patterns of FILD with the aim of providing substantial evidence as to the potential role of lung sounds as a screening and monitoring tool in ILD. Lung sounds were digitally recorded from subjects immediately prior to undergoing clinically indicated HRCT. Audio files were independently assessed by two chest physicians and both full volume and single HRCT sections corresponding to the recording sites were extracted. The relationship between audible "Velcro-type" crackles and radiologic HRCT patterns or individual features of pulmonary fibrosis was investigated using multivariate regression models.

Methods
Study population and data collection
A total of 254 subjects referred to undergo HRCT scan of the chest for various clinical indications were consecutively recruited at the Radiology Units of the University Hospitals of Modena and Parma, Italy, between January 2013 and February 2015. Patients were considered eligible if they were aged 18 years or over with capacity to provide valid informed consent.

Demographics, smoking history and family history for respiratory disorders were collected. The clinical indication for performing the HRCT scan was also collected when available as reported on slips or letters from the general practitioner or respiratory consultants. However, since patients were referred from several different physicians and centres, it was not feasible to collect further data from the following diagnostic workup. Just prior to the HRCT, lung sounds were recorded sequentially at six anatomical sites identified, based on the guidelines for Computerized Respiratory Sounds Analysis (CORSA) [11], on the posterior chest as indicated in Fig. 1a. Sounds were recorded for ten seconds at each site, a time sufficient to record a minimum of two full breathing cycles, using an electronic stethoscope (Littmann 3200, 3 M, USA). After each recording, a small, radio-opaque metallic mark (a bio-compatible electrocardiography electrode) was applied to the skin to allow visualization and hence correlation of the recording sites on the HRCT (Fig. 1b). The recordings were transferred to the Littmann StethAssist software (3 M, USA) via Bluetooth technology, and exported in the wav format (sampled at 4 kHz with a resolution of 16-bit). The study was approved by the local ethics committee of Modena and Parma (Italy). Written informed consent was collected from all participants.

Radiologic review
Full volume scans and single HRCT sections corresponding to the visible marked sites of recording were extracted for each study participant. After randomization, single HRCT sections were blindly reviewed by two other thoracic radiologists (D.M.H., and N.S.) with 28 and 12 years' experience and semi-quantitatively scored on 3 different features: 1) the presence or absence of pulmonary fibrosis 2) HRCT patterns of reticulation, honeycombing, ground glass and emphysema, as defined in the Fleischner society glossary of thoracic imaging [12] and 3) severity of traction bronchiectasis. This semi-quantitative scoring system was similar to those used in previous studies [13, 14]. For reticulation, honeycombing, ground glass and emphysema the scores were defined by the proportion of bronchopulmonary segments involved (absence = 0; ≤ 25% = 1; > 25% and ≤ 50% = 2; > 50 and < 75% = 3; ≥ 75% = 4). Traction bronchiectasis was assigned with a categorical "severity" score (none = 0, mild = 1, moderate = 2, severe = 3) that accounted for the average degree of airway dilatation within areas of fibrosis as well as the extent of traction bronchiectasis throughout the lobe. Qualitative scores for

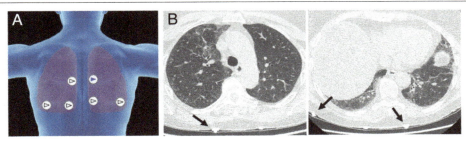

Fig. 1 Recording sites selected in the study. Per each side of the chest, two recordings were performed at the lung bases at seven cm below the scapular angle, at both two and five cm from the paravertebral line respectively; another recording was taken from mid chest in correspondence of the fourth or fifth intercostal space, at two cm from the paravertebral line (**a**). Metallic marks were applied to the posterior chest of the patient and were visible at HRCT (black arrows, (**b**)

pulmonary fibrosis were combined by an independent researcher (G.S.), who adjudicated an image as fibrotic in case of disagreement between the two observers. The semi-quantitative scores for individual features were averaged between the two observers. 76 Cases were identified based on the evidence of pulmonary fibrosis at one of the HRCT sections. 72 age and sex-matched controls were then selected from the remaining subjects showing no signs of fibrosis on the HRCT. As such, 148 subjects formed the final study population.

An expert thoracic radiologist (S.L.F.W.) with 10 years' experience blindly reviewed the full volume HRCT scans of cases and controls for the radiologic evidence of a diffuse fibrosing lung disease. Scans adjudicated as FILD were further classified as Usual Interstitial Pneumonia (UIP), possible UIP or inconsistent with UIP according to validated radiologic criteria [15].

Assessment of "Velcro-type" crackles

Two expert ILD physicians, blind to the clinical and radiology data, qualitatively assessed sound recordings for the presence of "Velcro-type" crackles. The sound files were played via personal computer using an open-source tool (Audacity software) and over-ear headphones (Sennheiser HD201 closed dynamic stereo). The sound files were randomized prior to assessment to avoid all files from the same subject being assessed consecutively. An independent researcher (G.S.) combined the scores of the two raters and adjudicated "Velcro-type" crackles as present when the physicians disagreed.

Correlation of acoustic and radiologic data

The relationships between "Velcro-type" crackles and individual features of pulmonary fibrosis were investigated by matching each recording with the corresponding HRCT section independently.

In order to determine the relationships between lung sounds and patterns on full volume HRCT, "Velcro-type" crackles were deemed as unilateral or bilateral in the individual patients according to their presence in the recordings from either one side or both sides of the chest, while they were considered absent when they could not be detected in any of the recordings from the same patient.

Statistical analysis

The collected data was entered into the SPSS software package (version 24, IBM, USA) for statistical analysis. Continuous and categorical data were summarized using means and standard deviations, or counts and percentages respectively. Nominal or ordinal data were contrasted using a Chi-squared test. The inter-rater agreement was calculated using weighted Cohen's kappa statistic (k_w), and categorized as follows: poor ($0 < k_w < 0.19$), fair ($0.20 < k_w < 0.39$), moderate ($0.40 < k_w < 0.59$), good ($0.60 < k_w < 0.79$), and optimal ($k_w > 0.81$) [16]. Univariate and multivariate logistic regression was used to estimate the relationships between the individual radiologic features and patterns (independent variables) and audible "Velcro-type" crackles (dependent variable). For all analyses, statistical significance was set at $p < 0.005$. Where applicable, models were adjusted for the number of images per patient, since not all subjects were represented by the same number of HRCT images and sound files in the data set.

Results

Characteristics of study groups

On full HRCT scan review, 66 subjects (44.6%) had radiologic findings consistent with FILD. 10 subjects (6.7%) who did not meet radiological criteria for FILD on full HRCT review had evidence of isolated pulmonary fibrosis on single HRCT sections. Demographic characteristics of the groups defined according to presence of FILD on full volume HRCT are reported in Table 1. FILD and non FILD subjects had a mean age (SD) of 71 (8.2) and 67.55 (8.96) years respectively. Subjects in both groups were predominantly males (65.2 and 54.9%, respectively) and had more frequently a positive smoking history (56.1 and 68.3%). While FILD subjects had been initially referred to HRCT mostly for suspect of ILD (69.7%), half (52.4%) of non FILD subjects were sent to

Table 1 Characteristics of study population. Data are expressed as counts (%) or mean with standard deviation (SD). FILD = Fibrotic Interstitial Lung Disease

	FILD (n = 66)	Non FILD (n = 82)
Age, years (SD)	71 (8.2)	67.55 (8.96)
Sex (%)		
Male	43 (65.2%)	45 (54.9%)
Female	23 (34.8%)	37 (45.1%)
Smoking history (%)		
Current/Former	37 (56.1%)	56 (68.3%)
Never smoker	29 (43.9%)	26 (31.7%)
Indication for HRCT (%)		
ILD	46 (69.7%)	19 (23.2%)
Other	14 (21.2%)	43 (52.4%)
Unknown	6 (9.1%)	20 (24.4%)
Family History (%)		
Pulmonary Fibrosis	3 (4.5%)	1 (1.2%)
Autoimmune disease	13 (19.7%)	10 (12.2%)
HRCT pattern (%)		
UIP	15 (22.7%)	N/A
Possible UIP	31 (47.0%)	
Inconsistent with UIP	20 (30.3%)	

HRCT for other reasons, including general symptoms such as dyspnoea and cough, chronic obstructive pulmonary disease, follow-up of lung nodules, or haemoptysis. Among subjects with FILD, 15 (22.7%) and 31 (47%) had a definite or a possible UIP pattern at HRCT, respectively; in the remaining 20 (30.3%) patients with FILD the pattern was not consistent with UIP.

Inter-rater agreement

On single HRCT sections, the inter-observer agreement between the thoracic radiologists was good for the qualitative evaluation of fibrosis ($k_w = 0.69$, 95% CI 0.65–0.73). Among the individual radiologic features, the level of agreement was good for honeycombing ($k_w = 0.71$, 95% CI 0.63–0.79) and reticular opacities (k_w 0.65, 95% CI 0.62–0.68), while it was moderate for traction bronchiectasis ($K_w = 0.51$, 95% CI 0.47–0.55), fair for emphysema ($K_w = 0.38$, 95% CI 0.31–0.44) and poor for ground glass opacities ($K_w = 0.28$, 95% CI 0.22–0.34). The level of agreement between chest physicians as to the presence of bilateral "Velcro-type" crackles was good ($k_w = 0.69$, 95% CI 0.57–0.82).

Relationships between "Velcro-type" crackles and patterns on full volume HRCT

The vast majority of subjects (81.1%) with "Velcro-type" crackles bilaterally on chest auscultation had a pattern consistent with FILD on subsequent HRCT scan. In contrast, FILD was present in only 26.8% of patients with unilateral "Velcro-type" crackles. Notably, 13 subjects (19.7%) with FILD on HRCT scan did not present "Velcro-type" crackles on chest auscultation. Of these, only one patient had a UIP pattern on HRCT, eight patients had possible UIP and four patients had a pattern inconsistent with UIP. On logistic regression analysis, the presence of bilateral "Velcro-type" crackles strongly predicted an FILD pattern (OR 13.46, 95% CI 5.85–30.96, $p < 0.001$), whilst unilateral "Velcro-crackles" were not significantly correlated (OR 0.58, CI 95% 0.29–1.16, $p = 0.2$) (Table 2). Different FILD patterns were independently associated with the presence of bilateral "Velcro-type" crackles on multivariate analysis, with the definite UIP pattern showing the strongest correlation (UIP: OR 19.8, 95% CI 5.28–74.25, $p < 0.001$; possible UIP: OR 13.09, 95% CI 4.87–35.2, $p < 0.001$; inconsistent with UIP: OR 10.8, 95% CI 3.85–32.85, $p < 0.001$).

Relationships between "Velcro-type" crackles and HRCT features

On univariate regression analysis of 805 images and corresponding sound files, the presence of "Velcro-type" crackles predicted the presence of signs of pulmonary fibrosis (Table 3). All the individual features of FILD on HRCT showed a significant association with "Velcro-type" sounds, with traction bronchiectasis showing the strongest correlation (OR 4.37, 95% CI 3.17–6.02, $p < 0.001$) (Table 3A). Multivariate regression analysis was performed in order to assess the independent relationship between the extent of individual radiologic features and the presence of "Velcro-type" crackles (Table 3B). Reticulation had the strongest relationship (OR 2.04, 95% CI 1.62–2.57, $p < 0.001$), followed by honeycombing (1.88, 95% CI 1.24–2.83, $p < 0.01$), ground glass opacities (OR 1.74, 95% CI 1.29–2.32, $p < 0.001$) and traction bronchiectasis (OR 1.55, 95% CI 1.03–2.32, $p < 0.05$).

Emphysema had a trend towards a negative association with the presence of "Velcro-type" crackles (OR 0.72, CI 95% 0.5–1.04, $p = 0.077$). To further investigate whether emphysema influences the transmission of lung sounds on chest auscultation in patients with coexisting fibrosis the mean scores for emphysematous alterations on single HRCT sections were compared between subgroups of FILD subjects with either bilateral, unilateral or absence of crackles on chest auscultation. Higher scores were found in patients with unilateral crackles (mean 0.3, SD 0.67) as compared to patients with bilateral or without crackles (mean 0.06, SD 0.23 and 0.11, SD 0.38), suggesting that in FILD subjects no clear link existed between the extent of emphysema and the absence of "Velcro-type" crackles.

Discussion

We have performed the first prospective, blinded study to investigate the relationship between "Velcro-type" crackles and radiologic patterns and features of FILD. We showed that bilateral crackles correlate with the presence of FILD, and most strongly predict the presence of a UIP pattern at HRCT. "Velcro-type" crackles

Table 2 Relationships between presence of unilateral or bilateral "Velcro-type" crackles and radiologic pattern on HRCT. Data expressed as Odds ratio (OR) with 95% Confidence Intervals (95% CI) and p value

HRCT pattern	Bilateral "Velcro-type" crackles		Unilateral "Velcro-type" crackles	
	OR (CI 95%)	p	OR (CI 95%)	p
FILD	13.46 (5.71–29.182)	< 0.001	0.58 (0.29–1.16)	0.12
Definite UIP	19.8 (5.28–74.25)	< 0.001	0.49 (0.14–1.66)	0.25
Possible UIP	13.09 (4.87–35.2)	< 0.001	0.55 (0.23–1.34)	0.19
Inconsistent with UIP	10.8 (3.85–32.85)	< 0.001	0.75 (0.26–2)	0.53

Table 3 Univariate (A) and multivariate (B) logistic regression of individual radiologic features on HRCT sections toward presence of "Velcro-type" crackles on corresponding recording sites. Data presented as odds ratios (OR) with 95% confidence intervals (CI) and p value

Feature	OR (95% CI)	p value
A		
Fibrosis	6.24 (4.5–8·66)	< 0.001
Ground glass opacities	2.13 (1.61–2.81)	< 0.001
Reticulation	2.57 (2.14–3.09)	< 0.001
Traction bronchiectasis	4.37 (3.17–6.02)	< 0.001
Honeycombing	2.39 (1.52–3.76)	< 0.001
Emphysema	0.72 (0.5–1.04)	0.077
B		
Ground glass opacities	1.74 (1.29–2.32)	< 0.001
Reticulation	2.04 (1.62–2.57)	< 0.001
Traction bronchiectasis	1.55 (1.03–2.32)	< 0.05
Honeycombing	1.88 (1.24–2.83)	< 0.01

correlated with the extent of specific interstitial abnormalities in the lung parenchyma underneath. Features representing advanced structural fibrotic alteration (such as honeycombing) and also those suggesting less advanced fibrosis (i.e. a range of extent of reticular and ground glass opacities) were independently associated with the presence of "Velcro-type" crackles. Our finding that early radiologic signs of pulmonary fibrosis such as ground glass change and reticulation generate "Velcro--type" crackles supports the concept that lung sounds could provide a tool for the early identification of FILD.

Corroborating a previous report on the association of "Velcro-type" crackles on standard chest auscultation and ILD patterns on HRCT [17], our unbiased approach highlight the importance of bilateral "Velcro-type" crackles in triggering further investigation, specifically chest HRCT, in patients presenting with chronic respiratory symptoms. Furthermore, the finding that bilateral "Velcro-type" crackles were most strongly associated with the UIP pattern support the international consensus guideline recommendation to consider IPF in patients presenting with bibasilar crackles. On the other hand, the finding that crackles were not heard in nearly 20% of patients with FILD would apparently disprove the utility of subjective chest auscultation as a screening tool. Nevertheless, among these patients only one had UIP on HRCT, suggesting that crackles are hardly missed when honeycombing – the hallmark of UIP and therefore IPF - is present. Having said that, it must be pointed out that this study was not designed for diagnostic testing purposes, and any conclusion regarding the yield of "velcro-type" crackles' assessment should not be drawn.

On individual HRCT sections the presence of pulmonary fibrosis was strongly associated with "Velcro-type" crackles. Extending this finding, multivariate analysis of individual radiologic features identified that reticulation, honeycombing, ground glass opacities and traction bronchiectasis were all independently associated with the presence of "Velcro-type" crackles in the lung parenchyma underneath. According to the stress-relaxation quadrupoles hypothesis developed through modeling by Fredberg in 1983 [18], crackles result from the acoustic energy produced by a change in elastic stress after a sudden opening or closing of distal airways. However, the pathological abnormalities underlying the generation of "Velcro-type" crackles and their pathologic significance have not been fully explored. The reticular pattern represents the hallmark of fibrotic interstitial lung disease at HRCT, correlating with a range of alterations from interlobular or intralobular thickening of the interstitial septa to the cyst walls of honeycombing [12]. The finding that the extent of reticular opacities is independently and strongly associated with "Velcro-type" crackles suggests that any degree of abnormal deposition of fibrotic tissue might cause the collapse of distal airways, according to the original theory of crackles generation [18]. Honeycombing is a term used to indicate the appearance of destroyed lung parenchyma and late stage fibrosis, presenting as piled, thick-walled cysts with a predominant distribution in the subpleural regions of the lungs. Assuming that airflow is maintained in these regions, it is likely that these dilated, distorted airspaces collapse during expiration and reopen during inspiration, causing the generation of the crackles. Ground glass opacities are areas of increased radiologic attenuation with preservation of bronchial and vascular margins, which may arise from partial filling of airspaces, increased capillary volume or interstitial intralobular thickening due to fluids or fibrosis [12]. The positive, independent association with "Velcro-type" crackles in this study strengthen the idea that even early stage interstitial involvement can be identified on chest auscultation. Traction bronchiectasis and bronchiolectasis represent abnormal bronchial and bronchiolar dilatation caused by surrounding fibrosis exerting a retractile force [12]. In the most peripheral regions, bronchiolectasis concurs to the architectural distortion of the lung parenchyma and may be actually seen as multiple cysts or microcysts, sometimes resembling honeycombing. As such, "Velcro-type" crackles might generate from these alterations as well following the same mechanisms.

Emphysema did not correlate with the presence of crackles, in keeping with the concept that destruction of alveolar walls result in a weaker transmission of lung sounds, either normal or adventitious [12]. In patients with coexisting fibrosis and emphysema it is possible that emphysema could mask "Velcro-type" crackles, thus decreasing the sensitivity of an acoustic assessment for fibrosis. To investigate this possibility, within this study we compared the emphysema scores between subgroups of FILD patients with different acoustic findings, and identified no evidence that emphysema reduces the sensitivity of auscultation to identify lung fibrosis.

This study has some points of strength. We recruited a large population of patients with a broad spectrum of lung pathologies. Lung sounds were recorded using a simple, point-of-care tool: an electronic stethoscope which is easily applicable in every clinical setting. The assessment of the recordings was performed by physicians blinded to any clinical information and unbiased towards their source (same or different patients). Lung sounds were paired with single HRCT slices: this approach allowed a precise matching with radiologic abnormalities in the lung parenchyma below the site of auscultation. Whilst lung sounds generated from a specific area might spread towards different regions of the same lung or to the other side of the chest, the transmission of "Velcro-type" crackles over different areas has been shown to be more limited than in other conditions such as chronic heart failure or pneumonia, supporting the rationale for the approach followed in this study [8]. The limitations of this study are mainly related to the research setting and cross-sectional design, which did not allow a comprehensive characterisation of the study population. The participants were not followed up and the final clinical diagnosis remained unknown in most cases. Physiology measurements and other clinical data were not collected, thereafter the relationships between "Velcro-type" crackles and clinical or functional deterioration were not addressed. Nevertheless, the study primarily focused on the validity of the subjective assessment of "Velcro-type" crackles against HRCT imaging, irrespectively of the clinical diagnosis or the functional status of the patients.

In conclusion, we identify that "Velcro-type" crackles not only predict the presence of FILD patterns at HRCT, but are also closely associated to the extent of different interstitial abnormalities in the lung parenchyma. Our finding that individual features of pulmonary fibrosis such as ground glass change and reticulation generate "Velcro-type" crackles warrants further investigation of the role of lung sounds as an early identification tool in FILD. The clinical utility of chest auscultation for assisting diagnosis and clinical management of ILD has been historically hampered by the subjectivity of standard chest auscultation and the poor signal transmission of standard stethoscopes [19]; if electronic auscultation were combined with computerized methods for lung sounds analysis and classification, this cost-effective approach might lead to the definition of an "acoustic signature" of FILD for both diagnostic and prognostic purposes, and this should be a focus of future studies.

Abbreviations
CORSA: Computerized Respiratory Sounds Analysis; FILD: Fibrotic Interstitial Lung Disease; HRCT: High Resolution Computed Tomography; IPF: Idiopathic pulmonary fibrosis; UIP: Usual Interstitial Pneumonia

Acknowledgments
We express our sincere gratitude to Professor David M Hansell who significantly contributed to the research by performing review of radiological data.

Funding
The conduction of the study was supported by funding from InterMune Europe and InterMune UK, the Wellcome Trust 100638/Z/12/Z (to MGJ) and 109682MA, and the NIHR Southampton Respiratory Biomedical Research Unit. Littmann 3200 electronic stethoscopes were provided by 3 M through an educational grant.
The sponsors funding the study did not provide any input or contributions in the development of the research and of the manuscript.

Authors' contributions
GS contributed to study conception and design, data acquisition, data analysis and interpretation, manuscript preparation and review, and approved the final version of the manuscript. SLFW contributed to study design, data analysis and interpretation, manuscript review, and approved the final version of the manuscript. NS contributed to data analysis, manuscript review, and approved the final version of the manuscript. SF contributed to data analysis, manuscript review, and approved the final version of the manuscript. SC contributed to study conception and design, data acquisition, data analysis, manuscript review, and approved the final version of the manuscript. BD contributed to data analysis and interpretation. DN and AB contributed to study design, data analysis, manuscript review, and approved the final version of the manuscript. FP and LL contributed to study design, data analysis, and approved the final version of the manuscript. FL contributed to study conception and design, manuscript review, and approved the final version of the manuscript. MGJ contributed to study design, data interpretation, manuscript review, and approved the final version of the manuscript. DD contributed to study design, data interpretation, and approved the final version of the manuscript. LR contributed to study conception and design, data interpretation, manuscript review, and approved the final version of the manuscript.

Competing interests

- Giacomo Sgalla: Dr. Sgalla reports grants from Roche (previously Intermune), during the conduct of the study; personal fees from Boheringer Ingelheim
- Simon Walsh: Dr. Walsh reports personal fees from Boehringer Ingelheim, personal fees from Boehringer Ingelheim, personal fees from Roche, personal fees from Roche, personal fees from Sanofi-Genzyme, outside the submitted work
- Nicola Sverzellati: Dr. Sverzellati reports personal fees from Roche, personal fees from Boehringer Ingelheim, outside the submitted work
- Sophie Fletcher: Dr. Fletcher reports personal fees Dr. Fletcher reports personal fees from Roche, InterMune, Boehringer Ingelheim, all outside the submitted work
- Stefania Cerri: Dr. Cerri reports grants from Roche (previously Intermune), during the conduct of the study; personal fees from Roche, personal fees from Boehringer Ingelheim, outside the submitted work
- Dragana Nikolic: Dr. Nikolic has nothing to disclose.
- Anna Barney: Dr. Barney has nothing to disclose.
- Fabrizio Pancaldi: Dr. Pancaldi has a patent "Sistema di auscultazione ed analisi dei suoni polmonari" pending
- Luca Larcher: Dr. Larcher has nothing to disclose

- Fabrizio Luppi: Dr. Luppi reports personal fees from Boehringer Ingelheim, grants and personal fees from Roche, during the conduct of the study. Dr. Luppi is currently acting as an associate editor for BMC Pulmonary Medicine.
- Mark G Jones: Dr. Jones has nothing to disclose.
- Donna Davies: Dr. Davies reports personal fees from Synairgen Research Ltd., other from synairgen Research Ltd., outside the submitted work
- Luca Richeldi: Dr. Richeldi reports grants and personal fees from InterMune, personal fees from Medimmune, personal fees from Biogen, personal fees from Sanofi-Aventis, personal fees from Roche, personal fees from ImmuneWorks, personal fees from Shionogi, personal fees from Boehringer Ingelheim, personal fees from Celgene, personal fees from Nitto, personal fees from FibroGen, outside the submitted work

Author details

[1]Division of Respiratory Medicine, University Hospital "A. Gemelli", Catholic University of Sacred Heart, Rome, Italy. [2]King's College Hospital, London, UK. [3]University Hospital of Parma, Parma, Italy. [4]National Institute for Health Research Southampton Respiratory Biomedical Research Unit and Clinical and Experimental Sciences, University of Southampton, Southampton, UK. [5]Centre for Rare Lung Disease, University Hospital of Modena, Modena, Italy. [6]Medical Statistics, Faculty of Medicine, University of Southampton, Southampton, UK. [7]Institute for Sound and Vibration Research, University of Southampton, Southampton, UK. [8]DISMI, University of Modena and Reggio Emilia, Reggio Emilia, Italy.

References

1. Richeldi L, Collard HR, Jones MG. Idiopathic pulmonary fibrosis. Lancet. 2017;389:1941–52.
2. Cottin V, Cordier JF. Velcro crackles: the key for early diagnosis of idiopathic pulmonary fibrosis? Eur Respir J. 2012;40:519–21.
3. Cordier JF, Cottin V. Neglected evidence in idiopathic pulmonary fibrosis: from history to earlier diagnosis. Eur Respir J. 2013;42:916–23.
4. Cottin V, Richeldi L. Neglected evidence in idiopathic pulmonary fibrosis and the importance of early diagnosis and treatment. Eur Respir Rev. 2014;23:106–10.
5. Bohadana A, Izbicki G, Kraman SS. Fundamentals of lung auscultation. N Engl J Med. 2014;370:744–51.
6. Forgacs P. Crackles and wheezes. Lancet. 1967;290:203–5.
7. Pasterkamp H, Brand PLP, Everard M, Garcia-Marcos L, Melbye H, Priftis KN. Towards the standardisation of lung sound nomenclature. Eur Respir J. 2016;47:724–32.
8. Vyshedskiy A, Bezares F, Paciej R, Ebril M, Shane J, Murphy R. Transmission of crackles in patients with interstitial pulmonary fibrosis, congestive heart failure, and pneumonia. Chest. 2005;128:1468–74.
9. Flietstra B, Markuzon N, Vyshedskiy A, Murphy R. Automated analysis of crackles in patients with interstitial pulmonary fibrosis. Pulm Med Hindawi Publishing Corporation. 2011;2011:590506.
10. Raghu G, Collard HR, Egan JJ, Martinez FJ, Behr J, Brown KK, et al. An official ATS/ERS/JRS/ALAT statement: idiopathic pulmonary fibrosis: evidence-based guidelines for diagnosis and management. Am. J. Respir. Crit. Care med. American thoracic Society. 2011;183:788–824.
11. Sovijärvi ARA, Vanderschoot J, Earis JE, Munksgaard. Computerized respiratory sound analysis (CORSA): recommended standards for terms and techniques : ERS task force report. Eur. Respir. Rev. Copenhagen: Munksgaard; 2000.
12. Hansell DM, Bankier AA, MacMahon H, McLoud TC, Müller NL, Remy J. Fleischner society: glossary of terms for thoracic imaging. Radiology. 2008;246:697–722.
13. Kazarooni EA, Martinez FJ, Flint A, Jamadar DA, Gross BH, Spizarny DL, et al. Thin-section CT obtained at 10-mm increments versus limited three-level thin-section CT for idiopathic pulmonary fibrosis: correlation with pathologic scoring. Am J Roentgenol. 1997;169:977–83.
14. Oda K, Ishimoto H, Yatera K, Naito K, Ogoshi T, Yamasaki K, et al. High-resolution CT scoring system-based grading scale predicts the clinical outcomes in patients with idiopathic pulmonary fibrosis. Respir Res. 2014;15:10.
15. Travis WD, Costabel U, Hansell DM, King TE, Lynch DA, Nicholson AG, et al. An official American Thoracic Society/European Respiratory Society statement: update of the international multidisciplinary classification of the idiopathic interstitial pneumonias. Am J Respir Crit Care Med. 2013;188:733–48.
16. Brennan P, Silman A. Statistical methods for assessing observer variability in clinical measures. Bmj. Arthritis and Rheumatism, Council Epidemiology Research Unit, University of Manchester. 1992;304:1491–4.
17. Sellarés J, Hernández-González F, Lucena CM, Paradela M, Brito-Zerón P, Prieto-González S, et al. Auscultation of Velcro crackles is associated with usual interstitial pneumonia. Medicine (Baltimore) 2016/02/06. From the Servei de Pneumologia, Hospital Clinic, IDIBAPS, Universitat de Barcelona, (JS, FH-G, CM feminineL, SC, AX); Centro de Investigacion Biomedica En Red-Enfermedades Respiratorias (CibeRes, CB06/06/0028) (JS, CM feminineL); Servei de Cirurgia Toraci; 2016;95:e2573.
18. Fredberg JJ, Holford SK. Discrete lung sounds: crackles (rales) as stress-relaxation quadrupoles. J Acoust Soc Am. 1983;73:1036–46.
19. Abella M, Formolo J, Penney DG. Comparison of the acoustic properties of six popular stethoscopes. J Acoust Soc Am Department of Internal Medicine, St John Hospital, Detroit, Michigan 48236. 1992;91:2224–8.

Profiling non-tuberculous mycobacteria in an Asian setting: characteristics and clinical outcomes of hospitalized patients in Singapore

Albert Y. H. Lim[1]*, Sanjay H. Chotirmall[2], Eric T. K. Fok[3], Akash Verma[1], Partha P. De[4], Soon Keng Goh[1], Ser Hon Puah[1], Daryl E. L. Goh[5] and John A. Abisheganaden[1]

Abstract

Background: Non-tuberculous mycobacteria (NTM) infection is an increasing problem worldwide. The epidemiology of NTM in most Asian countries is unknown. This study investigated the epidemiology, and clinical profile of inpatients in whom NTM was isolated from various anatomical sites in a Singaporean population attending a major tertiary referral centre.

Methods: Demographic profile, clinical data, and characteristics of patients hospitalized with NTM isolates at a major tertiary hospital over two-year period were prospectively assessed (2011–2012). Data collected included patient demographics, ethnicity, smoking status, co-morbidities, NTM species, intensive care unit (ICU) treatment, and mortality.

Results: A total of 485 patients (62.1% male) with 560 hospital admissions were analysed. The median patient age was 70 years. Thirteen different NTM species were isolated from this cohort. *Mycobacterium abscessus (M. abscessus)* (38.4%) was most frequently isolated followed by *Mycobacterium fortuitum (M. fortuitum)* (16.6%), *Mycobacterium avium complex (MAC)* (16.3%), *Mycobacterium kansasii (M. kansasii)* (15.4%), and *Mycobacterium gordonae (M. gordonae)* (6.8%). Most (91%) NTM was isolated from the respiratory tract. The three most common non-pulmonary sites were; blood (2.7%), skin wounds and abscesses (2.1%), and gastric aspirates (1.1%). A third (34.4%) of the study population had prior pulmonary tuberculosis (PTB). There was a significant association between isolated NTM species, and patient age ($p = 0.0002$). Eleven (2.2%) patients received intensive care unit (ICU) treatment during the study period and all cause mortality within 1 year of the study was 16.9% ($n = 82$). Of these, 72 (87.8%) patients died of pulmonary causes.

Conclusions: The profile of NTM species in Singapore is unique. *M. abscessus* is the commonest NTM isolated, with a higher prevalence in males, and in the elderly. High NTM prevalence is associated with high rates of prior PTB in our cohort.

Keywords: Non-tuberculous mycobacteria, Bronchiectasis, Tuberculosis, Epidemiology, *Mycobacterium abscessus*

Background

Non-tuberculous mycobacteria (NTM) are ubiquitous environmental organisms particularly in water and soil [1]. Their survival in water drainage, hospital water systems, and haemodialysis centres are attributable to its inherent resistance to high temperatures, low pH, and antibiotics [2–4].

NTM Infections are increasing exponentially in their global prevalence, morbidity and mortality [5]. The trend is partially attributed to the availability of improved molecular diagnostic testing [6], improved physicians' awareness, and a greater number of susceptible hosts. NTM incidence ranges between 7.2 and 13.6 per 100,000 persons [7, 8]. It is however difficult to determine the prevalence and incidence of infection accurately as its isolation microbiologically does not always equate to or even indicate clinical infection.

* Correspondence: albert_ly_hou@ttsh.com.sg
[1]Department of Respiratory and Critical Care Medicine, Tan Tock Seng Hospital, 11 Jalan Tan Tock Seng, Singapore 308433, Singapore
Full list of author information is available at the end of the article

A wide spectrum of NTM infections is reported including pulmonary, bone, eye, ear, and that affecting the central nervous system. Lymphadenitis, skin abscesses and disseminated infection, the latter in immuno-compromised individuals are also described [9]. The risk factors for NTM infections are varied and include genetic susceptibility, structural lung damage, autoimmune disease, acquired immunodeficiency states including AIDS, malignancy, and solid organ transplants [10]. Use of immunosuppressive drugs such as tumour necrosis factor (TNF) –α blockers also predispose to NTM infection [11, 12].

It is reported that more than 90% of the NTM positive cultures are pulmonary in origin [13]. The reported prevalence of NTM pulmonary infections in the USA varies between 4.1 and 14.1 per 100,000 [14]. NTM pulmonary infections are most common in females and those older than 65. Geographic and ethnic variations are also observed with NTM pulmonary infection [15]. For instance, in a study of NTM species from respiratory specimens of 20,182 patients in 30 countries across six continents, the most common NTM species identified was *Mycobacterium avium complex* (*MAC*), followed by *Mycobacterium gordonae* (*M. gordonae*), *Mycobacterium xenopi* (*M. xenopi*) and *Mycobacterium kansasii* (*M. kansasii*) [16]. In the same study, it was noted that although *MAC* is the commonest overall, its prevalence is higher in Asian countries [16]. In Singapore, a key South-East Asian island state, the distribution of NTM species is largely unknown and hence we studied the NTM profiles, clinical characteristics and outcomes in a large inpatient Asian cohort attending a major tertiary referral centre.

Methods

This prospective observational study included all adult patients where NTM was isolated on at least one specimen during a hospital admission at Tan Tock Seng Hospital, Singapore between January 2011 and December 2012 (2-year period). Patient demographics, ethnicity, smoking status, co-morbidities, and NTM species isolated were obtained from the computerized patient support system (CPSS) and collated for analysis. All data complied with the Singapore Personal Data Protection Act (PDPA) 2012 and the Institutional Review Board (IRB) of the National Healthcare Group approved the study protocol.

NTM specimens from pulmonary and non-pulmonary sites were analysed. The specimens obtained from 'pulmonary sites' included sputum, bronchoalveolar lavage (BAL), pleural biopsies and fluid. The 'non-pulmonary' site specimens included skin abscess fluid, skin wound swabs, blood, urine, and bone biopsy specimens. All specimens were stained by the Ziehl-Neelsen method according to the American Thoracic Society guidelines [17]. *Mycobacterium tuberculosis* (MTB) and NTM isolates were distinguished by their growth rate, colonial morphology, pigmentation, and by negative DNA probe (AccuProbe; Gen-Probe Inc., San Diego, CA) and NAP (p-nitro-α-acetylamino-β-hydroxy-propiophenone) tests for MTB. NTM species were identified by DNA reverse hybridization (INNO-LiPA MYCOBACTERIA v2, Innogenetics NV, Ghent, Belgium) and high-performance liquid chromatography. Further identifications were performed by 16S ribosomal RNA sequencing using primers 16S-27F (5′-AGA GTT TGA TCM TGG CTC AG-3′) and 16S-907R (5′-CCG TCA ATT CMT TTR AGT TT-3′).

Patient demographics are presented as summary statistics. Categorical variables were compared using Chi-squared analysis or Fisher's exact test. If continuous data were normally distributed, unpaired t-tests were used, and if non-normal, the Mann-Whitey rank sum test employed. For all statistical analysis, $p < 0.05$ was considered statistically significant.

Results

Characteristics of the study population

A total of 485 adult patients (62% male) with 560 NTM isolates were studied. The median (IQR) age and body mass index (BMI) of the study population were 70 (58–82) years and 19 (16–23) respectively. The majority were of Chinese descent (82%), followed by Malay (8%), Indian (4%) and other ethnicities including Eurasians (6%). Ninety five (19.5%) were current smokers. Bronchiectasis (28.7%) was the commonest underlying pulmonary disease, followed by chronic obstructive pulmonary disease (COPD) (14.2%). The three commonest non-pulmonary co-morbidities were hypertension (32.2%), hyperlipidaemia (25.8%), and diabetes mellitus (17.9%). Fifty two (10.7%) had human immunodeficiency virus (HIV) infection (Table 1).

NTM species and isolation sites

A total of 13 species of NTM were identified in this study. The five most frequently isolated NTM were *M. abscessus* (215 isolates; 38.4%), *M. fortuitum* (93 isolates; 16.6%), *MAC* (91 isolates; 16.3%), *M. kansasii* (86 isolates; 15.4%), and *M. gordonae* (38 isolates; 6.8%). These five species accounted for 93.5% of all NTM species isolated (Table 2). Five hundred and eleven (91%) of all the NTM isolates were from pulmonary sites. The three most common non-pulmonary sites were; blood specimens (15 isolates; 2.7%), skin wounds and abscesses (12 isolates; 2.1%), and gastric aspirates (6 isolates; 1.1%) (Table 3). *M. abscessus* was the most frequently isolated NTM species from pulmonary specimens (202 isolates; 39.5%), whilst *MAC* (14 isolates; 28.6%) was the most frequently NTM species isolated from non-pulmonary specimens, closely followed by *M. abscessus* (13 isolates; 26.5%) (Table 3).

Table 1 Demographics and clinical characteristics of the study population (n = 485)

Age (years): median (IQR)	70 (58–82)
Gender (male): n (%)	301 (62.1%)
BMI (kg/m^2): median (IQR)	19.4(16.4–23)
Smoking status: n (%)	
Current smoker	95 (19.6%)
Ex- smoker	94 (19.4%)
Never	296 (61%)
Previous history of PTB: n (%)	167 (34.4%)
Active PTB: n (%)	3 (0.6%)
Co-morbidities (pulmonary): n (%)	
Bronchiectasis	139 (28.7%)
COPD	69 (14.2%)
Asthma	32 (6.6%)
Pulmonary fibrosis	18 (3.7%)
Co-morbidities (non- pulmonary): n (%)	
Hypertension	156 (32.2%)
Hyperlipidaemia	125 (25.8%)
Diabetes mellitus	87 (17.9%)
Coronary artery disease	63 (12.9%)
HIV infection	52 (10.7%)
Psychiatry disorder	38 (7.8%)
Malignancy	29 (6%)
Cerebrovascular disease	23 (4.7%)
Chronic renal impairment	16 (3.3%)
Rheumatoid arthritis	11 (2.2%)
Prevalence of isolates per 100,000 hospital admissions	511/100,000

Table 2 Frequency of NTM species isolated during the study period (n = 650)

NTM species	N (%)
Mycobacterium abscessus	215 (38.4%)
Mycobacterium fortuitum complex	93 (16.6%)
Mycobacterium avium complex	91 (16.3%)
Mycobacterium kansasii	86 (15.4%)
Mycobacterium gordonae	38 (6.8%)
Mycobacterium chelonae	9 (1.6%)
Mycobacterium lentiflavum	8 (1.4%)
Mycobacterium scrofulaceum	6 (1.0%)
Mycobacterium haemophilum	4 (0.7%)
Mycobacterium simiae	3 (0.5%)
Mycobacterium szulgai	3 (0.5%)
Mycobacterium terrae complex	2 (0.4%)
Mycobacterium mucogenicum	2 (0.4%)

Association of gender, age, and NTM isolates

Most NTM isolates were found in male patients and those aged above 50 years (Table 4). There was a significant association between NTM isolation and patients' age ($p = 0.0002$). On subgroup analysis, M. abscessus (81.8%), M. fortuitum (96.3%), and MAC (84.5%) were commonly isolated from patients aged above 50. Contrary to the other species, M. abscessus was the only NTM species to be identified in younger patients (below age 30) (13 patients; 6%) (Table 4). There was no statistically significant difference noted among the NTM species isolated across the other age groups (Table 4).

Pulmonary tuberculosis, bronchiectasis and NTM isolates

Three patients were found to have co-infection with pulmonary tuberculosis (PTB) and M. abscessus during the study period. A third (34.4%) of the study population had prior PTB. Previous PTB accounted for the underlying aetiology in 88 (18.1%) of those with bronchiectasis described in this cohort. Among patients with bronchiectasis ($n = 139$), the three commonest NTM isolates were M. abscessus (41.7%; 58/139), MAC (15.8%, 22/139), and M. fortuitum (12.9%, 18/139). There was a preponderance for NTM in females in patients with bronchiectasis (52% vs. 32.4% respectively, $p < 0.0001$) in contrast to the male preference overall as reported above.

Intensive care treatment, mortality and NTM isolates

Eleven (2.2%) patients received intensive care unit (ICU) treatment during the study period and 82 (16.9%) patients died during the course of the study. Of these deaths, 72 (87.8%) were due to pulmonary causes. M. abscessus was the most frequently isolated NTM species in those who required ICU treatment or died (Table 5).

Discussion

We demonstrate a unique profile of NTM species in Singapore, a Southeast Asian city state. M. abscessus was the commonest NTM isolated, with a higher prevalence in males and the elderly. We further illustrated a high prevalence of NTM in hospitalised patients. Most significantly however, M. abscessus was the commonest of the 13 NTM species isolated and accounted for approximately a third of all the isolates followed by M. fortuitum (16.6%) and MAC (16.3%). This suggests a unique Asian profile in the spectrum of isolated NTM from hospitalised inpatients. Furthermore, half (53%) of our study population had an underlying pulmonary disorder with bronchiectasis being most common (28.7%). Interestingly, over one third of the cohort had prior PTB which in a large proportion accounted for the aetiology of their detected bronchiectasis.

In a small Singapore study published more than two decades ago, Teo and Lo [18] found that MAC was the

Table 3 Distribution of NTM species by isolation sites

	Pulmonary sites (n = 511)	Skin and soft tissues (n = 12)	Blood (n = 15)	Gastric aspirate (n = 6)	Urine (n = 4)	Liver (n = 4)	Other (n = 8)
M. abscessus – n (%)	202 (39.5%)	7 (58%)	2 (13.3%)	3 (50%)	1 (25%)	0 (0)	0 (0)
M. fortuitum – n (%)	85 (16.6%)	1 (8.3%)	0 (0)	0 (0)	2 (50%)	2 (50%)	3 (37.5%)
M. avium – n (%)	77 (15.1%)	0 (0)	10 (66.7%)	0 (0)	1 (25%)	0 (0)	3 (37.5%)
M. kansasii – n (%)	79 (15.5%)	2 (16.7%)	1 (6.7%)	1 (16.7%)	0 (0)	2 (50%)	1 (12.5%)
M. gordonae – n (%)	36 (7%)	0 (0)	0 (0)	2 (33.3%)	0 (0)	0 (0)	0 (0)
M. chelone – n (%)	9 (1.8%)	0 (0)	0 (0)	0 (0)	0 (0)	0 (0)	0 (0)
M. lentifalvum – n (%)	8 (1.6%)	0 (0)	0 (0)	0 (0)	0 (0)	0 (0)	0 (0)
M. scrolaceum – n (%)	6 (1.2%)	0 (0)	0 (0)	0 (0)	0 (0)	0 (0)	0 (0)
M. haemophilum – n (%)	0 (0)	2 (16.6%)	1 (6.7%)	0 (0)	0 (0)	0 (0)	1 (0)
M. szulgai – n (%)	3 (0.6%)	0 (0)	0 (0)	0 (0)	0 (0)	0 (0)	0 (0)
M. simiae – n (%)	3 (0.6%)	0 (0)	0 (0)	0 (0)	0 (0)	0 (0)	0 (0)
M. terrae – n (%)	2 (0.4%)	0 (0)	0 (0)	0 (0)	0 (0)	0 (0)	0 (0)
M. mucogenicum – n (%)	1 (0.2%)	0 (0)	1 (6.7%)	0 (0)	0 (0)	0 (0)	0 (0)

most common NTM isolated. The difference in their NTM profile from ours may be due to their small sample size of the older study. Other factors may be the improvement in laboratory techniques in diagnosing rapidly growing mycobacteria (RGM) over the intervening period as well as the emergence of RGM, especially M. abscessus as a human pathogen in the region.

NTM related disease has gained much attention due to its increasing prevalence globally and the improved ability for its isolation [15, 19–21]. There is geographic variation in the NTM species isolated with similar differences observed in disease manifestations [15, 16, 22]. MAC has been reported as the commonest NTM species isolated worldwide, followed by M. gordonae, and M. xenopi [16]. In the case of pulmonary NTM disease while MAC is generally the universal preponderant species, there is much regional variation with regard to other commonly encountered NTM species; in the USA and Japan M. kansasii is the next most common species, in South Korea it is M. abscessus, and in France M. Xenopi [17, 23–26].

Our finding of predominant M. abscessus is novel and likely unique in an East Asian context. The existing literature includes a recent study on 20,182 patients by the NTM-Network European Trials Group (NET) who reported that MAC species were the commonest (47%) NTM species isolated worldwide [16]. In the same study, RGM such as M. abscessus and M. fortuitum made up only 10–20% of all the NTM isolates described, in contrast to our dataset. Interestingly however, these isolates originated predominantly from Asian countries including Taiwan and South Korea. We believe our NTM profile is unique, dominated with M. abscessus followed by M. fortuitum and MAC. Likely reasons for the high prevalence of M. abscessus in our study population remains unclear, however

Table 4 Prevalence of NTM isolates by gender and age

	M. abscessus (n = 195)	M. fortuitum (n = 83)	M. avium (n = 78)	Other NTM (n = 129)	M. fortuitum	M. avium	Other NTM
	N (%)				OR (95%CI)		
Male	120 (62)	45 (54)	54 (69)	82 (64)	0.74 (0.44–1.24)	1.40 (0.80–2.46)	1.09 (0.6–1.73)
Age (years)							
< 30	10 (5)	0 (0)	0 (0)	0 (0)	0.11 (0.01–1.83)[a]	0.11 (0.01–1.95)	0.07 (0.01–1.18)[b]
31–50	25 (13)	5 (6)	9 (12)	17 (13)	0.44 (0.16–1.18)	0.89 (0.39–1.99)	1.03 (0.53–1.99)
51–70	73 (37)	34 (41)	29 (37)	43 (33)	1.16 (0.69–1.96)	0.99 (0.58–1.70)	0.83 (0.52–1.33)
> 70	87 (45)	44 (56)	40 (51)	69 (54)	1.12 (0.68–1.83)	1.31 (0.77–2.21)	1.43 (0.91–2.23)

[a] M. abscessus vs. M. fortuitum, p = 0.04
[b] M. abscessus vs. Other NTM, p = 0.007

Table 5 Intensive care unit treatment, mortality and NTM isolates

	Overall event rate	Species				
		M. abscessus	M. kansasii	MAC	M. fortuitum	M. gordonae
ICU admissions	11 (2.2%)	3 (27.3%)	3 (27.3%)	2 (18.2%)	2 (18.2%)	1 (9%)
Mortality						
- All cause	82 (16.9%)	38 (46.3%)	13 (15.9%)	17 (20.7%)	6 (7.3%)	3 (3.7%)
- Pulmonary cause	72 (14.8%)	35 (48.6%)	13 (18.1%)	14 (19.4%)	5 (6.9%)	2 (2.8%)

geographical, climatic, host and genetic factors have all been previously proposed [27].

There are a number of potential explanations for our findings in relation to past PTB in one third of those where NTM was isolated. Firstly, the incidence of TB is modest between 35 to 45 cases per 100,000 in Singapore. PTB also causes structural and functional lung damage including bronchiectasis, airway stenosis, bronchovascular distortion, and fibrosis that facilitate NTM growth [28]. Secondly, on Ingenuity Pathway Analysis (IPA) of gene to gene relationships, it is described that focus genes such as the Toll Like Receptor-2 (*TLR2*), Interleukin12 (*IL12*), and Interferon-gamma (*IFNG*) all play important roles in the innate and adaptive immune response and where genetic polymorphisms are present leads to an increased risk of both TB and NTM infection [29]. Thirdly, from network genes analysis, nuclear factor-κB (*NFκB*) complex, ERK1/2, and p38MAPK (mitogen-activated protein kinase) pathways all affect disease survival where both TB and NTM are implicated. Defects in these pathways increase the risk of both TB and NTM infections [30–32]. Prior studies also demonstrate that vitamin deficiencies (e.g. vitamins A, B, C, D, E, K, and lycopene) alter immune regulation and increase the risk of mycobacterial infection. Vitamin deficiencies are common in the Asian population and could explain our findings of high PTB and NTM prevalence [29].

In a study of 2548 patents with pulmonary NTM in the USA, Adjemain et al. found a higher prevalence of pulmonary NTM in the Asian and Pacific Islander population with a male predominance, in contrast with the white population where the prevalence is lower and female patients form the predominant group [15]. This preponderance of male patients infected with NTM disease is similarly seen in our study population which comprises various Asian ethnicities. In their work, the interactions of genetic, behavioural and environmental factors were cited as possible causes for this difference in the prevalence between ethnic groups.

In our study we found a high prevalence of NTM isolates among the elderly (median age 70 years); this is consistent with recent reports from USA and South Korea [19, 25]. Ageing and the increased incidence of co-morbidities in the elderly may play an important role in the acquisition and subsequent persistence of NTM. NTM isolation increases with age and most of these developed pulmonary NTM [25, 27]. As the population of Singapore aged 65 and above is expected to double by 2030, it is important to recognise NTM infection and particularly its association with age as an important public health issue with potential significant consequences for affected patients and use of healthcare resources. An important shortcoming of this study is the study of the profile of NTM isolates over a 2 year period which may not be long enough to determine associated trends particularly the development of active NTM pulmonary infection. Follow-up studies over longer periods may overcome this limitation, and likely provide additional and important information on trend and factors that may predict onset of active NTM pulmonary infection. Additionally, we only curated a number of clinical variables in this Asian-based assessment of NTM and lacked a comparator non-Asian group. Addressing these in future studies will likely provide a more comprehensive dataset permitting a greater degree of clinical relevance in the Asian context to be established.

The clinical outcomes of our study population were poor, further highlighting the importance of recognising NTM infection. Likely explanations for the poor prognosis include older patient age and associated co-morbidities and the predominance of *M. abscessus*, which in itself is associated with multi-drug resistance and accelerated declines in lung function [33].

Conclusion

In summary, our study demonstrates a unique profile of NTM species in Singapore. *M. abscessus* was the commonest NTM isolated, with higher prevalence in males and the elderly. A high prevalence of NTM is associated with a high burden of past PTB likely explained by PTB related pulmonary damage thus increasing the risk of acquiring NTM, or alternatively a strong genetic susceptibility to both MTB and NTM infection amongst the Asian population. In addition, the higher prevalence of NTM infection among our older population is significant particularly in the context of the anticipated rise in global ageing which necessitates the need to better understand epidemiological trends, clinical consequences, and economical burden of NTM infection across both Asia and internationally.

Acknowledgments
We thank Liew Hong Yin, Senior Medical Technologist, Laboratory Information System (LIS) for acquisition of the NTM data.

Authors' contributions
AYHL contributed to the conception and design of the study, analysis and interpretation of the data, and drafted the manuscript. SHC and AV contributed to the interpretation of the data, and drafting of the manuscript. ETKF contributed to the acquisition of the data and data analysis. DELG contributed to data analysis and helped in drafting of the manuscript. PDP, SKG, SHP, and JAA involved in analysis and interpretation of the data, critical reviewed of the contents and drafting of the manuscript. All authors read and approved the final version of the manuscript.

Competing interests
Sanjay H. Chortirmall is a member of the editorial board (Section Editor). All other authors declare that they have no competing interests.

Author details
[1]Department of Respiratory and Critical Care Medicine, Tan Tock Seng Hospital, 11 Jalan Tan Tock Seng, Singapore 308433, Singapore. [2]Lee Kong Chian School of Medicine, Translational Respiratory Research laboratory, Nanyang Technological University, Clinical Sciences Building, 11 Mandalay Road, Singapore 308232, Singapore. [3]Yong Loo Lin School of Medicine, National University of Singapore, 12 Science Drive 2, Singapore 117549, Singapore. [4]Department of Laboratory Medicine, Tan Tock Seng Hospital, 11 Jalan Tan Tock Seng, Singapore 308433, Singapore. [5]Dalhousie Medical School, Dalhousie University, 1459 Oxford Street, Halifax, NS B3H 4R2, Canada.

References
1. Falkinham JO 3rd. Environmental sources of nontuberculous mycobacteria. Clin Chest Med. 2015;36:35–41.
2. Bodmer T, Miltner E, Bermudez LE. Mycobacteria avium resists exposure to the acidic conditions of the stomach. FEMS Microbiol Lett. 2000;182:45–9.
3. Kirschner RA Jr, Parker BC, Falkinham JO 3rd. Epidemiology of infection by nontuberculous mycobacteria. Mycobacterium avium, Mycobacterium intracellulare, and Mycobacterium scrofulaceum in acid, brown-water swamps of southeastern United States and their association with environmental variables. Am Rev Respir Dis. 1992;145:271–5.
4. Falkinham JO 3rd. Growth in catheter biofilms and antibiotic resistance of Mycobacterium avium. J Med Microbiol. 2007;56:250–4.
5. Mirsaeidi M, Machado RF, Garcia JGN, Schraufnagel DE. Nontuberculous mycobacterial disease mortality in the United States, 1999–2010: a population-based comparative study. PLoS One. 2014;9(3):e91879.
6. Blackwood KS, He C, Gunton J, Turenne CY, Wolfe J, Kabani AM. Evaluation of recA sequences for identification of Mycobacterium species. J Clin Microbiol. 2000;38(8):2846–52.
7. Cassidy PM, Hedberg K, Saulson A, McNelly E, Winthrop KL. Non-tuberculous mycobacterial disease prevalence and risk factors: a changing epidemiology. Clin Infect Dis. 2009;49:e124–9.
8. Thomson RM. Changing epidemiology of pulmonary nontuberculous mycobacteria infections. Emerg Infect Dis. 2010;16:1576–83.
9. Jarand J, Levin A, Zhang L, Huitt G, Mitchell JD, Daley CL. Clinical and microbiologic outcomes in patients receiving treatment for mycobacterium abscessus pulmonary disease. Clin Infect Dis. 2011;52:565–71.
10. Henkle E, Winthrop KL. Nontuberculous mycobacteria infections in immunosuppressed hosts. Clin Chest Med. 2015;36:91–9.
11. Winthrop KL, Baxter R, Liu L, Varley CD, Curtis JR, Braddley JW, McFarland B, Austin D, Radcliffe L, Suhler E, et al. Mycobacterial diseases and antitumour necrosis factor therapy in USA. Ann Rheum Dis. 2013;72:37–42.
12. Brode SK, Jamieson FB, Ng R, Campitelli MA, Kwong JC, Paterson JM, Li P, Marchand-Austin A, Bombardier C, Marras TK. Increased risk of mycobacterial infections associated with anti-rheumatic medications. Thorax. 2015;70:677–82.
13. O'Brien RJ, Geiter LJ, Snider DE Jr. The epidemiology of nontuberculous mycobacterial diseases in the United States. Results from a national survey. Am Rev Respir Dis. 1987;135:1007–14.
14. Kendall BA, Winthrop KL. Update on the epidemiology of pulmonary nontuberculous mycobacterial infections. Semin Respir Crit Care Med. 2013;34:87–94.
15. Adjemian J, Olivier KN, Seitz AE, Holland SM, Prevots DB. Prevalence of nontuberculous mycobacterial lung disease in U.S. Medicare beneficiaries. Am J Respir Crit Care Med. 2012;185:881–6.
16. Hoefsloot W, van Ingen J, Andrejak C, Angeby K, Bauriaud R, Bemer P, Beylis N, Boeree MJ, Cacho J, Chihota V, et al. The geographical diversity of nontuberculous mycobacteria isolated from pulmonary samples: an NTM-NET collaborative study. Eur Respir J. 2013;42:1604–13.
17. American Thoracic Society. Diagnostic standards and classification of tuberculosis in adults and children. Am J Respir Crit Care Med. 2000;161:1376–95.
18. Teo SK, Lo KL. Nontuberculous mycobacterial disease in Singapore. Singap Med J. 1992;33:464–6.
19. Prevots DR, Shaw PA, Strickland D, et al. Nontuberculous mycobacterial lung disease prevalence at four integrated health care delivery systems. Am J Respir Crit Care Med. 2010;182(7):970–6.
20. Chu H, Zhao L, Xiao H, Zhang Z, Zhang J, Gui T, Gong S, Xu L, Sun X. Prevalence of nontuberculous mycobacteria in patients with bronchiectasis: a meta-analysis. Arch Med Sci. 2014;10(4):661–8.
21. Marras TK, Chedore P, Ying AM, Jamieson F. Isolation prevalence of pulmonary non-tuberculous mycobacteria in Ontario, 1997-2003. Thorax. 2007;62:661–6.
22. Tang SS, Lye DC, Jureen R, Sng LH, Hsu LY. Rapidly growing mycobacteria in Singapore, 2006–2011. Clin Microbiol Infect. 2015;21:236–41.
23. Tsukamura M, Kita N, Shimoide H, et al. Studies on the epidemiology of nontuberculous mycobacteriosis in Japan. Am Rev Respir Dis. 1988;137:1280–4.
24. Maiz L, Giron R, Olveria C, Vendrell M, Nieto R, Martinez-Garcia MA. Prevalence and factors associated with nontuberculous mycobacteria in non-cystic fibrosis bronchiectasis: a multicentre observational study. BMC Infect Dis. 2016;16:437–44.
25. Koh WJ, Kwon OJ, Jeon K, Kim TS, Lee KS, Park YK, Bai GH. Clinical significance of nontuberculous mycobacteria isolated from respiratory specimens in Korea. Chest. 2006;129:341–8.
26. Dailloux M, Abalain ML, Laurain C, Lebrun L, Loos-Ayav C, LozniewskiA MJ, the French Mycobacteria Study Group. Respiratory infections associated with nontuberculous mycobacteria in non-HIV patients. Eur Respir J. 2006;28:1211–5.
27. Simons SO, van Ingen J, Hsueh PR, et al. Nontuberculous mycobacteria in respiratory tract infections, eastern Asia. Emerg Infect Dis. 2011;7:343–9.
28. Chakaya J, Kirenga B, Getahun H. Long term complications after completion of pulmonary tuberculosis treatment: a quest for a public health approach. J Clin Tuber Other Mycobact Dis. 2016;3:10–2.
29. Lipner EM, Garcia BJ, Strong M. Network analysis of human genes influencing susceptibility to mycobacterial infections. PLoS One. 2016;11(1):e0146585.
30. Bai X, Feldman NE, Chmura K, Ovrutsky AR, Su W-L, Griffin L, et al. Inhibition of nuclear factor- kappa B activation decreases survival of mycobacterium tuberculosis in human macrophages. PLoS One. 2013;8(4):e61925.
31. Xia Z, Dickens M, Raingeaud JL, Davis RJ, Greenberg ME. Opposing effects of ERK and JNK-p38 MAP kinase on apoptosis. Science. 1995;270(5240):1326–31.
32. Pearson G, Robinson F, Beers Gibson T, Xu B-E, Karandikar M, Berman K, et al. Mitogen-activated protein (MAP) kinase pathways: regulation and physiological functions. Endocr Rev. 2001;22(2):152–83.
33. Esther CR Jr, Esserman DA, Gilligan P, Kerr A, Noone PG. Chronic mycobacterium abscessus infection and lung function decline in cystic fibrosis. J Cyst Fibrosis. 2010;9:117–23.

Anti-IL-5 therapy in patients with severe eosinophilic asthma – clinical efficacy and possible criteria for treatment response

Nora Drick[1*], Benjamin Seeliger[1], Tobias Welte[1,2], Jan Fuge[1,2] and Hendrik Suhling[1]

Abstract

Background: Interleukin-5 (IL-5) antibodies represent a promising therapeutic option for patients with severe eosinophilic asthma. To date, no official treatment response criteria exist. In this study, simple criteria for treatment response applicable to all asthma patients were used to evaluate clinical efficacy and predictors for treatment response in a real-life setting.

Methods: Data from 42 patients with severe eosinophilic asthma treated with mepolizumab for at least six months were analysed. Simple criteria to assess treatment response in clinical practice were used: increase of $FEV_1 \geq 12\%$ or ≥ 200 ml, reduction of blood eosinophils (< 150/μl or < 80% from baseline) and improvement of subjective condition (patient-judged subjective improvement or worsening following therapy). Patients were considered treatment responders if two criteria were fulfilled.

Results: Thirty-two out of 42 patients (76% [61–87%]) were classified as responders. Within the groups (responder vs non-responder), treatment with mepolizumab led to significant increase in FEV_1 (+ 600 ml vs -100 ml, $p = 0.003$), oxygenation (+ 8 mmHg vs -3 mmHg, $p = 0.001$), quality of life (visual analogue scale; + 28% vs − 5%, $p = 0.004$) and Asthma Control Test (+ 8 vs + 1 points, $p = 0.002$). In the responder group a significant decrease in the exacerbation rate over 12 months (1.45 vs 0.45, $p = 0.002$) was observed. Baseline characteristics (sex, BMI, smoking history, allergies, baseline level of eosinophils) did not predict treatment response.

Conclusion: Using improvement of lung function, decrease of eosinophils and improvement of subjective condition as response criteria, 76% of treated patients could be classified as treatment responders, demonstrating the efficacy of anti-IL-5 therapy in clinical practice.

Keywords: Severe eosinophilic asthma, Mepolizumab, Treatment response, IL-5, Lung function

Background

Asthma is a common chronic disease and affects approximately 315 million people worldwide [1]. About 3–10% of all asthma patients suffer from severe asthma which is defined as asthma remaining uncontrolled despite treatment with high-dose inhaled glucocorticoids combined with other controllers (long-acting β2-agonist, long-acting antimuscarinic agent, leukotriene receptor antagonist or theophylline) and/or treatment with systemic corticosteroids for at least 6 months [2, 3]. Despite the rather small percentage, patients with severe asthma are responsible for up to 50% of the direct and indirect costs associated with bronchial asthma [4]. Due to distinct symptoms, frequent exacerbations and numerous medication side effects, severe asthma represents a substantial burden for affected patients [5].

The first IL-5 antibody mepolizumab has been approved for over two years and has since become an established therapy for patients with uncontrolled severe asthma caused mainly by type 2 inflammation. Type 2 inflammation is characterized by the presence of IL-4, IL-5 and IL-13, produced by helper T cells leading to production, recruitment and activation of eosinophil granulocytes [6].

---
* Correspondence: Drick.Nora@mh-hannover.de
[1]Department of Respiratory Medicine, Hannover Medical School, Carl-Neuberg-Str.1, 30625 Hannover, Germany
Full list of author information is available at the end of the article

In large placebo-controlled trials, treatment with mepolizumab was well tolerated, resulting in a significant reduction of exacerbations and intake of oral corticosteroids (OCS) [7–9]. Meanwhile, another IL-5 antibody (reslizumab), differing from mepolizumab by the route of administration and an IL-5 receptor antibody (benralizumab) are available [10, 11]. Besides reduction of exacerbation rates and OCS dosages, all anti-IL-5 treatments led to a small but partly significant improvement of lung function [10, 12, 13]. As IL-5 functions as a central cytokine for activation and recruitment of eosinophils, it is not surprising that the number of eosinophil granulocytes in peripheral blood has been shown to be a predictor of clinical efficacy in targeted anti-IL-5 treatment with a greater reduction of exacerbations in patients with an eosinophil blood count of ≥150/μl [14]. So far this is the only available biomarker for selection of patients who are most likely to benefit from anti-IL-5 treatment [15]. The percentage of severe asthma patients presenting with high numbers of eosinophils is unknown, but studies of mild to severe asthma suggest approximately 50% [16]. Besides the initial studies which led to approval of the drugs, experience in clinical practice and efficacy is scarce. Especially, distinct definitions of treatment response to anti-IL-5 therapy remain to be elaborated. The *National Institute for Health and Care Excellence* (NICE) has published recommendations, defining the reduction of the exacerbation rate by at least 50% or a clinically reduced dose of continuous OCS as adequate response [17]. These criteria are not applicable to all patients with severe asthma, as not all patients require continuous OCS treatment or suffer from frequent exacerbations. We propose treatment response criteria, which are easy to assess and applicable to all patients as a continuous OCS therapy as well as frequent exacerbations are not required. Based on our treatment response criteria, we report the clinical efficacy of anti-IL-5 treatment in real-life setting and analyse potential predictors for treatment response.

Methods

In this single-centre, retrospective analysis, clinical efficacy of IL-5 antibody therapy with mepolizumab and potential predictors for treatment response in patients with severe eosinophilic asthma were examined. All patients were treated with high-dose inhaled glucocorticoids and a long-acting β2-agonist, partially with a second or third controller and partially with additional OCS therapy. Documentation of eosinophil counts of ≥300 cells/μl in peripheral blood within the past 12 months had to be present. All patients included received mepolizumab subcutaneously once every 4 weeks for at least 6 months. All patients under follow-up at our asthma outpatient clinic provided written informed consent and all retrospective analyses were performed with approval of the local institutional review board.

Treatment response criteria

According to the following treatment response criteria, patients were divided into two groups: responder and non-responder. To be classified as responder, at least two out of the three criteria had to be fulfilled. According to the *Global Initiative for Asthma* (GINA) the long-term goal of asthma treatment is represented by the control of symptoms and reduction of disease burden. In comparison to patients with mild Asthma, patients with severe Asthma face additional burdens influencing quality of life such as medication side effects, comorbidities or severe exacerbations leading to hospitalization [18]. To include all different aspects influencing daily life of patients with severe asthma, we included the overall term of *improvement of subjective condition* as the primary criterion. During interview patients were asked by the physician whether their subjective condition under therapy had improved or worsened (yes / no question). For their answer, patients were asked to consider asthma-related symptoms, quality of life (QoL), number of exacerbations and improvement of physical fitness.

Improvement of lung function is one central aspect of bronchial asthma therapy and for anti-IL-5 therapies improvement of FEV1 could be shown [19]. Therefore, improvement of lung function presents the second treatment response criterion (increase of forced expiratory volume in one second - FEV1 ≥ 12% or ≥ 200 ml). Values were chosen by analogy to the cut-offs used by the *Global Lung Initiative* [20].

Higher levels of eosinophils correlate with degree of airflow obstruction and disease severity as demonstrated by *Hancox* et al. [21]. Further, in severe asthma the extent of reduction in sputum eosinophils correlated with better asthma control [22]. Given these observations, we selected reduction of eosinophils in peripheral blood as third criterion (decrease in peripheral eosinophil blood count < 150/μl or less than 80% from baseline, by analogy to the mepolizumab approval studies [23]).

Follow-up and work-up

Routine follow-up in our outpatient clinic includes spirometry or body plethysmography standardized to ERS/ATS guidelines, blood gas analysis, and laboratory testing if indicated. Structured questionnaires, assessing for exacerbation rate, physical fitness (measured by flights of stairs), asthma control (Asthma Control Test - ACT), quality of life (EQ-5D-3 L and visual analogue scale [VAS]) and subjective condition are completed at each attendance. QoL was assessed using the EQ-5D-3 L visual analogue scale ranging from 0% (worst imaginable health state) to 100% (best imaginable health state) [24, 25]. The

ACT consists of 5 questions assessing asthma control in the previous 4 weeks inquiring the following asthma-related symptoms and items: shortness of breath, use of rescue inhaler, awakening at night due to wheezing, cough, shortness of breath, chest tightness or pain, activity limitation and self-perception of asthma control. The score ranges on a scale from 1 (poorly controlled) to 5 (well controlled), with a maximum score of 25. The ACT cut-off for GINA-defined uncontrolled asthma is ≤19; the recommendation for patients with severe asthma is ≤16 [26]. Exacerbations were defined as worsening of asthma symptoms requiring OCS or an increase in the OCS dose.

Assessment of treatment response

Data for analysis was assessed before treatment initiation (baseline) and at the latest follow-up appointment. The first follow-up appointment to assess treatment response was scheduled after 6 months. If responder criteria were not fulfilled, possible reasons for treatment non-responsiveness were evaluated. If the lack of response was attributable to an acute exacerbation or pulmonary infection or if the patient merely described a slow improvement but did not yet fulfil criteria, treatment was continued for another 3 months. If lack of response could not be explained by pulmonary infection or acute exacerbation and/or patients describe worsening of symptoms, IL-5 treatment was stopped. Follow-up evaluation is illustrated in Fig. 1.

Statistical analysis

IBM SPSS Statistics 25.0 (IBM Corp, USA) and STATA 13.0 (State Corp LP, USA) statistical software were used for univariate analysis. Categorical variables are stated as numbers (n) and percentages (%). Continuous variables are shown as mean ± SD (if normally distributed) or median and interquartile ranges unless indicated otherwise. For group comparisons (responder vs non-responder), Fisher's exact test, Chi-squared test, two-sided independent t-test or Mann-Whitney-U-test were used as appropriate. Logistic Regression models were created to determine effects on outcomes and in order to identify possible independent baseline characteristics having an effect on outcome, receiver operated characteristics (ROC) curves were drawn and the area under the curve (AUC) was calculated. All reported p-values are two-side. P-values < 0.05 were considered statistically significant. Dot-plots were created using Prism 7.04 (GraphPad, USA).

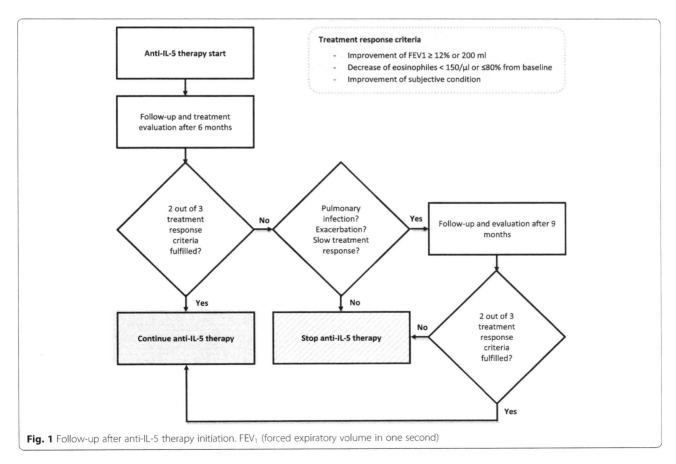

Fig. 1 Follow-up after anti-IL-5 therapy initiation. FEV_1 (forced expiratory volume in one second)

Results

Data from 42 patients with severe eosinophilic asthma and treatment with mepolizumab were analysed. Patient characteristics with group differences are displayed in Table 1.

Treatment response criteria

Thirty-two out of 42 patients (76%) were classified as treatment responders (95% confidence interval 61–87%). Median treatment time evaluated in the responder group was 12 months [IQR 8–15]. An improvement of subjective condition could be seen in all responders. A decrease of eosinophils (< 150/µl or less than 80% of baseline) was found in all patients except one (97%). Improvement of lung function was seen in 26/32 patients (81%). Ten patients did not fulfil response criteria and were classified as non-responders, accordingly. Anti-IL-5 therapy in these patients was discontinued after a median time of 9 months [IQR 6–12]. In the non-responder group, a decrease of eosinophils was observed in 8/10 patients (80%). There was no reported improvement of subjective condition, nor measured improvement in lung function in the non-responder-group. Response criteria and characteristics at follow-up visit are shown in Table 2.

Changes in lung function, oxygenation, asthma control and quality of life

In the responder group a significant improvement in lung function with increase of FEV_1, increase of forced vital capacity (FVC) and decrease of residual volume (RV) at control visit could be shown compared to the non-responder group (Fig. 2). The FEV_1 showed a median increase of 600 ml in the responder group whereas in the non-responder group a decrease of 100 ml could be measured (p = 0.003). Furthermore, oxygenation in capillary blood gas analysis was improved by 8 mmHg [IQR 4–15] in responder group and worsened by – 3 mmHg [IQR – 5-3] in the non-responder group (p = 0.001). Corresponding to the improvement of lung function and oxygenation patients in the responder group stated a significantly higher QoL according to VAS (improvement of 28% [IQR 6–50] vs. -5% [IQR -28-13], p = 0.004) as well as a significant higher score on the ACT compared to non-responder patients (improvement of 5 points [IQR 3–10] vs. 1 [IQR -2-5], p = 0.013). Within the responder-group, there was significant improvement in ACT, with a median of 12 points at baseline and 17 points at follow-up (p < 0.001). Non-responder patients improved by 1 point from 11 to 12 points.

Table 1 Demographics at baseline

Characteristic	All (n = 42)		Anti-IL-5 therapy responder (n = 32)		Anti-IL-5 therapy non-responder (n = 10)		p-value
Age (years), median (IQR)	51	(45–59)	51	(44–60)	50	(44–58)	0.456
Female, n (%)	19	(45)	16	(50)	3	(30)	0.267
Allergies, n (%)	24	(57)	17	(53)	7	(70)	0.347
Smoking history, n (%)							
active smoker	1	(2)	1	(3)	0	(0)	
ex-smoker	20	(48)	14	(44)	6	(60)	
non-smoker	21	(50)	17	(53)	4	(40)	0.432
Pack years, median (IQR)	20	(10–33)	15	(7–35)	20	(10–20)	0.708
Body mass index, median (IQR)	28	(24–34)	28	(24–31)	31	(27–36)	0.078
Lung function, median (IQR)							
FEV_1% of predicted	56	(41–71)	55	(46–67)	69	(39–80)	0.635
FEV_1 (l)	1.8	(1.4–2.4)	1.8	(1.3–2.3)	1.8	(1.5–2.7)	0.322
FVCex % of predicted	82	(72–98)	78	(71–93)	94	(82–101)	0.108
RV % of predicted	136	(119–174)	139	(122–174)	122	(107–162)	0.419
TLC % of predicted	100	(95–110)	101	(94–111)	98	(93–107)	0.737
Laboratory, median (IQR)							
Blood eosinophils (%)	7	(5–10)	7	(5–10)	6	(4–12)	0.589
Eosinophils absolute (cells/µl)	0.6	(0.4–0.8)	0.6	(0.4–0.8)	0.5	(0.4–1.0)	0.228
IgE (IE/ml)	128	(77–1222)	123	(66–1487)	298	(84–1362)	0.966
Continuous OCS therapy prior to IL-5 therapy, n (%)	23	(57)	17	(53)	6	(60)	0.703
Number of exacerbations per year prior to anti-IL-5 therapy, mean (±SD)	1.60	(±1.70)	1.78	(±1.77)	1.0	(±1.33)	0.208

BMI body mass index, *OCS* oral corticosteroids, *IgE* immunoglobulin E, *FEV_1* forced expiratory volume in one second, *FVC* forced vital capacity, *RV* residual volume. For comparisons, Fisher's exact test, Chi-squared test, Mann–Whitney U test or two-sided paired t-test were used as appropriate

Table 2 Therapy status at follow-up

Characteristic	All (n = 42)		Anti-IL-5 therapy responder (n = 32)		Anti-IL-5 therapy non-responder (n = 10)		p-value
Anti-IL-5 therapy in month, median (IQR)	12	(7–15)	12	(8–15)	9	(6–12)	0.146
Anti-IL-5 therapy response criteria, n (%)							
lung function (FEV$_1$)	26	(62)	26	(81)	0	(0)	
eosinophils	39	(93)	31	(97)	8	(80)	
subjective condition	32	(76)	32	(100)	0	(0)	
OCS therapy after anti-IL-5 therapy initiation							
Continuous OCS therapy at baseline – mg/d, median (IQR)	5	(5–10)	5	(5–10)	5	(5–12.5)	0.821
Continuous OCS therapy at follow-up, mg/d, median (IQR)	5	(4–12.5)	4.5	(3.3–5)	10	(5–17.5)	0.080
OCS therapy discontinued at follow-up, n (%)	10	(24)	9	(28)	1	(10)	0.240

OCS oral corticosteroids, *FEV$_1$* forced expiratory volume in one second. For comparisons, Fisher's exact test, Chi-squared test, Mann–Whitney U test or two-sided paired t-test were used as appropriate

Exacerbation rates

In the responder group a significant difference in the exacerbation rate 12 months prior to anti-IL-5 therapy (1.45 ± 1.77) and post treatment initiation (0.45 ± 0.75) could be seen ($p = 0.002$). No prediction concerning the non-responder group could be made and no comparison between the responder and non-responder-group could be performed due to the small number of non-responder patients receiving anti-IL-5 therapy for 12 months.

Oral corticosteroids

At baseline, 23/42 patients (57%) received continuous OCS, with similar dosages in both groups (5 mg [IQR 5–10] in the responder group, 5 mg [IQR 5–12,5] in the non-responder group). OCS dosages were reduced at follow-up in the responder group (4.5 mg [IQR 3.3–5]) and tended to increase in the non-responder group (10 mg [IQR 5–17.5], $p = 0.080$). Nine responder patients (28%) subsequently discontinued OCS versus one non-responder patient (10%, $p = 0.240$). Details are shown in Table 2.

Prediction of treatment response

No significant differences could be shown between the groups concerning levels of eosinophils at treatment initiation with a median of 600 cells/µl in the responder group and 500 cells/µl in the non-responder group, respectively ($p = 0.228$). No significant differences between the groups could be shown concerning history of smoking (pack years), and existence of allergies or immunoglobulin E (IgE)-levels. There was no difference in the body mass index at treatment initiation (Table 1). Using univariate logistic regression, neither sex, body weight, IgE-level, level of eosinophils at baseline, allergy status

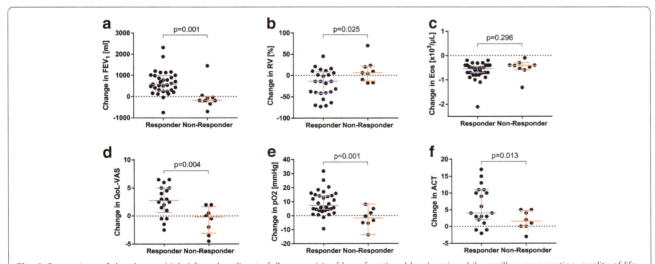

Fig. 2 Comparison of the change (delta) from baseline to follow-up visit of lung function, blood eosinophils, capillary oxygenation, quality of life and asthma control test between both groups (responder vs non-responder). Percentages are stated as % of predicted. **a** FEV$_1$, forced expiratory volume in one second; **b** *RV* residual volume; **c** *Eos* eosinophils; **d** *QoL* quality of life, *VAS* visual analogue scale; **e** *pO2* partial pressure of oxygen; **f** *ACT* asthma control test

nor lung function influenced allocation to treatment response groups (Fig. 3).

Assessment of treatment response
At initial follow-up (median 6 months), 32/42 patients were grouped as responders and 10 patients did not fulfil response criteria; 4/10 patients without signs of acute exacerbation or pulmonary infection were classified as non-responders and therapy was discontinued. Of the remaining 6 patients who initially did not fulfil response criteria, therapy was discontinued due to lack of efficacy after 9 months ($n = 4$) and 12 months ($n = 2$).

Side effects
In our cohort, no serious side effects leading to discontinuation of anti-IL-5 therapy occurred. The most common side effects were mild headache (7%), followed by injection-site reaction (5%), arthralgia (5%) and nausea (2%).

Discussion
This study aimed to identify response criteria for treatment with mepolizumab and to evaluate clinical efficacy of anti-IL-5 therapy in clinical practice. Furthermore, potential predictors of treatment response were analysed.

Since the approval of mepolizumab as the first available IL-5 antibody, official treatment response criteria remain to be defined [6, 27]. Based on placebo-controlled phase III-studies [8, 9], recommendations published by NICE define the reduction of the exacerbation rate by at least 50% or a clinically significant reduced dose of continuous OCS as adequate response criteria [8, 9, 17]. In accordance with the literature, treatment with mepolizumab led to a significant reduction of asthma exacerbations in the responder group of our cohort. No prediction could be made concerning the definite exacerbation rate in non-responder patients as treatment in all but 2 patients

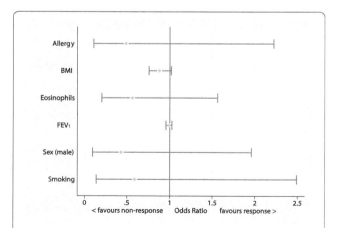

Fig. 3 Analysis of potential predictors for treatment response. BMI, body mass index; FEV₁, forced expiratory volume in one second

was stopped before reaching the 12 months interval. As exacerbations mainly occur during winter, assessment of at least 12 months is mandatory to truly reflect the exacerbation rate [28]. Furthermore, exacerbations are common in patients with severe asthma, but are not an ubiquitous feature [29]. Therefore, while prevention of exacerbation represents a hallmark treatment goal, the exacerbation rate by itself hardly represents a valid criterion for treatment response in routine clinical practice. Similarly, only approximately 30% of patients with severe asthma are dependent on additional OCS treatment with many patients using OCS on demand rather than continuously [30]. In our cohort 55% of patients were receiving continuous OCS at baseline, rendering the reduction of OCS as an ineligible treatment response criterion in this study.

As the exacerbation rate as well as OCS treatment shows a close correlation to asthma-related QoL, we chose improvement of subjective condition ("subjective treatment response") as one treatment response criterion [5, 31]. QoL and asthma control as traditional parameters were assessed separately with validated questionnaires, however, QoL is influenced by numerous aspects unrelated to asthma and the ACT has known limitations in severe asthma. *Korn* et al. recommended reducing the ACT cut-off for uncontrolled asthma in severe asthma to 16 [26]. Despite reduction of asthma-related symptoms following treatment, an ACT score remaining below 16 points indicates poorly controlled asthma where often there is no further option for therapy escalation. When asked about the effects of mepolizumab treatment, 32/42 patients (76%) in our cohort stated improvement of subjective condition. All 32 patients fulfilled at least two response criteria and were therefore grouped as responders, while in the non-responder group, no patient reported subjective improvement.

Given the type-2 immunologic pathway underlying eosinophilic asthma and the IL-5 antagonizing effects of mepolizumab, reduction of eosinophils as proof of interference with one main inflammatory mechanism was chosen as a second criterion for treatment response [32]. As IL-5 antibodies are approved for patients with blood eosinophils of ≥150 cells/μL at screening or ≥ 300 cells/μL within 12 months prior to treatment by the FDA (*Food and Drug Administration*) and EMA (*European Medicines Agency*), the blood eosinophil count had to be < 150 cells/μl or less than 80% from baseline to count as treatment responder in this category. A reduction to < 150 eosinophils or less than 80% from baseline could be seen in all responders except one. Interestingly, all non-responder patients except 2 dropped with eosinophil blood counts below 150/μl but did not show subjective improvement or improvement in lung function. This highlights that disease activity in refractory cases of eosinophilic asthma cannot be solely accounted for by eosinophilic inflammation.

Some patients with severe asthma present with combined neutrophilic and eosinophilic inflammation of the airways detectable in sputum [33]. These patients with a phenotype of a mixed inflammatory response appear to have the greatest disease burden and airway limitation, necessitating further research for treatment strategies for neutrophilic or mixed inflammation in asthma [34].

Price et al. could show that patients with higher blood eosinophils are more likely to benefit from anti-IL-5 therapy but whether the statement "the higher the better" is true is not universally agreed [35]. Post-hoc-analysis of the phase III *calima* and *sirocco* studies showed that improvement of lung function in patients with benralizumab treatment was proportional to the extent of blood eosinophilia [36]. In the real-life scenario presented herein, this could not be reproduced by allocation to response groups as reduction of eosinophil count was present in both groups without significantly differing magnitude. As the blood eosinophil count represents the only available biomarker for initiation of anti-IL-5 therapy, little conclusion can be drawn from eosinophils regarding clinical response. Therefore, identification and validation of possible new biomarkers are highly desirable.

All patients with severe asthma at least intermittently show an impaired lung function with obstructive patterns. As improvement in lung function was frequently observed alongside subjective improvement and decline in eosinophil counts, we decided to include the improvement of lung function as a third response criterion using a slightly modified version of the approved bronchodilator criteria [37]. In our cohort 26 patients (79%) showed improvement of FEV_1 of 12% or ≥ 200 ml. None of the non-responder patients showed improvement of lung function.

With these suggested response criteria 76% of our patients treated with mepolizumab could be classified as treatment responders. Treatment led to significant improvement in lung function, oxygenation, QoL and asthma control in responder vs. non-responder patients. Overall, anti-IL-5 therapy shows a favourable efficacy in patients with eosinophilic asthma in routine clinical practice.

Nevertheless, a quarter of patients with indication for anti-IL-5 therapy did not respond to treatment. In case of treatment failure, comorbidities as well as aggravating factors for severe eosinophilic asthma (such as allergic bronchopulmonary aspergillosis, bronchiectasis or eosinophilic granulomatosis with polyangiitis) should be ruled out. Demonstrated in family studies, there is increasing evidence that genetic abnormalities play a role in the pathogenesis of severe asthma [38]. Up to now, genetic testing is however not endorsed by international guidelines in these patients. Given the fixed mepolizumab dosage, under-dosing in obese patients should be considered, considering non-responders switching to intravenous anti-IL-5 agent allowing for individual dosing. Post-hoc analysis of the *Dose Ranging Efficacy And safety with Mepolizumab* (Dream)-study revealed similar reduction rates for exacerbations in obese and non-obese patients, but a recently published study demonstrated that in mepolizumab non-responders switch to intravenous, weight-adapted reslizumab can be beneficial [23, 39]. To account for overlap phenotypes with chronic obstructive pulmonary disease (COPD) and allergic bronchial asthma, we analysed smoking history and occurrence of allergies but no impact on treatment response was evident. Prior to anti-IL-5 therapy, 5 non-responder patients were eligible and received omalizumab therapy, but none of the patients responded to treatment. There was also no significant impact by body weight in our cohort.

Studies defining the appropriate follow-up schedule or the overall duration of anti-IL-5 therapy are missing. Mainly based on the approval studies, a treatment duration for initially 12 months is recommended due to the possibility of delayed treatment response [39]. In our cohort however, we did not observe any delayed treatment response in patients who failed to respond early after therapy initiation. Especially in regard to high treatment costs, regular assessment seems mandatory to detect treatment non-responders early [40]. When to delay or discontinue treatment with anti-IL-5 antibodies, is also still under debate. In patients with hypereosinophilic syndrome withdrawal of anti-IL-5 therapy led to a rebound of eosinophilia after 60–90 days [41]. In asthma patients a relapse of eosinophils to baseline could be seen after 6 months with a significant increase in exacerbations after 12 months [42]. Based on current available data, anti-IL-5 treatment should be regarded as long-term treatment.

Limitations

There are important limitations to this analysis, mainly inherent by its retrospective design. This especially limits conclusion about exacerbation rates as exacerbations were only reported 12 months prior to treatment initiation. Value of the data and conclusions regarding the predictive power of the assessed factors are partly limited due to the small number of patients especially in the non-responder group. With the criterion of subjective treatment response, we used a non-validated assessment tool.

Conclusion

Treatment with mepolizumab shows good efficacy and excellent safety in routine clinical practice. Using improvement of lung function, improvement of subjective condition and decrease of eosinophils in peripheral blood as treatment criteria, 3/4 of treated patients in our cohort can be classified as treatment responders. Anti-IL-5 therapy leads to significant increase in lung function, oxygenation, QoL and asthma control. Further research is needed to identify predictors for treatment response and to determine treatment duration.

Abbreviations
ACT: Asthma control test; BMI: Body mass index; Eos: Eosinophils; FEV_1: Forced expiratory volume in one second; FVC: Forced vital capacity; GINA: Global Initiative for Asthma; IgE: Immunoglobulin E; IL: Interleukin; NICE: National Institute for Health and Care Excellence; OCS: Oral corticosteroids; QoL: Quality of life; RV: Residual volume; VAS: Visual analogue scale

Funding
This study was funded by internal resources of Hannover Medical School.

Authors' contributions
ND wrote the paper, collected and analyzed the data; BS contributed to data interpretation, revised the manuscript; JF analyzed the data; TW contributed to data interpretation, revised the manuscript HS: revised the manuscript; collected data. All authors approved of the final version of the manuscript.

Competing interests
The authors declare that they have no competing interests.

Author details
[1]Department of Respiratory Medicine, Hannover Medical School, Carl-Neuberg-Str.1, 30625 Hannover, Germany. [2]Biomedical Research in End-Stage and Obstructive Lung Disease Hannover (BREATH), Member of the German Centre for Lung Research (DZL), Hannover, Germany.

References
1. To T, Stanojevic S, Moores G, Gershon AS, Bateman ED, Cruz AA, Boulet L-P. Global asthma prevalence in adults: findings from the cross-sectional world health survey. BMC Public Health. 2012;12:204. https://doi.org/10.1186/1471-2458-12-204.
2. Chung KF, Wenzel SE, Brozek JL, Bush A, Castro M, Sterk PJ, et al. International ERS/ATS guidelines on definition, evaluation and treatment of severe asthma. Eur Respir J. 2014;43:343–73. https://doi.org/10.1183/09031936.00202013.
3. Hekking P-PW, Wener RR, Amelink M, Zwinderman AH, Bouvy ML, Bel EH. The prevalence of severe refractory asthma. J Allergy Clin Immunol. 2015;135:896–902. https://doi.org/10.1016/j.jaci.2014.08.042.
4. Braman SS. The global burden of asthma. Chest. 2006;130:4S–12S. https://doi.org/10.1378/chest.130.1_suppl.4S.
5. Hyland ME, Whalley B, Jones RC, Masoli M. A qualitative study of the impact of severe asthma and its treatment showing that treatment burden is neglected in existing asthma assessment scales. Qual Life Res. 2015;24:631–9. https://doi.org/10.1007/s11136-014-0801-x.
6. Israel E, Reddel HK. Severe and difficult-to-treat asthma in adults. N Engl J Med. 2017;377:965–76. https://doi.org/10.1056/NEJMra1608969.
7. Bel EH, Wenzel SE, Thompson PJ, Prazma CM, Keene ON, Yancey SW, et al. Oral glucocorticoid-sparing effect of mepolizumab in eosinophilic asthma. N Engl J Med. 2014;371:1189–97. https://doi.org/10.1056/NEJMoa1403291.
8. Pavord ID, Korn S, Howarth P, Bleecker ER, Buhl R, Keene ON, et al. Mepolizumab for severe eosinophilic asthma (DREAM): a multicentre, double-blind, placebo-controlled trial. Lancet. 2012;380:651–9. https://doi.org/10.1016/S0140-6736(12)60988-X.
9. Ortega HG, Liu MC, Pavord ID, Brusselle GG, FitzGerald JM, Chetta A, et al. Mepolizumab treatment in patients with severe eosinophilic asthma. N Engl J Med. 2014;371:1198–207. https://doi.org/10.1056/NEJMoa1403290
10. Castro M, Zangrilli J, Wechsler ME, Bateman ED, Brusselle GG, Bardin P, et al. Reslizumab for inadequately controlled asthma with elevated blood eosinophil counts: results from two multicentre, parallel, double-blind, randomised, placebo-controlled, phase 3 trials. Lancet Respir Med. 2015;3:355–66. https://doi.org/10.1016/S2213-2600(15)00042-9.
11. Nair P, Wenzel S, Rabe KF, Bourdin A, Lugogo NL, Kuna P, et al. Oral glucocorticoid-sparing effect of Benralizumab in severe asthma. N Engl J Med. 2017;376:2448–58. https://doi.org/10.1056/NEJMoa1703501.
12. Chupp GL, Bradford ES, Albers FC, Bratton DJ, Wang-Jairaj J, Nelsen LM, et al. Efficacy of mepolizumab add-on therapy on health-related quality of life and markers of asthma control in severe eosinophilic asthma (MUSCA): a randomised, double-blind, placebo-controlled, parallel-group, multicentre, phase 3b trial. Lancet Respir Med. 2017;5:390–400. https://doi.org/10.1016/S2213-2600(17)30125-X.
13. FitzGerald JM, Bleecker ER, Nair P, Korn S, Ohta K, Lommatzsch M, et al. Benralizumab, an anti-interleukin-5 receptor α monoclonal antibody, as add-on treatment for patients with severe, uncontrolled, eosinophilic asthma (CALIMA): a randomised, double-blind, placebo-controlled phase 3 trial. Lancet. 2016;388:2128–41. https://doi.org/10.1016/S0140-6736(16)31322-8.
14. Ortega HG, Yancey SW, Mayer B, Gunsoy NB, Keene ON, Bleecker ER, et al. Severe eosinophilic asthma treated with mepolizumab stratified by baseline eosinophil thresholds: a secondary analysis of the DREAM and MENSA studies. Lancet Respir Med. 2016;4:549–56. https://doi.org/10.1016/S2213-2600(16)30031-5.
15. Yancey SW, Keene ON, Albers FC, Ortega H, Bates S, Bleecker ER, Pavord I. Biomarkers for severe eosinophilic asthma. J Allergy Clin Immunol. 2017;140:1509–18. https://doi.org/10.1016/j.jaci.2017.10.005.
16. Woodruff PG, Modrek B, Choy DF, Jia G, Abbas AR, Ellwanger A, et al. T-helper type 2-driven inflammation defines major subphenotypes of asthma. Am J Respir Crit Care Med. 2009;180:388–95. https://doi.org/10.1164/rccm.200903-0392OC.
17. National Institute for Health and Care Excellence (NICE). Mepolizumab for treating severe refractory eosinophilic asthma. 25.01.2017. https://www.nice.org.uk/guidance/ta431 [Assessed 25 Jan 2017].
18. Hyland ME, Jones RC, Lanario JW, Masoli M. The construction and validation of the severe asthma questionnaire (SAQ). Eur Respir J. 2018; https://doi.org/10.1183/13993003.00618-2018.
19. Farne HA, Wilson A, Powell C, Bax L, Milan SJ. Anti-IL5 therapies for asthma. Cochrane Database Syst Rev. 2017;9:CD010834. https://doi.org/10.1002/14651858.CD010834.pub3.
20. Quanjer PH, Stanojevic S, Cole TJ, Baur X, Hall GL, Culver BH, et al. Multi-ethnic reference values for spirometry for the 3-95-yr age range: the global lung function 2012 equations. Eur Respir J. 2012;40:1324–43. https://doi.org/10.1183/09031936.00080312.
21. Hancox RJ, Pavord ID, Sears MR. Associations between blood eosinophils and decline in lung function among adults with and without asthma. Eur Respir J. 2018; https://doi.org/10.1183/13993003.02536-2017.
22. Mukherjee M, Aleman Paramo F, Kjarsgaard M, Salter B, Nair G, LaVigne N, et al. Weight-adjusted intravenous Reslizumab in severe asthma with inadequate response to fixed-dose subcutaneous Mepolizumab. Am J Respir Crit Care Med. 2018;197:38–46. https://doi.org/10.1164/rccm.201707-1323OC.
23. Ortega H, Li H, Suruki R, Albers F, Gordon D, Yancey S. Cluster analysis and characterization of response to mepolizumab. A step closer to personalized medicine for patients with severe asthma. Ann Am Thorac Soc. 2014;11:1011–7. https://doi.org/10.1513/AnnalsATS.201312-454OC.
24. Pickard AS, Wilke C, Jung E, Patel S, Stavem K, Lee TA. Use of a preference-based measure of health (EQ-5D) in COPD and asthma. Respir Med. 2008;102:519–36. https://doi.org/10.1016/j.rmed.2007.11.016.
25. EuroQol--a new facility for the measurement of health-related quality of life. Health Policy. 1990;16:199–208.
26. Korn S, Both J, Jung M, Hübner M, Taube C, Buhl R. Prospective evaluation of current asthma control using ACQ and ACT compared with GINA criteria. Ann Allergy Asthma Immunol. 2011;107:474–9. https://doi.org/10.1016/j.anai.2011.09.001.
27. Fajt ML, Wenzel SE. Development of new therapies for severe asthma. Allergy Asthma Immunol Res. 2017;9:3–14. https://doi.org/10.4168/aair.2017.9.1.3.
28. Gerhardsson de verdier M, Gustafson P, McCrae C, Edsbäcker S, Johnston N. Seasonal and geographic variations in the incidence of asthma exacerbations in the United States. J Asthma. 2017;54:818–24. https://doi.org/10.1080/02770903.2016.1277538
29. Miller MK, Lee JH, Miller DP, Wenzel SE. Recent asthma exacerbations: a key

predictor of future exacerbations. Respir Med. 2007;101:481–9. https://doi.org/10.1016/j.rmed.2006.07.005.
30. Sullivan PW, Ghushchyan VH, Globe G, Schatz M. Oral corticosteroid exposure and adverse effects in asthmatic patients. J Allergy Clin Immunol. 2018;141:110–116.e7. https://doi.org/10.1016/j.jaci.2017.04.009.
31. Luskin AT, Chipps BE, Rasouliyan L, Miller DP, Haselkorn T, Dorenbaum A. Impact of asthma exacerbations and asthma triggers on asthma-related quality of life in patients with severe or difficult-to-treat asthma. J Allergy Clin Immunol Pract 2014;2:544–52.e1–2. https://doi.org/10.1016/j.jaip.2014.02.011.
32. Stein ML, Villanueva JM, Buckmeier BK, Yamada Y, Filipovich AH, Assa'ad AH, Rothenberg ME. Anti-IL-5 (mepolizumab) therapy reduces eosinophil activation ex vivo and increases IL-5 and IL-5 receptor levels. J Allergy Clin Immunol. 2008;121:1473–83, 1483.e1–4. https://doi.org/10.1016/j.jaci.2008.02.033.
33. Simpson JL, Scott R, Boyle MJ, Gibson PG. Inflammatory subtypes in asthma: assessment and identification using induced sputum. Respirology. 2006;11:54–61. https://doi.org/10.1111/j.1440-1843.2006.00784.x.
34. Moore WC, Hastie AT, Li X, Li H, Busse WW, Jarjour NN, et al. Sputum neutrophil counts are associated with more sszsevere asthma phenotypes using cluster analysis. J Allergy Clin Immunol. 2014;133:1557. https://doi.org/10.1016/j.jaci.2013.10.011.63.e5.
35. Price DB, Rigazio A, Campbell JD, Bleecker ER, Corrigan CJ, Thomas M, et al. Blood eosinophil count and prospective annual asthma disease burden: a UK cohort study. Lancet Respir Med. 2015;3:849–58. https://doi.org/10.1016/S2213-2600(15)00367-7.
36. FitzGerald JM, Bleecker ER, Menzies-Gow A, Zangrilli JG, Hirsch I, Metcalfe P, et al. Predictors of enhanced response with benralizumab for patients with severe asthma: pooled analysis of the SIROCCO and CALIMA studies. Lancet Respir Med. 2018;6:51–64. https://doi.org/10.1016/S2213-2600(17)30344-2.
37. Selection of reference values and interpretative strategies. American Thoracic Society. Am Rev Respir Dis. Lung function testing, 1991:144–1202–18. https://doi.org/10.1164/ajrccm/144.5.1202.
38. Poon AH, Hamid Q. Severe asthma: have we made progress? Ann Am Thorac Soc. 2016;13(Suppl 1):S68–77. https://doi.org/10.1513/AnnalsATS.201508-514MG.
39. Haldar P. Patient profiles and clinical utility of mepolizumab in severe eosinophilic asthma. Biologics. 2017;11:81–95. https://doi.org/10.2147/BTT.S93954.
40. Basu A, Dalal A, Canonica GW, Forshag M, Yancey SW, Nagar S, Bell CF. Economic analysis of the phase III MENSA study evaluating mepolizumab for severe asthma with eosinophilic phenotype. Expert Rev Pharmacoecon Outcomes Res. 2017;17:121–31. https://doi.org/10.1080/14737167.2017.1298444.
41. Kim Y-J, Prussin C, Martin B, Law MA, Haverty TP, Nutman TB, Klion AD. Rebound eosinophilia after treatment of hypereosinophilic syndrome and eosinophilic gastroenteritis with monoclonal anti-IL-5 antibody SCH55700. J Allergy Clin Immunol. 2004;114:1449–55. https://doi.org/10.1016/j.jaci.2004.08.027.
42. Haldar P, Brightling CE, Singapuri A, Hargadon B, Gupta S, Monteiro W, et al. Outcomes after cessation of mepolizumab therapy in severe eosinophilic asthma: a 12-month follow-up analysis. J Allergy Clin Immunol. 2014;133:921–3. https://doi.org/10.1016/j.jaci.2013.11.026.

A modified risk score in one-year survival rate assessment of group 1 pulmonary arterial hypertension

Wei Xiong[1,2†], Yunfeng Zhao[3], Mei Xu[4,5†], Bigyan Pudasaini[2], Xuejun Guo[1*] and Jinming Liu[2*]

Abstract

Background: Risk assessment of pulmonary arterial hypertension (PAH) contributes to its management. Unfortunately, the existing risk assessment approaches are defective for clinicians to practice in daily clinical settings to some extent.

Methods: We designed a modified Risk Assessment Score of PAH (mRASP) comprising four non-invasive variables which were World Health Organization functional class(WHO FC), 6-min walk distance (6MWD), N-terminal of the pro-hormone brain natriuretic peptide(NT-pro BNP), and right atrial area(RAA), then validated it in the prediction of one-year survival rate for patients with PAH by contrast with the REVEAL risk score.

Results: For the validation cohort($n = 216$), the predicted one-year survival rate were 95–100%, 90–95%, and < 90% in the mRASP risk score strata of 0–2, 3–5, and 6–8, respectively; meanwhile, the observed one-year survival rates were 97.1, 92.6, and 52.2%, in each corresponding stratum, respectively. The mRASP (c-index = 0.727) demonstrated similar predictive power in contrast with the REVEAL risk assessment score (c-index = 0.715) in the prediction of one-year survival rate.

Conclusion: The mRASP is an eligible risk assessment tool for the prognostic assessment of PAH. In contrast with the REVEAL score, it demonstrated similar predictive power and accuracy, with extra simplicity and convenience.

Keywords: Pulmonary arterial hypertension, Group 1, Risk assessment score, Survival rate, Modified, REVEAL

Background

Pulmonary arterial hypertension is a pathophysiological disorder complicating both of cardiovascular and respiratory diseases. It is defined by a mPAP ≥ 25 mmHg, a pulmonary artery wedge pressure (PAWP) ≤ 15 mmHg and a pulmonary vascular resistance(PVR) > 3 Wood units (WU) without other causes of pre-capillary PH [1, 2].

The 2015 ESC/ERS(European Society of Cardiology/European Respiratory Society) PH guidelines strongly recommend a comprehensive regular assessment of patients with PAH since there is no single variable that provides sufficient diagnostic and prognostic information instead of a multidimensional approach [1, 3]. Based on the evaluation of multiple variables, PAH patients can be categorized as low, intermediate or high risk with estimated one-year mortality of < 5%, 5–10% and > 10%, respectively [3]. The basic program should include the functional class(FC) and at least one measurement of exercise capacity. It is also recommended to obtain some information on right ventricular (RV) function [1].

However, an individual patient is unlikely to have all variables indicative of merely one strata, thus the physician's decision on the overall risk is subjective and the assessment could vary between different physicians [3]. One approach which can distinctly classify the risk strata of PAH is the French registry risk equation, which unfortunately concerns sex, 6MWD and cardiac output merely [3, 4]. Another one is the risk assessment score of Registry to Evaluate Early and Long-Term Pulmonary

---

* Correspondence: guoxuejun@xinhuamed.com.cn; xiongyifan200716@wo.cn; jinmingliu2013@126.com
†Wei Xiong and Mei Xu contributed equally to this work.
[1]Department of Respiratory Medicine, Xinhua Hospital, Shanghai Jiaotong University School of Medicine, 1665, Kongjiang Road, Shanghai 200092, China
[2]Department of Cardiopulmonary Circulation, Shanghai Pulmonary Hospital, Tongji University School of Medicine, Shanghai, People's Republic of China
Full list of author information is available at the end of the article

Arterial Hypertension Disease Management (REVEAL) which is a simplified risk score based on the prognostic equation, and is designed to be simple and easy enough to be adopted in everyday clinical practice, compared with the relatively complex REVEAL risk equation [5]. However, RHC is not readily available or accessible or suitable or acceptable for every patient anytime. Besides, regardless of the right atrial pressure(RAP), cardiac index (CI) and mixed venous oxygen saturation (SvO2) assessed by right heart catheterization (RHC) being the most robust indicators of RV function and prognosis, and providing important prognostic information both at the time of diagnosis and during follow-up, whereas mPAP in RHC provides little prognostic information [6–10]. In addition, some of the variables in the REVEAL risk score, such as age and PAH etiology, are not modifiable offsetting the change of modifiable variables, and potentially leading to an inaccurate evaluation of the patient's prognosis [3]. The last but not least, the variable of vital signs such as resting systolic BP and heart rate in the REVEAL risk score is inconsistent and unreliable. Consequently, we postulated whether a modified risk assessment score could be the better approach for the prognostic assessment of PAH.

Methods
Study design
This study was launched in May, 2016. The eligible patients registered between May, 2014 and May, 2015 of Department of Cardiopulmonary Circulation, Shanghai Pulmonary Hospital were enrolled into the establishment cohort which was used to establish the model of mRASP by means of retrospectively corresponding the patients' score of the mRASP in May, 2015 to the actually observed survival rate between May, 2015 and May, 2016. After the establishment of the model of mRASP, all eligible patients registered between May, 2015 and May, 2016 were enrolled into the validation cohort which was assessed by the mRASP score in May, 2016 and the REVEAL score in May, 2016, respectively and simultaneously. Patients in the validation cohort were predicted to be in certain risk strata by both risk assessment scores, then were prospectively followed up and observed for all-cause mortality in the coming 12 months till May, 2017. During the follow-up, as per their condition, all patients received at least one of the specific drug therapies available in Chinese market including: endothelin receptor antagonists: ambrisentan, bosentan; phosphodiesterase type 5 inhibitors: sildenafil, tadalafil; prostacyclin analogues: treprostinil; and calcium channel blockers(for responders of acute vasodilator testing), on the basis of supportive therapies such as oral anticoagulants, diuretics, oxygen therapy, digoxin, etc., according to the guidelines [1]. After the follow-up, for patients in each stratum stratified with the risk assessment score, the predicted one-year survival rates were validated by contrast with the actually observed one-year survival rates to explore the goodness of fit between them. Meanwhile, the predictive efficiency was compared between the mRASP score and the REVEAL score. All variables in the assessment were obtained within 3 months prior to the time point of assessment. The death of the patients who died out of hospital was confirmed by telephone follow-up at the end of every month. This protocol was approved by the Institutional Review Board of Shanghai Pulmonary Hospital. Written informed consents were obtained from all eligible patients enrolled in this study.

Study population
All eligible patients were enrolled according to the inclusion and exclusion criteria. Inclusion criteria:1) age ≥ 18 years; 2) a diagnosis of PH on the presence of mPAP ≥ 25 mmHg and PAWP ≤15 mmHg and a PVR > 3 Wood units (WU) in RHC. Exclusion criteria: 1)a diagnosis of PH in Group 2, Group 3, Group 4, and Group 5 according to classifications in 2015 ESC/ERS PH guidelines [1]; 2) co-morbidity with other severe cardiopulmonary diseases; 3)absence of any variables involved in risk assessment; 4) no adherence to PAH-specific therapy; 4) loss to follow-up.

Risk assessment tools
The REVEAL risk assessment score
Variables independently associated with increased mortality by physical examination or laboratory tests: men aged > 60 years, PAH associated with portal hypertension, PAH associated with connective tissue disease, family history of PAH, modified New York Heart Association (NYHA)/World Health Organization (WHO) functional class III or IV, renal insufficiency, resting systolic BP < 110 mmHg, heart rate > 92 beats/min, mean RAP > 20 mmHg, 6MWD < 165 m, NT-pro BNP > 1500 pg/mL, PVR > 32 WU, % predicted diffusing capacity of lung for carbon monoxide (Dlco) ≤32%, and the presence of pericardial effusion on echocardiogrphy. Risk strata are indicated by the lines: predicted one-year survival is 95 to 100% in the low-risk group, 90 to 95% in the average-risk group, 85 to 90% in the moderately high-risk group, 70 to 85% in the high-risk group, and < 70% in the very high-risk group.The average predicted one-year survival is 95 to 100% (low-risk) for patients with risk scores of 0 to 7. Similarly, the ranges specified for average-risk, moderately high-risk, high-risk, and very high-risk correspond to risk scores of 8, 9, 10 to 11, and ≥ 12, respectively [5].

The modified risk assessment score
We conducted an univariate and then a multivariate analysis between all the determinants in the TABLE 13 of 2015 ESC/ERS PH guidelines and the risk of one-year

mortality. The results showed that one-year mortality was mostly correlated with 4 noninvasive variables which were WHO FC, 6MWD, NT-pro BNP, and right atrial area(RAA) in echocardiography. Figure 1 The modified risk assessment score of PAH (mRASP) consists of four variables which are WHO FC, 6MWD, NT-pro BNP, and right atrial area(RAA) in echocardiography. For each variable, the specification was derived from the variable in the TABLE 13 of 2015 ESC/ERS PH guidelines [1]. The specific feature of mRASP is that each column of low-risk, intermediate-risk, and high-risk in it account for a score of 0 point, 1 point, and 2 points, respectively. The total score of mRASP ranged between a minimum of 0 and a maximum of 8. The algorithm of the mRASP was generated by retrospectively corresponding the patients' score of the mRASP to the actually observed survival rate in the establishment cohort. The results showed that the risk score stratum of 0–2, 3–5, and 6–8 in mRASP corresponded to the low-risk class in which survival rate was 95 to 100%, intermediate-risk class in which survival rate was 90 to 95%, and high-risk class in which survival rate was < 90%, respectively. The mRASP form is illustrated in Table 1.

Overall, REVEAL score comprises 9 variables including non-modifiable one such as etiological subgroup, invasive one such as RHC, and some inconsistent one such as vital signs, whereas mRASP score comprises 4 noninvasive variables in REVEAL score: WHO FC, 6MWD, NT-pro BNP and echo. WHO FC was assessed by the patients' attending physicians who had abundant clinical experience in the management of PAH. 6MWD and echocardiography were performed by professional personnel under standard operating procedure.NT-pro BNP was assayed with AQT90 FLEX rapid immune analyzer of Radiometer Medical ApS. Echocardiography was conducted with GE VIVID i color Doppler ultrasonography.

Statistical analysis

On the basis of the prevalence of group 1 PAH in China, to obtain a two-sided 95% confidence interval of 2.5% for the prevalence of group 1 PAH, we estimated that a sample size of 200 patients with group 1 PAH should be required. Calibration plot was used as an approach to show agreement between the mean predicted one-year survival rates beforehand and the actually observed survival rates afterwards in the validation cohort to validate the validity of risk assessment score. The mean predicted one-year survival rate was defined as the mean value of each risk stratum. That is to say, for mRASP score, the mean predicted survival rates were 97.5, 92.5 and 45.0% in low-risk, intermediate-risk and high-risk stratum, respectively. Likewise, for the REVEAL score, the mean predicted survival rates were 97.5, 92.5, 87.5, 77.5, and 35.0% in low-risk, average-risk, moderately high-risk, high-risk, and very high-risk stratum, respectively. Comparison of predictive power between the mRASP score and the REVEAL score was assessed by c-index which means the probability of concordance signifying an approach of how significant the predictive model distinguishes patients who survive from who die, and of how much the chance that the patient with lower predicted risk score will survive longer. A p-value < 0.05 was considered to have statistical significance.

Results

Demographics and characteristics of patients in two cohorts

By the time of May, 2015, 108 patients with PAH from May, 2014 to May, 2015 was determined to be the establishment cohort. Between May, 2015 and May, 2016, 18 patients died and 5 patients lost to follow-up in this cohort. For the validation cohort, it comprised 216 patients besides 7 cases who were lost to the follow-up between May, 2016 and May, 2017. The mean age, proportion of female patients, 6MWD, NT-pro BNP, and proportion of WHO FC III or IV of establishment cohort and validation cohort were 52.8 and 54.6(p = 0.088), 71.3 and 73.6%(p = 0.123), 338 m and 309 m(p = 0.019), 3268 pg/mL and 3497 pg/mL(p = 0.066), 63.9% and 72.2%(p = 0.005), respectively. The demographics and characteristics of patients in the establishment cohort and the validation cohort are summarized in Table 2.

Model establishment of the mRASP

The model of modified risk assessment score of PAH was established by using the establishment cohort. The score of mRASP of establishment cohort had a minimum risk score of 0, a maximum risk score of 8, and a mean risk score of 4.5. After the retrospective correspondence between the risk score and the observed survival rates in the establishment cohort, a score of 0–2, 3–5, and 6–8 were corresponded to the low-risk stratum in which survival rate was 95 to 100%, the intermediate-risk stratum in which survival rate was 90 to 95%, and the high-risk stratum in which survival rate was < 90%, respectively Fig. 2.

Validation of the mRASP

In the validation cohort, the observed mean overall one-year survival rate was 81.5%. In total of 40 patients died in the follow-up. Among all the deceased, 29 cases died of aggravation of right ventricular failure during hospitalization, 11 cases died of sudden death out of hospitalization.

On the basis of the patients' mRASP scores being 0–2, 3–5, and 6–8, they were stratified into low-risk stratum, intermediate-risk stratum and high-risk stratum in which the predicted one-year survival rates were expected to be

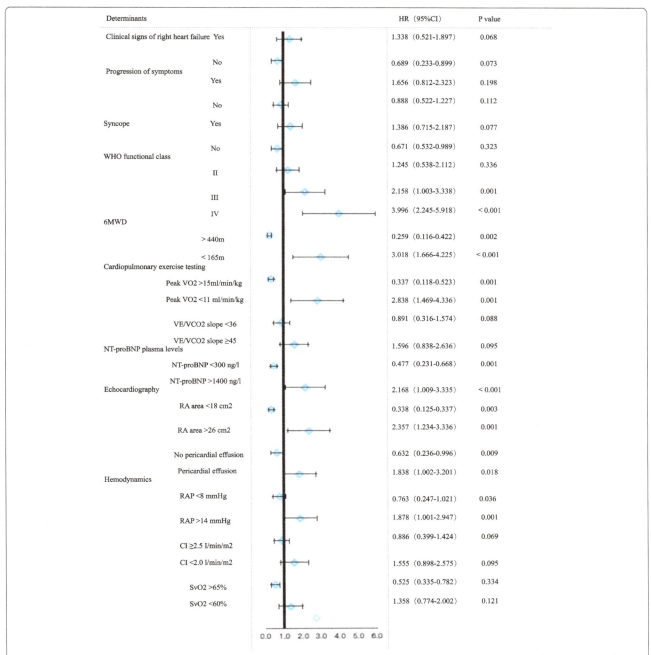

Fig. 1 The multivariate analysis between all the risk assessment determinants in 2015 ESC/ERS PH guidelines and the risk of one-year mortality in the establishment cohort

95–100%, 90–95%, and 0–90%, respectively. The number of patients in low-risk stratum, intermediate-risk stratum, and high-risk stratum in the validation cohort were 68, 81, and 67 presenting in normal distribution. During the follow-up, the number of the deceased patients in each risk stratum were 2, 6, and 32, respectively. The observed one-year survival rates in each risk stratum were 97.1, 92.6, and 52.2%, respectively. The observed survival rates fell within the range of the pre-estimated risk strata. Calibration plot between the predicted mean one-year survival rates by the mRASP score and the actually observed survival rates in the validation cohort is illustrated in Fig. 3.

For the REVEAL score, the number of patients stratified into the REVEAL score strata of 0–7, 8, 9, 10–11,

Table 1 The modified risk assessment score of PAH

Determinants of prognosis	Score 0	Score 1	Score 2
WHO functional class	I, II	III	IV
6MWD	> 440 m	165-440 m	< 165 m
NT-proBNP	NT-proBNP < 300 ng/l	NT-proBNP 300–1400 ng/L	NT-proBNP > 1400 ng/L
Echocardiography	RA area < 18 cm^2	RA area 18–26 cm^2	RA area > 26 cm^2
Total score	0–2 → Low-risk stratum → One-year survival rate 95–100%		
	3–5 → Intermediate-risk stratum → One-year survival rate 90–95%		
	6–8 → High-risk stratum → One-year survival rate < 90%		

PAH pulmonary arterial hypertension, WHO world health organization, 6MWD 6-min walking distance, BNP brain natriuretic peptide, RA right atrial

Table 2 Characteristics of patients in two cohorts

Characteristics	Establishment cohort ($n = 108$)	Validation cohort ($n = 216$)	p Value
Age-years	52.8 ± 14.9	54.6 ± 17.2	0.088
Female-no.(%)	77 (71.3)	159 (73.6)	< 0.001(0.123)
WHO group 1 subgroup-no.(%)			
Idiopathic PAH	48 (44.4)	100 (46.3)	< 0.001(0.147)
Associated with CTD	35 (32.4)	62 (28.7)	< 0.001(0.007)
Associated with CHD	10 (9.3)	25 (11.6)	< 0.001(0.358)
Associated with PoPH	7 (6.5)	10 (4.6)	0.086(0.414)
Familial PAH	3 (2.8)	6 (2.8)	< 0.001(0.95)
Other	5 (4.6)	13 (6.0)	< 0.001(0.27)
WHO functional class-no.(%)			
I	9 (8.3)	21 (9.7)	< 0.001(0.33)
II	30 (27.8)	39 (18.1)	0.046(0.007)
III	55 (50.9)	131 (60.6)	< 0.001(0.025)
IV	14 (13.0)	25 (11.6)	< 0.001(0.259)
Systolic BP-mm Hg	122 ± 23	115 ± 19	0.005
Heart rate-beats/min	85 ± 15	88 ± 17	0.151
6MWD-m	338 ± 119	309 ± 125	0.019
N-terminal proBNP -pg/mL	3268 ± 2431	3497 ± 2896	0.066
Renal insufficiency(yes)-no.(%)	11 (10.2)	19 (8.8)	0.006(0.382)
DLco of predicted in PFT -%	53.8 ± 24.9	49.7 ± 22.3	0.024
Peak VO2 in CPET -ml/min/kg	14.4 ± 9.2	12.8 ± 8.6	0.036
Echocardiography			
Right atrial area-cm^2	21.6 ± 14.9	23.1 ± 16.7	0.188
Pericardial effusion(yes)-no.(%)	28 (25.9)	66 (30.6)	< 0.001(0.033)
Right heart catheterization			
Right atrial pressure-mm Hg	9.7 ± 5.2	10.6 ± 5.8	0.234
Mean pulmonary artery pressure-mm Hg	45.2 ± 12.8	46.7 ± 13.4	0.371
Pulmonary vascular resistance-WU	10.5 ± 5.1	11.2 ± 6.3	0.565
Death -no.(%)	18(16.7)	40(18.5)	< 0.001(0.096)
Loss to follow-up -no.(%)	5(4.6)	7(3.2)	0.071(0.122)

WHO world health organization, PAH pulmonary arterial hypertension, CTD connective tissue diseasem, CHD congenital heart disease, PoPH portal pulmonary hypertension, 6MWD 6-min walking distance, BNP brain natriuretic peptide, DLco diffusing capacity of lung for carbon monoxide, PFT pulmonary function test, VO2 volume of oxygen, CPET cardiopulmonary exercise testing, WU Wood units

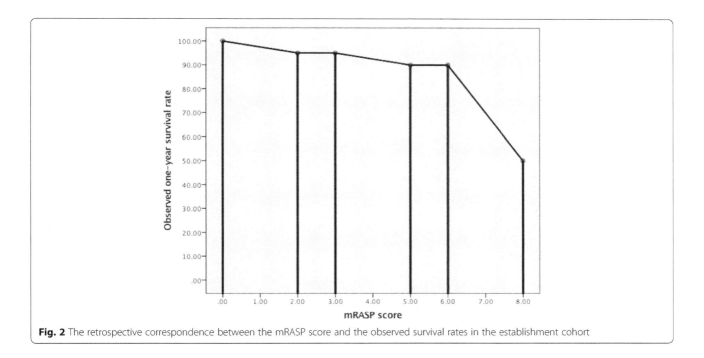

Fig. 2 The retrospective correspondence between the mRASP score and the observed survival rates in the establishment cohort

and ≥ 12 in the validation cohort were 62, 26, 36, 52, and 40, respectively. During the follow-up, the number of the deceased patients in each risk stratum were 2, 2, 5, 12 and 19, respectively. The observed one-year survival rates were 96.8, 92.3, 86.1, 76.9 and 52.5% in each risk stratum, respectively. The observed survival rates all fell within the range of the pre-estimated risk stratum 95–100%, 90–95%, 85–90%, 70–85%, and < 70%. Calibration plot between the predicted mean one-year survival rates by the REVEAL score and the actually observed survival rates in the validation cohort is illustrated in Fig. 4.

Comparison of predictive power between the REVEAL score and the mRASP score

The bias-corrected c-index for the mRASP score in the validation cohort was calculated to be 0.727. The

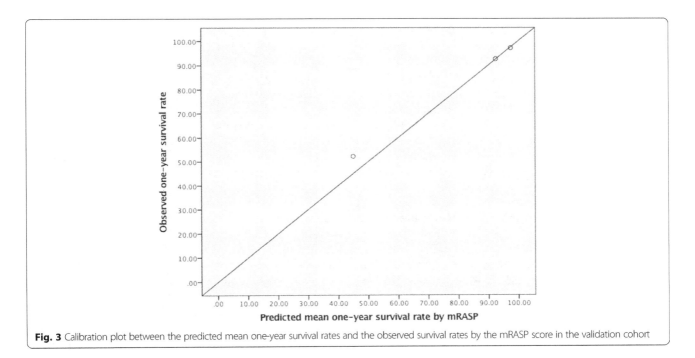

Fig. 3 Calibration plot between the predicted mean one-year survival rates and the observed survival rates by the mRASP score in the validation cohort

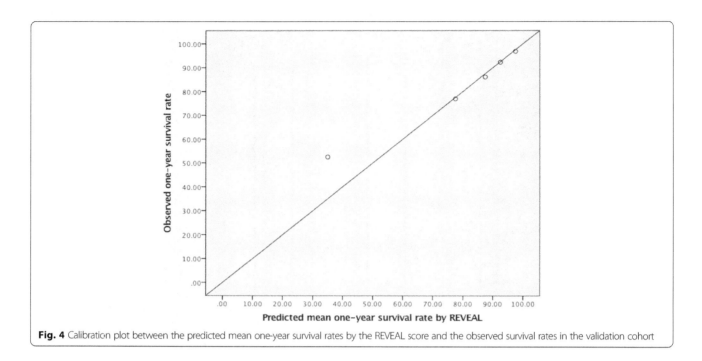

Fig. 4 Calibration plot between the predicted mean one-year survival rates by the REVEAL score and the observed survival rates in the validation cohort

bias-corrected c-index for the REVEAL score in the validation cohort was 0.715. That is to say, patients with lower predicted risk score of the mRASP and the REVEAL will have 72.7 and 71.5% chances to survive longer, respectively(p = 0.666). The similar c-index of both risk scores indicated that the mRASP score had similar discriminatory ability with the REVEAL score.

Discussion

Clinical daily assessment is a critical method to evaluate patients with PH, for determining disease severity and prognosis as well as disease management, and should be performed regularly with a combination of variables [1, 3]. Although the existing risk assessment approaches have been validated to be valid in predicting survival rates in multiple cohorts [4, 5, 11], there are still some defectives which reserved potential rooms for improvement. In consequence, this study was aimed at developing a modified risk assessment score of PAH. For the model establishment of this modified risk assessment score of PAH, we deliberated our desirable determinants on the principle of validity, accuracy, simplicity and convenience. The incentives that we applied those four determinants to be the variables of our modified risk assessment score was not only that they were the basic program most frequently used in PH centers [1], but also they were qualified to be mostly correlated with mortality in a multivariate analysis. Also the score provided quantitative assessments rather than qualitative ones, since the latter might vary dramatically between physicians [12].

WHO FC is one of the most valid predictors of survival, for both diagnosis and follow-up notwithstanding its variability [6, 7, 13, 14]. A deteriorating FC is one of the most serious sign of disease progression [7, 8]. 6MWD is the result of 6-min walking test (6MWT) which is a sub-maximal exercise test. It is the most inexpensive and familiar exercise test frequently used in PH centers. The overall treatment goal for patients with PAH is to achieve a low-risk status which usually means being in WHO-FC II, mostly together with a normal or near normal 6MWD [1, 15–20]. BNP/NT-proBNP levels represent myocardial dysfunction and provide prognostic information at the time of diagnosis or during follow-up [21]. NT-proBNP is regarded as a stronger predictor of prognosis compared with BNP [22]. Echocardiography is an important follow-up approach due to RV function is a crucial determinant of outcome in PH [1]. On the contrary, clinical signs of right heart failure, progression of symptoms, syncope and pericardial effusion of echocardiography in which all the severity are difficult to stratify were excluded from the mRASP in order to improve accuracy. Since life expectancy has been improved for patients with PAH warranting noninvasive approaches for prognostic assessment, and there has been no evidence that receiving regular RHC is associated with better outcomes than a non-invasive follow-up strategy [1], HC was not included in the mRASP. The reason we did not use the serial risk score assessments was that it involved the variables of two different time points resulting in the poor feasibility of the assessment of newly diagnosed patients or patients whose last assessment scores are not available [23].

The results of the present study demonstrated that the one-year survival rates predicted by the mRASP matched the actually observed ones. This validated the validity of mRASP which was derived from the establishment cohort for assessing one-year survival rates in the validation cohort. In our opinion, a valid risk assessment score of PAH should have excellent applicability, generalizability and adaptability for PAH cohorts with various characteristics, and outstanding discriminatory power to distinguish the potential survival from mortality. We noticed that patients in the validation cohort appeared to be more severe than those in the establishment cohort in regard to WHO FC, and believed that it was due to the validation cohort had more newly diagnosed patients who had never received any PAH-specific therapy than the establishment cohort. Nevertheless, from another perspective, it reveals the excellent applicability, generalizability and adaptability of the mRASP in different cohorts with different severity. It is worth noting that otherwise than the study of Benza et al. [5] there is a plunge of survival rate between the intermediate-risk stratum and the high-risk stratum in the validation cohort similar to what happened in the establishment cohort. Between score of 5 points and 6 points, the survival rate descends from more than 90% to almost its half, meanwhile, the mortality rate ascends approximately 6 folds. It may suggest that a score of 6 points could potentially be a cutoff value which implies the prognosis may deteriorate dramatically if patients' risk scores exceed it, distinctly differentiating the potential survival from mortality.

The next comparison showed that the predictive efficacy for one-year survival rate by the mRASP score was similar to that by the REVEAL score. In the study of Benza et al. in 2012 [5], the REVEAL simplified risk score calculator were demonstrated to have good discriminatory power in patients with PAH. Afterwards, this risk assessment tool has been validated to be effective in the prediction of survival in several cohorts, demonstrating its prognostic generalizability in different PAH populations [4, 11]. It is the mostly recognized risk assessment score for PAH to date. Nevertheless, due to some problematic issues we encountered in the application of REVEAL score such as the poor accessibility of RHC, instability of vital signs, non-modifiable determinants, inspiring us to search for some solution through this study. The conception of the mRASP was an overlapping of determinants in the TABLE 13 of 2015 ESC/ERS PH guidelines and the score calculator of the REVEAL score. The original purpose of designing was aimed to inherit their pros and discard their cons to generate a simplified standardized algorithm which could be highly applicable and valid under most circumstances by means of validating the generalizability of those cut-off values in parameters from expert opinion or consensus which might be highly representative. Also the four selected variables was validated to be mostly correlated with mortality in a multivariate analysis. Since finally the two risk assessment tools did not display much distinction on validity from each other, the mRASP could be regarded as a risk assessment model with noninvasiveness, accuracy, simplicity, and convenience comparable with the REVEAL score.

Regardless of the advantages that the mRASP has, several issues must be addressed for its clinical application. It is noteworthy that since RHC is absent in the mRASP, clinicians should apply it with discretion whilst therapeutic decisions can be generated from the results [1]. It also should be noted that even though the mRASP may provide prognostic information to guide therapeutic decisions, the individual application must be performed carefully in light of that it is too population-based to precisely predict individual patient, being similar to the REVEAL score or French risk equation. In other words, when it comes to an individual patient, all risk assessments should be applied under the circumstances of considering the patient's history and the corresponding PAH-specific therapy. Another important issue is that patients should not calculate their risk themselves for avoiding the misinterpretation. It is the responsibility of medical professionals to discuss the results of risk assessment and to consider the next steps [3]. Another issue that cannot be overlooked is that even though we endeavored to optimize the designing of mRASP as much as possible, it is potentially possible that other designs can achieve the same or even better assessment effect. For example, recently Boucly et al. built a risk assessment model composed of the following determinants: WHO FC I or II, 6MWD > 440 m, RAP < 8 mmHg and CI $\geq$ 2.5 L·min^{-1}·m^{-2}, which could accurately predict the prognosis of incident PAH in a retrospective study [24]. However, as said in the article, it remained unknown whether the addition of echocardiography or cardiopulmonary exercise testing to their criteria could further improve the prognostic power [24]. In another study, Hoeper et al. validated the validity of risk assessment strategy in 2015 European PH guidelines with a model composed of WHO FC, 6MWD, BNP or NT-pro BNP, right atrial pressure, cardiac index and mixed venous oxygen saturation [25]. However, this model is still invasive not being suitable for daily clinical practice. In any case, novel assessment models invariably require prospective validation. As our recognition and management of PAH advances, predictive tools will need updating to reflect current practice [4].

The strength of this study is that we prospectively validated the validity of the newly designed risk score, by contrast with the REVEAL score. Nevertheless, limitations also exist in this study. First of all, the sample volume is not very large. The validation of the mRASP in another large cohort is warranted in the future. Secondly, in the development of mRASP score by retrospectively reviewing the establishment cohort, the risk score-related assessments were not performed at mandatory visits undermining the quality of the study more or less. Thirdly, since this study did not involve the predictive efficacy of the mRASP for the survival rate beyond 1 year or for the survival rate in other groups of PH, we have no comments to make on it. The study regarding the long-term risk assessment of PAH or of other groups of PH with the mRASP is warranted in the future. The last but not least, since all patients assessed in our cohorts were all of Chinese population, this risk assessment score may not be applicable for other races.

Conclusions

In conclusion, under the circumstances of existing risk assessment approaches for PAH having limitations in daily clinical practice, a modified risk assessment score of PAH was designed in order to improve it. The mRASP was validated to be an eligible risk assessment tool for the prognostic assessment of PAH. It demonstrated the similar predictive power to the REVEAL score in the validation of predicting one-year survival rates for patients with newly and previously diagnosed PAH. Along with its noninvasiveness, accuracy, simplicity and convenience, the mRASP may be a substitute for the REVEAL score under some circumstances. Although the mRASP still needs to further prove its consistency and stability in the future, we hope that it would at least contribute an inspiration to clinicians in the risk assessment of PAH.

Abbreviations
6MWD: 6 min walk distance; CAT: COPD assessment test; CPET: Cardiopulmonary exercise test; CTEPH: Chronic thromboembolic pulmonary hypertension; mPAP: Mean pulmonary arterial pressure; mPAP: Mean pulmonary arterial pressure; NT-proBNP: N-terminal pro-brain natriuretic peptide; PAH: Pulmonary arterial hypertension; PAH: Pulmonary arterial hypertension; PAWP: Pulmonary artery wedge pressure; Peak VO$_2$: peak oxygen consumption; PFT: Pulmonary function test,; RBT: Routine blood test; RHC: Right heart catheterization; RV: Right ventricular

Acknowledgements
We sincerely thank Dr. Lan Wang, Dr. Jian Guo, Dr. Sugang Gong, Dr. Jing He, Dr. Qinhua Zhao, Dr. Rong Jiang, Dr. Cijun Luo, Dr. Hongling Qiu, Dr. Wenhui Wu, Dr. Minqi Liu, Dr. Tianxiang Chen, Dr. Xingxing Sun, and Dr. Chuanyu Wang of Department of Cardiopulmonary Circulation, Shanghai Pulmonary Hospital, Tongji University School of Medicine, Shanghai, China, for their assistance in this study.

Funding
This work was supported by the following funds: The Program of Shanghai Natural Science Foundation (16ZR1429000), from Shanghai Science and Technology Commission; The Program of Development Center for Medical Science and Technology(ZX-01-C2016144), from National Health and Family Planning Commission of the People's Republic of China.

Authors' contributions
WX conceived of the study, and participated in its design, performance, statistics, coordination, drafting and revising of the manuscript. YFZ conceived of the study, and participated in its design, statistics, coordination, and revising of the manuscript. MX conceived of the study, and participated in its design, statistics, coordination, drafting and revising of the manuscript. BP participated in its design, statistics, performance, coordination, drafting and revising of the manuscript. XJG participated in its design, statistics, coordination, and revising of the manuscript. JML conceived of the study, and participated in its design, coordination and revising of the manuscript. All authors read and approved the final manuscript.

Competing interests
The authors declare that they have no competing interests.

Author details
[1]Department of Respiratory Medicine, Xinhua Hospital, Shanghai Jiaotong University School of Medicine, 1665, Kongjiang Road, Shanghai 200092, China. [2]Department of Cardiopulmonary Circulation, Shanghai Pulmonary Hospital, Tongji University School of Medicine, Shanghai, People's Republic of China. [3]Department of Respiratory Medicine, Punan Hospital, Pudong New District, Shanghai, China. [4]Department of Pediatrics, Kongjiang Hospital, Yangpu District, Shanghai, China. [5]Department of Pediatrics, Shanghai Dinghai Community Health Service Center, Tongji University School of Medicine, Yangpu District, Shanghai, China.

References
1. Galiè N, Humbert M, Vachiery J-L, Gibbs S, Lang I, Torbicki A, et al. ESC/ERS guidelines for the diagnosis and treatment of pulmonary hypertension. Eur Respir J. 2015;46:879–82.
2. Hoeper MM, Bogaard HJ, Condliffe R, Frantz R, Khanna D, Kurzyna M, et al. Definitions and diagnosis of pulmonary hypertension. J Am Coll Cardiol. 2013;62(Suppl):D42–50.
3. Raina A, Humbert M. Risk assessment in pulmonary arterial hypertension. Eur Respir Rev. 2016;25:361–3.
4. Sitbon O, Benza RL, Badesch DB, Barst RJ, Elliott CG, Gressin V, et al. Validation of two predictive models for survival in pulmonary arterial hypertension. Eur Respir J. 2015;46:152–64.
5. Benza RL, Gomberg-Maitland M, Miller DP, Frost A, Frantz RP, Foreman AJ, et al. The REVEAL registry risk score calculator in patients newly diagnosed with pulmonary arterial hypertension. Chest. 2012;141:354–62.
6. Sitbon O, Humbert M, Nunes H, Parent F, Garcia G, Hervé P, et al. Long-term intravenous epoprostenol infusion in primary pulmonary hypertension: prognostic factors and survival. J Am Coll Cardiol. 2002;40:780–8.
7. Nickel N, Golpon H, Greer M, Knudsen L, Olsson K, Westerkamp V, et al. The prognostic impact of follow-up assessments in patients with idiopathic pulmonary arterial hypertension. Eur Respir J. 2012;39:589–96.
8. Benza RL, Miller DP, Gomberg-Maitland M, Frantz RP, Foreman AJ, Coffey CS, et al. Predicting survival in pulmonary arterial hypertension: insights from the registry to evaluate early and long-term pulmonary arterial hypertension disease management (REVEAL). Circulation. 2010;122:164–72.
9. McLaughlin V, Sitbon O, Badesch DB, Barst RJ, Black C, Galiè N, et al. Survival with first-line bosentan in patients with primary pulmonary hypertension. Eur Respir J. 2005;25:244–9.
10. Sitbon O, McLaughlin V, Badesch DB, Barst RJ, Black C, Galiè N, et al. Survival in patients with class III idiopathic pulmonary arterial hypertension treated with first line oral bosentan compared with an historical cohort of patients started on intravenous epoprostenol. Thorax. 2005;60:1025–30.
11. Sitbon O, Jaïs X, Savale L, Cottin V, Bergot E, Macari EA, et al. Upfront triple combination therapy in pulmonary arterial hypertension: a pilot study. Eur Respir J. 2014;43:1691–7.
12. Lee KL, Pryor DB, Harrell FE Jr, Califf RM, Behar VS, Floyd WL, et al. Predicting outcome in coronary disease. Statistical models versus expert clinicians. Am J Med. 1986;80:553–60.
13. Taichman DB, McGoon MD, Harhay MO, Archer-Chicko C, Sager JS, Murugappan M, et al. Wide variation in clinicians' assessment of New York heart association/World Health Organization functional class in patients with pulmonary arterial hypertension. Mayo Clin Proc. 2009;84:586–92.
14. Barst RJ, Chung L, Zamanian RT, Turner M, McGoon MD. Functional class improvement and 3-year survival outcomes in patients with pulmonary arterial hypertension in the REVEAL registry. Chest. 2013;144:160–8.
15. Waxman AB, Farber HW. Using clinical trial end points to risk stratify patients with pulmonary arterial hypertension. Circulation. 2015;132:2152–61.
16. Wensel R, Opitz CF, Anker SD, Winkler J, Höffken G, Kleber FX, et al. Assessment of survival in patients with primary pulmonary hypertension: importance of cardiopulmonary exercise testing. Circulation. 2002;106:319–24.

17. Wensel R, Francis DP, Meyer FJ, Opitz CF, Bruch L, Halank M, et al. Incremental prognostic value of cardiopulmonary exercise testing and resting haemodynamics in pulmonary arterial hypertension. Int J Cardiol. 2013;167:1193-8.
18. Blumberg FC, Arzt M, Lange T, Schroll S, Pfeifer M, Wensel R. Impact of right ventricular reserve on exercise capacity and survival in patients with pulmonary hypertension. Eur J Heart Fail. 2013;15:771-5.
19. Diller GP, Dimopoulos K, Okonko D, Li W, Babu-Narayan SV, Broberg CS, et al. Exercise intolerance in adult congenital heart disease: comparative severity, correlates, and prognostic implication. Circulation. 2005;112:828-35.
20. Arena R, Lavie CJ, Milani RV, Myers J, Guazzi M. Cardiopulmonary exercise testing in patients with pulmonary arterial hypertension: an evidence-based review. J Heart Lung Transplant. 2010;29:159-73.
21. Warwick G, Thomas PS, Yates DH. Biomarkers in pulmonary hypertension. Eur Respir J. 2008;32:503-12.
22. Leuchte HH, El Nounou M, Tuerpe JC, Hartmann B, Baumgartner RA, Vogeser M, et al. N-terminal pro-brain natriuretic peptide and renal insufficiency as predictors of mortality in pulmonary hypertension. Chest. 2007;131:402-9.
23. Benza RL, Miller DP, Foreman AJ, Frost AE, Badesch DB, Benton WW, et al. Prognostic implications of serial risk score assessments in patients with pulmonary arterial hypertension: a registry to valuate early and long-term pulmonary arterial hypertension disease management (REVEAL) analysis. J Heart Lung Transplant. 2015;34:356-61.
24. Boucly A, Weatherald J, Savale L, Jaïs X, Cottin V, Prevot G, et al. Risk assessment, prognosis and guideline implementation in pulmonary arterial hypertension. Eur Respir J. 2017;50:1700889.
25. Hoeper MM, Kramer T, Pan Z, et al. Mortality in pulmonary arterial hypertension: prediction by the 2015 European pulmonary hypertension guidelines risk stratification model. Eur Respir J. 2017;50:1700740.

Real-world treatment patterns for patients 80 years and older with early lung cancer: a nationwide claims study

Kyungjong Lee[1†], Hye Ok Kim[2†], Hee Kyoung Choi[2] and Gi Hyeon Seo[2*]

Abstract

Background: Old age is an important factor that could affect the treatment of early-stage lung cancer. In this study, we evaluated the treatment patterns and outcomes of patients over the age of 80 years who had been diagnosed with early-stage lung cancer in real-world practice.

Methods: Elderly patients who were diagnosed with early-stage lung cancer between 2008 and 2016 were identified using claims data provided by the Health Insurance Review and Assessment Service. The proportion of patients who underwent surgical resection or stereotactic body radiation therapy (SBRT), practice pattern trends, and overall survival (OS) were analyzed from the population-based data.

Results: Over 9 years, 1,684 patients underwent surgical resection (74.9%) or SBRT (25.1%) as a localized treatment. From 2008 to 2016, the treatment modality changed: the percentage of patients who underwent surgical resection decreased from 90.6 to 71.4%, and those who underwent SBRT increased from 9.4 to 28.6%. The percentage of patients treated with SBRT increased over time ($p < 0.001$). The median OS was 56.4 months in the surgery group and 35.5 months in the SBRT group. The SBRT group showed worse OS compared with the surgery group (Adjusted hazard ratio, 1.44; 95% confidence interval, 1.21–1.72; $p < 0.001$).

Conclusion: Changes in local treatment patterns in elderly lung cancer patients were observed and SBRT increased its role in this population. Surgical resection or SBRT should be considered the treatment of choice in elderly patients with localized lung cancer. Further prospective studies are required to elucidate the benefits of surgery and SBRT.

Keywords: Radiosurgery, Thoracic surgery, Treatment trends, Lung neoplasms

Background

Lung cancer is the leading cause of cancer-related deaths in South Korea, although the 5-year survival rate has increased from 11.3 to 25.1% [1]. Lung cancer develops two or three times more frequently in individuals 70 years and older than in younger individuals, and it is the leading cause of cancer-related deaths in those aged 80 years and older [2]. Because the incidence of cancer is expected to increase among the elderly [3], it will be important to improve patient survival, especially in this population.

* Correspondence: seogihyeon@hira.or.kr
†Kyungjong Lee and Hye Ok Kim contributed equally to this work.
[2]Health Insurance Review and Assessment Service, 60 Hyeoksin-ro (Bangok-dong), Wonju-si, Gangwon-do 26465, South Korea
Full list of author information is available at the end of the article

Surgical resection for early-stage lung cancer is the best treatment to improve survival. However, elderly patients (> 80 years old) with comorbidities do not easily receive surgery due to concerns about surgery-related mortality and morbidity [4–6]. Additionally, patients at this age often abandon the opportunity to cure early-stage non-small-cell lung cancer (NSCLC) due to the number of comorbidities, which increase proportionally with age [7, 8]. Stereotactic body radiation therapy (SBRT) is an alternative treatment modality that destroys lesions by delivering a high dose of radiation to the target site. SBRT showed a high local control rate comparable to lobectomy in early-stage NSCLC patients who were not eligible for surgery, with tolerable toxicities in patients with underlying emphysema and vascular diseases [9, 10]. The excellent local control and lower complication rates of SBRT may lead to changes in practical treatment patterns in patients with early-stage lung cancer who are not suitable for surgery or refuse treatment due to concerns over surgical complications. Toxicity issues associated with the treatment of early-stage NSCLC in the elderly remain, although previous studies have suggested that SBRT is safe and tolerable in elderly populations [11]. A recent study reported that the practice pattern and treatment outcomes have changed in elderly stage I lung cancer patients since the introduction of SBRT in the United States [12]. However, there was no report of annual survival outcomes for surgery and SBRT in a limited cohort of 80 years and older patients with early-stage lung cancer using a population-based database from South Korea.

This study evaluated the trends in practice patterns and survival outcomes over 9 years in patients 80 years and older diagnosed with early-stage lung cancer and compared the overall survival (OS) rates of those who underwent surgery and SBRT. We used a national claims database provided by the Health Insurance Review and Assessment service (HIRA).

Methods
Data source
The HIRA database, a nationwide claims database, covers the claims of 100% of the South Korean population. The HIRA database includes patient demographics and the record of diagnosis (as determined by the International classification of Disease, Tenth Revision), interventions, and prescriptions. The HIRA service provided the data after patient de-identification, in accordance with the Act on the Protection of Personal Information maintained by public agencies. This study was conducted in accordance with the Declaration of Helsinki. The Institutional Review Board of Samsung Medical Center approved this retrospective cohort study (Approval no. 2018-02-023); informed consent from patients was waived by the Board.

Patient selection
Patients 80 years and older with a new diagnosis of lung cancer between January 2008 and December 2016 were collected from the HIRA database for possible inclusion. Lung cancer outcomes were identified on the basis of insurance claims data selected as the major diagnosis code in in-patient records (C34). Patients 80 years and older who underwent lung cancer surgery (lobectomy, segmentectomy, or wedge resection) or SBRT were included. Patients who underwent both surgery and SBRT, and who had a history of chemotherapy before SBRT or surgery were excluded. Patients who received any type of chemotherapy within 90 days after surgery or SBRT were also excluded. It was possible to retrieve only the HIRA data of patients who claimed treatments for lung cancer. We could not identify patients who had lung cancer with no treatments. Early-stage lung cancer was defined as cases of surgery or SBRT only without neoadjuvant/adjuvant treatment. The index date was defined as the first recorded date of surgery or SBRT. Cancer-directed treatment was regarded when the treatment occurred within 3 months after the diagnosis of lung cancer.

Statistical analysis
Descriptive statistical analyses were performed on all patients. Continuous and categorical variables are presented as the mean ± standard deviation (SD) and numbers (%). Baseline characteristics among the two groups (operation vs. SBRT) were compared using the t-test for continuous variables and Pearson's χ^2 test for categorical variables. Univariate and multivariate Cox proportional hazard models were used to reveal the association between clinical variables and survival outcomes. These results are reported as hazard ratios (HRs) with 95% confidence intervals (CIs). Survival curves were calculated using the Kaplan-Meier method and were compared using the log-rank test. A two-tailed p-value of < 0.05 was considered to indicate statistical significance. All statistical analyses were performed using R program version 3.4.0.

Results
Patient characteristics
In total, 1,684 patients diagnosed with early-stage lung cancer from 2008 to 2016 and who met the inclusion criteria were eligible for this study. Of those, 1,262 (74.9%) patients underwent surgical resection and 422 (25.1%) underwent SBRT. The clinical characteristics are summarized in Table 1. The mean age at lung cancer diagnosis was 82.0 ± 2.2 years in the surgery group and 83.2 ± 3.1 years in the SBRT group. Males accounted for 71.6% of the subjects in the surgery group and 71.8% in the SBRT group. In total, 91.3% of patients in the surgery group and 91.9% of patients in the SBRT group did not receive any type of chemotherapy during the entire follow-up period. Only 8.7% of individuals in the surgery group and 8.1% of individuals in the SBRT group received chemotherapy after 3 months of local treatment. There was no significant difference in clinical treatment failure represented as additional chemotherapy between the two groups ($p = 0.750$). The median length of follow-up was 20.4 months (interquartile range [IQR], 7.4–40.3 months) for the surgery group and 16.8 months (IQR, 6.9–30.0 months) for the SBRT group.

Temporal changes in local treatment patterns
During the study period, the use of local treatment increased among the elderly patients with early-stage lung cancer from 64 patients in 2008 to 364 patients in 2016.

Table 1 Demographics of very elderly (≥80 years old) lung cancer patients

Characteristic	Treatment, No. (%)		
	Total (N = 1,684)	Surgery (N = 1,262)	SBRT (N = 422)
Mean age, years	82.3 ± 2.5	82.0 ± 2.2	83.2 ± 3.1
Sex			
Male	1,207 (71.7)	904 (71.6)	303 (71.8)
Female	477 (28.3)	358 (28.4)	119 (28.2)
Chemotherapy[a]			
No	1,540 (91.4)	1,152 (91.3)	388 (91.9)
Yes	144 (8.6)	110 (8.7)	34 (8.1)
Year of treatment			
2008	64	58 (90.6)	6 (9.4)
2009	83	72 (86.7)	11 (13.3)
2010	105	89 (84.8)	16 (15.2)
2011	111	90 (81.1)	21 (18.9)
2012	186	139 (74.7)	47 (25.3)
2013	219	154 (70.3)	65 (29.7)
2014	255	188 (73.7)	67 (26.3)
2015	297	212 (71.4)	85 (28.6)
2016	364	260 (71.4)	104 (28.6)
Follow-up, months			
Median	19.4	20.4	16.8
IQR	7.2–36.5	7.4–40.3	6.8–30.0
Median OS, months			
Median	49.8	56.4	35.5
95% CI	44.7–56.3	49.1–66.5	28.9–41.7
30-day mortality			
No. (%)	36 (2.2)	30 (2.4)	6 (1.5)
95% CI	1.5–2.9	1.6–3.3	0.3–2.6

[a]Defined as patients who received any type of chemotherapy after 3 months of local treatment
All values are presented as the number (%). N number, OS overall survival, CI confidence interval, SBRT stereotactic body radiation therapy

The trends in treatment practice change between 2008 and 2016 are shown in Fig. 1. The proportion of patients who underwent surgery declined continuously from 90.6 to 71.4%; however, the use of SBRT increased from 9.4% in 2008 to 28.6% in 2016 ($p < 0.001$).

Survival outcomes and predictive factors for elderly lung cancer

Compared with the SBRT group, OS was higher in the surgery group (2-year OS, 72.2% for the surgery group vs. 62.6% for the SBRT group, $p = 0.005$). The median survival time was 56.4 months in the surgery group and 35.5 months in the SBRT group. Post-treatment mortality at 30 days was 2.4% for the surgery group and 1.5% for the SBRT group. At 6 months after local treatment, the rate of mortality was 11.0% in the surgery group and 10.7% in the SBRT group. The comparison of OS between the surgery and SBRT groups from 2008 to 2016 is presented in Fig. 2. To determine the predictive factors for survival in elderly lung cancer patients, a Cox's regression analysis was performed using clinical factors. Clinical variables for the univariate and multivariate analyses are listed in Table 2. According to the univariate analysis, male sex, chemotherapy after 3 months of local treatment, and SBRT were associated with decreased OS. However, patient age in the elderly population (> 80 years) was not a predictive factor. Sex, chemotherapy after 3 months of local treatment, and SBRT remained significantly associated with OS after the multivariate analysis. In terms of treatment modality, the adjusted HR for SBRT was 1.44 (95% CI, 1.21–1.72) with a reference to surgery.

Discussion

In this population-based study, we uncovered temporal practice changes in patients 80 years and older diagnosed with early-stage lung cancer between 2008 and 2016 in real practice in South Korea. Although most patients received surgical resection (74.9%), there were significant changes in treatment trends at the time of the study period. Compared to 2008, the rate of surgical resection decreased gradually from 90.6 to 71.4%. However, the rate of SBRT increased over time from 9.4% in 2008 to 28.6% in 2016. The standard treatment for early-stage lung cancer is surgical resection with lobectomy [13]. However, in cases of poor surgical candidates with old age and comorbidities, it is not easy to perform surgical resection because of the high risk of complications. Since the introduction of SBRT for non-operable lung cancer due to comorbidities such as severe emphysema or heart disease [14], it has been adopted in clinical practice as an alternative to surgery accompanied by expected high risks of complications in patients with early-stage lung cancer. Practice pattern changes in elderly stage I NSCLC patients in which SBRT replaced surgery based on older age is now recognized in the United States [12]. Our data also suggest that SBRT increased its proportion substantially in elderly early-stage lung cancer patients in South Korea.

In our study, the median OS and 5-year survival rate in patients 80 years and older was 49.8 months and 44.8% with local treatment for early-stage lung cancer, respectively. A large population-based study analyzed 101,844 cases of lung cancer registered in the California Cancer Center for 4 years; stage 1 lung cancer was diagnosed in 19,702 patients. Of these, 7.3% of patients did not receive surgery or any type of radiation or chemotherapy. In this untreated group, the median OS and 5-year survival rate was 9 months and 6%, respectively [15]. In particular, lung cancer in the elderly has shown increased mortality, regardless of stage [16]. Therefore,

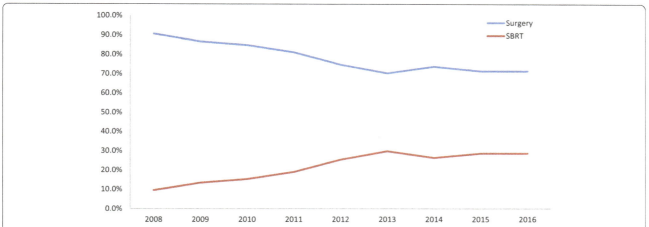

Fig. 1 Practice changes in local treatment patterns in very elderly (≥80 years old) patients diagnosed with early-stage lung cancer. The proportion of patients who underwent stereotactic body radiation therapy (SBRT) increased gradually as a local treatment modality in the old age group over the year ($p < 0.001$)

screening for lung cancer with low-dose computed tomography [17] may be considered for those older than 80 years to reduce mortality in at-risk patients, although the evidence is not sufficient. However, there are concerns that old age makes treatment decisions difficult due to increased comorbidities and decreased physiologic performance. In advanced-stage NSCLC, a substantial number of patients were not treated and older patients were more likely to not receive any treatment [18]. Patients 80 years and older are less likely to be subjected to local treatment compared to younger patients; this results in a poor survival rate in older patients with lung cancer. Although we were unable to compare the survival rate between patients who received treatment and those who did not, definitive local treatment with surgery or SBRT should be performed in patients 80 years and older to increase the survival rate.

Our study shows that surgical resection had higher survival outcomes compared with SBRT after adjusting for variables using these population-based data. However, this result does not represent the head-to-head comparison of OS between the two treatment modalities. SBRT is generally adopted for patients who are not surgically suitable. In any nationwide claims study, selection bias is inevitable because it is impossible to obtain information regarding stage I or II cases, Eastern Cooperative Oncology Group (ECOG) performance, and factors related to surgical risk. Comorbidities increase with age and are the major reason for elderly patients with increased comorbidities to be precluded from surgical resection in cases of early-stage lung cancer [19].

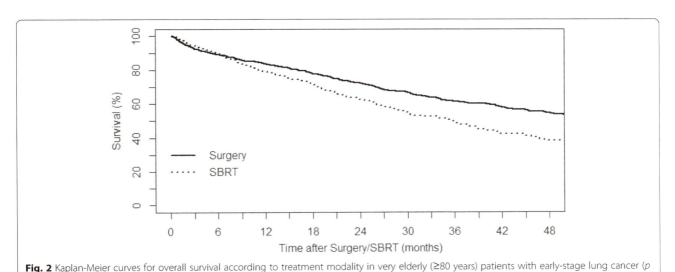

Fig. 2 Kaplan-Meier curves for overall survival according to treatment modality in very elderly (≥80 years) patients with early-stage lung cancer ($p < 0.001$, log-rank test). SBRT, stereotactic body radiation therapy

Table 2 Hazard model of survival outcomes in patients with early-stage lung cancer

Variable	Univariate analysis			Multivariate analysis		
	HR	95% CI	p-value	HR	95% CI	p-value
Age, years						
80–84	Reference					
85–90	1.12	0.90–1.40	0.302			
> 90	1.11	0.67–1.86	0.686			
Sex						
Male	Reference			Reference		
Female	0.42	0.34–0.52	< 0.001	0.41	0.33–0.50	< 0.001
Treatment year						
2008	1.36	0.83–2.22	0.225			
2009	1.49	0.94–2.39	0.091			
2010	1.75	1.23–2.73	0.013			
2011	1.15	0.73–1.82	0.548			
2012	1.15	0.74–1.77	0.532			
2013	1.44	0.95–2.19	0.089			
2014	1.07	0.69–1.64	0.769			
2015	0.97	0.62–1.51	0.882			
2016	Reference					
Chemotherapy						
No	Reference			Reference		
Yes	1.92	1.47–2.26	< 0.001	1.95	1.54–2.39	< 0.001
Treatment modality						
Surgery	Reference			Reference		
SBRT	1.44	1.21–1.72	< 0.001	1.44	1.21–1.72	< 0.001

HR hazard ratio, *CI* confidence interval, *SBRT* stereotactic body radiation therapy

Published surgical mortality and morbidity rates in patients 80 years and older range from 2.0 to 3.6% and 8.4 to 46%, respectively [4, 5, 20]. Although the Radiation Therapy Oncology Group confirmed SBRT as an alternative treatment modality for inoperable early-stage lung cancer [9], there are concerns about the safety and efficacy of SBRT in patients 80 years and older. A multicenter study reported that grade 2 radiation pneumonitis (RP) developed in 34.5% of patients and non-RP related toxicity was reported in 12.1%; however, no grade 4 or 5 toxicity was reported in the group who underwent SBRT for early-stage lung cancer (median age, 84.9 years) [21]. Another study regarding the safety of definitive SBRT in patients more than 80 years old suggested its high efficacy and tolerability [11]. Of interest, a prior study that investigated the effectiveness of SBRT at a single center reported that the OS rates for patients over 75 years were 86% at 1 year, 57.5% at 3 years, and 39.5% at 5 years [22], which is comparable to the survival rates of 79.1% at 1 year, 61.3% at 3 years, and 32.4% at 5 years in our patients who underwent SBRT.

Local relapse or distant metastasis is an important issue in early-stage lung cancer with definitive local treatment. The overall recurrence (local/regional/distant) reported in previous studies for elderly patients with SBRT was 30–40% [21, 23]. Therefore, the 8–9% rate of systemic chemotherapy after 3 months of local treatment in our study may be relatively low, in which surgery or SBRT revealed no significant difference in systemic chemotherapy after 3 months of definitive local treatment. This relatively low chemotherapy rate may be explained by old age-related comorbidities or poor ECOG performance. Although it should not be interpreted as a parameter of recurrence, we may indirectly estimate the rate of systemic chemotherapy as treatment failure after local control and suggest similar rates of treatment failure between the two modalities.

Our study has several limitations. A major limitation of nationwide claims data is the lack of clinical information. We could not obtain information related with performance status, underlying lung function with chronic obstructive pulmonary disease, interstitial lung disease, and accompanied comorbidities. Second, lung cancer stage (I or II) was not clearly divided in this study. The HIRA database contains only information related to claims covered by national insurance. Therefore, it was impossible to stratify the lung cancer staging according to the clinical information. Based on the claims database, we could retrieve early-stage lung cancer data only indirectly using patients who underwent surgical resection only or stereotactic body radiation therapy (SBRT) with no neoadjuvant treatment or adjuvant chemotherapy within 3 months after local treatment. Finally, local recurrence and distant metastasis could not be measured. Only data regarding chemotherapy 3 months later could be obtained; therefore, the rate of treatment failure may be underestimated.

Conclusions

The rate of SBRT increased gradually in patients 80 years and older with early-stage lung cancer, in contrast with the decrease in surgical resection. Surgical resection or SBRT is a reasonable treatment choice for elderly patients with early-stage lung cancer and should be adopted in light of multifactorial decision making.

Abbreviations
ECOG: Eastern Cooperative Oncology Group; HIRA: Health insurance review and assessment service; HRs: Hazard ratios; NSCLC: Non-small-cell lung cancer; OS: Overall survival; SBRT: Stereotactic body radiation therapy

Authors' contributions
GHS had full access to all of the data in the study, and takes responsibility for the integrity of the data and the accuracy of the data analysis. Consception and design: KL, HOK Drafting of the manuscript: KL, HOK Critical revision of the manuscript: KL, HOK, HKC, GHS. All authors have read and approved the final manuscript.

Competing interests
The authors declare that they have no competing interests.

Author details
[1]Department of Medicine, Division of Pulmonary and Critical Care Medicine, Samsung Medical Center, Sungkyunkwan University School of Medicine, Seoul, South Korea. [2]Health Insurance Review and Assessment Service, 60 Hyeoksin-ro (Bangok-dong), Wonju-si, Gangwon-do 26465, South Korea.

References
1. Jung KW, Won YJ, Oh CM, Kong HJ, Lee DH, Lee KH. Cancer statistics in Korea: incidence, mortality, survival, and prevalence in 2014. Cancer Res Treat. 2017;49(2):292–305.
2. Siegel RL, Miller KD, Jemal A. Cancer statistics, 2017. CA Cancer J Clin. 2017;67(1):7–30.
3. Smith BD, Smith GL, Hurria A, Hortobagyi GN, Buchholz TA. Future of cancer incidence in the United States: burdens upon an aging, changing nation. J Clin Oncol. 2009;27(17):2758–65.
4. Okami J, Higashiyama M, Asamura H, Goya T, Koshiishi Y, Sohara Y, et al. Pulmonary resection in patients aged 80 years or over with clinical stage I non-small cell lung cancer: prognostic factors for overall survival and risk factors for postoperative complications. J Thorac Oncol. 2009;4(10):1247–53.
5. Berry MF, Onaitis MW, Tong BC, Harpole DH, D'Amico TA. A model for morbidity after lung resection in octogenarians. Eur J Cardiothorac Surg. 2011;39(6):989–94.
6. Owonikoko TK, Ragin CC, Belani CP, Oton AB, Gooding WE, Taioli E, et al. Lung cancer in elderly patients: an analysis of the surveillance, epidemiology, and end results database. J Clin Oncol. 2007;25(35):5570–7.
7. Shirvani SM, Jiang J, Chang JY, Welsh J, Likhacheva A, Buchholz TA, et al. Lobectomy, sublobar resection, and stereotactic ablative radiotherapy for early-stage non-small cell lung cancers in the elderly. JAMA Surg. 2014;149(12):1244–53.
8. Husain ZA, Kim AW, Yu JB, Decker RH, Corso CD. Defining the high-risk population for mortality after resection of early stage NSCLC. Clin Lung Cancer. 2015;16(6):e183–7.
9. Timmerman R, Paulus R, Galvin J, Michalski J, Straube W, Bradley J, et al. Stereotactic body radiation therapy for inoperable early stage lung cancer. JAMA. 2010;303(11):1070–6.
10. Navarro-Martin A, Aso S, Cacicedo J, Arnaiz M, Navarro V, Rosales S, et al. Phase II trial of SBRT for stage I NSCLC: survival, local control, and lung function at 36 months. J Thorac Oncol. 2016;11(7):1101–11.
11. Kreinbrink P, Blumenfeld P, Tolekidis G, Sen N, Sher D, Marwaha G. Lung stereotactic body radiation therapy (SBRT) for early-stage non-small cell lung cancer in the very elderly (>/=80years old): extremely safe and effective. J Geriatr Oncol. 2017;8(5):351–5.
12. Dalwadi SM, Szeja SS, Bernicker EH, Butler EB, Teh BS, Farach AM. Practice patterns and outcomes in elderly stage I non-small-cell lung cancer: a 2004 to 2012 SEER analysis. Clin Lung Cancer. 2018;19(2):e269–e76.
13. Ettinger DS, Wood DE, Aisner DL, Akerley W, Bauman J, Chirieac LR, et al. Non-small cell lung cancer, version 5.2017, NCCN clinical practice guidelines in oncology. J Natl Compr Cancer Netw. 2017;15(4):504–35.
14. Timmerman RD, Kavanagh BD, Cho LC, Papiez L, Xing L. Stereotactic body radiation therapy in multiple organ sites. J Clin Oncol. 2007;25(8):947–52.
15. Raz DJ, Zell JA, Ou SH, Gandara DR, Anton-Culver H, Jablons DM. Natural history of stage I non-small cell lung cancer: implications for early detection. Chest. 2007;132(1):193–9.
16. Shin A, Oh CM, Kim BW, Woo H, Won YJ, Lee JS. Lung cancer epidemiology in Korea. Cancer Res Treat. 2017;49(3):616–26.
17. Chin J, Syrek Jensen T, Ashby L, Hermansen J, Hutter JD, Conway PH. Screening for lung cancer with low-dose CT--translating science into Medicare coverage policy. N Engl J Med. 2015;372(22):2083–5.
18. David EA, Daly ME, Li CS, Chiu CL, Cooke DT, Brown LM, et al. Increasing rates of no treatment in advanced-stage non-small cell lung cancer patients: a propensity-matched analysis. J Thorac Oncol. 2017;12(3):437–45.
19. Girones R, Torregrosa D, Gomez-Codina J, Maestu I, Tenias JM, Rosell R. Prognostic impact of comorbidity in elderly lung cancer patients: use and comparison of two scores. Lung Cancer. 2011;72(1):108–13.
20. Mun M, Kohno T. Video-assisted thoracic surgery for clinical stage I lung cancer in octogenarians. Ann Thorac Surg. 2008;85(2):406–11.
21. Cassidy RJ, Patel PR, Zhang X, Press RH, Switchenko JM, Pillai RN, et al. Stereotactic body radiotherapy for early-stage non-small-cell lung cancer in patients 80 years and older: a multi-center analysis. Clin Lung Cancer. 2017;18(5):551–8.e6.
22. Brooks ED, Sun B, Zhao L, Komaki R, Liao Z, Jeter M, et al. Stereotactic ablative radiation therapy is highly safe and effective for elderly patients with early-stage non-small cell lung cancer. Int J Radiat Oncol Biol Phys. 2017;98(4):900–7.
23. Ricardi U, Frezza G, Filippi AR, Badellino S, Levis M, Navarria P, et al. Stereotactic ablative radiotherapy for stage I histologically proven non-small cell lung cancer: an Italian multicenter observational study. Lung Cancer. 2014;84(3):248–53.

Impact of multidrug-resistant bacteria on outcome in patients with prolonged weaning

Johannes Bickenbach[1*], Daniel Schöneis[1], Gernot Marx[1], Nikolaus Marx[2], Sebastian Lemmen[3] and Michael Dreher[2]

Abstract

Background: Pneumonia and septic pneumonic shock are the most common indications for long-term mechanical ventilation and prolonged weaning, independent of any comorbidities. Multidrug resistant (MDR) bacteria are emerging as a cause of pneumonia or occur as a consequence of antimicrobial therapy. The influence of MDR bacteria on outcomes in patients with prolonged weaning is unknown.

Methods: Patients treated in a specialized weaning unit of a university hospital between April 2013 and April 2016 were analyzed. Demographic data, clinical characteristics, length of stay (LOS) in the intensive care unit (ICU) and weaning unit, ventilator-free days and mortality rates were determined in prolonged weaning patients with versus without MDR bacteria (methicillin-resistant *Staphylococcus aureus* bacteria, [MRSA]; extended spectrum beta lactamase [ESBL]- and Gyrase-producing gram negative bacteria resistant to three of four antibiotic groups [3 MRGN]; panresistant *Pseudomonas aeruginosa* and other carbapenemase-producing gram-negative bacteria resistant to all four antibiotic groups [4 MRGN]). Weaning failure was defined as death or discharge with invasive ventilation.

Results: Of 666 patients treated in the weaning unit, 430 fulfilled the inclusion criteria and were included in the analysis. A total of 107 patients had isolates of MDR bacteria suspected as causative pathogens identified during the treatment process. Patients with MDR bacteria had higher SAPS II values at ICU admission and a significantly longer ICU LOS. Four MRGN *P. aeruginosa* and *Acinetobacter baumanii* were the most common MDR bacteria identified. Patients with versus without MDR bacteria had significantly higher arterial carbon dioxide levels at the time of weaning admission and a significantly lower rate of successful weaning (23% vs 31%, $p < 0.05$). Mortality rate on the weaning unit was 12.4% with no difference between the two patient groups. There were no significant differences between patient groups in secondary infections and ventilator-free days.

Conclusions: In patients with pneumonia or septic pneumonic shock undergoing prolonged weaning, infection with MDR bacteria may influence the weaning success rate but does not appear to impact on patient survival.

Keywords: Multidrug resistance, Mechanical ventilator weaning, Bacterial pneumonia, Survival

Background

Prolonged weaning from mechanical ventilation (MV) with ≥3 spontaneous breathing trials (SBTs) or ≥ 7 days of ventilation defines a group of patients who require complex and protracted treatment to achieve discontinuation of ventilation [1]. Ventilator-associated pneumonia (VAP) and/or pneumonic septic shock are the most common causes of prolonged weaning and are associated with significantly longer length of stay (LOS) in the intensive care unit (ICU) and increased mortality rates [2].

Despite the introduction of care bundles for the prevention of VAP [3], mortality rates still remain high [4] with an incidence of approximately 6 per 1000 ventilator days. In addition, the development of increasing antibiotic resistance, especially among gram-negative (GN) pathogens in VAP, presents a significant challenge in ICU patients. This makes it even more difficult to break

---

* Correspondence: jbickenbach@ukaachen.de
[1]Department of Intensive Care Medicine, Medical Faculty, RWTH Aachen University, Pauwelsstr. 30, D-52074 Aachen, Germany
Full list of author information is available at the end of the article

the cycle of VAP treatment, prolonged MV and weaning from the ventilator, and improve patient outcomes.

It has previously been shown that the presence of GN, multidrug resistant (MDR) bacteria predicts mortality, pneumonia per se and the complexity of treatment, and that the severity of a critical illness may also be associated with worse outcome [5]. Data from a meta-analysis of 21 studies in patients with MDR versus non-MDR infections showed that the presence of MDR and inadequate treatment of MDR were predictors of mortality [5]. These findings illustrate the clinical relevance of MDR bacteria. However, it is difficult to determine whether it is inappropriate treatment measures that resulted in MDR bacteria or that the MDR bacteria themselves that are the most important factors in contributing to worse outcomes.

Another complicating factor is that patients with prolonged weaning often have important co-morbidities (e.g. chronic obstructive pulmonary disease [COPD], chronic cardiac insufficiency), have received prolonged ICU-based treatment after acute conditions (e.g. septic or cardiogenic shock, acute respiratory failure), and/or have severe weakness of respiratory muscles, fluid overload and recurrent infections. They often require intensive speech and physical therapy, but isolation measures due to the presence of MDR bacteria may influence routine daily care strategies.

Although there are differences between weaning centers due to local circumstances, management and facilities, these centers should all be able to monitor and treat mechanically ventilated patients. The 18-bed weaning unit where this study was conducted is a closed unit that meets all criteria for a fully equipped ICU with respect to patient monitoring, treatment of invasively and non-invasively ventilated patients, and staffing. There is at least one certified doctor in attendance 24 h a day (two assistant doctors and one senior physician during the day and one assistant doctor during the night), nurses (nurse-patient ratio of 1:2), physiotherapists (therapist-patient ratio of 1:6 and a warranted treatment option of 2/day), one speech therapist, and one psychologist.

There is currently a lack of clinical data investigating the effects of MDR bacteria on outcome in patients with prolonged weaning. Several studies have demonstrated an association between MDR bacteria-related VAP and prolonged ICU treatment [6, 7]. However, characteristics of pathogens during the course of treatment and the impact of MDR bacteria on the outcome of prolonged weaning are not known. Therefore, the aim of this study was to assess the prevalence of MDR pathogens and their resistance profile in prolonged weaning patients, and to determine the effects of MDR pathogens on patient outcome.

Methods
Study design
This observational study received approval from the Institutional Review Board for Human Studies at the Medical Faculty of the University Hospital Aachen, Germany, and need for informed consent was waived. All analyses were conducted according to the principles of the Declaration of Helsinki.

Study population
All patients with prolonged weaning treated in the weaning unit over the period April 2013 to April 2016 were eligible. Inclusion criteria were at least one episode of VAP (diagnosed using the Clinical Pulmonary Infection Score [CPIS] [8]) and/or septic pneumonic shock (according to the American College of Chest Physicians [ACCP]/Society of Critical Care Medicine [SCCM] consensus criteria [9]) in the ICU, requiring long-term ventilation, followed by prolonged weaning (≥3 spontaneous breathing trials [SBT] or ≥ 7 days of ventilation) [1]). Patients with community-acquired pneumonia (CAP) and patients with other causes for prolonged weaning, those without prolonged weaning, and patients being admitted from external hospitals were excluded (Fig. 1). In eligible patients, the presence of MDR bacteria was assessed invasively and two groups were defined based on the presence or absence of MDR bacteria.

The primary endpoint was mortality rate on the weaning unit. Secondary endpoints were weaning success rate and ventilator-free days.

Data collection
Data were retrieved from an electronic patient record system (medico//s, Siemens, Germany) and from an online patient data documentary system (IntelliSpace Critical Care and Anesthesia, ICCA Rev. F.01.01.001, Philips Electronics, the Netherlands). Data on age, sex, pre-existing COPD, pre-existing coronary artery disease (CAD), need for renal replacement therapy (RRT), antibiotic therapy, Simplified Acute Physiology Score (SAPS II) at ICU admission, ICU LOS before admission to the weaning unit, and time on MV before admission to the weaning unit were documented. The following data about treatment in the weaning unit were also extracted: SAPS II at discharge; blood gas analysis on admission; and duration of MV and ventilator-free days. At the time of discharge, patients were classified into the three subgroups of prolonged weaning (weaning category 3) as defined by the German S2 k-guideline [10]:

- 3a: Successful weaning after at least 3 failed SBT or MV longer than 7 days after the first failed SBT without the use of non-invasive ventilation (NIV);

- 3b: Successful weaning after at least 3 failed SBT or MV longer than 7 days after the first failed SBT in

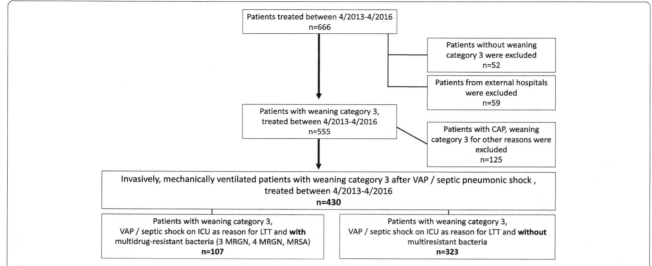

Fig. 1 Inclusion and exclusion criteria for the retrospective data analysis. The weaning categories were based on those described previously by Boles et al. [1]. Patients without category 3 ($n = 52$), patients from external hospitals ($n = 59$), and patients with community acquired pneumonia as reason for the initial ICU admission, and patients with other reasons for prolonged weaning were excluded ($n = 125$). CAP, community-acquired pneumonia, VAP, ventilator-associated pneumonia, ICU, intensive care unit, LTT, long-term treatment.

combination with NIV; if necessary, continued into out-of-hospital (home) MV;

- 3c: Death or discharge with invasive MV via tracheostomy.

MDR bacteria were categorized into three groups: methicillin-resistant *Staphylococcus aureus* (MRSA); extended spectrum beta lactamase (ESBL)- and Gyrase-producing GN bacteria resistant to three of four antibiotic groups (3 MRGN); and panresistant *Pseudomonas aeruginosa* and other carbapenemase-producing GN bacteria resistant to all four antibiotic groups (4 MRGN) [11, 12].

All MDR bacteria as causative pathogens were isolated from blood probes (and positively identified by at least 1 positive blood culture) or from at least one respiratory specimen (including sputum and tracheobronchial aspirates in MV patients or flexible bronchoscopy with bronchoalveolar lavage [BAL]). Typical contaminants, such as coagulase-negative staphylococci, enterococci or candida spp., were not considered as true pathogens.

Statistical analysis

Continuous variables were reported as mean values with standard deviations, or medians with interquartile range when data were not distributed normally. Differences between continuous variables were tested using Student's t-test and Kruskal-Wallis test. Categorical variables were tested using Chi-squared test and McNemar's test, as appropriate. Ventilator-free days were modelled using a generalized linear model with the logarithmic link function. MDR group was used as the independent variable.

In an adjusted model, age (years, continuous), SAPS II (continuous), preexisting pulmonary disease (yes/no), RRT (yes/no) and length of stay (days, continuous) were considered as additional independent variables. Interaction terms were not used. Mortality on the weaning unit was analyzed using separate survival curves for patients in the MDR and non-MDR groups. To compare survival rates in the two patient groups, a Cox proportional hazard model with independent variables MDR group (yes/no), age (years, continuous), SAPS II (continuous), coronary artery disease (CAD) (yes/no), preexisting pulmonary disease (yes/no), and RRT (yes/no) was used. Interactions were not considered. Hazard ratio (HR) and 95% confidence interval (CI) values were estimated.

Results

A total of 666 patients were treated in the weaning unit over the study period; 430 tracheotomized patients with prolonged weaning from invasive MV met the inclusion criteria and were analyzed (Table 1). There were 107 patients with isolates of MDR bacteria as the causative pathogens for pneumonia/septic shock during the course of treatment. Patients from the MDR group were significantly younger and had a lower incidence of CAD. In addition, MDR versus non-MDR patients had significantly higher SAPS II values at the time of ICU admission (39 ± 9.3 vs. 35.9 ± 8.5, $p = 0.03$) and greater ICU LOS (25.3 ± 17.3 vs. 19.5 ± 12.8, $p = 0.01$). RRT was needed in 25.2% (MDR) and 33.1% (non-MDR) of cases, without no significant difference between the groups.

Table 1 Demographic and clinical characteristics of patients with and without multidrug (MDR) bacteria who had prolonged weaning during the intensive care unit stay

Variable	Patients with MDR bacteria (n = 107)	Patients without MDR bacteria (n = 323)	p-value
Age, years	63 ± 15	69 ± 11	< 0.001
Male, n (%)	71 (66.3)	213 (65.9)	0.94
Pre-existing COPD, n (%)	39 (36.4)	98 (30.3)	0.24
Pre-existing CAD, n (%)	28 (26.2)	151 (46.7)	< 0.001
SAPS II at ICU admission	39.0 ± 9.3	35.9 ± 8.5	0.03
Renal replacement therapy during ICU stay, n (%)	27 (25.2)	107 (33.1)	0.127
Days of MV in the ICU	18.1 ± 11.8	17.1 ± 11.4	0.36
ICU LOS, days[a]	25.3 ± 17.3	19.5 ± 12.8	0.01

Data are given as mean ± standard deviation or number of patients (%)
CAD Coronary artery disease; *COPD* Chronic obstructive pulmonary disease; *ICU* Intensive care unit; *LOS* Length of stay; *MV* Mechanical ventilation; *SAPS II* Simplified Acute Physiology Score II
[a]41 data sets of non-MDR patients missing

The proportion of patients with MDR bacteria during ICU and weaning unit stays was 23.8% and 26.9%, respectively. The presence of MRSA in blood culture or respiratory specimens was confirmed in 21 patients during ICU stay (4.8%) and this increased to 39 positive results (9.1%) during time in the weaning unit ($p = 0.006$, McNemar's test). The chronological distribution of the most relevant 3 MRGN and 4 MRGN strains in the ICU and weaning unit is shown in Fig. 2. In general, there was a marked increase in panresistant bacteria, particularly *P. aeruginosa* and *Acinetobacter baumanii* during time spent in the weaning unit.

At the time of admission to the weaning unit, arterial carbon dioxide (p_aCO_2) was significantly higher in MDR patients ($p < 0.001$) (Table 2); there were no other significant between-group differences in clinical parameters. Recurrent respiratory infection was documented in 37.4% of cases in the MDR group and 43.9% of cases in the non-MDR group.

Overall mean LOS in the weaning unit was 23.2 ± 21.7 days, with no significant difference between patient groups. Weaning success rates were lower in MDR patients, shown by the smaller proportion of patients in category 3a (defined as patients successfully weaned without any respiratory support) and the higher proportion in category 3c (defined as patients who were in need of invasive home mechanical ventilation or died) compared with the non-MDR group ($p = 0.05$) (Table 2).

There was no significant between-group difference in the number of ventilator-free days in patients with and without MDR bacteria. Based on an unadjusted model, there were an estimated 7.2 and 7.4 ventilator-free days in the MDR and non-MDR groups, respectively (the coefficient of multidrug resistance was – 0.03, 95% CI –0.34,

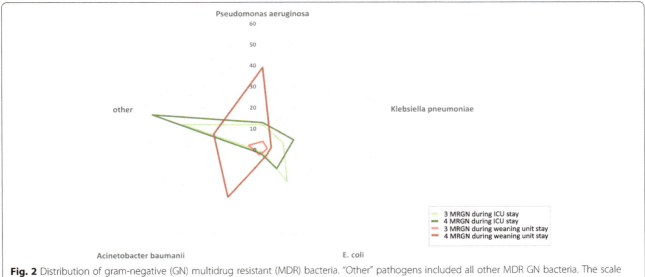

Fig. 2 Distribution of gram-negative (GN) multidrug resistant (MDR) bacteria. "Other" pathogens included all other MDR GN bacteria. The scale shows the number of pathogens identified

Table 2 Differences between patients with and without multidrug resistant (MDR) bacteria with prolonged weaning during stay in the weaning unit

Variable	Patients with MDR bacteria (n = 107)	Patients without MDR bacteria (n = 323)	p-value
p_aO_2 at weaning unit admission, mmHg	87.7 ± 42.2	88.6 ± 27.8	0.83
p_aCO_2 at weaning unit admission, mmHg	42.6 ± 9.6	39.6 ± 8.5	< 0.001
pH at weaning unit admission	7.44 ± 0.06	7.44 ± 0.06	0.29
Lactate at weaning unit admission, mmol/L	0.9 ± 0.41	0.9 ± 0.42	0.87
Secondary respiratory infection in the weaning unit[a], n (%)	40 (37.4)	142 (43.9)	0.28
Days of MV in the weaning unit	15.4 ± 15.8	16.9 ± 22.8	0.31
Weaning unit LOS, days	24.2 ± 26.8	22.9 ± 19.8	0.21
SAPS II at weaning unit discharge	28.3 ± 12.3	29.9 ± 11.5	0.24
Weaning category at discharge[b]			0.05
3a	65 (60.7)	229 (72.0)	
3b	9 (8.4)	13 (4.1)	
3c	33 (30.9)	76 (23.2)	

Data are given as mean ± standard deviation or number of patients (%)
MV Mechanical ventilation; *p_aCO_2* Arterial carbon dioxide pressure; *p_aO_2* Arterial oxygen pressure; *SAPS II* Simplified Acute Physiology Score II
Weaning categories were based on the German guidelines for prolonged weaning [10]
[a]Defined as ventilator-associated pneumonia, ventilator-associated tracheobronchitis, pneumonic septic shock
[b]Calculated for n = 318, weaning category not defined in 5 data sets of patients without MDR bacteria

0.24). The distribution of ventilator-free days is shown in Fig. 3.

The overall crude mortality rate in the weaning unit for the study population was 12.4%. An adjusted Cox model with consideration of potential coefficients (Table 3) did not show any association between the presence of MDR bacteria and survival, but both age and SAPS were independent predictors of mortality. The survival curve is shown in Fig. 4. In the adjusted Cox model, there were no significant differences in survival between patients with or without MDR bacteria (Fig. 4).

Discussion

In this study, approximately one-quarter of infections in patients with prolonged weaning after pneumonia and/or septic pneumonic shock were caused by MDR bacteria, with a marked increase of panresistant bacteria, especially *P. aeruginosa* and *A. baumanii*, during the course of MV. Although there was no difference in mortality rates and ventilator-free days between patients with an without MDR bacteria, those with infections due to MDR bacteria had higher SAPS II at the time of ICU admission, higher p_aCO_2 at the time of admission to the weaning unit, and lower rates of successful prolonged weaning at the time of weaning unit discharge.

VAP is the most common complication in patients needing MV [13] and may further prolong MV requirement and the weaning process. Our study included a sick group of prolonged weaning patients, as demonstrated by high SAPS II, need for RRT in approximately one-third of patients, and the number of MV days in the ICU before transfer to the weaning unit. This is consistent with previous data on ICU LOS, days on MV and SAPS II in another cohort of long-term mechanically ventilated patients where the most likely reason for prolonged weaning was also the occurence of pneumonia [14].

Our patients with MDR bacteria were significantly younger and had a lower rate of pre-existing CAD compared to those without MDR bacterial infection. However, significantly higher SAPS II suggests that the MDR group

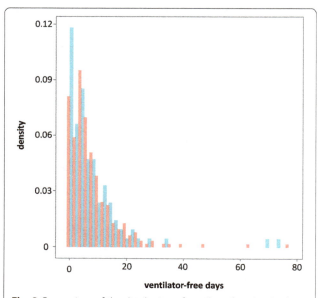

Fig. 3 Comparison of the distribution of ventilator-free days in the weaning unit between multidrug resistant (MDR; blue columns) and non-MDR (red columns) patients with prolonged weaning

Table 3 Summary of analysed coefficents for an adjusted Cox model

Variable	coef	HR	95% CI		p-value
Age	0.04	1.04	1.00	1.07	0.03
SAPS II at admission to the weaning unit	0.04	1.04	1.00	1.07	0.03
Pre-existing COPD and/or emphysema	0.10	1.10	0.61	1.98	0.74
Pre-existing CAD	0.13	1.14	0.64	2.03	0.66
Need for renal replacement therapy during the course of treatment	0.13	1.14	0.62	2.09	0.68
MDR bacteria	−0.07	0.93	0.46	1.89	0.84

CI Confidence interval; *coef*, coefficient; *COPD* Chronic obstructive pulmonary disease; *CAD* Coronary artery disease; *HR* Hazard ratio; *MDR* Multidrug resistant; *SAPS II* Simplified Acute Physiology Score II

was more severely ill during the course of treatment. In addition, significantly higher p_aCO_2 in the group with MDR bacteria at the time of weaning unit admission suggest that the weaning process was less advanced, which resulted in a significantly lower rate of complete weaning success at weaning unit discharge. This is in congruence to other studies who could demonstrate that hypercapnia is associated with weaning failure [15] and prolonged weaning, respectively [16]. In our study, one further, potential explanation for higher p_aCO_2 is that a high load of MDR bacteria in respiratory specimens could lead to greater secretions or mucus, which would in turn have a negative impact on the weaning process. Another possibility is that co-existing peripheral wounds and skin lesions, which require complex care, might be more extensive in the group with MDR bacteria. These important issues need to be further investigated to facilitate understanding of MDR bacteria-related factors that could influence weaning success rate.

Data on the prevalence of infections with MDR bacteria in patients with prolonged weaning are scarce. In our study, the overall prevalence of MDR bacterial infections was 24.8%, including MRSA, 3 MRGN and 4 MRGN. Increases in MRSA infection rates over time are often seen, most likely due to long-term treatment and repeated courses of antibiotics. A large surveillance study of nearly 150 Spanish ICUs reported that prolonged care and colonisation with several different MDR pathogens were significant, independent risk factors for MRSA colonisation or infection [17]. It is worth noting that MRSA accounted for only 20% of MDR bacteria, and the remaining 80% comprised 3 MRGN and 4 MRGN species. Despite their increasing relevance, there is wide variability in definitions of GN bacteria, making comparison of clinical studies difficult [12]. We particularly noted an increase in 4 MRGN *P. aeruginosa* and *A. baumanii* in the weaning unit over time, which can be seen both as a result of long-term treatment with inappropriate duration antibiotic therapy and as evidence for increasing bacterial virulence. A sub-analysis of the PNEUMA trial showed that the existence of GN bacteria increased infection recurrence, which is consistent with

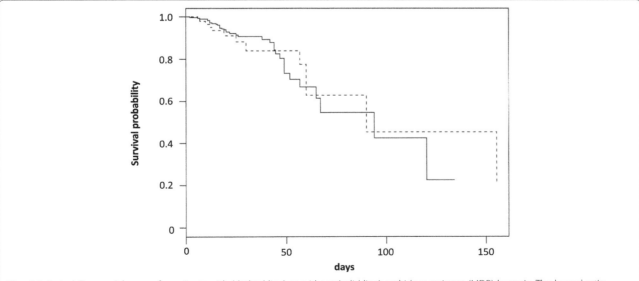

Fig. 4 Adjusted Cox model curves for patients with (dashed line) or without (solid line) multidrug resistant (MDR) bacteria. The hazard ratio estimate (0.98, 95% confidence interval 0.49; 1.98) suggests no association between the presence of MDR bacteria and survival

our findings [18]. In our study, 37.4% of patients with MDR bacterial infection and 43.9% of those not infected with MDR pathogens developed secondary respiratory infections. The between-group difference was not statistically significant, but these high recurrence rates again emphasize the severity of illness in the study population. This makes it difficult to determine whether high mortality rates are attributable to the high pathogenicity of bacteria, inappropriate anitibiotic treatment, or other factors relating to ICU treatment.

In contrast to other studies [19, 20], we did not find any statistically significant difference in mortality rates between patients with or without MDR bacteria. One explanation could be the complexity of patients with prolonged weaning and long-term treatment leading to comparable pathogen-host interactions.

The overall crude mortality rate of 12.4% in our study is similar to that reported by Peñuelas et al. [14], although variations may be due to differences in patient groups (e.g. medical vs. surgical) and institutions [21]. We should point out that our weaning unit is physically separate from the ICU, but has the same monitoring, medical devices and nurse-patient ratio. This enables a systematic, focussed approach to the process of ventilator discontinuation and a procedure of hygiene measures [12] with high adherence to local standards resulting in comparable outcomes in the two patient groups in this study. In addition, the comparability of our unit to an ICU might explain the high illness severity of patients being treated in our weaning unit. Under these conditions, our findings suggest that parameters other than the presence of MDR bacteria appear to have a more dominant influence on survival, as seen in the adjusted Cox model.

Several limitations need to be mentioned when interpreting the results of this study. Firstly, data were obtained retrospectively from a single center. Secondly, the study design only allowed us to examine the distribution of MDR bacteria. These were considered as causative pathogens because they were detected at high concentrations in blood cultures and respiratory specimens. However, it cannot definitively be stated that all MDR pathogens were the source of infection. Finally, we analyzed ventilator-free days and weaning unit mortality, but do not have any data on long-term outcomes in our patients.

Conclusion

We have shown for the first time the potential impact of infection with MDR bacteria in patients with prolonged weaning. After long-term, complex ICU and weaning unit treatment, mortality rates are quite high but hospital mortality was not affected by the presence of MDR bacteria in our patients. However, MDR bacteria did influence weaning outcome because patients with MDR bacteria had lower rates of successful prolonged weaning. Further prospective studies are needed to analyze infections with MDR bacteria and clinical parameters in this patient group.

Abbreviations
BAL: Bronchoalveolar lavage; CAP: Community acquired pneumonia; COPD: Chronic obstructive pulmonary disease; CPIS: Clinical pulmonary infection score; GN: Gram negative; ICU: Intensive care unit; LOS: Length of stay; MDR: Multi-drug resistant; MRGN: Multi-resistant gram negative; MV: Mechanical ventilation; RRT: Renal replacement therapy; SAPS: Simplified acute physiology score; SBT: Spontaneous breathing trial; VAP: Ventilator associated pneumonia; WEA: Weaning unit

Acknowledgements
English language editing assistance was provided by Nicola Ryan, independent medical writer.

Funding
This research did not receive any specific grant from funding agencies in the public, commercial, or not-for-profit sectors.

Authors' contributions
JB, and MD have made substantial contributions to the study, regarding study design, statistics and data analysis. JB, SB and MD contributed to study realization and draft of the manuscript. DS contributed to data acquisition and analysis. GM and NM supported the study design and execution of the study. All authors critically proof-read the final manuscript. No financial support was supported to any individual being involved to the study.

Competing interests
The authors declare that they have no competing interests.

Author details
[1]Department of Intensive Care Medicine, Medical Faculty, RWTH Aachen University, Pauwelsstr. 30, D-52074 Aachen, Germany. [2]Department of Cardiology, Pneumology, Angiology and Intensive Care Medicine, Medical Faculty, RWTH Aachen University, Aachen, Germany. [3]Department of Infection Control and Infectious Diseases, Medical Faculty, RWTH Aachen University, Aachen, Germany.

References
1. Boles JM, Bion J, Connors A, Herridge M, Marsh B, Melot C, et al. Weaning from mechanical ventilation. Eur Respir J. 2007;29:1033–56.
2. Safdar N, Dezfulian C, Collard HR, Saint S. Clinical and economic consequences of ventilator-associated pneumonia: a systematic review. Crit Care Med. 2005;33:2184–93.
3. Rello J, Afonso E, Lisboa T, Ricart M, Balsera B, Rovira A, et al. A care bundle approach for prevention of ventilator-associated pneumonia. Clin Microbiol Infect. 2013;19:363–9.
4. Sinuff T, Muscedere J, Cook DJ, Dodek PM, Anderson W, Keenan SP, et al. Implementation of clinical practice guidelines for ventilator-associated pneumonia: a multicenter prospective study. Crit Care Med. 2013;41:15–23.
5. Vardakas KZ, Rafailidis PI, Konstantelias AA, Falagas ME. Predictors of mortality in patients with infections due to multi-drug resistant gram negative bacteria: the study, the patient, the bug or the drug? J Inf Secur. 2013;66:401–14.
6. Arvanitis M, Anagnostou T, Kourkoumpetis TK, Ziakas PD, Desalermos A, Mylonakis E. The impact of antimicrobial resistance and aging in VAP outcomes: experience from a large tertiary care center. PLoS One. 2014;9: e89984.
7. Micek ST, Wunderink RG, Kollef MH, Chen C, Rello J, Chastre J, et al. An international multicenter retrospective study of Pseudomonas aeruginosa nosocomial pneumonia: impact of multidrug resistance. Crit Care. 2015;19:219.

8. Pugin J, Auckenthaler R, Mili N, Janssens JP, Lew PD, Suter PM. Diagnosis of ventilator-associated pneumonia by bacteriologic analysis of bronchoscopic and nonbronchoscopic "blind" bronchoalveolar lavage fluid. Am Rev Respir Dis. 1991;143:1121-9.
9. Dellinger RP, Levy MM, Rhodes A, Annane D, Gerlach H, Opal SM, et al. Surviving Sepsis campaign: international guidelines for management of severe sepsis and septic shock, 2012. Intensive Care Med. 2013;39:165-228.
10. Schönhofer B, Geiseler J, Dellweg D, Moerer O, Barchfeld T, Fuchs H, et al. S2k-guideline "prolonged weaning". Pneumologie. 2015;69:595-607.
11. Ruscher C. Recommendations for prevention and control of methicillin-resistant staphylococcus aureus (MRSA) in medical and nursing facilities. Bundesgesundheitsbl Gesundheitsforsch Gesundheitsschutz. 2014;57: 696-732.
12. Hygiene measures for infection or colonization with multidrug resistant gram-negative bacilli. Commission recommendation for hospital hygiene and infection prevention (KRINKO) at the Robert Koch Institute (RKI). Bundesgesundheitsblatt Gesundheitsforschung Gesundheitsschutz. 2012;55: 1311-54.
13. Vora CS, Karnik ND, Gupta V, Nadkar MY, Shetye JV. Clinical profile of patients requiring prolonged mechanical ventilation and their outcome in a tertiary care medical ICU. J Assoc Physicians India. 2015;63:14-9.
14. Peñuelas O, Frutos-Vivar F, Fernández C, Anzueto A, Epstein SK, Apezteguía C, et al. Characteristics and outcomes of ventilated patients according to time to liberation from mechanical ventilation. Am J Respir Crit Care Med. 2011;184:430-7.
15. Raurich JM, Rialp G, Ibáñez J, Ayestarán I, Llompart-Pou JA, Togores B. Hypercapnia test and weaning outcome from mechanical ventilation in COPD patients. Anaesth Intensive Care. 2009;37(5):726-32.
16. Raurich JM, Rialp G, Ibáñez J, Llompart-Pou JA, Ayestarán I. CO2 response and duration of weaning from mechanical ventilation. Respir Care. 2011; 56(8):1130-6.
17. Callejo-Torre F, Eiros Bouza JM, Olaechea Astigarraga P, Coma Del Corral MJ, Palomar Martínez M, et al. Risk factors for methicillin-resistant Staphylococcus aureus colonisation or infection in intensive care units and their reliability for predicting MRSA on ICU admission. Infez Med. 2016;24:201-9.
18. Combes A, Luyt CE, Fagon JY, Wolff M, Trouillet JL, Chastre J. Early predictors for infection recurrence and death in patients with ventilator-associated pneumonia. Crit Care Med. 2007;35:146-54.
19. Magret M, Lisboa T, Martin-Loeches I, Manez R, Nauwynck M, Wrigge H, et al. Bacteremia is an independent risk factor for mortality in nosocomial pneumonia: a prospective and observational multicenter study. Crit Care. 2011;15:R62.
20. Agbaht K, Diaz E, Munoz E, Lisboa T, Gomez F, Depuydt PO, et al. Bacteremia in patients with ventilator-associated pneumonia is associated with increased mortality: a study comparing bacteremic vs. nonbacteremic ventilator-associated pneumonia. Crit Care Med. 2007;35: 2064-70.
21. Funk GC, Anders S, Breyer MK, Burghuber OC, Edelmann G, Heindl W, et al. Incidence and outcome of weaning from mechanical ventilation according to new categories. Eur Respir J. 2010;35:88-94.

# The long-term rate of change in lung function in urban professional firefighters

Flynn Slattery[1*], Kylie Johnston[2], Catherine Paquet[3], Hunter Bennett[1] and Alan Crockett[1]

Abstract

Background: Despite the known occupational hazards, it is not yet clear whether long-term career firefighting leads to a greater rate of decline in lung function than would normally be expected, and how this rate of change is affected by firefighting exposures and other risk/protective factors.

Methods: A systematic search of online electronic databases was conducted to identify longitudinal studies reporting on the rate of change in the forced expiratory volume in one second (FEV_1) of forced vital capacity (FVC). Included studies were critically appraised to determine their risk of bias using the Research Triangle Institute Item Bank (RTI-IB) on Risk of Bias and Precision of Observational Studies.

Results: Twenty-two studies were identified for inclusion, from four different countries, published between 1974 and 2016. Examined separately, studies were categorised by the type of firefighting exposure. Firefighters experienced variable rates of decline in lung function, which were particularly influenced by cigarette smoking. The influence of routine firefighting exposures is unclear and limited by the methods of measurement, while firefighters exposed to 'non-routine' severe exposures unanimously experienced accelerated declines.

Conclusions: The data provided by longitudinal studies provide an unclear picture of how the rate of change in lung function of firefighters relates to routine exposures and how it compares to the rate of change expected in a working-age population. Non-smoking firefighters who routinely wear respiratory protection are more likely than otherwise to have a normal rate of decline in lung function. Exposure to catastrophic events significantly increases the rate of decline in firefighter lung function but there is limited evidence detailing the effect of routine firefighting. Future studies will benefit from more robust methods of measuring exposure.

Keywords: Firefighters, Firefighting, Spirometry, Lung function, Exposure, Longitudinal, Systematic review

Background

The risks to firefighters' respiratory health are well known. Reductions in lung function, increases in airway hyper-responsiveness, and the onset of other symptoms of respiratory illness have been reported in firefighters following exposures during firefighting duties [1–6].

Other reports indicate that firefighters have better lung function than the general population in both FEV_1 and FVC: likely due to a strong healthy worker effect [7–10]. This makes the routine comparison of these values to a reference standard following a single pulmonary function test more challenging, and may serve to misclassify some firefighters' lung function. For example, a firefighter with an FEV_1 of 5.0 l (and 130% of predicted) could lose more than 1 litre before being below 100% of predicted normal, and more than two litres before being below the lower limit of normal (LLN) [11]. Serial measurements and subsequent analyses of the rate of change

*Correspondence: f.ynn.slattery@mymail.unisa.edu.au
[1]Alliance for Research in Exercise, Nutrition and Activity, Sansom Institute for Health Research, School of Health Sciences, Universitiy of South Australia, Adelaide, Australia
Full list of author information is available at the end of the article

in lung function may represent the most useful way of monitoring firefighter respiratory health.

The long-term rate of change in FEV_1 in healthy, non-smoking adults of working age was initially reported by Fletcher and Peto as − 36 mL/yr [12]. Further studies have reported rates of change ranging from around − 20 to − 38 mL per year [13–21], and as much as 56 mL per year [22]. Despite the known occupational hazards, it is not yet clear whether long-term routine firefighting leads to a greater rate of decline in lung function than would normally be expected. This review aims to answer the following questions: 1) What is the rate of change of lung function in professional urban firefighters? 2) How is this rate of change influenced by level of exposure to routine firefighting and non-routine firefighting (i.e. catastrophic events) and protective or deleterious factors? 3) How is the rate of change in lung function measured/calculated and reported in studies of professional firefighters?

Methods

This systematic review was conducted in accordance with the Preferred Reporting Items for Systematic Reviews and Meta-Analyses (PRISMA) Statement guidelines [23], and the protocol was registered on the International Prospective Register of Systematic Reviews (PROSPERO) (registration number CRD42017058499).

Selection of studies

Studies selected for review had to satisfy three conditions: 1) FEV_1 and/or FVC had to be measured in the same individuals on more than one occasion (if not using regression techniques), with a minimum observation period of 12 months; 2) The rate of change in either FEV_1 or FVC had to be available directly or calculable from the presented data; and 3) Participants had to be adult (≥ 18 years of age) full-time professional urban firefighters; excluding part-time, volunteer and country/wildland firefighters. There was no restriction placed on publication date or language.

Search strategy

Relevant publications were initially sought with a systematic search conducted on March 8 2017, using the online electronic databases CINAHL, Embase, Medline, Medline (Epub ahead of print), Scopus and Web of Science. Under the advice of an academic librarian, the following keyword string was used to find candidate papers: (("fire fighter*" or firefighter* or firem#n or "fire m#n") or (fire [within three words] personnel)) AND (("lung* function" or "pulmonary function" or respiratory) or (FEV* or "forced expiratory volume*" or FVC* or "vital capacit*" or spirometr*)). When available, the following subject headings were also combined with the keyword search (Firefighters/) AND (Lung/ or spirometry/ or vital capacity or forced vital capacity or forced expiratory volume or respiratory airflow). Two authors independently conducted all searches, collated all returned titles and abstracts and removed duplicate items.

Title and abstract screening

All titles and abstracts were independently screened to assess each item's suitability for full-text review. When the title or abstract provided insufficient information to make a decision, the full-text paper was retrieved. The authors then independently reviewed all selected full-text papers and selected eligible papers for inclusion. Reference lists and citations (Google Scholar search March 29 2017) of eligible papers were then screened and the full-texts of relevant papers were examined: eligible papers were then included for review. Discrepancies were resolved at each stage of the selection process by discussion between the two authors, with a third author available for adjudication in case of disagreement.

Data extraction

Data from each included paper were independently entered into a database by two authors. Extracted information included, but was not limited to, the characteristics of the cohort(s) studied, study methodology and results. When the data were only reported graphically, they were extracted using an online tool [24]. When the rate of change in FEV_1 and/or FVC was not reported and unavailable from the authors, it was calculated (and rounded to the nearest whole millilitre) as the difference between baseline and follow-up value divided by the time interval (or when more than two data points were available: calculated by using simple linear regression). When available, the respective rates of change were reported stratified by smoking status as well as for the entire cohort. When stratified data were not available, and the average rate of change for the entire cohort was reported alone, as well as the cohort's smoking rate.

Quality assessment

Included studies were critically appraised to determine their risk of bias using the Research Triangle Institute Item Bank (RTI-IB) on Risk of Bias and Precision of Observational Studies [25], which provides a means to assess the quality of studies related to exposure outcomes. The RTI-IB is one of the only quality appraisal scoring tools available for observational studies, providing a comprehensive list of 29 questions covering a range of categories of bias [26]. The authors recommend the tool be modified based on its appropriateness to the literature. For this reason, questions 8, 12, 26 and 27 of the tool were omitted, due to their inapplicability to the topic, while a "cannot determine" response was added to question 13. The critical appraisal was carried out independently by two authors, with discrepancies being resolved by discussion. Each study was given a score based on the number of applicable RTI-IB items met and subsequently graded, based on previous publications [27–29] as low (0–.40), moderate (.41–.70), or high (.71–1) methodological quality/risk of bias.

Data analysis
A descriptive analysis was conducted due to the large heterogeneity of the included studies in terms of their population characteristics, type of assessment of exposure, and reporting of outcome measures.

Results
The searches yielded a total of 788 unique articles, including eight that were identified through reference checking (Fig. 1). Following the screening and review process, a total of 22 papers met the eligibility criteria and were included for review.

Characteristics of included studies
Descriptive information about the included studies is summarised in Table 1 and includes study location and dates, the baseline characteristics of the study population and the methods of conducting spirometry and measuring exposure.

Within the 22 studies, all published between 1974 and 2016, there were 11 distinct firefighter populations: one from each of Australia [8] and South Korea [30], two from England [31, 32] and the remaining seven from the USA. These seven populations consisted of firefighters from Baltimore [33], Boston in both the 1960/1970s [34–37] and 1990s [38], Houston [39] and Phoenix [40–43], as well as New York firefighters exposed [44–48] or not-exposed to 9/11 [9]. The average age of active firefighters at study commencement ranged from 26.1 to 43.6 years, while recently-retired firefighters of one study

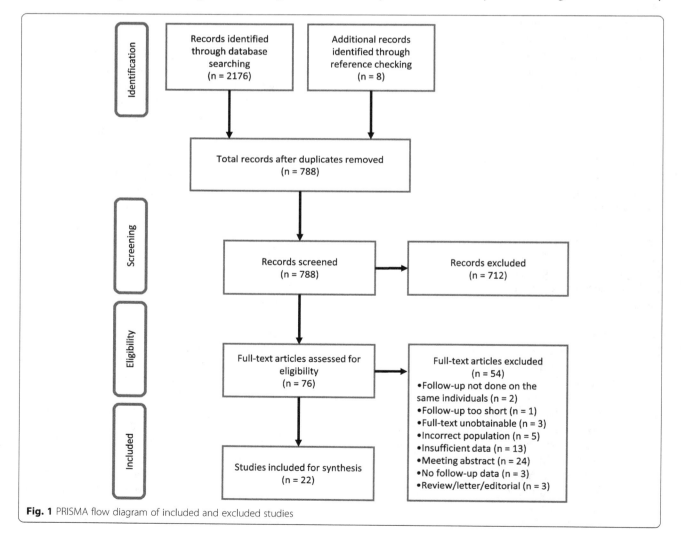

Fig. 1 PRISMA flow diagram of included and excluded studies

Table 1 Descriptive information. Studies are ordered by population type and year of publication

Author & Year [Ref]	Location and period	Population (n=)	Baseline age (years)	Race (%)	Sex (%)	Standardisation of spirometry	Measurement of exposure (main index)
Populations exposed to routine firefighting							
Peters et al. 1974 [37]	Boston, USA 1970 to 1972	Firefighters (1430)	43.13	NR	M	Average of best 3 of 5 trials	Interview using structured questionnaire (fires fought in previous 12 months)
Musk et al. 1977 [35]	Boston, USA 1970 to 1974	Firefighters (1146)	41.9	NR	M[a]	Average of best 3 of 5 trials	Interview using structured questionnaire and BFD records (fires fought in previous 12 months, service time)
Musk et al. 1977 [36]	Boston, USA 1970 to 1975	Retired firefighters (109)	54.5	NR	M[a]	Average of best 3 of 5 trials	Interview using structured questionnaire (fires fought in 12 month period, service time)
Musk et al. 1982 [34]	Boston, USA 1970 to 1976	Firefighters (951)	40.9 (9.4)	W	M[a]	Mean of best 3 of 5 satisfactory (within 5% of best trial) trials	Interview using structured questionnaire and BFD records (fires fought in previous 12 months)
Douglas et al. 1985 [31]	London, England 1976 to 1977	Firefighters (890)	25–29[b]	NR	M	≥ 5 FVC manoeuvres, mean of the last 3 values used for analysis	Self-report questionnaire (service time, absence from work after exposure)
Tepper et al. 1991 [33]	Baltimore, USA 1974–77 to 1983–84	Firefighters (628)	38.2 (10)	C (86)	M	ATS 1978	Estimated from fire department records (years spent in exposed jobs before baseline, number of emergency responses before baseline) and self-report questionnaire (previous exposure to ammonia/chlorine)
Kales et al. 1997 [38]	Boston, USA 1992–93 to 1995	HAZMAT firefighters (37)	36.8 (5.9)	NR	M	ATS 1979	NR
Burgess et al. 2004 [40]	Phoenix, USA 1988 to 1999	Firefighters (1204)	34.6 (8.9)	W (75), H (16), B (6), O (3)[c]	M (96) F (4)	No info available; retrospective analysis of existing database.	None. Retrospective analysis of existing database.
Josyula et al. 2007 [41]	Phoenix, USA 1998 to 2005	Firefighters (67)	38.6 (7.8)	W (78), H (10), AA (6), O (6)	M (96) F (4)	ATS 1987	Self-report questionnaire (not used in analysis)
Yucesoy et al. 2008 [42]	Phoenix, USA 1988 to 2003	Firefighters (374)	M: 31.9 (6.4) F: 29.7 (3.9)	M: NHW (76.4), HW (19.5), AA (4.1). F: NHW (100)	M (97.3) F (2.7)	ATS 1987	None
Populations exposed to routine firefighting with non-firefighter controls							
Sparrow et al. 1982 [10]	Boston, USA 1963–68 to 1968–1973	Firefighters (168)[d] GP controls (1474)[d]	NR	NR	M	Best 1 of 3 'acceptable' tracings (≥4 s with maximal effort)	Self-report questionnaire (service time)
Horsfield et al. 1988 [32]	West Sussex, England NR	Firefighters (96) GP controls (69)	32.5 [Range 18–54][e] 39.5 [Range 16–63]	NR	M	NR	None
Hnizdo 2012 [43]	Phoenix, USA 1989 to 2000	Firefighters (965) Paper-pulp mill workers (1286) Construction workers (460)	36.3 (9.3) 36.4 (8.4) 35.4 (8.8)	NR	M	ATS 1994	None. Retrospective analysis of existing database.

Table 1 Descriptive information. Studies are ordered by population type and year of publication (Continued)

Author & Year [Ref]	Location and period	Population (n=)	Baseline age (years)	Race (%)	Sex (%)	Standardisation of spirometry	Measurement of exposure (main index)
Aldrich et al. 2013 [9]	New York, USA 2003–06 to 2011	Firefighters (940) EMS controls (97)	26.1 (3.3) 27.6 (7.0)	B (6), W (94) B (52), W (48)	M	≥ 3 acceptable efforts with standardised criteria	None
Schermer et al. 2013 [8]	Adelaide, Australia 2000–08 to 2003–2011	Firefighters (254) GP controls (678)	43.5 (8.0) 43.4 (9.8)	C (99.6) C (95.5)	M	Firefighters: ATS/ERS 2005 Controls: ATS 1987	Self-report questionnaire (use of respiratory protection)
Choi et al. 2014 [30]	Daegu, Korea 2008 to 2011	Firefighters (322) Non-firefighter controls (107)	43.6 (6.9) 44.1 (10.1)	NR	NR	≥ 3 acceptable efforts with standardised criteria	Interview by physician using structured questionnaire (active/inactive firefighting status)
Populations exposed to non-routine firefighting							
Unger et al. 1980 [39]	Houston, USA 1987 to 1989	Firefighters exposed to major chemical warehouse fire (20)	27.2 (5.36)[f]	B, W	M	Best of 3 trials	Self-report questionnaire at 6-week follow-up
Banauch et al. 2006 [44]	New York, USA 1997 to 2002	9/11-exposed FDNY firefighters & EMS workers (11766)	39.7 (7.7)[g]	W (85.6)	M (95.6), F (3.4)	ATS 1994	Self-reported arrival time at WTC site
Aldrich et al. 2010 [45]	New York, USA NR to 2008	9/11-exposed firefighters (10870) 9/11-exposed EMS workers (1911)	40.8 [CI, 40.6–40.9][g] 37.1 [CI, 36.7–37.5][g]	W (94), B (2.5) W (49.7), B (22.2)	M (99.8), F (0.2) M (75.6), F (24.4)	ATS/ERS 2005	Self-reported arrival time at WTC site
Banauch et al. 2010 [48]	New York, USA 2001 to 2005	9/11-exposed firefighters (90)	40.7 (7.1)[g]	W (86)	M (98), F (2)	ATS/ERS 2005	Self-reported arrival time at WTC site
Aldrich et al. 2016 [46]	New York, USA 2000 to 2014	9/11-exposed firefighters (10641)	41.4 [Range 21.3–74.6][g]	W (97.4), AA (2.6)	M (99.8), F (0.2)	ATS/ERS 2005	Self-reported arrival time at WTC site
Aldrich et al. 2016 [47]	New York, USA 2000 to 2014	9/11-exposed firefighters (173)	42.6 (7)[g]	W (95.4), AA (4.6)	M	NR	Self-reported arrival time at WTC site

Values are means (SD), unless stated otherwise. 9/11 = World Trade Center disaster on September 11, 2001, AA African-American, ATS American Thoracic Society, B Black, BFD Boston Fire Department, C Caucasian, CI = 95% Confidence interval, EMS Emergency Medical Services, ERS European Respiratory Society, F Female (s), FDNY Fire Department of New York, GP General population, HAZMAT Hazardous materials, HW Hispanic white, LFB London Fire Brigade, M Male(s), N = Total number of participants used in the rate of change analysis, NHW Non-Hispanic white, NR Not reported, NWAHS North-West area health study, PFT Pulmonary function test, ROD Rate of decline, USA The United States of America, W White, WTC World Trade Center. [a]Inferred based on timeframe of study, [b]Median age range (reported in 5-yr intervals), [c]Estimated based on frequencies within 1400 Phoenix firefighters at the time of the study, [d]Normative Ageing Study, [e]Mean of n = 101 firefighters measured at follow-up (96 of whom were included for analysis), [f]Mean of n = 24 firefighters measured at baseline (20 of whom followed-p and included in analysis, [h]Age on 9/11

[36] had an average age of 54.5 years. Seven studies involved both sexes (the highest proportion of female firefighters was 4%) and the remaining included males only. Eleven studies reported the proportions of different racial groups, with the majority of firefighters in each study (76.4 to 100%) being Caucasian/white and the rest being reported as African-American/black (0 to 6%), Hispanic (0 to 19.5%) or unspecified (0 to 14.4%). Two studies reported race without specifying proportions and nine did not report any racial information. Average follow-up time ranged from one to 12.2 years and each study measured lung function at least once, with the highest average number of measures reported being 10.3. Ten studies performed standardised spirometry based on published criteria, nine performed standardised spirometry (usually best or average of three trials) but not according to published standards and three did not report information on spirometry standardisation. The most common method of estimating firefighting exposure was self-report questionnaire ($n = 15$), and three of these studies combined this with an estimate of exposure based on fire department records (one of which did not use these data during analysis). One study obtained information by interview using a structured questionnaire and the remaining six either did not measure exposure, or did not report any measurement.

The rate of change in FEV_1 and FVC
Routine firefighting
Sixteen studies reported on firefighter populations involved in routine firefighting (Table 2). Among nine studies reporting FEV_1 change without stratifying by smoking status (smokers and non-smokers pooled together), six observed declines of between − 24.99 and − 39.6 mL/yr. [33, 35, 40–43] while the remaining three showed declines of − 68.2 to − 110 mL/yr. [30, 31, 37]. Within these nine studies, four included smoking status in their regression modelling: two studies observed significantly greater declines in both ever-smokers relative to never-smokers (additional 4.7 mL/yr. decline, $p = 0.042$) [42] and current smokers relative to non-smokers (Actual difference and p value not reported) [31], while the two others reported no significant effect [40, 41]. One study reported different rates of decline when stratified by occupational exposure, but observed no significant differences in smoking habits between the groups [37] while the remaining four studies did not report on the longitudinal effect of smoking on lung function [30, 33, 35, 43]. Five studies reported on the rate of change in FVC without stratifying by smoking status, observing declines of − 16.55 (66.75) [33], -40 [35], -76.7 [37], -103 [30] and − 107 [31] mL/yr. (SD (where available)). Among these studies, one reported significantly greater declines in current smokers relative to non-smokers (p value not reported) [31].

Six studies reported changes in lung function in firefighters involved in routine firefighting stratified by smoking status. Two studies observed significantly less negative rates of change in FEV_1 in never smokers than other smoking groups [36, 38] and four studies found no significant differences [8–10, 32]. One study reported an FVC decline in never smokers of − 10 mL/yr. [36], significantly less negative than current smokers, while four others reported rates of change in FVC of − 19 [9], -27 (52) [34], -66, [32] -76.8 (10.7) [10], and + 11.2 (140.3) [8] mL/yr. (SD), with no significant differences compared to other smoking groups.

Six studies compared lung function changes in firefighters involved in routine firefighting to non-firefighter controls [8–10, 30, 32, 43]. One study showed a significantly greater rate of FEV_1 decline in firefighters vs. industrial workers [30], one showed a significantly greater rate of decline in general population controls vs. firefighters [32], and four did not report any significant differences in changes in FEV_1 compared to general population controls [8, 10], emergency medical workers [9] or paper-pulp mill and construction workers [43]. Five studies compared changes in the FVC of firefighters vs non-firefighters with two showing significantly greater FVC declines in firefighters [10, 30], one showing significantly greater FVC declines in non-firefighters [32], and two showing no significant differences [8, 9].

Non-routine firefighting
Six studies reported changes in lung function of firefighters exposed to non-routine firefighting [39, 44–48]. Firefighters involved in one study were exposed to smoke during a chemical warehouse fire [39], and experienced declines in FEV_1 and FVC of − 81.3 and − 41.33 mL/yr., respectively, in the time between measurements after exposure and 18 months later. The remaining five studies reported on the changes in FEV_1 observed in a cohort of New York firefighters following World Trade Centre site exposure after the terrorist attacks of September 11, 2001 (9/11). The pre-9/11 rate of change in FEV_1 in firefighters and Emergency Medical Service (EMS) workers was reported as − 31 mL/yr. [44], while each group lost an average of 383 [95% CI, 374–393] mL and 319 [299–340] mL, respectively, in the first year following the disaster. In the 7 years after the initial reduction, the rate of change in FEV_1 (adjusted for age, height, race and sex) of never-smoking firefighters was − 26 [95% CI, 20–31] mL/yr.: less than that of former or current smokers and significantly different from the − 40 [38–42] mL/yr. observed in never-smoking EMS workers [45]. A similar rate FEV_1 decline of − 26.4 mL/yr. was observed in a follow-up study of the never-smoking

Table 2 Rate of decline in FEV_1. Studies are ordered by population type and year of publication. Values are means (SD), medians [IQR] or means [95% CI]

Author [Ref]	Group	Follow-up (yr)	No. measures	Calculation of rate of change (no. adjusted variables)	Whole-group baseline FEV_1 (L)	Smoking Status [% smokers]	Rate of change in FEV_1 mL/yr	Effect of exposure	Effect of risk/protective factors
Populations exposed to routine firefighting only									
Peters et al. 1974 [37]	Firefighters	1	2	Δvalue/Δtime	3.578	Mix [NR]	−68.2	Significant difference in FEV_1 changes when stratified by exposure (no. of fires fought in previous 12 months): FEV_1 change (mL/yr): 1–40 fires; −49, 41–99 fires; −71, ≥100 fires; −109 ($p < 0.02$).	No apparent differences in age, height, smoking habits, race when compared between groups stratified by exposure.
Musk et al. 1977 [35]	Firefighters	3.4	3	Δvalue/Δtime[a]	3.62	Mix [NR]	−30	No significant relationship between FEV_1 change and estimated (by fire department records or firefighter) fires fought in previous 12 months. No relationship between FEV_1 change and fires fought when stratified by age, smoking status or service time. Significantly greater FEV_1 decline in firefighters who fought fewer fires in 1973 vs. 1970 than those who fought the same number or more ($p < 0.05$). Firefighters who fought no fires experienced greatest decline.	No significant relationship between FEV_1 decline and age.
Musk et al. 1977 [36]	Retired firefighters	4.4	3	Δvalue/Δtime[a]	3.19	Nev For Cur Total: Mix [31]	−30 −30 −100* ($p < .05$ relative to Nev & For) Total: −50	No significant difference between FEV_1 change of retired firefighters who were active vs inactive (during 1970) prior to retirement. No significant difference in FEV_1 decline when stratified by years of service.	Greater FEV_1 decline in current vs never or ex-smokers ($p < .05$).
Musk et al. 1982 [34]	Firefighters	6	2	Δvalue/Δtime[b]	3.68 (0.64)	Nev For Cur Cur/For cigar/pipe Total: Mix [NR]	−33 (44) −33 (39) −47 (45) −31 (44) Total: −36	Amongst active firefighters; no relationship between FEV_1 decline and either calculated[c] or estimated[d] number of fires fought in previous 12 months Inactive (fought no fires in	No correlation between change in FEV_1, or FVC between 1970 and 1976 and the initial level of FEV_1 in 1970 ($r = 0.10$ for FEV_1). No relationship between annual change in FEV_1 and the stated tendency

Table 2 Rate of decline in FEV_1. Studies are ordered by population type and year of publication. Values are means (SD), medians [IQR] or means [95% CI] (Continued)

Author [Ref]	Group	Follow-up (yr)	No. measures	Calculation of rate of change (no. adjusted variables)	Whole-group baseline FEV_1 (L)	Rate of change in FEV_1 Smoking Status [% smokers]	Rate of change in FEV_1 mL/yr	Effect of exposure	Effect of risk/protective factors
									of the subjects to voluntarily wear protective breathing apparatus.
Douglas et al. 1985 [31]	Firefighters	1	2	NR	NS	Mix [NR]	-92	Only cross-sectional effect of exposure reported. Change in FEV_1 unrelated to service time, or to absence from work after exposure to smoke.	Statistically significant greater FEV_1 decline among current smokers (Actual difference and p value not reported).
Tepper et al. 1991 [33]	Repeating[e] firefighters ($n = 492$)	6–10	2	Δvalue/Δtime	3.83 (0.68)	Mix [Cur, 50]	−24.99 (61.23)*	Significantly greater adjusted (multiple linear regression[2, 4, 14, 15, 18, 21]) FEV_1 decline in active vs inactive repeating[e] firefighters (−29.33 vs 0.30 mL/yr) ($p < .01$), but not non-repeaters[e]. Non-significant trend of greater adjusted FEV_1 decline in those who reported ever vs never being exposed to ammonia (−38.82 vs −23.16 mL/yr) ($p = .06$) (amongst all firefighters), but no differences based on past chlorine exposure. No significant relationship between adjusted FEV_1 decline and years spent in exposed jobs before baseline or number of firefighting responses before baseline.	Greater adjusted FEV_1 decline in those who reported never vs ever using a mask while extinguishing fires, but only significant in non-repeaters[e] (−68.44 vs −30.90 mL/yr) ($p = .01$). No significant difference in FEV_1 decline based on mask-use during fire overhaul.
	Non-repeating[e] firefighters ($n = 136$)					Mix [Cur, 45]	−34.79 (40.00)* ($p = .03$)		
Kales et al. 1997 [38]	HAZMAT firefighters	2.58	2	Δvalue/Δtime	NR	Nev Cur or For Total: Mix [Ev, 38]	−40.69[f] −68.6[f] ($p = .27$) Total: -51	NR	No significant difference in FEV_1 changes between smokers and former/current smokers, or between younger (≤35 years) and older (> 35 years) firefighters.

Table 2 Rate of decline in FEV_1. Studies are ordered by population type and year of publication. Values are means (SD), medians [IQR] or means [95% CI] (Continued)

Author [Ref]	Group	Follow-up (yr)	No. measures	Calculation of rate of change (no. adjusted variables)	Whole-group baseline FEV_1 (L)	Smoking Status [% smokers]	Rate of change in FEV_1 mL/yr	Effect of exposure	Effect of risk/protective factors
Burgess et al. 2004 [40]	Firefighters	≥5	≥6	Simple linear regression	4.27 (0.66)	Mix [Ev, 28]	−34 (43)	NR	Rate of FEV_1 decline increased significantly with baseline FEV_1 ($p < .001$) and age (relative to reference group ≤30 yrs. of age: 31–40 yrs. ($p = .006$), 41–50 yrs. and >50 ($p < .001$), but no significant effect of smoking (never vs ever) or sex. TT genotype at IL-10 SNP 1668 was associated with a significantly lower rate of FEV_1 decline, compared to the AA genotype ($p = 0.023$) (based on a subsample of firefighters with IL-10 SNP information; $n = 379$) (ANOVA[2, 3, 17, 18]).
Josyula et al. 2007 [41]	Firefighters	7	≥4	Simple linear regression	4.16 (0.70)	Mix [For, 18, Ev; 12] (100% CurNS)	−33 (59)	NR	Greater baseline FEV_1 and asthma associated with greater FEV_1 decline ($p = .002$ and $p = .0023$, respectively). Weight gain was close to being significantly associated with FEV_1 decline ($p = .05$). No significant relationship between FEV_1 change and gender, baseline age, height, baseline body mass index, race or smoking status. Mean FEV_1 decline significantly lower in those possessing the TT genotype of the IL-10 (819) polymorphism [n = 3, −125 (27) mL/yr], vs. the CC [n = 33, −20 (61)] or CT genotypes [n = 3), −38 (51)] ($p = .009$). Increased IL-1RA associated with slower FEV_1 decline ($p = .025$) (Multiple regression[1, 2, 3, 13, 17, 18, 22]).

Table 2 Rate of decline in FEV_1. Studies are ordered by population type and year of publication. Values are means (SD), medians [IQR] or means [95% CI] (Continued)

Author [Ref]	Group	Follow-up (yr)	No. measures	Calculation of rate of change (no. adjusted variables)	Whole-group baseline FEV_1 (L)	Rate of change in FEV_1 Smoking Status [% smokers]	Rate of change in FEV_1 mL/yr	Effect of exposure	Effect of risk/protective factors
Yucesoy et al. 2008 [42]	Firefighters	M: 11.8 (2.5) F: 11.6 (2.3)	M: 10.3 (2.1) F: 10.3 (2.2)	Simple linear regression	M: 4.39 (0.63) F: 3.60 (0.43)	M: Mix [19.8] F: Mix [30]	M: −34 (27) F: −38 (20) Total: −34 (30)	NR	Lower rate of FEV_1 decline in the presence of the TGFβ1−509 TT genotype ($p = .043$) (multiple linear regression[2, 3, 13, 16, 17, 18, 25]). Carrying an A allele at TNFα-308 ($p = 0.010$) and GG genotype at TNFα-238 ($p = 0.028$) was associated with a more rapid rate of FEV_1 decline. The TNFα-308A/−238G haplotype was associated with an increased rate of decline compared with the other haplotypes. Ever-smokers had a significantly greater rate of decline (−4.7 mL/yr) compared with never smokers ($p = .042$). FEV_1 changes not significantly different by race or gender.
Populations exposed to routine firefighting only with use of non-firefighter controls									
Sparrow et al. 1982 [10]	Firefighters[9]	5	2	Δvalue/Δtime	4.08 (0.073) (Nev)	Nev For Cur	−81.2 (19.2) −68.2 (8.7) −77.9 (8.5)	Non-significant trend of greater FEV_1 decline (additional 12 ml/yr) in firefighters vs controls ($p = .054$). No significant relationship between years of employment and FEV_1 decline.	Greater FEV_1 decline in current vs never smokers ($p < .001$), adjusted for firefighting status. Non-significant difference in FEV_1 decline in former smokers vs never ($p = .530$). Greater age and baseline FEV_1 as well as lesser height were associated with greater rates of FEV_1 decline ($p < .001$).
	GP controls[9]				3.93 (0.029) (Nev)	Nev For Cur	−64.1 (3.9) −62.8 (3.7) −65.2 (3.2)		
Horsfield et al. 1988 [32]	Firefighters	1−4	4−8	Simple linear regression	NR	Nev For Cur	−66.5* ($p < .05$) −53.8* ($p < .05$) −70.5 Total: −65.4* ($p < .01$)	Compared to GP CON, the rate of change in FEV_1 was significantly less negative in all firefighters ($p < .01$) and never and former smoking firefighters ($p < .05$).	No significant difference in rate of change in FEV_1 between firefighting smoking groups.
	GP controls					Nev	−100.3* (All p values relative to GP controls)		

Table 2 Rate of decline in FEV_1. Studies are ordered by population type and year of publication. Values are means (SD), medians [IQR] or means [95% CI] (Continued)

Author [Ref]	Group	Follow-up (yr)	No. measures	Calculation of rate of change (no. adjusted variables)	Whole-group baseline FEV_1 (L)	Smoking Status [% smokers]	Rate of change in FEV_1 mL/yr	Effect of exposure	Effect of risk/protective factors
Hnizdo 2012 [43]	Firefighters	8–11	≥4	Simple linear regression	4.39 (0.64)	Mix [≈5]	−39.6 (29.5)	NR	NR
	Paper-pulp mill workers				4.33 (0.60)	Nev	−34.3 (33.5)		
					4.11 (0.68)	Mix [60]	−45.2 (32.2)[h]		
	Construction workers				4.10 (0.7)	Mix [NR]	−48.7 (50.1)		
Aldrich et al. 2013 [9]	Firefighters	5	5	Linear mixed effects modelling (5[2, 8, 13, 21, 22])	4.4 (0.6)	Nev	−344.8 [CI, −347.3 to −342.3][i]	No significant difference in FEV_1 change between Firefighters and controls: average difference (Fire − EMS) 0.2 mL/yr. (CI −9.2 to 9.6).	Weight gain and service time independently associated with increased rate of FEV_1 decline (p value not reported). No difference in FEV_1 decline in ever vs never smokers.
						Nev	−337.6 [CI, −340.4 to −334.8]		
						Ev	−336 [CI, −341 to −332]		
	EMS control				3.9 (0.7)	Nev	−44.6 [CI, −53.2 to −35.5][i]		
						Nev	−33.8 [CI, −43.7 to −23.8]		
						Ev	−29 [CI, −38 to −19]		
Schermer et al. 2013 [8]	Firefighters	2.9 (0.3)	2	Δvalue/Δtime	4.51 (0.66)	CurNS	+15.6 (104.0)[j]	The difference in the annual change in FEV_1 between the younger and older age categories differed between the firefighters and controls (interaction term stage cohort age category: $p = .040$). Firefighters had a lower odds of accelerated FEV_1 decline compared with population controls (OR = 0.60, CI 0.44–0.83; $p = .002$) (Logistic regression analysis[2, 9, 18]).	Firefighters who reported never or rarely using their respiratory protection during fire knockdown had a higher odds of accelerated FEV_1 decline compared with those who used it often or frequently (OR = 2.20, CI 1.02–4.74; $p = .044$)
	GP controls	3.5 (1.1)			3.73 (0.70)	CurNS	−27.8 (78.6)[j]		
Choi et al. 2014 [30]	Firefighters	3	2	NR	NR	Mix [Cur, 11.8]*	−110*	No significant difference between active and non-active firefighters (RMA-NOVA[2, 7, 8, 12, 18]), FEV_1 decline was significantly greater in firefighters compared to non-firefighters ($p < .001$).	NR
	Non-firefighter controls					Mix [Cur, 42.9]* ($p < .001$)	−67* ($p < .01$)		

The long-term rate of change in lung function in urban professional firefighters   179

Table 2 Rate of decline in FEV$_1$. Studies are ordered by population type and year of publication. Values are means (SD), medians [IQR] or means [95% CI] *(Continued)*

Author [Ref]	Group	Follow-up (yr)	No. measures	Calculation of rate of change (no. adjusted variables)	Whole-group baseline FEV$_1$ (L)	Smoking Status [% smokers]	Rate of change in FEV$_1$ mL/yr	Effect of exposure	Effect of risk/protective factors
Populations exposed to non-routine firefighting									
Unger et al. 1980 [39]	Exposed firefighters	Post exposure: 1.5	2	ROD not reported[f]	Post exposure: 4.003 (0.633)	Mix [NR]	-81.3[f]	NR. No pre-exposure measurements, no comparison to un-exposed controls.	NR
Banauch et al. 2006 [44]	9/11-exposed FDNY firefighters & EMS workers	Pre 9/11: 5 Post 9/11: 1	1–7	Linear random-effects modelling (5[2, 8, 13, 17, 18])	4.30 [IQR, 3.80–4.80]	Mix [29]	Pre-9/11 (Fire & EMS) -31 Post-9/11: Fire; -383 ml [CI, -393 to -374] EMS; -319 ml [CI, -340 to -299]	Significant difference in pre and post-9/11 FEV$_1$, within arrival time-based exposure groups ($p < .001$). Trans-9/11 FEV$_1$ decline by exposure group: high-intensity exposure; -388 ml (CI, -370 to -406), intermediate-intensity; -372 ml (CI, -363 to -381), low-intensity; -357 ml (CI, -339 to -374) (Significant linear trend in exposure intensity-response, $p = .048$). Significant differences in trans 9/11 loss, according to work assignment (Fire vs EMS) ($p < .001$).	Significant difference in reported 'frequent' use of protective mask on arrival day between exposure groups ($p < .001$); no observed protective effect of mask use frequency on adjusted average post 9/11 FEV$_1$.
Aldrich et al. 2010 [45]	9/11-exposed firefighters	Post 9/11: 6.1 [IQR, 5.2–6.6]*	5 [IQR, 4–7]	Linear mixed models (4[2, 8, 13, 17])	Nev: 4.54[k] For: 4.48[k] Cur: 4.46[k]	Nev[l] For[l] Cur[m]	Post-9/11 -26 [CI, -31 to -20]* -38[k] -43[k]	FEV$_1$ decline 6 months post 9/11: FIRE; -355 ml [CI, -352 to -359], EMS; -272 ml [CI, -268 to -276] ($p = 0.004$). FEV$_1$ decline 12 months post 9/11: FIRE; -439 ml [CI, -408 to -471], EMS; -267 ml [CI, -263 to -271] ($p = 0.003$). Firefighters, but not EMS workers, with heaviest dust exposure had significantly larger declines of -371 ml (CI, -362 to -380) during the first 6 months and -585 ml (CI, -515 to -656) during the first	NR
	9/11-exposed EMS workers	6.4 [IQR, 5.9–6.7]* ($p < .001$)			Nev: 3.90[k] For: 3.90[k] Cur: 3.80[k]	Nev[k] For[k] Cur[k]	-40 [CI,42 to -38]* ($p < .001$) -38[k] -42[k]		

Table 2 Rate of decline in FEV_1. Studies are ordered by population type and year of publication. Values are means (SD), medians [IQR] or means [95% CI] (Continued)

Author [Ref]	Group	Follow-up (yr)	No. measures	Calculation of rate of change (no. adjusted variables)	Whole-group baseline FEV_1 (L)	Smoking Status [% smokers]	Rate of change in FEV_1 mL/yr	Effect of exposure	Effect of risk/protective factors
								year than did the other members of the cohort. Last FEV_1 in the final 2 years for workers who had never smoked, there was a non-significant trend toward an association between the number of months of work at the WTC site after 9/11 and the FEV_1 value, a decline of 4 ml per month of work ($p = .07$).	
Banauch et al. 2010 [48]	9/11-exposed firefighters	Pre-9/11: 3 Post-9/11: 4	2–10	Mixed linear random effects modelling (9[2, 8, 10, 11, 13, 17, 18, 23, 24])	Pre-9/11 4.19 (0.68)	Mix [NR]	Post 9/11: No AAT-deficiency: -37 (SE -28 to -45[k]) (adjusted)	Average FEV_1 reduction of -370 mL due to 9/11 exposure.	Comparing firefighters with different AAT phenotype combinations: Significantly greater rate of post-9/11 FEV_1 decline in firefighters with mild (-69 [SE -41 to -97[k]] mL/yr) and moderate (-147 [SE -110 to -184[k]]) AAT-deficiency compared to normal ($p = .011$). Significant trend for decline rate acceleration by AAT phenotype combination ($p = .003$). Significantly greater rate of post-9/11 FEV_1 decline in Firefighters with Low AAT serum level (-86 [SE -66 to -107[k]]) vs normal ($p = .027$).
Aldrich et al. 2016 [46]	9/11-exposed firefighters	Post 9/11: 12.2 [IQR, 11.6–12.6][q]	9 [IQR, 7–10]	Linear mixed models (5[2, 8, 13, 17, 21])	Nev: 4.59[k] For[n]: 4.61[k] For[o]: 4.52[k] For[p]: 4.45[k] Cur: 4.55[k]	Nev For[n] For[o] For[p] Cur	Post-9/11: -26[k] -31[k] -33[k] -37[k] -48[k]	Among never smokers, firefighters arriving the morning of September 11 had slightly lower average FEV_1 than lesser exposed firefighters; this difference remained significant during most of follow-up ($p < .05$ for most 6-monthly time intervals)	Body weight at the time of PFT was associated with FEV_1 ($p < .05$); for each pound of body mass gained, FEV_1 decline averaged 3.93 mL. FEV_1 change differed significantly by smoking status ($p < .001$). After first 3 years of follow-up, never smokers had significantly greater FEV_1 than

Table 2 Rate of decline in FEV$_1$. Studies are ordered by population type and year of publication. Values are means (SD), medians [IQR] or means [95% CI] (Continued)

Author [Ref]	Group	Follow-up (yr)	No. measures	Calculation of rate of change (no. adjusted variables)	Whole-group baseline FEV$_1$ (L)	Rate of change in FEV$_1$ — Smoking Status [% smokers]	Rate of change in FEV$_1$ — mL/yr	Effect of exposure	Effect of risk/protective factors
									current smokers and former smokers who quit after September 11. During last time interval, FEV$_1$ significantly greater in non-smokers and those who quit before 9/11 than current or former smokers who quit after 9/11. Firefighters quitting smoking before March 10, 2008, had significantly greater FEV$_1$ than current smokers during most of the post-September 11 follow-up.
Aldrich et al. 2016 [47]	9/11-exposed firefighters	Post-9/11: 11.5 (0.5)	Pre-9/11: 1 Post-9/11: 2	Δvalue/Δtime	4.28 (0.67)[q]	Mix [Cur 6.4, For 17.9]	Post-9/11: -32 (unadjusted) -36.78 (adjusted in multiple regression model)	Effect of 9/11 exposure on FEV$_1$ decline post-9/11 not investigated. Average reduction in FEV$_1$ across 9/11–399 (468.3) mL.	15.39 mL/year more rapid FEV$_1$ decline in those with BHR at follow-up, compared with those without BHR ($p = .0104$). Use of steroids associated with a 13.01 mL/year slower rate of decline, compared with those who never used steroids ($p = .0197$).

AAT Alpha-1 antitrypsin, *BHR* Bronchial hyper-reactivity, *CI* = 95% Confidence interval, *Cur* Current smokers, *CurNS* Current non-smokers, *EMS* Emergency medical services, *Ev* Ever smokers, *FEV$_1$* Forced expiratory volume in one second, *FIRE* Firefighters, *For* Former smokers, *FVC* Forced vital capacity, *Gp* General population, *IL-10* Interleukin-10, *IL-1RA* Interleukin-1 receptor antagonist, *IQR* Interquartile range, *Knockdown* Fire suppression, *Nev* Never smokers, *OR* Odds ratio, *Overhaul* Clean-up following fire suppression, *RMANOVA* Repeated measures analysis of variance, *SE* Standard error, *SNp* Single nucleotide polymorphism, *TGFβ1* Transforming growth factor β1, *TNFα* Tumor necrosis factor-α. Adjusted variables: [1]Asthma status, [2]Age, [3]Baseline lung function, [4]Blood type, [5]Body mass index, [6]Bronchial hyper-reactivity, [7]Duration of exposure, [8]Height, [9]History of chronic respiratory conditions, [10]Interaction of smoking with AAT deficiency, [11]Length of FDNY tenure, [12]Physical activity, [13]Race, [14]Respiratory protection, [15]Respiratory symptoms, [16]Root mean square error term, [17]Sex, [18]Smoking, [19]Steroid use, [20]Trans-9/11 change, [21]Weight, [22]Weight change, [23]Work assignment on September 11, 2001, [24]WTC exposure intensity, [25]Years of follow-up. *Significant difference between groups. [a]Baseline and final follow-up used for calculation of rate of decline, [b]Longitudinal results of study reported, [c]Calculated based on fire department records, [d]Estimated by firefighter, [e]Firefighters with repeatable/non-repeatable spirometry reported separately. Repeater is defined as an individual whose two highest values for both FEV$_1$ and FVC agreed within one-tenth litre or 5% of the highest value at both the baseline and follow-up studies, [f]Calculated as ΔFEV$_1$/ΔTime by review authors, [g]Study data obtained from the Normative Ageing Study, [h]Total among all paper-pulp mill workers, [i]Unadjusted for weight-gain, [j]Values reported by authors upon request, [k]Extracted from graph, [l]Smoked before 9/11, [m]Smoked after 9/11, [n]Quit before 9/11/2001, [o]Quit between 9/11/2001 and 3/10/08, [p]Quit after 3/10/08, [q]Last pre-9/11 measure (Fire and EMS)

firefighters after 13 years [46]. Compared to continuing smokers, the rate of change in FEV_1 of former smokers who quit before or after 9/11 was significantly less negative. Two small subgroups of 9/11-responding firefighters were also studied, observing post-9/11 FEV_1 declines of − 36.7 mL/yr. (adjusted for age, bronchial hyper-reactivity, height, race, steroid use and the initial loss of lung function related to 9/11 exposure) [47] and 37 mL/yr. (adjusted for age, height, interaction of smoking with AAT deficiency, length of FDNY tenure, race, sex, smoking, work assignment on 9/11 and WTC exposure intensity) [48].

In summary, most studies of non-smoking firefighters exposed to routine firefighting showed negative rates of change in FEV_1 and FVC that were analogous to the rates observed in longitudinal studies of healthy non-smokers in the general population [12–22]. Those that showed greater rates of decline than would normally be expected were either less than [32] or not significantly different to [10] general population controls in direct comparisons, or were particularly limited by a lack of information on smoking status [30, 31, 37]. Firefighters exposed to non-routine events experienced significant reductions in lung function in the initial year after exposure, with long-term rates of change representing normal decline without recovery.

Influence of firefighting and protective or deleterious factors

Influence of firefighting exposure level

In their 1974 report of Boston firefighters, Peters and colleagues showed significant inverse relationships between self-reported fire exposure over a 12-month period and changes in FEV_1 and FVC [37]. However, no significant relationship was observed in three [35] and six-year [34] follow-up studies on the same population, using self-reported exposure and estimates derived from fire department records. A significantly greater FEV_1 decline was observed in active vs inactive firefighters in one study [33] but is contrasted by two others which showed trends of higher rates of decline in inactive vs active firefighters [34, 35], while a further study showed no difference [30]. No studies identified a relationship between service time and rate of change in FEV_1 or FVC [10, 30, 31, 33, 35, 36]. One study reported significantly greater rates of FEV_1 decline in firefighters who reported previous exposure to ammonia, however past chlorine exposure had no apparent effect [33].

Firefighters responding to the 9/11 disaster experienced dramatic declines in FEV_1 in the first year following exposure [44–48]. Measured by self-reported arrival time, a significant dose-response relationship was observed between exposure intensity and loss of FEV_1 [44]. Firefighters that reported the greatest dust exposure (those arriving earliest) also experienced the greatest rate of FEV_1 decline in the subsequent 7 and 13-year follow-ups [45, 46].

The included studies show a dose-response relationship between changes in lung function and exposure level in non-routine severe firefighting events, but results were inconsistent regarding the presence of such an effect of exposure level in routine firefighting.

Influence of respiratory protection

Four studies investigated the effect of respiratory protection on changes in FEV_1. In one study, firefighters who reported 'never or rarely' using their respiratory protection during fire knockdown had higher odds of 'accelerated' FEV_1 decline (greater than 50 mL/yr) compared with those who used it 'often or frequently' (Odds Ratio = 2.20, 95% Confidence Interval = 1.02–4.74, $p = .044$) [8]. Another study observed a greater FEV_1 decline in firefighters who reported 'never' vs 'ever' using a mask while extinguishing fires (− 68.44 vs − 30.90 mL/yr), but the association was only significant in those with non-repeatable spirometry [33]. There was no significant difference in changes of FEV_1 based on mask-use during fire overhaul (clean-up). A further study showed no relationship between the rate of change in FEV_1 and the stated tendency of firefighters to wear protective respiratory apparatus [34] while there was also no identifiable protective effect of using any type of protective mask during the response to the 9/11 disaster [44].

Influence of other factors

In the five studies that included covariates in their models to estimate changes in lung function, four included race, sex and smoking status as well as baseline age and height [44–46, 48], while one included only race as well as baseline age and height: due to the absence of females and separate analyses with smokers [9]. Three of these studies included weight at baseline [9, 45, 46] with one also including weight change in a separate model [9]. These five variables as well as a further 20 were included in subsequent modelling to investigate factors that affect the rate of change in lung function (all variables listed in Table 2). Overall, noteworthy predictors included weight gain, which was associated with a significantly greater decline in FEV_1 in two studies [9, 46] and close to being significant in another [41], while four studies observed significantly increased or decreased rates of FEV_1 decline based on different variations in gene expressions [40–42, 48]. One study associated the development of bronchial hyper-reactivity with a significant increase in FEV_1 decline in 9/11-exposed firefighters, while the use of steroids was associated with a less negative rate of change in FEV_1 [47].

Calculation/measurement and reporting of the rate of change in FEV$_1$ and FVC

Eight studies calculated the rate of change in FEV$_1$ and/or FVC as the change in volume divided by the change in time using data from two time-points [8, 10, 33–37, 47]: four of which had measured lung function on more than two occasions [34–36]. Five studies used simple linear regression [32, 40–43], five used linear mixed models [9, 44–46, 48], while a further four did not report on the rate of change, or did not report their method of calculation [30, 31, 38, 39]. There was no apparent indication that any technique was more biased toward positive, negative or null results.

Six studies reported on the proportion of firefighters with a decline in FEV$_1$ or FVC that was greater than a particular cut-off: often referred to as an 'accelerated' or 'greater than expected' decline. The cut-offs (proportion of firefighters above cut-off) were set at declines of > 50 mL/yr. (Fire: 26%, Controls: 39%) [8], > 60 mL/yr. (18.4% [42], 23% [40]), > 64 mL/yr. (19.5%) [46], ,> 75 mL/yr. (50.8%) [38] and > 90 mL/yr. (4.8%) [43], with the latter study also using a relative cut-off of > 2.1% per year (5.6%) [43]. One study also reported on FVC declines of greater than 75 mL/yr. (35.1%) [38].

Quality assessment/risk of bias

Two articles were rated as high quality/low risk of bias, 12 as moderate quality/moderate risk of bias, and eight as low quality/high risk of bias (Table 3).

The most evident biases were performance bias, information bias and attrition bias. Studies generally failed to use valid and reliable means of measuring exposures and did not report them with great detail in respect to the measurement and reporting of confounding variables. Seven studies reported loss to follow-up of greater than 30%, yet none investigated any potential effect of this through sensitivity analyses or other adjustment methods.

Biases that were the most unclear were selection bias/confounding, detection bias, performance bias and precision. The most common issues were around the clarity of inclusion/exclusion criteria, the lack of clarity in reporting blinding of assessors to exposure status as well as the appropriateness of statistical techniques: although this was mainly a reflection of the age of the studies.

Discussion

To our knowledge, this is the first study to systematically review the literature measuring longitudinal changes in lung function of professional urban firefighters and its associations with occupational exposure. Among firefighters exposed to routine firefighting, the reported rates of change in lung function were variable and ranged from normal rates of decline to what could be considered accelerated: particularly among current smokers. There is a general lack of evidence of a relationship between measures of routine firefighting exposure and long-term changes in lung function: though this

Table 3 Summary of individual study quality/risk of bias assessment using the RTI-IB. Studies are ordered by population type and year of publication

may be primarily due to limitations in exposure measurement itself. In contrast, exposure to non-routine disastrous events is more clearly related to reductions in lung function.

The large variability in the reported rates of change in lung function of firefighters exposed to routine firefighting make definitive conclusions difficult. Most observations among never-smokers were consistent with other longitudinal studies of the general population, or were at least no more negative than non-firefighter general population controls. However, the range of findings and low rating in quality assessments among included studies, and the fact that there is no clear upper limit of normal lung function decline, precludes any definitive conclusions about the risks of accelerated longitudinal declines in lung function of professional urban firefighters in relation to routine firefighting.

Among studies of routine firefighters, the study with the highest score (0.63) in the quality rating/lowest risk of bias assessment consisted of 5 years of annual measurements and provides the best evidence of the effect of contemporary firefighting on lung function [9]. Firefighters in this study experienced a longitudinal rate of change in FEV_1 of -45 mL/yr. which was equal to that of unexposed controls. While this is greater than the rate of decline reported in most longitudinal studies of healthy adult non-smokers, it is still less than is reported by others such as Tashkin et al. [22] This highlights the difficulties associated with comparing rates of change in lung function between studies of different periods, which utilised different recruitment strategies as well as different equipment and standards of lung function testing. For these reasons, studies that make direct comparisons to a well-matched (yet unexposed) reference group who are sampled in the same way, are particularly valuable, but equally scarce.

One of the few studies employing a control population made a surprising observation of an increase in FEV_1 and FVC in non-smoking firefighters concurrent to a decline in age-matched, non-smoking general population controls [8]. Although this may be somewhat influenced by the inclusion of younger firefighters whose lungs may still be maturing, the mean changes in FEV_1 and FVC for firefighters aged 36–45 years were positive. This is contradictory to the notion that lung function declines after peaking during in the third decade of life [15, 21, 49–51]. Caution, though, is needed in interpreting these results, as this study would have benefited from further follow-up in order to reduce any possible effect of statistical regression to the mean.

In attempting to quantify the effect of routine firefighting exposures on changes in lung function, multiple different strategies have been employed, each with limited success. The number of responses to fires has not been meaningfully associated with negative changes in FEV_1 or FVC, either through estimates based on fire department records (FDR) or recalled by firefighters themselves [33–36]. Musk et al. [35] also reported a poor correlation between the two methods, which may suggest that firefighters cannot accurately recall their exposures over a twelve-month period, that the FDR method of estimation was unreliable, or both. Service/employment time has also been a poor index of exposure [10, 31, 33, 35, 36], and has questionable validity given the way in which firefighters can move between active and inactive roles throughout their careers. This movement of workers also undermines any assumptions that active firefighters have had greater exposures than inactive firefighters, given that firefighters may self-select out of active roles as a direct result of poor health following work-related exposure. Further crude indices of exposure have included self-reported heavy smoke exposure, informally described as "shellackings" [35, 37], "lungers" or "pastings" [34], as well as absence from work following exposure to smoke [31], showing no significant associations with changes in lung function.

Examined separately from studies of firefighters exposed to routine firefighting, studies investigating changes in lung function following severe exposure reveal consistent outcomes of accelerated declines in lung function. Observing firefighters immediately following exposure to a chemical warehouse fire, Unger et al. [39] reported a high average rate of decline in FEV_1 over the subsequent 18 months. While a lack of pre-exposure data is a limitation of the study, the rate of decline may have even been underestimated, if there were cases of lung function recovery, over the course of follow-up. This may provide an example of how studies involving 'non-routine events' could bias the estimate of the rate of change in lung function following the event and supports the separate interpretation of the results in this review. This issue also applies to the studies which followed firefighters after 9/11 [44–48]. In addition, some of these studies included firefighters who retired during follow-up and thereby removing them from firefighting exposures which may further affect estimates of the rate of change in lung function. Notwithstanding these issues, these studies were among the highest quality rated studies with the lowest risk of bias and have benefitted from the presence of several years of pre-exposure data. They provide unequivocal evidence of the dramatic long-term negative effect of this exposure on lung function and highlight the importance of routine lung function surveillance in firefighters.

Among all studies included in the review that made the comparison, most studies observed greater rates of decline in never-smoking firefighters compared to current-smoking firefighters. Although the significance of this difference was not always tested statistically, the excess declines in current smokers were comparable to those observed in general smoking population [52, 53]. Cigarette smoking has the potential to be particularly dangerous to firefighters, given that it has been linked with reductions in immune responses [54], which may leave them more vulnerable to the dangers of fire smoke. Based on the information available in this review, however, it was not possible to speculate any further than this.

Along with smoke exposure, both from fires and cigarettes, one of the most important variables affecting firefighter lung function trajectories is the use of respiratory protection, which has undergone many changes across the time periods of the included studies. The US-based National Fire Protection Association (NFPA) produced its first *Standard for Respiratory Protective Equipment for Firefighters* (*NFPA 19B*) in 1971, with the aim of prohibiting filter-type canister masks for firefighters and permitting only self-contained breathing apparatus (SCBA) [55]. The regularly updated standard has overseen improvements in technology that are likely to have influenced the frequency with which SCBA is utilised by firefighters, which may have implications on respiratory health. In their pioneering studies of the early 1970s Boston, Musk et al... found no relationship between firefighters' "self-stated tendency" to use respiratory protection and changes in FEV_1, but provided no further information on the frequency of use [34]. Tepper and colleagues later compared changes in the FEV_1 of firefighters who reported 'never' vs 'ever' using a mask while extinguishing fires, showing little association [33]. This method, though, may lack sensitivity due to the use of the broad term 'ever', which may have grouped together those who have used it once only, or at every response. Two decades later, Schermer et al [8] showed that firefighters who reported 'never or rarely' using respiratory protection during fire suppression were significantly more likely than others to experience greater declines in FEV_1. They were also less likely to not use respiratory protection during fire overhaul: the period following extinguishment of visible flame, when exposures are still dangerous [56, 57]. These firefighters were also more likely to be older, suggesting a possible cohort effect whereby use of respiratory protection increases with each new generation of firefighters. Among responders to the 9/11 disaster in New York in 2001, there was no identifiable protective effect of using any type of protective mask [44]. However, this is likely due to the fact that most firefighters were entirely unprotected, or wore only a disposable mask in the first 2 days of the event [58].

Studies that received the highest quality assessment/lowest risk of bias scores tended to be among the most recently published studies, and employed more contemporary statistical methods of analysis [9, 44–48]. Among the remaining studies, there was no discernible relationship between publication date and quality. Mixed models approaches offer several advantages over other 'pre-post' analyses, with the latter being more susceptible to influence by measurement error. Further, given the natural variability in lung function measurements, studies with more than two measures of lung function over five or more years of follow-up can more precisely and reliably evaluate the rate of change in lung function [18]. Those studies that met this criterion tended to report normal rates of decline in FEV_1 or FVC. None of the included studies assessed for non-linear changes in lung function.

A limitation of this review was the absence of meta-analytical techniques, which were precluded by the lack of homogeneity across studies published over several decades. The review may also be limited by publication bias, as it did not include evidence that was unpublished or pending publication. Additionally, the minimum follow-up time for studies to be included was 1 year. Given the value of repeated measurements over long periods [18], approximately half of the studies included may be too short to provide truly meaningful insights into the way lung function changes over time. Further, due to the manner in which published data were reported, some data were estimated from graphical figures using computer software, or calculated from the data that were available and this may have reduced the precision of estimates of rate of change. Moreover, the focus of this review was on professional urban firefighters, whose exposures may differ in type, intensity and duration to those of wildland firefighters. Although exposure to wildland firefighting has produced cross-shift [59] and cross-seasonal [60] reductions in lung function, further studies are needed to investigate the long-term effects of such firefighting.

Conclusions

The data provided by longitudinal studies, which were mostly concerned with FEV_1, are highly variable and provide an unclear picture of how the rate of change in lung function of firefighters relates to routine exposures and how it compares to the rate of change expected in a non-exposed working-age population. Firefighters who abstain from cigarette smoking and who routinely wear respiratory protection are more likely than otherwise to have a normal rate of decline in lung function. Exposure to catastrophic events, such as 9/11, significantly increases the rate of decline in lung function but there is limited evidence detailing the effect of routine firefighting and future studies will benefit from more robust methods of measuring exposure.

Abbreviations

9/11: World Trade Center disaster on September 11, 2001; AA: African-American; AAT: Alpha-1 antitrypsin; B: Black; BHR: Bronchial hyper-reactivity; C: Caucasian; CI: 95% Confidence Interval; Cur: Current smokers; CurNS: Current non-smokers; EMS: Emergency Medical Services; ERS: European Respiratory Society; Ev: Ever smokers; F: Female(s); FDNY: Fire department New York; FDR: Fire department records; FEV_1: Forced Expiratory Volume in one second; FIRE: Firefighters; For: Former smokers; FVC: Forced vital capacity; GP: General population; HAZMAT: Hazardous materials; HW: Hispanic White; IL-10: Interleukin-10; IL-1RA: Interleukin-1 receptor antagonist; IQR: Inter-quartile range; Knockdown: Fire suppression; LFB: London fire brigade; LLN: Lower limit of normal; NFPA: National Fire Protection Association; NR: Not reported; NWAHS: North-West area health study; OR: Odds ration; Overhaul: Clean-up following fire suppression; PFT: Pulmonary function test; PRISMA: Preferred Reporting Items for Systematic Reviews and Meta-Analyses; PROSPERO: International Prospective Register of Systematic Reviews; RMANOVA: Repeated measures analysis of variance; ROD: Rate of decline; RTI-IB: Research Triangle Institute Item Bank; SCBA: Self-contained breathing apparatus; SD: Standard deviation; SE: Standard error; SNP: Single nucleotide polymorphism; $TG\beta1$: Transforming growth factor $\beta1$; $TNF\alpha$: Tumour necrosis factor-α; USA: The United States of America; W: White; WTC: World Trade Center

Funding

This research was supported by the South Australian Metropolitan Fire Service and an Australian Government Research Training Program (RTP) Scholarship (FS).

Authors' contributions

FS was involved in the conception and design of this research, article searching and screening, data extraction and analysis, as well as manuscript drafting and revision. KJ was involved in the conception and design of this research, data extraction and analysis, as well as manuscript drafting and revision. CP was involved in manuscript drafting and revision. HB was involved in article searching and screening, as well as manuscript drafting and revision. AC was involved in the conception and design of this research as well as manuscript drafting and revision. All authors read and approved the final manuscript.

Competing interests

The authors declare that they have no competing interests.

Author details

[1]Alliance for Research in Exercise, Nutrition and Activity, Sansom Institute for Health Research, School of Health Sciences, Universitiy of South Australia, Adelaide, Australia. [2]School of Health Sciences, Sansom Institute for Health Research, University of South Australia, Adelaide, Australia. [3]Centre for Population Health Research, Sansom Institute for Health Research, School of Health Sciences, University of South Australia, Adelaide, Australia.

References

1. Greven FE, Krop EJ, Spithoven JJ, Burger N, Rooyackers JM, Kerstjens HA, et al. Acute respiratory effects in firefighters. Am J Ind Med. 2012;55:54–62. https://doi.org/10.1002/ajim.21012.
2. Sheppard D, Distefano S, Morse L, Becker C. Acute effects of routine firefighting on lung function. Am J Ind Med. 1986;9:333–40. https://doi-org.access.library.urisa.edu.au/10.1002/ajim.4700090404.
3. Sherman CB, Barnhart S, Miller MF, Segal MR, Aitken M, Schoene R, et al. Firefighting acutely increases airway responsiveness. Am Rev Respir Dis. 1989;140:185–90. https://doi.org/10.1164/ajrccm/140.1.185.
4. Chia KS, Jeyaratnam J, Chan TB, Lim TK. Airway responsiveness of firefighters after smoke exposure. Br J Ind Med. 1990;47:524–7. http://dx.doi.org/10.1136/oem.47.8.524.
5. Banauch GI, Alleyne D, Sanchez R, Olender K, Cohen HW, Weiden M, et al. Persistent hyperreactivity and reactive airway dysfunction in firefighters at the world trade center. Am J Respir Crit Care Med. 2003;168:54–62. https://doi.org/10.1164/rccm.200211-1329OC.
6. Brandt-Rauf PW, Cosman B, Fallon LF Jr, Tarantini T, Idema C. Health hazards of firefighters: acute pulmonary effects after toxic exposures. Br J Ind Med. 1989;46:209–11. https://doi.org/10.1002/ajim.21012.
7. Schermer TR, Malbon T, Morgan M, Briggs N, Holton C, Appleton S, et al. Lung function and health status in metropolitan fire-fighters compared to general population controls. Int Arch Occup Environ Health. 2010;83:715–23. https://doi.org/10.1007/s00420-010-0528-0.
8. Schermer TR, Malbon W, Adams R, Morgan M, Smith M, Crockett AJ. Change in lung function over time in male metropolitan firefighters and general population controls: a 3-year follow-up study. J Occup Health. 2013; https://doi.org/10.1539/joh.12-0189-O
9. Aldrich TK, Ye F, Hall CB, Webber MP, Cohen HW, Dinkels M, et al. Longitudinal pulmonary function in newly hired, non-world trade center-exposed fire department city of New York firefighters: the first 5 years. Chest. 2013;143:791–7. https://doi.org/10.1378/chest.12-0675.
10. Sparrow D, Bosse R, Rosner B, Weiss ST. The effect of occupational exposure on pulmonary function: a longitudinal evaluation of fire fighters and nonfire fighters. Am Rev Respir Dis. 1982;125:319–22. https://doi.org/10.1164/arrd.1982.125.3.319.
11. Quanjer PH, Stanojevic S, Cole TJ, Baur X, Hall GL, Culver BH, et al. Multi-ethnic reference values for spirometry for the 3–95-yr age range: the global lung function 2012 equations. Eur Respir J. 2012;40:1324–43. https://doi.org/10.1183/09031936.00080312.
12. Fletcher C, Peto R. The natural history of chronic airflow obstruction. Br Med J. 1977;1:1645–8. https://doi.org/10.1136/bmj.1.6077.1645.
13. Tager IB, Segal MR, Speizer FE, Weiss ST. The natural history of forced expiratory volumes. Effect of cigarette smoking and respiratory symptoms. Am Rev Respir Dis. 1988;138:837–49. https://doi.org/10.1164/ajrccm/138.4.837.
14. Lange P, Groth S, Nyboe G, Mortensen J, Appleyard M, Jensen G, et al. Effects of smoking and changes in smoking habits on the decline of FEV_1. Eur Respir J. 1989;2:811–6. http://erj.ersjournals.com/content/2/9/811.article-info.
15. Sherrill D, Lebowitz M, Knudson R, Burrows B. Continuous longitudinal regression equations for pulmonary function measures. Eur Respir J. 1992;5:452–62.
16. Rodriguez BL, Masaki K, Burchfiel C, Curb JD, Fong K-O, Chyou P-H, et al. Pulmonary function decline and 17-year total mortality: the Honolulu heart program. Am J Epidemiol. 1994;140:398–408.
17. James AL, Palmer LJ, Kicic E, Maxwell PS, Lagan SE, Ryan GF, et al. Decline in lung function in the Busselton health study the effects of asthma and cigarette smoking. Am J Respir Crit Care Med. 2005;171:109–14. https://doi.org/10.1164/rccm.200402-230OC.
18. Wang ML, Avashia BH, Petsonk EL. Interpreting periodic lung function tests in individuals: the relationship between 1-to 5-year and long-term FEV_1 changes. Chest. 2006;130:493–9. https://doi.org/10.1378/chest.130.2.493.
19. Wang ML, Avashia BH, Petsonk EL. Interpreting longitudinal spirometry: weight gain and other factors affecting the recognition of excessive FEV_1 decline. Am J Ind Med. 2009;52:782–9. https://doi.org/10.1002/ajim.20727.
20. Abramson MJ, Kaushik S, Benke GP, Borg BM, Smith CL, Dharmage SC, et al. Symptoms and lung function decline in a middle-aged cohort of males and females in Australia. Int J Chron Obstruct Pulmon Dis. 2016;11:1097–103. https://doi.org/10.2147/COPD.S103817.
21. Kohansal R, Martinez-Camblor P, Agustí A, Buist AS, Mannino DM, Soriano JB. The natural history of chronic airflow obstruction revisited: an analysis of the Framingham offspring cohort. Am J Respir Crit Care Med. 2009;180:3–10. https://doi.org/10.1164/rccm.200901-0047OC.
22. Tashkin DP, Clark VA, Coulson AH, Simmons M, Bourque LB, Reems C, et al. The UCLA population studies of chronic obstructive respiratory disease: VIII. Effects of smoking cessation on lung function: a prospective study of a free-living population 1–3. Am Rev Respir Dis. 1984;130:707–15.
23. Moher D, Liberati A, Tetzlaff J, Altman DG, Group P. Preferred reporting items for systematic reviews and meta-analyses: the PRISMA statement. PLoS Med. 2009;6:e1000097. https://doi.org/10.1136/bmj.b2535.
24. Rohatgi A. WebPlotDigitizer version 4.0. Austin; 2017. Available from: https://zenodo.org/record/1039373#.W4CqYugzaUk.
25. Viswanathan M, Berkman ND. Development of the RTI item bank on risk of bias and precision of observational studies. J Clin Epidemiol. 2012;65:163–78. https://doi.org/10.1016/j.jclinepi.2011.05.008.

26. Margulis AV, Pladevall M, Riera-Guardia N, Varas-Lorenzo C, Hazell L, Berkman ND, et al. Quality assessment of observational studies in a drug-safety systematic review, comparison of two tools: the Newcastle-Ottawa scale and the RTI item bank. Clin Epidemiol. 2014;6:359–68. https://doi.org/10.2147/CLEP.S66677.
27. Fuentes JP, Armijo Olivo S, Magee DJ, Gross DP. Effectiveness of interferential current therapy in the Management of Musculoskeletal Pain: a systematic review and meta-analysis. Phys Ther. 2010;90:1219–38. https://doi.org/10.2522/ptj.20090335.
28. Fuentes CJ, Armijo-Olivo S, Magee DJ, Gross DP. Effects of exercise therapy on endogenous pain-relieving peptides in musculoskeletal pain: a systematic review. Clin J Pain. 2011;27:365–74. https://doi.org/10.1097/AJP.0b013e31820d99c8.
29. Al-Saleh MA, Armijo-Olivo S, Thie N, Seikaly H, Boulanger P, Wolfaardt J, et al. Morphologic and functional changes in the temporomandibular joint and stomatognathic system after transmandibular surgery in oral and oropharyngeal cancers: systematic review. J Otolaryngol Head Neck Surg. 2012;41:345–60. https://scinapse.io/papers/2344114275.
30. Choi J-H, Shin J-H, Lee M-Y, Chung I-S. Pulmonary function decline in firefighters and non-firefighters in South Korea. Ann Occup Environ Med. 2014;26:1. https://doi.org/10.1186/2052-4374-26-9.
31. Douglas DB, Douglas RB, Oakes D, Scott G. Pulmonary function of London firemen. Br J Ind Med. 1985;42:55–8. https://doi.org/10.1136/oem.42.1.55.
32. Horsfield K, Guyatt A, Cooper FM, Buckman MP, Cumming G. Lung function in West Sussex firemen: a four year study. Br J Ind Med. 1988;45:116–21. https://doi.org/10.1136/oem.45.2.116.
33. Tepper A, Comstock GW, Levine M. A longitudinal study of pulmonary function in fire fighters. Am J Ind Med. 1991;20:307–16. https://doi.org/10.1002/ajim.4700200304.
34. Musk AW, Peters JM, Bernstein L, Rubin C, Monroe CB. Pulmonary function in firefighters: a six-year follow-up in the Boston fire department. Am J Ind Med. 1982;3:3–9. https://doi.org/10.1002/ajim.4700030103.
35. Musk AW, Peters JM, Wegman DH. Lung function in fire fighters, I: a three year follow-up of active subjects. Am J Public Health. 1977;67:626–9. https://doi.org/10.2105/ajph.67.7.626.
36. Musk AW, Petters JM, Wegman DH. Lung function in fire fighters, II: a five year follow-up fo retirees. Am J Public Health. 1977;67:630–3. https://doi.org/10.2105/ajph.67.7.630.
37. Peters JM, Theriault GP, Fine LJ, Wegman DH. Chronic effect of fire fighting on pulmonary function. N Engl J Med. 1974;291:1320–2. https://doi.org/10.1056/NEJM197412192912502.
38. Kales SN, Polyhronopoulos GN, Christiani DC. Medical surveillance of hazardous materials response fire fighters: a two-year prospective study. J Occup Environ Med. 1997;39:238–47. https://journals.lww.com/joem/pages/articleviewer.aspx?year=1997&issue=03000&article=00014&type=abstract.
39. Unger KM, Snow RM, Mestas JM, Miller WC. Smoke inhalation in firemen. Thorax. 1980;35:838–42. https://doi.org/10.1136/thx.35.11.838.
40. Burgess JL, Fierro MA, Lantz RC, Hysong TA, Fleming JE, Gerkin R, et al. Longitudinal decline in lung function: evaluation of interleukin-10 genetic polymorphisms in firefighters. J Occup Environ Med. 2004;46:1013–22. https://doi.org/10.1097/01.jom.0000141668.70006.52.
41. Josyula AB, Kurzius-Spencer M, Littau SR, Yucesoy B, Fleming J, Burgess JL. Cytokine genotype and phenotype effects on lung function decline in firefighters. J Occup Environ Med. 2007;49:282–8. https://doi.org/10.1097/JOM.0b013e3180322584.
42. Yucesoy B, Kurzius-Spencer M, Johnson VJ, Fluharty K, Kashon ML, Guerra S, et al. Association of cytokine gene polymorphisms with rate of decline in lung function. J Occup Environ Med. 2008;50:642–8. https://doi.org/10.1097/JOM.0b013e31816515e1.
43. Hnizdo E. The value of periodic spirometry for early recognition of long-term excessive lung function decline in individuals. J Occup Environ Med. 2012;54:1506–12. https://doi.org/10.1097/JOM.0b013e3182664811.
44. Banauch GI, Hall C, Weiden M, Cohen HW, Aldrich TK, Christodoulou V, et al. Pulmonary function after exposure to the world trade center collapse in the new York City fire department. Am J Respir Crit Care Med. 2006;174:312–9. https://doi.org/10.1164/rccm.200511-1736OC.
45. Aldrich TK, Gustave J, Hall CB, Cohen HW, Webber MP, Zeig-Owens R, et al. Lung function in rescue workers at the world trade center after 7 years. N Engl J Med. 2010;362:1263–72. https://doi.org/10.1056/NEJMoa0910087.
46. Aldrich TK, Vossbrinck M, Zeig-Owens R, Hall CB, Schwartz TM, Moir W, et al. Lung function trajectories in WTC-exposed NYC firefighters over 13 years: the roles of smoking and smoking cessation. Chest. 2016;149:1419–27.
47. Aldrich TK, Weakley J, Dhar S, Hall CB, Crosse T, Banauch GI, et al. Bronchial reactivity and lung function after world trade center exposure. Chest. 2016;150:1333–40. https://doi.org/10.1016/.chest.2016.07.005.
48. Banauch GI, Brantly M, Izbicki G, Hall C, Shanske A, Chavko R, et al. Accelerated spirometric decline in new York City firefighters with alpha(1)-antitrypsin deficiency. Chest. 2010;138:1116–24. https://doi.org/10.1378/chest.10-0187.
49. Brändli O, Schindler C, Künzli N, Keller R, Perruchoud A. Lung function in healthy never smoking adults: reference values and lower limits of normal of a Swiss population. Thorax. 1996;51:277–83.
50. Van Pelt W, Borsboom G, Rijcken B, Schouten JP, Van Zomeren BC, Quanjer PH. Discrepancies between longitudinal and cross-sectional change in ventilatory function in 12 years of follow-up. Am J Respir Crit Care Med. 1994;149:1218–26.
51. Knudson RJ, Lebowitz M, Holberg C, Burrows B. Changes in the normal maximal expiratory flow-volume curve with growth and aging. Am Rev Respir Dis. 1983;127:725–34. https://doi.org/10.1164/arrd.1983.127.6.725.
52. Kerstjens H, Rijcken B, Schouten JP, Postma DS. Decline of FEV_1 by age and smoking status: facts, figures, and fallacies. Thorax. 1997;52:820–7. https://doi.org/10.1136/thx.52.9.820.
53. James AL, Palmer LJ, Kicic E, Maxwell PS, Lagan SE, Ryan GF, et al. Decline in lung function in the Busselton health study: the effects of asthma and cigarette smoking. Am J Respir Crit Care Med. 2005;171:109–14.
54. Sopori M. Effects of cigarette smoke on the immune system. Nat Rev Immunol. 2002;2:372–7. https://doi.org/10.1038/nri803.
55. NFPA 1981. Standard on open-circuit self-contained breathing apparatus (SCBA) for emergency services. Quincy: National Fire Protection Association; 2007. p. 119.
56. Bolstad-Johnson DM, Burgess JL, Crutchfield CD, Storment S, Gerkin R, Wilson JR. Characterization of firefighter exposures during fire overhaul. AIHAJ. 2000;61:636–41. https://asu.pure.elsevier.com/en/publications/characterization-of-firefighter-exposures-during-fire-overhaul.
57. Burgess JL, Nanson CJ, Bolstad-Johnson DM, Gerkin R, Hysong TA, Lantz RC, et al. Adverse respiratory effects following overhaul in firefighters. J Occup Environ Med. 2001;43:467–73. https://journals.lww.com/joem/pages/articleviewer.aspx?year=2001&issue=05000&article=00007&type=abstract.
58. Feldman DM, Baron SL, Bernard BP, Lushniak BD, Banauch G, Arcentales N, et al. Symptoms, respirator use, and pulmonary function changes among new York City firefighters responding to the world trade center disaster. Chest. 2004;125:1256–64.
59. Gaughan DM, Piacitelli CA, Chen BT, Law BF, Virji MA, Edwards NT, et al. Exposures and cross-shift lung function declines in wildland firefighters. J Occup Environ Hyg. 2014;11:591–603. https://doi.org/10.1080/15459624.2014.895372.
60. Liu D, Tager IB, Balmes JR, Harrison RJ. The effect of smoke inhalation on lung function and airway responsiveness in wildland fire fighters. Am Rev Respir Dis. 1992;146:1469–73. https://doi.org/10.1164/ajrccm/146.6.1469.

Albuminuria in patients with chronic obstructive pulmonary disease: a cross-sectional study in an African patient cohort

Festo K. Shayo[1,2,3]* and Janet Lutale[1,2]*

Abstract

Background: Cardiovascular disease (CVD) is remarkably frequent in patients with chronic obstructive pulmonary disease (COPD). Albuminuria is a marker of vascular endothelial dysfunction and predictor of CVD events. Albuminuria is prevalent in patients with COPD as it has been shown in Caucasian and Oriental populations with COPD. The objective of this study was to determine the prevalence of Albuminuria and COPD severity correlates among black patients with chronic obstructive pulmonary disease in order to see whether a similar trend of albuminuria is also prevalent in this population.

Methods: A total of 104 COPD patients were enrolled in the study. Lung functions were assessed by means of the Easy One™ spirometer. Albuminuria defined by urine albumin to creatinine ratio (ACR) was tested using CYBOW 12MAC microalbumin strips in a random spot urine collection. SPSS version 20 was used for data analysis.

Results: In the studied population, 25/104 (24%) patients had albuminuria and 16/104 (15.4%) patients had CVD. Abnormal urine albumin (Albuminuria and Proteinuria) was present in all patients with CVD. In the subset of 46 COPD patients assessed for severity, 60.9% (95%CIs 46.1–73.9) had moderate COPD and 30.4% (95% CIs, 17.9–49.0) severe COPD. Albuminuria was moderately significantly associated with COPD severity, $p = 0.049$; $(0.049 < p < 0.05)$. Participants who ever smoked cigarettes had significantly likelihood of severe and very severe COPD (OR 11.5; 95% CIs, 1.3, 98.4) however, the significance was lost when adjusted for age and gender.

Conclusion: Albuminuria was prevalent in patients with COPD and it had a significant association with COPD severity.

Keywords: Cardiovascular disease, Albuminuria, Chronic obstructive pulmonary disease

Background

The chronic obstructive pulmonary disease is currently the 4th cause of death worldwide; projected the 3rd by 2020 [1]. COPD has potential extra-pulmonary effects but it can be prevented and treated, however, no cure has been established. Cardiovascular disease is the most common extra-pulmonary presentation of COPD and therefore patients are at increased risk of morbidity and mortality due to acute cardiovascular events [2]. Different studies have shown that cardiovascular disease is common in COPD and likely to add to the complexity of the disease [3]. For instance; in the USA, the prevalence of cardiovascular disease in COPD patients was reported to be 22% versus 9% in non-COPD patients. In the UK, the relative risks of angina and myocardial infarction were 1.67 and 1.75, respectively, versus subjects without COPD [4]. A CONSISTE study in Spain showed that patients with COPD had a significantly higher prevalence of ischemic heart disease, cerebrovascular disease, and peripheral vascular disease compared non-COPD group [5].

Albuminuria is known to be a sensitive biomarker of endovascular dysfunction and a significant predictor of cardiovascular events and all-cause mortality in the general population. Vascular endothelial dysfunction is evident in patients with chronic obstructive pulmonary

* Correspondence: feca_sha@yahoo.co.uk; janet.lutale@yahoo.com
[1]Department of Internal Medicine, Muhimbili University of Health and Allied Sciences, P.O BOX 65001 Dar es Salaam, Tanzania
Full list of author information is available at the end of the article

disease [6]. Presence of albuminuria indicates a state of generalized endothelial dysfunction and therefore it is a screening tool for early cardiovascular disease prevention [2]. Albuminuria is common in COPD patients and it independently correlates significantly with hypoxemia [2, 6, 7]. The aim of this study was to determine the prevalence of albuminuria and chronic obstructive pulmonary disease severity correlates in patients with COPD of African cohort. The results from this study will provide an insight on the prevalence of albuminuria in black population with COPD.

Methods
Study design and setting
This was a hospital-based cross-sectional study. It was carried out in outpatient pulmonology clinic at Muhimbili National Hospital, Dar es Salaam, Tanzania from July 2016 to December 2016. Study participants were consecutively recruited from the Muhimbili national hospital pulmonology clinic. Patients with clinical diagnosis of COPD made by the attending physician/pulmonologist, underwent spirometry examination to confirm COPD diagnosis. A total of 117 patients were assessed for the study eligibility; of these, 58 were known COPD on follow up the clinic and 59 were new clinically diagnosed COPD patients. All known COPD patients underwent repeated spirometry without bronchodilator to re-confirm COPD diagnosis, of which all 58 were re-confirmed. The new clinically diagnosed COPD patients underwent both pre and post-bronchodilator to confirm COPD diagnosis, of which 46 were confirmed COPD diagnosis. Hence a total of 104 confirmed COPD cases were enrolled for the study (see Fig. 1). Inclusion criteria were (1) Patients with confirmed COPD defined FEV1/FVC < 70% of post-bronchodilator and pre-bronchodilator spirometry for new and previous cases respectively and (2) Age 18 years and above. Exclusion criteria were patients with urinary tract infection (UTI). The study was approved by the Muhimbili University of Health and Allied Sciences Senate Research and Publication Committee. The written consent was given by study participants.

A structured questionnaire was used to collect all important information from the study participants. These included a history of symptoms suggestive of COPD; progressive dyspnoea, chronic cough and chronic sputum production and history of cigarette smoking and biomass fuel exposure. Also, a history of any known associated co-morbidities like renal, cardiovascular disease, hypertension and malignancy condition were obtained. Baseline clinical parameters; blood pressure, respiratory rate, oxygen saturation and anthropometrics; body weight, height, and BMI were measured.

Assessment of lung functions
Lung functions were assessed by means of the Easy One™ spirometer available at the clinic, manufactured by ndd Medizintechnik-Switzerland which complies with the 2005 American Thoracic Society/European Respiratory Society (ATS/ERS) spirometry standards and does not need daily calibration [8–10]. Spirometry was performed without a nose clip. Disposable mouthpieces (spirettes) were used and discarded after single use. COPD was classified as per 2015 GOLD guidelines.

Assessment of albuminuria
The urinary albumin was screened using CYBOW 12MAC microalbumin strips in a random spot urine collection. These strips were available in a local market, manufactured by DFI CO., Ltd. 542–1 Daman Ri, Jinrye-Myun Gimhae-City Gyung-Nam Korea and have been approved by Food and Drug Authority (FDA). The reagent strip is a multi-strip for rapid determination of 12 components

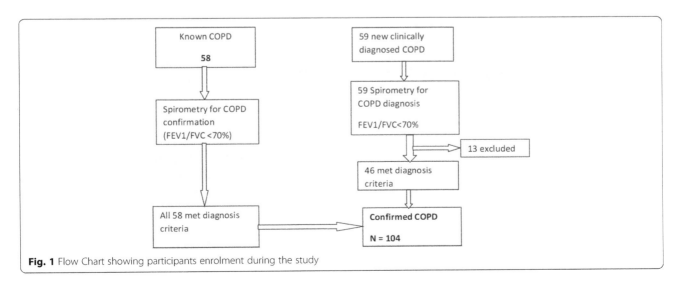

Fig. 1 Flow Chart showing participants enrolment during the study

including protein, microalbumin, creatinine, nitrite, and leucocytes. CYBOW 12MAC reagent strips are both qualitative and semi-quantitative dip strips [11]. The earlier product of the strips (CYBOW 2MAC) has been used in some studies to assess for urinary albumin [12]. The sensitivity of this test ranged from 10 mg/L to150mg/L for microalbumin and 0.9 to 26.5 mmol/L for urine creatinine. Albumin-creatinine ratio (ACR) was then calculated to determine the level of albuminuria and expressed as mg/mmol. ACR < 2 mg/mmol for male and < 2.8 mg/mmol for female defined normoalbuminuria, ACR ≥ 2.5–29.9 mg/mmol for male and ≥ 3.5–29.9 mg/mmol for female defined albuminuria and ACR ≥ 30 mg/mmol for both male and female defined macroalbuminuria/proteinuria.

Statistical analysis
The collected data were entered into EpiData 3.1 sheet and cleaned. Chi-square test and logistic regression were employed to ascertain the measure of statistical association by using SPSS version 20. The results were expressed as absolute numbers, mean plus or minus standard deviation (SD), and percentages. A p-value of < 0.05 was taken as statistically significant.

Results
A total of 104 study participants were analysed. The mean age was 58.6 ± 14.2 (SD) years, males constituted 56.7% of the study population. More than one-third of the study participants were of age range 42–83 years. More than half 56(53.8%) of study participants were smokers. Among smokers a large proportion 60.7% were heavy smokers; smoked > 10 pack year. A significant number of participants had a history of exposure to biomass fuel (firewood) and kerosene as cooking fuels; 40(38.5%) and 63 (60.6%) respectively, (Table 1).

A chronic cough and progressive dyspnoea were the most mentioned COPD related symptoms; 102/104 (98.1%) and 46/104 (44.2%) respectively. A small proportion 16/104 (15.4%) of the study participants had comorbid CVD by history. About one-third of the participants were overweight 32/104 (30.8%), and 12/104 (11.5%) obese. The proportion of study participants with elevated blood pressure on single reading was 39/104 (37.5%). (Table 2).

COPD severity
Of the 46 COPD patients assessed for COPD severity; 60.9% (95%CIs 46.1–73.9) had moderate COPD and 30.4% (95%CIs, 17.9–49.0) severe COPD (Table 3).

Predictors of COPD severity
In unadjusted regression model participants who ever smoked cigarette was significantly likely to have severe and very severe COPD (OR 11.5; 95% CI 1.3, 98.4; $p < 0.05$), however, the significance was lost when adjusted for age and gender. The participants who were; currently smokers, heavy smokers, and with a history of CVD had a non-significant increased the likelihood of severe and very severe COPD. (Table 4).

Albuminuria
All 104 study participants underwent a dipstick urinalysis test using CYBOW 12MAC strips. Out of 104 participants 31 (29.8%) had proteinuria, 25 (24.0%) albuminuria, and 48(46.2%) normoalbuminuria. No urine sample had features of urinary tract infections. Therefore, the prevalence of albuminuria was 24%. Abnormal urine albumin (albuminuria and proteinuria) was prevalent in all study participants with CVD (Table 5).

Table 1 Social demographic characteristics of study participants ($N = 104$)

Variables		n (%)
Age groups (yrs.)		
28–41		11 (10)
42–55		33 (32)
56–69		35 (34)
70–83		22 (21)
> 84		3 (3)
Mean Age (SD)		58.63 ± 14.192
Sex		
Females		45 (43.3)
Males		59 (56.7)
Marital Status		
Single		10 (10)
Married		82 (79)
Divorced		1 (1)
Widow/Widower		11 (10)
Occupation		
Domestic/office work		40 (38.5)
Farmers/peasants		43 (41.3)
Industry		20 (19.2)
Others		1 (1.0)
Cigarette smoking:	Yes	56 (53.8)
Pack year	≤ 10 pack year	22 (39.3)
	> 10 pack year	34 (60.7)
Biomass fuel exposure:	Firewood	40 (38.5)
	Charcoal	34 (32.7)
	Kerosene	63 (60.6)

Table 2 Clinical characteristics of the study participants (N = 104)

Variables	Categories	n (%)
History suggestive of COPD	Progressive dyspnoea	46 (44.2)
	Chronic cough	102 (98.1)
	Chronic sputum production	13 (12.5)
History of Co-morbidities	Hypertension	1 (0.96)
	Cardiovascular disease	16 (15.4)
[b]Body Mass Index (BMI) in Kg/M^2	Underweight (< 18.8)	10 (9.6)
	Normal weight (18.5–24.9)	50 (48.1)
	Overweight (25–29.9)	32 (30.8)
	Obesity (> 30)	12 (11.5)
[a]Blood pressure(mmHg): Systolic BP	Elevated (> 140)	21 (20.2)
Diastolic BP	Elevated (> 90)	18 (17.3)
Oxygen saturation %	Normal (92–100)	104 (100)

[a]BP is based on a single reading and therefore not diagnostic for hypertension
[b]Anthropometrics measured and categorized according to WHO

COPD severity and albuminuria

Of the 46 participants assessed for COPD severity, albuminuria moderately significantly associated with COPD severity or with the lower level of FEV1% predicted, $p = 0.049$; ($0.049 < p < 0.05$). (Table 6).

Discussion

This was a hospital-based cross-section study of 104 black Africans patients with COPD determining the prevalence of albuminuria and COPD severity correlates. Regarding COPD severity in the current study, a large proportion of study participants had moderate to severe COPD according to GOLD classification; 60.9% (95% [CI], 17.9–49.0] and 30.4, 95% [CI], 46.1–73.9) respectively. In a study by *Mehmood K* et al. the COPD was also classified according to GOLD criteria and the majority of study participants were in stage III (severe) and above; 55.7% [2]. This discrepancy can be accounted for by differences in study design and characteristics of study population between the two studies in respect to cigarette smoking. In the current study, the proportion of cigarette smoking was 53.8% while in the study by Mehmood K et al. all study participants were heavy smokers of >10pack year.

Albuminuria prevalence in the current study was 24% (95% [CI], 17.0–33.0) while abnormal urine albumin

Table 3 Post bronchodilator Spirometry assessing COPD severity (N = 46)

Variables (FEV1)	n (%)	95%CI
Mild (FEV1 ≥ 80%)	2 (4.3)	0–10.4
Moderate (50 ≤ FEV1 < 80%)	28 (60.9)	46.1–73.9
Severe (30 ≤ FEV1 < 50%)	14 (30.4)	17.9–49.0
Very severe (FEV1 < 30%)	2 (4.3)	0–14.7

(albuminuria and proteinuria) was prevalent in all study participants with CVD. The presence of CVD was assessed through history alone. Of 104 study participants, 16/104 (15.5%) had CVD, of which 12 participants had the coronary arterial disease, 3 resolved stroke, and 1 hypertensive heart disease. More extra-pulmonary co-morbidities could have been detected if laboratory markers were to be used, which was not the case in the current study. In a prospective cohort study conducted in India by *Mehmood K* et al. on albuminuria and hypoxemia in patients with COPD in 97 COPD smokers versus 94 non-COPD smokers as a controls over a period of 2 years; albuminuria was found to be more frequent in COPD smokers compared to smokers without COPD (20.6%versus 7.4% $p = 0.007$). The confounding co-morbidities like renal disease, diabetes, and cardiovascular disease were excluded using laboratory biomarkers and relevant history [2]. In the current study comorbid CVD, renal and diabetes were excluded by history only and hence might explain the differences in albuminuria prevalence.

The prevalence of albuminuria in the current study was similar to the prevalence of albuminuria found in a study done in Spain by *Ciro Casanova* et al. on albuminuria and hypoxemia in COPD patients (129 COPD cases versus 51 controls). In that study, the prevalence of albuminuria was 24% in patients with COPD and smoking history versus 6% in non-COPD smokers control; ($p = 0.005$), and all confounding co-morbidities were excluded using history and laboratory biomarkers [13].

In the current study, the COPD severity and albuminuria were significantly inversely related; the risk of albuminuria increased moderately significantly with COPD severity or the lower level of FEV1% predicted, ($p = 0.049$). All COPD patients with normoalbuminuria

Table 4 Predictors of severe and very severe COPD among study participants assessed for COPD severity (N = 46)

Predictors	Test group	Comparative	OR	95% CI	P value
Smoking History	Ever smoker	Never smoker	11.5	1.3–98.4	0.026
Smoking status	Currently smoker	Former smoker	1.7	0.4–6.9	0.465
Pack-years smok.	≥10 - Heavy smoker	< 10- non-heavy	2.0	0.3–12.9	0.466
History of CVD	Yes	No	2.2	0.5–10.2	0.327

had GOLD stage I (mild) and II (moderate). A 12-year follow-up study in Norway by *Solfrid Romundstad* et al. on COPD and albuminuria in 53,129 patients showed that the risk for albuminuria increased significantly at lower levels of FEV1% predicted ($p = 0.001$). The majority (95.3%) of COPD patients without albuminuria had less severe COPD stages (GOLD stage of I and II) which is comparable to the findings in the current study [14].

Albuminuria in patients with COPD is also common in other associated co-morbidities including Chronic kidney disease (CKD), Pulmonary arterial hypertension (PAH), and atherosclerosis as a result of systemic endothelial dysfunction. Patients with COPD have shown to have endothelial injury pathways in the lungs and kidneys [15]. One study reported the evidence of the glomerular damage by increased ACR; (0.80 mg/mmol versus 0.46 mg/mmol) in COPD and non-COPD patients respectively [16].

Studies elsewhere have shown a significantly increased frequency of renal injury in COPD population compared to the non-COPD population. CKD comorbidity occurs frequently in COPD patients. For instance, one case-control study reported a significant CKD prevalence in COPD compared to non-COPD groups; (31% vs 8% $p < 0.001$) based on estimated glomerular filtration rate (eGFRCr), and (53% vs 15% $p < 0.001$) based on estimated cystatin C levels (eGFRCys). The odds ratio was 4.91 (95% CI, 1.94–12.46, $P = 0.0008$) and 6.30 (95% CI, 2.99–13.26, $P = 0.0001$) based on eGFRCr and eGFRCys respectively [17]. A systematic review and meta-analysis of observational studies reported increased odds of developing CKD (OR 2.20; 95% CI 1.83, 2.65) among COPD subjects compared to non-COPD subjects [18].

In this current study, the blood biomarkers for CKD, and other comorbidities were not carried out to ascertain their presence in COPD patients. A longitudinal study with thorough screening for these co-morbidities in order to explain their temporal association with COPD in the context of African patient cohort population is necessary, however.

This paper addressed the presence of albuminuria among African COPD patient cohort. COPD racial differences have not been well elucidated in the racial context. Literature is uncertain about COPD racial disparity due to differences in socioeconomic determinants risks for COPD. Limited available evidence reported that African-American with COPD is significantly younger and are less smoker. However, Africa-Americas have less emphysema than non-Hispanic Whites (NHW) but the same degree of airway disease. Furthermore, women of Africa-America ethnicity appear to be at higher risk of developing COPD than whites [19, 20].

It is common for people in low and middle-income countries including Africa to be exposed to biomass fuel/indoor pollution since childhood. Hence the mean age of COPD presentation in Africa is at the younger age some studies reported 35–45 years but also can be detected as early as the late teenage years. Women are the main cooks in the family and therefore are potentially vulnerable to particulate matters from biomass combustions. Young children less than 5 years of age do spend much time with their mothers hence are relatively equally exposed to biomass combustions [21–24]. Exposure to biomass fuel combustions is associated with increased prevalence of respiratory symptoms, reduced lung function and development COPD [25–27]. The domestic exposure to biomass fuel smoke in Tanzania and other African countries is alarmingly high. For instance, in Sub-Saharan Africa, the percentage of households using wood fuel varies from 86 to 99% in rural areas and 26–96% in urban areas. Overall 94% of African rural and 73% urban population used wood fuel (firewood and charcoal) as the primary source of energy [28].

Table 5 Prevalence of albuminuria (ACR) and its association with CVD among the study participants (N = 104)

		Urine albumin to creatinine ratio (ACR)			
		Normoalbuminuria	Albuminuria	Proteinuria	
		48 (46.2)	25 (24)	31 (29.8)	$p < 0.001$
		CI (36.2–55.5)	CI (17–33)	CI (21.5–37.5)	
History of CVD	Yes 16(100)	0 (0.0)	3 (18.8)	13 (81.2)	
	No 88(100)	48 (54.5)	22 (25.0)	18 (20.5)	

Table 6 Association between albuminuria and COPD severity of the 46 participants assessed for COPD severity (N = 46)

VARIABLES	Total n (%)	Urine albumin to creatinine ratio (ACR)			P-value
		Normal n (%)	Micro n (%)	Macro n (%)	
Mild FEV1 ≥ 80%)	2 (4.3)	1 (50.0)	0 (0.0)	1 (50.0)	0.049
Moderate 50 ≤ FEV1 < 80%)	28 (60.9)	12 (42.9)	12 (42.9)	4 (14.3)	
Severe (30 ≤ FEV1 < 50%)	14 (30.4)	0 (0.0)	10 (71.4)	4 (28.6)	
Very severe (FEV1 < 30%)	2 (4.3)	0 (0.0)	2 (100.0)	0 (0.0)	
TOTAL n (%)	46	13	24	9	

Tanzania energy balance is dominated by biomass-based fuels, especially wood fuel (firewood and charcoal) which accounts for > 90% of primary energy supply [28]. More than 9 in 10 households (94%) use biomass fuels for cooking, heating, and lighting. Regarding tobacco use, less than 1 % of women (0.6%) smoke any tobacco while 14% of men smoke tobacco of which most of them smoke cigarettes on a daily basis [29]. Therefore, apart from tobacco smoking, the use of biomass fuels may be one of the important risk factors for COPD in Tanzania. The prevalence of COPD in Tanzania was conducted among 496 participants aged > 35 years in a rural setting by using spirometry diagnosis. Indoor and outdoor carbon monoxide (CO) levels from biomass fuel combustions were also measured. The overall prevalence of COPD was 17.5% of which 21.7% in males and 12.9% in females [30].

Study limitations

The study had the following limitations; first, Chronic obstructive pulmonary disease severity classification was done only in newly diagnosed patients; this could underestimate it association with albuminuria in the context of sample size studied. For known COPD patients, it was difficult to stop their medications and arrange consecutively 2 days' visits for assessing disease severity. Second, the use of history alone to describe the existence of comorbidity might have underestimated the existence of other conditions may cause albuminuria. A budget was not sufficient to cater for blood biomarker analysis.

Conclusion

A large proportion of study participants who were assed for COPD severity had moderate and severe COPD. Albuminuria was prevalent in patients with chronic obstructive pulmonary disease and it increased significantly with COPD severity. All study participants with CVD had abnormal urine albumin (albuminuria and proteinuria). Screening for albuminuria in COPD patients can be used as an early marker of CVD risk and therefore prevention strategies can be planned. A longitudinal study to further explain the pattern of albuminuria among the black population is highly needed in order to have a better comparison with previous studies done among Caucasian and Oriental populations.

Abbreviations

ACR: Albumin Creatinine ratio; ATS: American Thoracic Society; BMI: Body Mass Index; BP: Blood Pressure; CKD: Chronic Kidney Disease; COPD: Chronic Obstructive Pulmonary Disease; CVD: Cardiovascular Disease; eGFRCr: Estimated Glomerular Filtration Rate; eGFRCys: Estimated Cystatin C; ERS: European Respiratory Society; FEV1: Forced Expiratory Volume in 1 second; FVC: Forced Vital Capacity; MI: Myocardial Infarction; MNH: Muhimbili National Hospital; PAH: Pulmonary arterial hypertension; SPSS: Statistical Package for the Social Sciences; UK: United Kingdom; USA: United State of America; UTI: Urinary Tract Infections

Acknowledgments

We are grateful to Almighty God for His Everlasting Mercy throughout the entire duration of this study. We are thankful to all study participants/patients who consented to the study. We thank all staffs of Internal Medicine of the Muhimbili University of Health and Allied Sciences, for their different opinions during results dissemination. We are thankful for the following for their technical assistance in this study; Dr. Simon Mamuya – Head department of environment science – school of public health and social sciences of the Muhimbili University of Health and Allied Sciences for lending us a spirometer, Dr. R. Mpembeni – Public health specialist and biostatistician at school of public health and social sciences of the Muhimbili University of Health and Allied Sciences and Mr. Amandus Kimario – independent statistician and mathematician – amanduskimario@gmail.com for their statistical assistance. We thank Dr. Hussein Mwanga – Occupational Health Physician at School of Public Health and Social Sciences of the Muhimbili University of Health and Allied Sciences, Dr. Paulina Chale – Pulmonologist at the Muhimbili National Hospital and Sr. Anneth Kweyunga – a nurse at pulmonary functions laboratory of the Muhimbili National Hospital.

Funding

I requested and granted a supporting fund during data collection and analysis from my employer - Muhimbili National Hospital, P.O Box 65000, Dar es Salaam, Tanzania.

Authors' contributions

Both authors have read and approved the manuscript. 1. FKS. This is my original work as a partial fulfillment of the requirements for the Degree of Master of Medicine (Internal Medicine) of Muhimbili University of Health and Allied Sciences. I fully involved in the conception, development, data collection, analysis and report writing of this study. My manuscript was selected for presentation at two scientific conferences; the Muhimbili university annual scientific conference of 2017, and the Tanzania health summit of 2017. 2. JL. She is a consultant physician/endocrinologist, and Professor of Medicine at the department of internal medicine of the Muhimbili University of Health and Allied Sciences. She was involved in study conception, methodology, and interpretation of the results. She was also involved in manuscript preparation.

Competing interests
The authors declare that they have no competing interests (declaration form are available for each author in case they are needed).

Author details
[1]Department of Internal Medicine, Muhimbili University of Health and Allied Sciences, P.O BOX 65001 Dar es Salaam, Tanzania. [2]Department of Internal Medicine, Muhimbili National Hospital, P.o box 14087 Dar es Salaam, Tanzania. [3]Tokyo Medical and Dental University, 1-5-45 Yushima, Bunkyo-ku, Tokyo 113-8510, Japan.

References
1. World Health Organization. World health statistics 2008. Geneva: World Health Organization; 2008. http://www.who.int/iris/handle/10665/43890.
2. Mehmood K, Sofi FA. Microalbuminuria and hypoxemia in patients with COPD. J Pulm Respir Med. 2015; https://doi.org/10.4172/2161-105X.1000280.
3. Barr RG, Celli BR, Mannino DM, Petty T, Rennard SI, Sciurba FC, et al. Comorbidities, patient knowledge, and disease management in a national sample of patients with COPD. Am J Med. 2009;122(4):348–55.
4. Anant RC, Patel JR, et al. Extrapulmonary comorbidities in chronic obstructive pulmonary disease: State of the art. Expert Rev Respir Med. 2011;5(5):647–62.
5. de Lucas-Ramos P, Izquierdo-Alonso JL, Rodriguez-Gonzalez Moro JM, Frances JF, Lozano PV, Bellón-Cano JM. Chronic obstructive pulmonary disease as a cardiovascular risk factor – result from a case control (CONSISTE study). Int J Chron Obstruct Pulmon Dis. 2012; https://doi.org/10.2147/COPD.S36222.
6. Casanova C, de Torres JP, Navarro J, Aguirre-Jaíme A, Toledo P, Cordoba E, et al. Microalbuminuria and hypoxemia in patients with chronic obstructive pulmonary disease. Am J Respir Crit Care Med. 2010;182(8):1004–10.
7. Kumar R. Study of Microalbuminuria in Patients with Stable COPD. Ann Int Med Dent Res. 2016; https://doi.org/10.21276/aimdr.2016.2.3.24.
8. Skloot GS, Edwards NT, Enright PL. Four-year calibration stability of the EasyOne portable spirometer. Respir Care. 2010;55(7):873–7.
9. Barr RG, Stemple KJ, Mesia-Vela S, Basner RC, Derk SJ, Henneberger PK, et al. Reproducibility and validity of a handheld spirometer. Respir Care. 2008; 53(4):433–41.
10. Walters JAE, Wood-Baker R, Walls J, Johns DP. Stability of the EasyOne ultrasonic spirometer for use in general practice. Respirology. 2006;11(3): 306–10.
11. DFI Care. www.dficare.com/en/bbs/board.php?bo_table=cybow_en&wr_id= 5. Accessed 18 July 2018.
12. Efundem NT, Assob JCN, Feteh VF, Choukem SP. Prevalence and associations of microalbuminuria in proteinuria-negative patients with type 2 diabetes in two regional hospitals in Cameroon: A cross-sectional study. BMC Res Notes. 2017;10(1):6–10. https://doi.org/10.1186/s13104-017-2804-5.
13. Casanova C, Celli BR. Microalbuminuria as a potential novel cardiovascular biomarker in patients with COPD. Eur Respir J. 2014;43(4):951–3.
14. Romundstad S, Naustdal T, Romundstad PR, Sorger H, Langhammer A. COPD and microalbuminuria: a 12-year follow-up study. Eur Respir J. 2014; 43(4):1042–50.
15. Polverino F, Celli BR, Owen CA. COPD as an endothelial disorder: endothelial injury linking lesions in the lungs and other organs. Pulm Circ. 2018;8(1):1–18.
16. John M, Hussain S, Prayle A, Simms R, Cockcroft JR, Bolton CE. Target renal damage: the microvascular associations of increased aortic stiffness in patients with COPD. Respir Res. 2013; https://doi.org/10.1186/1465-9921-14-31.
17. Yoshizawa T, Hosokawa Y, Hashimoto S, Okada K, Furuichi S, Ishiguro T, et al. Prevalence of chronic kidney diseases in patients with chronic obstructive pulmonary disease: assessment based on glomerular filtration rate estimated from creatinine and cystatin C levels. Int J Chron Obstruct Pulmon Dis. 2015;10:1283–9.
18. Gaddam S, Gunukula SK, Lohr JW, Arora P. Prevalence of chronic kidney disease in patients with chronic obstructive pulmonary disease: a systematic review and meta-analysis. BMC Pulm Med. 2016;16(1):158.
19. Hansel NN, Washko GR, Foreman MG, Han MK, Hoffman EA, Demeo DL, et al. Racial differences in CT phenotypes in COPD. COPD J Chronic Obstr Pulm Dis. 2013;10(1):20–7.
20. Kamil F, Pinzon I, Foreman MG. Sex and race factors in early-onset COPD. Curr Opin Pulm Med. 2013;19(2):140–4.
21. Gordon S, Bruce N, Grigg J, Hibberd P, Kurmi O, Lam K, et al. Respiratory risks from household air pollution in low and middle income countries. Lancet Respir Med. 2014;2(10):823–60.
22. Van Gemert F, Kirenga B, Chavannes N, Kamya M, Luzige S, Musinguzi P, et al. Prevalence of chronic obstructive pulmonary disease and associated risk factors in Uganda (FRESH AIR Uganda): a prospective cross-sectional observational study. Lancet Glob Health. 2015;3(1):e44–51.
23. Salvi S. The silent epidemic of COPD in Africa. Lancet Glob Health. 2015;3(1): e6–7. https://doi.org/10.1016/S2214-109X(14)70359-6.
24. Kurmi OP, Devereux GS, Smith WCS, Semple S, Steiner MFC, Simkhada P, et al. Reduced lung function due to biomass smoke exposure in young adults in rural Nepal. Eur Respir J. 2013;41(1):25–30.
25. da Silva LFF, Saldiva SRDM, Saldiva PHN, Dolhnikoff M. Impaired lung function in individuals chronically exposed to biomass combustion. Environ Res. 2012;112:111–7.
26. Kilabuko JH, Nakai S. Effects of cooking fuels on acute respiratory infections in children in Tanzania. Int J Environ Res Public Health. 2007;4(4):283–8.
27. Hu G, Zhou Y, Tian J, Yao W, Li J, Li B, et al. Risk of COPD from exposure to biomass smoke: A metaanalysis. Chest. 2010;138(1):20–31. https://doi.org/10.1378/chest.08-2114.
28. Lusambo LP. Household Energy Consumption Patterns in Tanzania. J Ecosyst Ecography. 2016;01 https://doi.org/10.4172/2157-7625.S5-007.
29. Ministry of Health, Community Development, Gender, Elderly and Children (MoHCDGEC) [Tanzania Mainland], Ministry of Health (MoH) [Zanzibar], National Bureau of Statistics (NBS), Office of the Chief Government Statistician (OCGS), and ICF. Tanzania Demographic and Health Survey and Malaria Indicator Survey (TDHS-MIS) 2015-16. Dar es Salaam, Tanzania, and Rockville, Maryland, USA: MoHCDGEC, MoH, NBS, OCGS, and ICF. 2016.
30. Magitta NF, Walker RW, Apte KK, Shimwela MD, Mwaiselage JD, Sanga AA, et al. Prevalence, risk factors and clinical correlates of COPD in a rural setting in Tanzania. Eur Respir J. 2018;51(2) https://doi.org/10.1183/13993003.00182-2017.

Adherence to inhaled therapy and its impact on chronic obstructive pulmonary disease (COPD)

Magdalena Humenberger[1,2], Andreas Horner[1,2]*, Anna Labek[3], Bernhard Kaiser[3], Rupert Frechinger[4], Constanze Brock[1], Petra Lichtenberger[1] and Bernd Lamprecht[1,2]

Abstract

Background: COPD is a treatable disease with increasing prevalence worldwide. Treatment aims to stop disease progression, to improve quality of life, and to reduce exacerbations. We aimed to evaluate the association of the stage of COPD on adherence to inhaled therapy and the relationship between adherence and COPD exacerbations.

Methods: A retrospective analysis of patients hospitalized for acute exacerbation of COPD in a tertiary care hospital in Upper Austria and discharged with a guideline conform inhaled therapy was performed. Follow-up data on medical utilization was recorded for the subsequent 24 months. Adherence to inhaled therapy was defined according to the percentage of prescribed inhalers dispensed to the patient and classified as complete (> 80%), partial (50–80%) or low (< 50%).

Results: Out of 357 patients, 65.8% were male with a mean age of 66.5 years and a mean FEV_1 of 55.0%pred. Overall, 35.3% were current smokers, and only 3.9% were never-smokers. In 77.0% inhaled triple therapy (LAMA + LABA + ICS) was prescribed. 33.6% showed complete adherence to their therapy (33.2% in men, 34.4% in women), with a mean age of 67.0 years. Mean medication possession ratio by GOLD spirometry class I – IV were 0.486, 0.534, 0.609 and 0.755, respectively ($p = 0.002$). Hence, subjects with complete adherence to therapy had a significantly lower FEV_1 compared to those with low adherence (49.2%pred. vs 59.2%pred., respectively; $p < 0.001$).
The risk of exacerbations leading to hospitalization was 10-fold higher in GOLD spirometry class IV compared to GOLD spirometry class I, which was even more evident in multivariate analysis (OR 13.62).

Conclusion: Complete adherence to inhaled therapy was only seen in 33.6% and was higher among those with more severe COPD.

Keywords: Chronic obstructive pulmonary disease, Adherence, Inhaled therapy

Background

Chronic obstructive pulmonary disease (COPD) is an underdiagnosed, preventable and treatable disease with increasing prevalence worldwide. It has been a major problem over decades and will be a challenge within the twenty-first century [1–4].

To reduce mortality in COPD patients, lower the economic and clinical burden and to improve quality of life, it is crucial to prevent disease progression, reduce exacerbation rates and focus on the treatment of comorbidities [5–9]. Adherence to inhaled therapy appears to have significant impact on treatment goals. Therefore, it is crucial to increase the patients' and physicians' awareness concerning this topic.

Only few data are available on adherence and influencing factors. A meta-analysis of over 50 years of research on adherence shows an association between adherence and social and emotional resources [10, 11]. In a study

---

* Correspondence: Andreas.Horner@kepleruniklinikum.at
[1]Department of Pulmonology, Kepler University Hospital, Krankenhausstrasse 9, A4021, Linz, Austria
[2]Faculty of Medicine, Johannes-Kepler-University, Linz, Austria
Full list of author information is available at the end of the article

of patients including those with COPD by Balkrishnan et al., the numbers of hospitalization rates and physician visits were reduced in patients who were adherent to prescribed therapy [12].

Nonadherence is a tremendous problem in the treatment of patients in general [13]. Furthermore, adherence in COPD patients is particularly poor and reported nonadherence rates range from 50 to 80% [14–16].

In patients with COPD, nonadherence to inhaled therapy is caused by several factors and could lead to high mortality and morbidity as well as hospitalizations and a reduced quality of life [14, 17–21]. Thus, the consequences of nonadherence, clinically and economically, are neither completely obvious nor fully understood, but there is an association between nonadherence and increasing healthcare costs [17, 19, 22, 23].

The aim of this retrospective data analysis was to evaluate the association of the stage of COPD on adherence and the relationship between adherence and COPD exacerbations. We hypothesized, that better adherence is associated with less COPD exacerbations leading to hospitalization.

Methods

The primary outcome parameter of this retrospective analysis was to describe the characteristics of an Upper Austrian COPD cohort based upon degree of adherence to inhaled therapy and its association with spirometrically defined COPD stages. Moreover, we explored adherence as a risk factor for the poor outcome of exacerbation risk and we described further influencing factors on adherence.

Data of patients hospitalized for COPD exacerbations at the department for pulmonology in a tertiary care hospital in Upper Austria and discharged with a guideline conform inhaled therapy in 2012 were analyzed. The following observation period was 24 months. Patients who died within the first six months of the observation period were excluded due to the short observation period. However, patients who died afterwards but during the observation period, were included until death. Hence, the observation period was shorter in these patients and it was assumed that these individuals would have continued with the same adherence routine prior to their death.

Inclusion criteria were age > 40 years, COPD diagnosis (GOLD spirometry class I – IV) based on lung function testing (post-bronchodilator $FEV_1/FVC < 70\%$) and a prescribed permanent inhaled therapy. Inhaled therapy was prescribed according to the risk assessment (A – D) as proposed in the GOLD report 2011 [24].

All patients discharged in 2012 were screened looking for a diagnosis with ICD-10-Code 44.0–44.9 at time of discharge. COPD diagnosis and stage were verified by the most recent lung function performed in 2012. Based on lung function criteria, patients with partial post-bronchodilator reversibility were included. However, patients with complete reversibility ($\Delta FEV_1 > 12\%$, or > 0.2 l) were excluded.

Adherence to inhaled therapy, based on the 24 months observation period, was defined according to the percentage of prescribed inhalers dispensed to the patient and classified as follows: Complete adherence (> 80%), partial adherence (50–80%) and low adherence (< 50%). 80% is a frequently used threshold for the differentiation of adherence (high or low) [23]. We decided to further divide the participants according to adherence into three groups to show more precise results in the low adherence group (partial and low adherence).

Additionally, adherence was reported as mean medication possession ratio (MPR) [25], and categorized by sex, $FEV_1\%pred$, smoking status and inhaled therapy. The MPR was calculated using the ratio of personal adherence months to the whole observation period of each participant.

For a permanent inhaled therapy, one medical prescription per month for each device was assumed for complete adherence. Complete data therefore was provided by the Upper Austrian Health Insurance (OÖGKK).

Statistical analysis was performed using SAS 9.3. Figures and tables were created with Microsoft Excel 2016. The adherence category (complete, partial, low) was the underlying and central variable in all statistical analyses performed in this study. The association between adherence and most important covariates (age, sex, $FEV_1\%pred$, smoking status) is shown in a descriptive overview using means and proportions.

Nonparametric Chi-square test, Mann-Whitney U test and t-test were used to investigate differences between groups according to adherence category.

COPD control was assessed using the rate of severe exacerbations leading to hospitalization per year. Concerning exacerbations leading to hospitalization a binary univariate and multivariate logistic regression analysis was performed, based on odds ratios, to determine the influence of several factors (age, sex, $FEV_1\%pred$, smoking status, adherence) on exacerbation rates.

Results are mainly expressed as frequencies or as mean. Statistical significance was defined as $p < 0.05$ for all analyses in this study.

Results

Out of 592 hospitalized patients with COPD and discharged with a guideline conform inhaled therapy in 2012, complete data was available of 476 cases in the database of the Upper Austrian Health Insurance

(OÖGKK). 54 subjects died within 6 months after discharge and 65 had no prescription for permanent inhaled medication and were therefore excluded (Fig. 1).

Out of 357 patients, 65.8% were male and 34.2% were female, with a mean age of 66.5 years and a mean FEV_1 of 55.0%pred. 55% had GOLD spirometry class I – II COPD and 45% had GOLD spirometry class III – IV COPD. Overall, 35.3% were current smokers, 57.4% former smokers and only 3.9% were never smokers. In 77.0% of all cases, inhaled triple therapy (LAMA + LABA + ICS) was prescribed at the time of discharge (for other inhaled therapies see Table 1). 74.2% had an additional prescription for SAMA and/or SABA, as inhaled therapy on demand. 17% of all subjects were on long-term oxygen therapy. There was no significant difference between men and women concerning age, FEV_1, smoking status or long-term oxygen therapy. However, significantly more male patients were treated with triple therapy (83.0% vs 65.6%; $p < 0.001$).

33.6% of 357 patients showed complete adherence to their therapy (33.2% in men, 34.4% in women), with a mean age of 67.0 years and a mean FEV_1 of 49.2% predSubjects with complete adherence to therapy had a significantly lower FEV_1 compared to those with low adherence (49.2%pred. vs 59.2%pred., respectively; $p < 0.001$). (for further baseline characteristics by adherence see Table 2).

Among all 357 patients, complete adherence was noted in 44.9% of GOLD spirometry category IV participants, while only 19.4% of GOLD spirometry category I were noted to be completely adherent (Fig. 2).

Using the medication possession ratio (MPR), to describe adherence, the overall mean MPR was 0.565. Hence, on average patients were adherent in 56.5% of all months during the observation period.

Male patient had slightly higher MPRs than females (0.568 vs 0.558, respectively; $p = 0.883$). MPRs by GOLD spirometry class I – IV were 0.486, 0.534, 0.609 and 0.755, respectively. These differences were statistically highly significant ($p = 0.002$). Former smokers had a higher mean

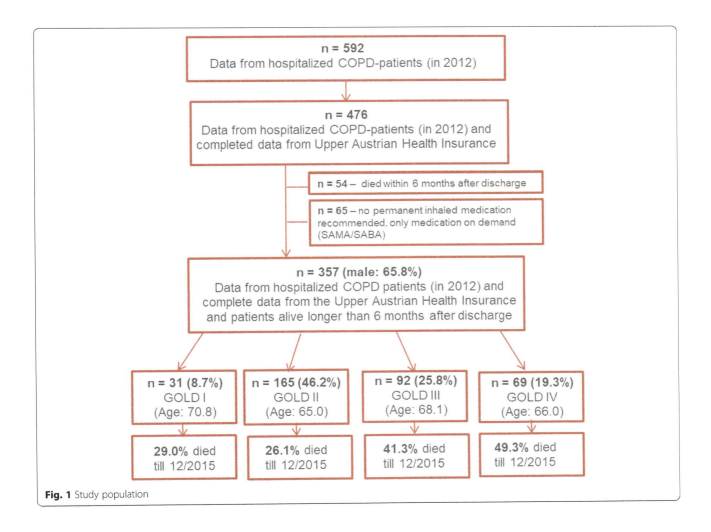

Fig. 1 Study population

Table 1 Characteristics of the participants at baseline

	All	Female	Male	p-value
n (%)	357	122 (34.2)	235 (65.8)	
Age in year, mean (SD)	66.5 (10.6)	66.1 (11.1)	66.7 (10.0)	0.580
FEV_1%pred., mean (SD)	55.0 (18.5)	58.0 (19.4)	53.4 (17.9)	0.067
Smoking status, n (%)				
Current smoker	126 (35.3)	43 (35.3)	83 (35.3)	0.982
Former smoker	205 (57.4)	67 (54.9)	138 (58.7)	0.471
Never smoker	14 (3.9)	8 (6.5)	6 (2.6)	0.065
No information	12 (3.4)	4 (3.3)	8 (3.4)	
Inhaled Therapy, n (%)				
LAMA only	10 (2.8)	3 (2.5)	7 (3.0)	0.777
LABA only	3 (0.8)	2 (1.6)	1 (0.4)	0.233
LABA + ICS	64 (17.9)	34 (27.9)	30 (12.8)	< 0.001
LAMA + LABA + ICS	275 (77.0)	80 (65.6)	195 (83.0)	< 0.001
LABA + LAMA	5 (1.4)	3 (2.5)	2 (0.9)	0.952
LTOT, n (%)	60 (17.0)	26 (21.5)	34 (14.7)	0.101

LAMA – long-acting muscarinic antagonist; LABA – long-acting beta-adrenoceptor agonist; ICS – inhaled corticosteroid; LTOT – long-term oxygen therapy

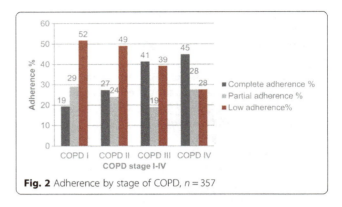

Fig. 2 Adherence by stage of COPD, n = 357

MPR (0.610) compared to smokers (0.510) and never smokers (0.464) (p = 0.021). Patients on triple therapy (LABA + LAMA + ICS) were, statistically not significant, more adherent compared to patients on other therapy regimes (0.584 vs 0.499, respectively; p = 0.089).

Table 3 shows the results of a binary univariate and multivariate logistic regression analysis of factors independently associated with exacerbations leading to hospitalizations during the observation period. The risk of exacerbations leading to hospitalization was 10-fold higher in GOLD stage IV compared to GOLD stage I (OR 10.69; CI 2.99; 38.24) in univariate analysis. In the univariate and multivariate analysis, an inverse association between adherence to therapy and exacerbations leading to hospitalization was observed. Subjects with low adherence had a reduced risk of exacerbations (not significant in multivariate analysis; OR 0.58; 95% CI (0.33; 1.02)); for details see Table 3.

Discussion

In our retrospective data analysis, we were able to show that adherence to inhaled therapy in COPD patients is generally low. Complete adherence to inhaled therapy was only seen in 33.6%. Factors associated with better adherence were age, former smoking, and more severe airflow limitation.

In prior studies adherence in COPD ranged between 70 to 90% in several clinical trials; however, in clinical practice, adherence is lower within the range of 10–40%, irrespective of the probable insufficient or incorrect use of the device [15, 26, 27].

We could show that adherence to inhaled therapy was higher in GOLD spirometry class III – IV COPD and was highest in patients with GOLD spirometry class IV COPD. This may be due to the fact, that with advanced disease and a higher burden of symptoms, the inhaled medication is perceived more necessary by the patient. The association between symptom relief and medication use may be a potent trigger for better adherence [16]. Contrariwise, lack of clinical symptoms can be

Table 2 Baseline characteristics of patients by adherence; n = 357

	Complete adherence (> 80%)	Partial adherence (50–80%)	Low adherence (< 50%)	All	p-value
n (%)	120 (33.6)	85 (23.8)	152 (42.6)	357	
Sex, n (%)					0.865
Female (%, n = 122)	42 (34.4)	27 (22.1)	53 (43.5)	122	
Male (%, n = 235)	78 (33.2)	58 (24.7)	99 (42.1)	235	
Age in years, mean (SD)	67.0 (9.2)	66.7 (9.9)	66.0 (11.5)	66.5 (10.4)	0.920
FEV_1%pred, mean (SD)	49.2 (17.6)	56.0 (18.3)	59.2 (18.2)	55.0 (18.5)	< 0.001
Smoking status, n (%)					0.081
Current smoker	33 (27.5)	31 (36.5)	62 (40.8)	126 (35.3)	
Former smoker	81 (67.5)	48 (56.5)	76 (50.0)	205 (57.4)	
Never smoker	3 (2.5)	3 (3.5)	8 (5.3)	14 (3.9)	
No information	3 (2.5)	3 (3.5)	6 (3.9)	12 (3.4)	

Table 3 Parameters independently associated with severe exacerbations/ hospitalizations; n = 357

	OR (95% CI) crude	OR (95% CI) adjusted
Gender		
Female	Reference	Reference
Male	0.89 (0.58; 1.38)	0.95 (0.57; 1.57)
Age (years)		
< 50	Reference	Reference
50–60	1.68 (0.56; 5.06)	0.87 (0.26; 2.90)
60–70	2.12 (0.74; 6.07)	1.00 (0.32; 3.13)
> 70	1.12 (0.39; 3.21)	0.71 (0.22; 2.24)
FEV_1		
> 80% pred.	Reference	Reference
50–80% pred.	0.86 (0.39; 1.88)	0.94 (0.40; 2.24)
30–50% pred.	2.09 (0.92; 4.75)	2.50 (1.02; 6.13)
< 30% pred.	10.69 (2.99; 38.24)	13.62 (3.11; 59.63)
Smoking status		
Current smoker	Reference	Reference
Former smoker	1.11 (0.71; 1.73)	1.19 (0.70; 2.02)
Never smoker	0.67 (0.21; 2.12)	0.82 (0.23; 2.92)
Adherence to therapy		
Complete (≥ 80%)	Reference	Reference
Partial (50–80%)	0.77 (0.44; 1.35)	0.95 (0.50; 1.78)
Low (< 50%)	0.44 (0.27; 0.71)	0.58 (0.33; 1.02)

misinterpreted and can lead to treatment interruption and cessation [26]. This is in accordance with previous studies, where adherence was better in patients with more severe disease [28, 29].

In our univariate and multivariate analysis, the risk of exacerbations leading to hospitalization was more than 10-fold higher in GOLD stage IV compared to GOLD stage I. Patients with low adherence tended to have a reduced risk for exacerbations leading to hospitalization (OR 0.58; 0.33, 1.02; not significant in multivariate analysis).

In previous research, better adherence in COPD patients was associated with a reduced risk for exacerbations and health care utilization [18, 30].

This paradoxical result may be caused by other influencing factors as this trend was considerably less pronounced and statistically not significant in multivariate compared to univariate analysis. Furthermore, the non-adherent patients predominately had GOLD spirometry class I – II COPD with less impairment of lung function, probably less symptoms and better quality of life.

Adherence in COPD patients is complex and multiple factors may be influencing. Parameters associated with poor adherence include the dosing regime, drug side effects, comorbidities, age and costs, the patient's disease perception but also social factors [14, 15, 23].

Possibilities to improve adherence include knowledge about self-management, overcoming misperceptions, close communication and shared decision-making between patients and their physicians, simple therapy regimes and low out-of-pocket costs for medications [13, 18, 23, 26, 31–33].

Limitations
Due to administrative limitations, we could only include patients insured by the Upper Austrian Health Insurance (OÖGKK). Therefore, we have no data for subjects insured by other health insurance companies. However, the Upper Austrian Health Insurance covers more than 80% of the general Upper Austrian population.

As a noninterventional study, we were not able to use electronically monitored inhalers, adherence scores or questionnaires to evaluate adherence. Although prescription refill rates are widely used in scientific literature, they may not perfectly reflect the electronically monitored inhaler use of COPD patients [34]. Moreover, refill rates might depend on social support and cognitive abilities of COPD patients [35–37]. Unfortunately, there is no data about the social framework of our patients available. As adherence was classified by dispensed inhalers, we are not able to evaluate if the patients have taken their medication correctly.

Conclusion
Complete adherence to inhaled therapy was only seen in about one third of subjects with a prior hospitalization due to a COPD exacerbation. Adherence was significantly higher among those with spirometrically more severe COPD.

Identifying reasons for and a better understanding of underlying causes of poor adherence are necessary and warrant further research.

Abbreviations
COPD: chronic obstructive pulmonary disease; FEV_1: forced expiratory volume in 1 s; FVC: forced vital capacity; GOLD: Global Initiative for Chronic Obstructive Lung Disease; ICD-10: 10th revision of the International Statistical Classification of Diseases; ICS: inhaled corticosteroid; LABA: long-acting beta-adrenoceptor agonist; LAMA: long-acting muscarinic antagonist; MPR: medication possession ratio; pred.: predicted; SABA: short-acting beta-adrenergic agonist; SAMA: short-acting muscarinic antagonist

Funding
The Upper Austrian Health Insurance supported the current work with an unrestricted grant. AL and BK are employees of and data on adherence was provided by the Upper Austrian Health Insurance. However, this funding source had no role in study design, data analysis, decision to publish, or preparation of the manuscript.

Authors' contributions
MH, AH, BK, AL and BL contributed to the study conception and design, data analysis and interpretation. MH, AH, PL and BL contributed to drafting the manuscript. RF, CB contributed to the data acquisition, data interpretation and critical revision of the manuscript for important intellectual content. All authors approved the final manuscript.

Competing interests

The authors declare that they have no competing interests. AL and BK are employees of the Upper Austrian Health Insurance.

Author details

[1]Department of Pulmonology, Kepler University Hospital, Krankenhausstrasse 9, A4021, Linz, Austria. [2]Faculty of Medicine, Johannes-Kepler-University, Linz, Austria. [3]Department of Health Economics, Upper Austrian Health Insurance, Linz, Austria. [4]Department of Medical Controlling, Kepler University Hospital, Linz, Austria.

References

1. Buist AS, McBurnie MA, Vollmer WM, Gillespie S, Burney P, Mannino DM, Menezes AM, Sullivan SD, Lee TA, Weiss KB, et al. International variation in the prevalence of COPD (the BOLD study): a population-based prevalence study. Lancet. 2007;370(9589):741–50.
2. Firlei N, Lamprecht B, Schirnhofer L, Kaiser B, Studnicka M. The prevalence of COPD in Austria--the expected change over the next decade. Wien Klin Wochenschr. 2007;119(17-18):513–8.
3. Lamprecht B, Scriano JB, Studnicka M, Kaiser B, Vanfleteren LE, Gnatiuc L, Burney P, Miravitlles M, Garcia-Rio F, Akbari K, et al. Determinants of underdiagnosis of COPD in national and international surveys. Chest. 2015;148(4):971–85.
4. Lopez-Campos JL, Tan W, Soriano JB. Global burden of COPD. Respirology. 2016;21(1):14–23.
5. Wouters EF. Economic analysis of the Confronting COPD survey: an overview of results. *Respir Med*. 2003;97(Suppl C):S3–14.
6. Anzueto A, Sethi S, Martinez FJ. Exacerbations of chronic obstructive pulmonary disease. Proc Am Thorac Soc. 2007;4(7):554–64.
7. Foster TS, Miller JD, Marton JP, Caloyeras JP, Russell MW, Menzin J. Assessment of the economic burden of COPD in the U.S.: a review and synthesis of the literature. COPD: J Chron Obstruct Pulmon Dis. 2009;3(4):211–8.
8. Beran D, Zar HJ, Perrin C, Menezes AM, Burney P. Forum of international respiratory societies working group c: Burden of asthma and chronic obstructive pulmonary disease and access to essential medicines in low-income and middle-income countries. Lancet Respir Med. 2015;3(2):159–70.
9. Lisspers K, Larsson K, Johansson G, Janson C, Costa-Scharplatz M, Gruenberger JB, Uhde M, Jorgensen L, Gutzwiller FS, Stallberg B. Economic burden of COPD in a Swedish cohort: the ARCTIC study. Int J Chron Obstruct Pulmon Dis. 2018;13:275–85.
10. DiMatteo MR. Variations in patients' adherence to medical recommendations: a quantitative review of 50 years of research. Med Care. 2004;42(3):200–9.
11. Tashkin DP. Multiple dose regimens. Impact on compliance. *Chest*. 1995; 107(5 Suppl):175S–82S.
12. Balkrishnan R, Christensen DB. Inhaled corticosteroid use and associated outcomes in elderly patients with moderate to severe chronic pulmonary disease. Clin Ther. 2000;22(4):452–69.
13. Yusuf S. Why do people not take life-saving medications? The case of statins. Lancet. 2016;388(10048):943–5.
14. Rand CS. Patient adherence with COPD therapy. Eur Respir Rev. 2005;14(96): 97–101.
15. Restrepo RD, Alvarez MT, Wittnebel LD, Sorenson H, Wettstein R, Vines DL, Sikkema-Ortiz J, Gardner DD, Wilkins RL. Medication adherence issues in patients treated for COPD. Int J Chron Obstruct Pulmon Dis. 2008;3(3):371–84.
16. George M. Adherence in asthma and COPD: new strategies for an old problem. Respir Care. 2018;63(6):818–31.
17. Ari A. Patient education and adherence to aerosol therapy. Respir Care. 2015;60(6):941–55 discussion 955-947.
18. Toy EL, Beaulieu NU, McHale JM, Welland TR, Plauschinat CA, Swensen A, Duh MS. Treatment of COPD: relationships between daily dosing frequency, adherence, resource use, and costs. Respir Med. 2011;105(3):435–41.
19. Ramsey SD. Suboptimal medical therapy in COPD: exploring the causes and consequences. Chest. 2000;117(2 Suppl):33S–7S.
20. Vestbo J, Anderson JA, Calverley PM, Celli B, Ferguson GT, Jenkins C, Knobil K, Willits LR, Yates JC, Jones PW. Adherence to inhaled therapy, mortality and hospital admission in COPD. Thorax. 2009;64(11):939–43.
21. Khdour MR, Hawwa AF, Kidney JC, Smyth BM, McElnay JC. Potential risk factors for medication non-adherence in patients with chronic obstructive pulmonary disease (COPD). Eur J Clin Pharmacol. 2012;68(10):1365–73.
22. Antoniu SA. Adherence to inhaled therapy in COPD: effects on survival and exacerbations. Expert Rev Pharmacoecon Outcomes Res. 2010;10(2):115–7.
23. van Boven JF, Chavannes NH, van der Molen T, Rutten-van Molken MP, Postma MJ, Vegter S. Clinical and economic impact of non-adherence in COPD: a systematic review. Respir Med. 2014;108(1):103–13.
24. Vestbo J, Hurd SS, Agusti AG, Jones PW, Vogelmeier C, Anzueto A, Barnes PJ, Fabbri LM, Martinez FJ, Nishimura M, et al. Global strategy for the diagnosis, management, and prevention of chronic obstructive pulmonary disease: GOLD executive summary. Am J Respir Crit Care Med. 2013;187(4):347–65.
25. Raebel MA, Schmittdiel J, Karter AJ, Konieczny JL, Steiner JF. Standardizing terminology and definitions of medication adherence and persistence in research employing electronic databases. Med Care. 2013;51(8 Suppl 3):S11–21.
26. Bourbeau J, Bartlett SJ. Patient adherence in COPD. Thorax. 2008;63(9):831–8.
27. Garcia-Aymerich J, Monso E, Marrades RM, Escarrabill J, Felez MA, Sunyer J, Anto JM, Investigators E. Risk factors for hospitalization for a chronic obstructive pulmonary disease exacerbation. EFRAM study. Am J Respir Crit Care Med. 2001;164(6):1002–7.
28. Cramer JA, Bradley-Kennedy C, Scalera A. Treatment persistence and compliance with medications for chronic obstructive pulmonary disease. Can Respir J. 2007;14(1):25–9.
29. Huetsch JC, Uman JE, Udris EM, Au DH. Predictors of adherence to inhaled medications among veterans with COPD. J Gen Intern Med. 2012;27(11): 1506–12.
30. Makela MJ, Backer V, Hedegaard M, Larsson K. Adherence to inhaled therapies, health outcomes and costs in patients with asthma and COPD. Respir Med. 2013;107(10):1481–90.
31. Vincken W, Dekhuijzen R, Barnes P. The ADMIT series — issues in inhalation therapy. 4 how to choose inhaler devices for the treatment of COPD. Prim Care Respiratory J. 2009;19(1):10–20.
32. Broeders ME, Sanchis J, Levy ML, Crompton GK, Dekhuijzen PR. The ADMIT series — issues in inhalation therapy. 2 improving technique and clinical effectiveness. Prim Care Respiratory J. 2009;18(2):76–82.
33. Han MK, Martinez CH, Au DH, Bourbeau J, Boyd CM, Branson R, Criner GJ, Kalhan R, Kallstrom TJ, King A, et al. Meeting the challenge of COPD care delivery in the USA: a multiprovider perspective. Lancet Respir Med. 2016; 4(6):473–526.
34. Moran C, Doyle F, Sulaiman I, Bennett K, Greene G, Molloy GJ, Reilly RB, Costello RW, Mellon L. The INCA(TM) (inhaler compliance assessment(TM)): a comparison with established measures of adherence. Psychol Health. 2017; 32(10):1266–87.
35. Trivedi RB, Bryson CL, Udris E, Au DH. The influence of informal caregivers on adherence in COPD patients. Ann behav med. 2012;44(1):66–72.
36. Sulaiman I, Cushen B, Greene G, Seheult J, Seow D, Rawat F, MacHale E, Mokoka M, Moran CN, Sartini Bhreathnach A, et al. Objective assessment of adherence to inhalers by patients with chronic obstructive pulmonary disease. Am J Respir Crit Care Med. 2017;195(10):1333–43.
37. Cushen B, Sulaiman I, Greene G, MacHale E, Mokoka M, Reilly RB, Bennett K, Doyle F, van Boven JFM, Costello RW: The clinical impact of different adherence behaviors in patients with severe chronic obstructive pulmonary disease. Am J Respir Crit Care Med 2018, 197(12):1630–1633.

Solid part size is an important predictor of nodal metastasis in lung cancer with a subsolid tumor

Jun Yeun Cho[1,2], Cho Sun Leem[1], Youlim Kim[1,2], Eun Sun Kim[1,2], Sang Hoon Lee[1,2], Yeon Joo Lee[1,2], Jong Sun Park[1,2], Young-Jae Cho[1,2], Jae Ho Lee[1,2], Choon-Taek Lee[1,2] and Ho Il Yoon[1,2]*

Abstract

Background: Candidates for preoperative or intraoperative nodal assessment among patients with non-small cell lung cancer (NSCLC) manifesting as a subsolid tumor are not established. The present study was conducted to demonstrate the distribution of nodal metastasis rate according to newly proposed T categories for subsolid tumors, and we further aimed to identify radiologic parameters that can be predictive of nodal metastasis.

Methods: We retrospectively reviewed cases of NSCLC manifesting as a subsolid tumor in computed tomography scans in a university-affiliated tertiary hospital between April 2013 and August 2016. All patients underwent mediastinal lymph node dissection during resection surgery. Multivariate analysis was performed among clinical and radiologic parameters.

Results: Of the 269 eligible patients, T-categories were classified as cTis ($n = 23$, 8.6%), cT1 ($n = 203$, 75.5%), and cT2 ($n = 43$, 16.0%). Ten patients (3.7%) had nodal metastasis: pN1 ($n = 5$, 1.9%), pN2 ($n = 5$, 1.9%). Nodal metastasis was not observed in tumors with a solid part ≤1.0 cm (cT1mi and cT1a) or in nonsolid tumors ≤3.0 cm (cTis). The nodal metastasis rate in cT1b, cT1c, and cT2 tumors was 6.1% (4/65), 8.3% (1/12), and 11.7% (5/43), respectively. Multivariate analysis showed that a solid part size > 1.5 cm [odds ratio, 5.89; 95% confidence interval, 1.25–27.68, $p = 0.025$] was significantly associated with nodal metastasis.

Conclusions: We observed nodal metastasis from cT1b tumors (solid part size > 1 cm) among proposed T categories for subsolid tumors and a solid part size is an important radiologic parameter predictive of nodal metastasis in NSCLC manifesting as a subsolid tumor. Considering the low rate of nodal metastasis, pathologic nodal assessment may be unnecessary in early T category tumors with a small solid part size.

Keywords: Risk factor, Non-small cell lung Cancer, Lymphatic metastasis

Background

The considerable increase in lung cancer screening has recently led to issues such as an increased number of lung nodules discovered via computed tomography (CT) and the management of these lesions. The subsolid nodule, defined as a well-demarcated lung lesion containing a ground-glass opacity, exhibits different behaviors from a solid nodule and accordingly, has garnered much attention. In 2013, the Fleischner Society recommendations emphasized that from a management perspective, both pure and part-solid ground-glass nodules are best considered as a category separate from purely solid lesions [1]. Subsequently, many studies have investigated subsolid nodules, and consequently, the recently proposed eighth tumor-node-metastasis staging system includes more detailed T1 categories of subsolid nodules, compared to previous versions [2].

Accurate nodal staging is fundamental in diagnosing and treating non-small cell lung cancer (NSCLC). Generally, the nodal metastasis rate in patients with NSCLC manifesting as a subsolid nodule has been known to be

---

* Correspondence: dextro70@gmail.com
[1]Division of Pulmonary and Critical Care Medicine, Department of Internal Medicine, Seoul National University Bundang Hospital, 82, Gumi-ro 173 Beon-gil, Bundang-gu, Seongnam-si, Gyeonggi-do 13620, Republic of Korea
[2]Department of Internal Medicine, Seoul National University College of Medicine, Seoul, Republic of Korea

low [3–5]. Therefore, it is questionable whether preoperative or intraoperative nodal assessment is needed. Recently updated National Comprehensive Cancer Network guidelines state that preoperative pathologic mediastinal evaluation is optional for solid tumors < 1.0 cm and purely non-solid tumors < 3.0 cm with radiologic negative mediastinum [6] because of the low rate of mediastinal metastasis. Intraoperative nodal assessment in this situation is also controversial, and there is no consensus. Currently, many clinicians conduct intraoperative nodal assessment based on their experiences.

Given this background, the present study was conducted to demonstrate the distribution of nodal metastasis rate according to newly proposed T categories for subsolid tumors. For selecting candidates for preoperative or intraoperative nodal assessment, we further aimed to identify radiologic parameters that can be predictive of nodal metastasis.

Methods

We selected patients with surgically resected NSCLC manifesting as a subsolid tumor on CT scans in a university affiliated-tertiary hospital from April 2013 to August 2016. All patients underwent mediastinal lymph node dissection (MLND) during resection surgery. The patient's clinical data, radiologic features, and pathologic results were retrospectively reviewed.

The definitions of nodal zone and nodal station were based on the International Association of the Study of Lung Cancer (IASLC) lymph node map [7]. The pathologic diagnoses were based on the 2011 IASLC classification [8]. Real-time endobronchial ultrasound (EBUS) was performed in selected patients. Rapid on-site evaluation was not conducted during EBUS procedure.

We described radiologic features of a subsolid tumor based on expert thoracic radiologists' reports. In the present study, we defined a subsolid tumor as a mass (> 3 cm) or nodule (≤3 cm) that contained ground-glass lesions on CT images. The total tumor (including ground glass portion around solid part) and solid part size were measured as the maximum diameters on the lung window setting. Subsolid tumors less than or equal to 3 cm were classified according to recently proposed T categories [2]. T categories were classified by the total tumor and solid part size; cTis (total tumor size of 0.6–3.0 cm with no solid part), cT1 (total tumor size of 0.6–3.0 cm with solid part size 0.6–3.0 cm) and cT2 (total tumor size of 3.0–7.0 cm with any solid part size).

If a total tumor measured 3 cm to 7 cm, it was categorized as cT2 regardless of the solid part size. Cases with multiple tumors were excluded. A tumor was considered central if it was visualized within the inner third of the lung field or abutted mediastinal structures on CT or positron emission tomography (PET) images. Radiologic N staging was determined from CT scans with or without PET findings. Lymph nodes with shortest diameters of > 1 cm on CT and/or a maximum standardized uptake value > 2.5 on PET were considered metastatic. Pathologic N stage was determined by the final pathologic report after surgery.

All data are presented as mean values (± standard deviations) for continuous variables and numbers (percentages) for categorical variables. Data were compared between defined groups using the Mann–Whitney test for continuous variables and Fisher's exact test for categorical variables. A linear-by-linear association was defined using Pearson's

Table 1 Clinical, radiologic and pathologic characteristics of patients

Characteristic	Total (n = 269)
Age, years	62.4 ± 10.4
Male sex	115 (42.8)
Former/Current smoker	90 (33.5)
Previous extra-thoracic malignancy	34 (12.6)
Previous lung cancer	6 (2.2)
Tumor centrality	14 (5.2)
Radiologic N stage	
N0	227 (84.4)
N1–2	42 (15.6)
T categories for subsolid tumor[a]	
cTis	23 (8.6)
cT1	203 (75.5)
cT2	43 (16.0)
EBUS	99 (36.8)
Operation extent	
Segmentectomy	41 (15.2)
Lobectomy	228 (84.8)
Pathology	
AAH/AIS	2 (0.7)
MIA	29 (10.8)
Invasive ADC	235 (87.4)
Invasive mucinous ADC	3 (1.1)
Pathologic N stage[b]	
N0	259 (96.3)
N1	5 (1.9)
N2	5 (1.9)

Data are presented as n (%) or mean ± standard deviation
AAH atypical adenomatous hyperplasia, *ADC* adenocarcinoma, *AIS* adenocarcinoma in situ, *EBUS* endobronchial ultrasound, *MIA* minimally invasive adenocarcinoma
[a]T categories were classified by the total tumor size (cm) and solid part size (cm). Total tumor size was defined as a size including ground glass around the solid part; cTis (total tumor size of 0.6–3.0 cm with no solid part), cT1 (total tumor size of 0.6–3.0 cm with solid part size 0.6–3.0 cm) and cT2 (total tumor size of 3.0–7.0 cm with any solid part size)
[b]Pathologic N stage was determined by the final pathologic report after surgery

coefficient and performed to test the trends of ordinal scales in categorical variables.

Significant variables from clinical and radiologic data identified in the univariate analysis were used for multivariate analysis to elucidate predictive factors of nodal metastasis. SPSS 22.0 (IBM, Armonk, NY, USA) was used for the statistical analyses. A p value < 0.05 was considered statistically significant.

Results

A total of 269 eligible patients were identified, and their baseline characteristics are summarized in Table 1. The patients had a mean age of 62.4 ± 10.4 years. One hundred fifteen patients (42.8%) were male, and 90 (33.5%) were former or current smokers. Fourteen (5.2%) patients had a centrally located tumor. The tumors were categorized into three groups: cTis (n = 25, 8.9%), cT1 (n = 212, 75.7%), and cT2 (n = 43, 15.4%). There were no cases presenting as a nonsolid tumor less than 0.5 cm. Ninety-nine (36.8%) patients underwent EBUS prior to resection surgery, and 228 patients (84.8%) underwent lobectomy. The most frequent tissue pathology was invasive adenocarcinoma (n = 235, 84.8%). We identified 10 patients with nodal metastasis: pN1 (n = 5, 1.9%) and pN2 (n = 5, 1.9%).

Patients with more advanced clinical T category frequently underwent EBUS and lobectomy (Table 2). In cT1 tumors, the pN1 and pN2 rates were 1.5 and 1.0%, respectively, whereas there was no nodal metastasis in cTis tumors. In cT2 tumors, the pN1 and N2 rates were 4.7 and 7.0%, respectively. More advanced T tumors had significantly more advanced nodal metastasis. In addition, invasive adenocarcinomas were frequently diagnosed in advanced T tumors.

The distribution of nodal metastasis in tumors classified by the proposed clinical T categories is detailed in Table 3. Nodal metastasis was observed in tumors in which the solid part was > 1.0 cm or total tumor size > 3.0 cm. There was no nodal metastasis in cTis, cT1mi, and cT1a tumors. The nodal metastasis rates in cT1b, cT1c, and cT2 tumors were 6.1% (4/65), 8.3% (1/12), and 11.7% (5/43), respectively. The mean solid part size in cT2 tumors (2 cases were nonsolid tumors) was 2.0 ± 1.0 cm.

The detailed information of patients with nodal metastasis is presented in Table 4. All patients had a solid part exceeding 1 cm. Only one patient had a centrally located tumor. Most cases of metastatic N1 involved a peribronchial node, and 3 of 5 cases of metastatic N2 involved a subcarinal node. Tumors with nodal metastasis were invasive adenocarcinoma with acinar, papillary, or solid subtype. Four patients with pN2 underwent EBUS prior to surgery. One patient (patient number 9) was diagnosed with pN2 disease by EBUS, and subsequently underwent surgery due to single N2. Other cases (patient number 7, 8, 10) were diagnosed with pN2 disease by surgery.

We performed a multivariate analysis to identify the risk factors predictive of nodal metastasis (Table 5). The multivariate analysis included variables that were identified as significant in the univariate analysis. A solid part

Table 2 Differences between cTis, cT1 and cT2 tumors

Variables	cTis (n = 23)	cT1 (n = 203)	cT2 (n = 43)	p Value
EBUS				0.000
Not performed	21 (91.3)	134 (66.0)	15 (34.9)	
Performed	2 (8.7)	69 (34.0)	28 (65.1)	
Operation extent				0.009
Segmentectomy	5 (21.7)	36 (17.7)	0 (0.0)	
Lobectomy	18 (78.3)	167 (82.3)	43 (100.0)	
Pathologic N stage				0.039
N0	23 (100.0)	198 (97.5)	38 (88.4)	
N1	0 (0.0)	3 (1.5)	2 (4.7)	
N2	0 (0.0)	2 (1.0)	3 (7.0)	
Pathology				0.002
AAH/AIS	0 (0.0)	2 (1.0)	0 (0.0)	
MIA	7 (30.4)	22 (10.8)	0 (0.0)	
Invasive ADC	16 (69.6)	176 (86.7)	43 (100.0)	
Invasive mucinous ADC	0 (0.0)	3 (1.5)	0 (0.0)	

Data are presented as n (%)

AAH atypical adenomatous hyperplasia, *ADC* adenocarcinoma, *AIS* adenocarcinoma in situ, *EBUS* endobronchial ultrasound, *MIA* minimally invasive adenocarcinoma

Table 3 Distribution of nodal metastasis in tumors classified by proposed clinical T categories[a]

Categories	Total tumor Size[b] (cm)	Solid part Size (cm)	pN0	pN1	pN2
cTis	0.6–3.0	0	23 (100.0)	0 (0.0)	0 (0.0)
cT1mi	≤3.0	≤0.5	46 (100.0)	0 (0.0)	0 (0.0)
cT1a	0.6–3.0	0.6–1.0	80 (100.0)	0 (0.0)	0 (0.0)
cT1b	1.1–3.0	1.1–2.0	61 (93.8)	3 (4.6)	1 (1.5)
cT1c	2.1–3.0	2.1–3.0	11 (91.7)	0 (0.0)	1 (8.3)
cT2[c]	3.0–7.0	Any	38 (88.4)	2 (4.7)	3 (7.0)

[a]The nodal metastasis rate was significantly different among classified T categories ($P = 0.033$)
[b]Defined as a size including ground glass portion around the solid part
[c]Two cases were nonsolid tumors, and the mean solid part size was 2.0 ± 1.0 cm

size > 1.5 cm [odds ratio (OR), 5.89; 95% confidence interval (CI), 1.25–27.68, $p = 0.025$] was found to associate significantly with nodal metastasis.

Discussion

In our cohort, the nodal metastasis rate was 3.7% (1.9% with both pN1 and pN2). Among part-solid nodules (cT1a-cT1c), the pN1 and pN2 rates were 1.5 and 1.0%, respectively, whereas there was no nodal metastasis in cTis (nonsolid nodule ≤3 cm). These findings of low incidence of nodal metastasis are consistent with previous studies [4, 5, 9].

When tumors were classified by the proposed new T categories, any nodal metastasis was observed from cT1b to cT2 tumors, in which the solid part size was > 1.0 cm or total tumor size > 3.0 cm. In the final pathologic reports, patients with nodal metastasis had adenocarcinoma with invasive subtypes. There was no early stage adenocarcinoma (e.g., adenocarcinoma in situ (AIS), minimally invasive adenocarcinoma (MIA), lepidic predominant adenocarcinoma (LPA)). These findings suggest that preoperative pathologic nodal evaluation or extended lymph node assessment might be unnecessary when early stage adenocarcinomas are suspected by radiologic features.

It is debatable whether extended lymph node assessment should be performed in patients with early stage NSCLC. As noted earlier, the incidence of nodal metastasis in NSCLCs manifesting as a subsolid tumor is lower than in NSCLCs with pure solid tumor. Furthermore, the extent of intraoperative node assessment (e.g., selective sampling vs. systematic dissection) in NSCLC patients remains controversial [10]. Although more extended node dissection has positive effects on clinical outcomes [11, 12], it is important to consider various procedure-related morbidities. Flores et al. compared 151 cases of NSCLC (subsolid nodules) with MLND and 52 cases of NSCLC without MLND [13]. They observed no differences in survival and asserted that performing MLND is not mandatory when screen-diagnosed NSCLC manifests as a subsolid nodule.

Currently available guidelines recommend that preoperative pathologic mediastinal evaluation (e.g., EBUS) should be considered regarding tumor size, radiologic N status, and tumor centrality [14, 15]. However, they do not suggest recommendations exclusively for subsolid tumors. In the

Table 4 Detailed characteristics of patients with nodal involvement[a]

Patient number	Total tumor size	Solid part size	T stage	Central Tumor	N Stage (CT)	N Stage (PET)	EBUS	pN stage	Involved N1	Involved N2	Pathology/Subtype
1	3.0	1.7	cT1b	No	0	0	Yes	pN1	Interlobar	–	ADC/papillary
2	1.8	1.4	cT1b	No	0	0	Yes	pN1	Peribronchial	–	ADC/solid
3	4.1	2.3	cT2	No	0	2	Yes	pN1	Peribronchial	–	ADC/acinar
4	3.2	3.1	cT2	No	0	0	Yes	pN1	Peribronchial	–	ADC/papillary
5	2.7	1.2	cT1b	No	0	0	Yes	pN1	Peribronchial	–	ADC/acinar
6	3.7	2.8	cT2	No	0	0	No	pN2	Peribronchial	2,3,4	ADC/papillary
7	3.2	1.3	cT2	Yes	0	0	Yes	pN2	–	6	ADC/acinar
8	5.4	2.0	cT2	No	0	2	Yes	pN2	Peribronchial	7	ADC/acinar
9	2.7	2.6	cT1c	No	1	0	Yes	pN2	Peribronchial	7	ADC/acinar
10	2.4	1.8	cT1b	No	0	0	Yes	pN2	–	7	ADC/papillary

ADC adenocarcinoma, *CT* computed tomography, *EBUS* endobronchial ultrasound, *PET* positron emission tomography
[a]Four patients with pN2 underwent EBUS prior to surgery. One patient (patient number 9) was diagnosed with pN2 disease by EBUS, and subsequently underwent surgery due to single N2. Other cases (patient number 7, 8, 10) were diagnosed with pN2 disease by surgery

Table 5 Risk factors predictive of nodal metastasis

Variables	Univariate		Multivariate		
	OR	95% CI	OR	95% CI	p Value
Total tumor size > 3 cm	5.81	1.61–21.05	2.46	0.57–10.50	0.226
Solid part size > 1.5 cm	8.66	2.17–34.57	5.89	1.25–27.68	0.025
Tumor centrality	2.10	0.25–17.87			
Radiologic nodal metastasis	2.42	0.60–9.75			

CI confidence interval, OR odds ratio

present study, multivariate regression analysis showed that solid part size (> 1.5 cm) is predictive of nodal metastasis. Previous studies focused on importance of solid consistency for predicting nodal metastasis in NSCLCs. Koike et al. suggested 89% solid consistency (proportion of solid part size in total tumor size including ground glass) as a cutoff value to predict mediastinal metastasis in clinical IA NSCLCs [16]. Gao et al. reported that an occult N2 risk was lower in tumors with a ground glass component than in tumors without, among T1–2 N0 NSCLCs determined by PET CT [17]. Ye et al. asserted that ground glass status (part solid or pure solid vs nonsolid) is more accurate predictor than tumor diameter in clinical IA adenocarcinoma [4]. However, these studies included numbers of pure solid tumors, not only subsolid tumors. Our study's strength is that only cases of NSCLC manifesting as subsolid tumors were included. This is an important finding because solid part size can be a determinant radiologic criterion when preoperative pathologic nodal assessments are performed.

Tumor size has been considered an important risk factor for predicting nodal metastasis, and preoperative pathologic nodal assessment was considered in cases of tumor exceeding 3 because of low negative predictive value of PET-CT for detecting mediastinal nodal metastasis [18, 19]. However, total tumor size including ground glass was not a significant predictive factor (Table 5). The relatively small number of cT2 cases might have contributed to this result. Moreover, data from Table 2 shows that the nodal metastasis rate was significantly higher in cT2 tumors than in cTis or cT1 tumors. We believe that total tumor size is still worthy as an important predictive radiologic factor, as well as solid part size.

In our study, we did not find an association between tumor centrality and nodal metastasis, although tumor location has been considered an important factor related to NSCLC. In a study by Lee et al. [20] of 221 patients with clinical IA NSCLC with a radiologically negative mediastinum, the frequency of central tumor location was 23%, with a higher incidence of pN2 disease relative to peripherally located tumors. However, only 5.2% of tumors in the present study were centrally located, and primary lung adenocarcinomas were generally located peripherally. Moreover, the term "tumor centrality" is vague even among radiologists. Hence, the ability of tumor centrality to predict nodal metastasis should be evaluated in future studies.

There are some limitations in our study. First, because of the retrospective design nature, selection bias may have affected the results. EBUS and lobectomy were performed more frequently in more advanced T categories (Table 2). Therefore, it is assumed that clinicians did not actively conduct preoperative or intraoperative nodal assessment in patients with early stage NSCLCs (AIS, MIA, and LPA). Indeed, we identified 376 surgically resected NSCLCs manifesting as a subsolid tumor during the study period and excluded 107 patients who did not undergo MLND. Second, the actual nodal metastasis rate was low because we included only subsolid tumors. Hence, logistic regression analysis showed widened confidence intervals for the odds ratios, subsequently indicating statistically weak data. Future studies correcting these limitations are needed.

Conclusions

Among the proposed T categories for subsolid nodules, we observed nodal metastasis from cT1b, in which the solid part size exceeded 1 cm. The nodal metastasis rate was 3.7%, and solid part size is an important radiologic parameter predictive of nodal metastasis in NSCLC manifesting as a subsolid tumor. Considering the low rate of nodal metastasis, pathologic nodal assessment may be unnecessary in early T category tumors with a small solid part size.

Abbreviations

AIS: Adenocarcinoma in situ; CI: Confidence interval; CT: Computed tomography; EBUS: Endobronchial ultrasound; IASLC: International Association of the Study of Lung Cancer; LPA: Lepidic predominant adenocarcinoma; MIA: Minimally invasive adenocarcinoma; MLND: Mediastinal lymph node dissection; NSCLC: Non-small cell lung cancer; OR: Odds ratio; PET: Positron emission tomography

Acknowledgements

The authors would like to thank all thoracic surgery staffs at Seoul National University Bundang Hospital for their contributions to lung cancer surgery.

Funding

There is no funding supports for this study.

Authors' contributions

JYC, HIY were involved in the design of this study; JYC, HIY, CSL, YLK, ESK were involved in participant recruitment and data collection; SHL, YJL, JSP, YJC were involved in sample processing; JYC, JHL, CTL, HIY were all involved in manuscript preparation and editing. All authors approved the final manuscript.

Competing interests

All authors declare that they have no competing interests.

References

1. Naidich DP, Bankier AA, MacMahon H, et al. Recommendations for the management of subsolid pulmonary nodules detected at CT: a statement from the Fleischner society. Radiology. 2013;266:304–17.
2. Travis WD, Asamura H, Bankier AA, et al. The IASLC lung Cancer staging project: proposals for coding T categories for subsolid nodules and assessment of tumor size in part-solid tumors in the forthcoming eighth edition of the TNM classification of lung cancer. J Thorac Oncol. 2016;11:1204–23.
3. Hattori A, Suzuki K, Matsunaga T, et al. Is limited resection appropriate for radiologically "solid" tumors in small lung cancers? Ann Thorac Surg. 2012;94:212–5.
4. Ye B, Cheng M, Li W, et al. Predictive factors for lymph node metastasis in clinical stage IA lung adenocarcinoma. Ann Thorac Surg. 2014;98:217–23.
5. Cho S, Song IH, Yang HC, Kim K, Jheon S. Predictive factors for node metastasis in patients with clinical stage I non-small cell lung cancer. Ann Thorac Surg. 2013;96:239–45.
6. Ettinger DS, Wood DE, Aisner DL, et al. Non–small cell lung Cancer, version 5. 2017, NCCN clinical practice guidelines in oncology. J Natl Compr Cancer Netw. 2017;15:504–35.
7. Rusch VW, Asamura H, Watanabe H, et al. The IASLC lung cancer staging project: a proposal for a new international lymph node map in the forthcoming seventh edition of the TNM classification for lung cancer. J Thorac Oncol. 2009;4:568–77.
8. Travis WD, Brambilla E, Noguchi M, et al. American Thoracic Society. International Association for the Study of Lung Cancer/American Thoracic Society/European Respiratory Society: international multidisciplinary classification of lung adenocarcinoma: executive summary. Proc Am Thorac Soc. 2011;8:381–5.
9. Lee SM, Park CM, Paeng JC, et al. Accuracy and predictive features of FDG-PET/CT and CT for diagnosis of lymph node metastasis of T1 non-small-cell lung cancer manifesting as a subsolid nodule. Eur Radiol. 2012;22:1556–63.
10. Lardinois D, De Leyn P, Van Schil P, et al. ESTS guidelines for intraoperative lymph node staging in non-small cell lung cancer. Eur J Cardiothorac Surg. 2006;30:787–92.
11. Lardinois D, Suter H, Hakki H, Rousson V, Betticher D, Ris H-B. Morbidity, survival, and site of recurrence after mediastinal lymph-node dissection versus systematic sampling after complete resection for non-small cell lung cancer. Ann Thorac Surg. 2005;80:268–75.
12. Doddoli C, Aragon A, Barlesi F, et al. Does the extent of lymph node dissection influence outcome in patients with stage I non-small-cell lung cancer? Eur J Cardiothorac Surg. 2005;27:680–5.
13. Flores RM, Nicastri D, Bauer T, et al. Computed tomography screening for lung Cancer: mediastinal lymph node resection in stage IA nonsmall cell lung Cancer manifesting as subsolid and solid nodules. Ann Surg. 2017;265:1025–33.
14. Murgu SD. Diagnosing and staging lung cancer involving the mediastinum. Chest. 2015;147:1401–12.
15. Stamatis G. Staging of lung cancer: the role of noninvasive, minimally invasive and invasive techniques. Eur Respir J. 2015;46:521–31.
16. Koike T, Yamato Y, Yoshiya K, Toyabe S. Predictive risk factors for mediastinal lymph node metastasis in clinical stage IA non-small-cell lung cancer patients. J Thorac Oncol. 2012;7:1246–51.
17. Gao SJ, Kim AW, Puchalski JT, et al. Indications for invasive mediastinal staging in patients with early non-small cell lung cancer staged with PET-CT. Lung Cancer. 2017;109:36–41.
18. Gómez-Caro A, Boada M, Cabañas M, et al. False-negative rate after positron emission tomography/computer tomography scan for mediastinal staging in cl stage non-small-cell lung cancer. Eur J Cardiothorac Surg. 2012;42:93–100.
19. Wang J, Welch K, Wang L. Negative predictive value of positron emission tomography and computed tomography for stage T1-2N0 non–small-cell lung cancer: a meta-analysis. Clin Lung Cancer. 2012;13:81–9.
20. Lee PC, Port JL, Korst RJ, Liss Y, Meherally DN, Altorki NK. Risk factors for occult mediastinal metastases in clinical stage I non-small cell lung cancer. Ann Thorac Surg. 2007;84:177–81.

Epidemiology of pulmonary disease due to nontuberculous mycobacteria in Southern China, 2013–2016

Yaoju Tan[1†], Biyi Su[1†], Wei Shu[2], Xingshan Cai[1], Shaojia Kuang[1], Haobin Kuang[1], Jianxiong Liu[1*] and Yu Pang[2*]

Abstract

Background: Pulmonary nontuberculous mycobacteria (NTM) disease is of increasing public health concern in China. Information is limited regarding risk factors associated with this disease in China. The objective of this study was to describe the epidemiology of pulmonary disease due to NTM in Southern China.

Methods: We retrospectively reviewed the medical records of pulmonary NTM patients registered in the Guangzhou Chest Hospital with positive mycobacterial cultures during 2013–2016. We described sex, age, residence, treatment history, laboratory examination results and comorbidities of pulmonary NTM patients.

Results: Among the 607 NTM cases, the most prevalent species were *Mycobacterium avium* complex (44.5%), *Mycobacterium abscessus* complex (40.5%), *Mycobacterium kansasii* (10.0%) and *Mycobacterium fortuitum* (2.8%). The male:female ratio was significantly lower among patients infected with rapidly growing mycobacteria (RGM) than among those with slowly growing mycobacteria (SGM). The risk of developing SGM disease significantly increased with advancing age. In addition, pulmonary RGM diseases were more common in migrant population than resident population. Notably, patients with pulmonary RGM diseases were significantly more likely to have bronchiectasis underlying noted than those with SGM diseases. No significant difference was observed in in vitro drug susceptibility among NTM species.

Conclusion: Our data illustrate that the *M. avium* complex is the most predominant causative agent of pulmonary NTM disease in Southern China. Female, migrant population, the presence of bronchiectasis are independent risk factors for pulmonary diseases due to RGM. In addition, the prevalence of SGM increases significantly with advancing age.

Keywords: Nontuberculous mycobacteria, Epidemiology, Slowly growing mycobacteria, Rapidly growing mycobacteria, Comorbidity

Background

Nontuberculous mycobacteria (NTM) are a heterogeneous group of species other than the *Mycobacterium tuberculosis* complex and *Mycobacterium leprae* [1]. As the etiologic agents, NTM have been found in a variety of environmental sources, such as soil, water and aerosols [2]. Despite being less pathogenic than *M. tuberculosis*, these environmental bacteria are associated with a wide array of clinical diseases, especially in HIV-infected patients or those with immunodeficiencies [3]. Notably, NTM disease incidence has increased significantly during the past decade [3], while this emerging disease is given a lower public health priority as compared with tuberculosis due to lack of definitive evidence of person-to-person transmission of NTM [4]. The most available data on NTM infections come from sentinel laboratory-based surveillance studies [5, 6], which makes it difficult to distinguish between colonizers and causative pathogens among these positive mycobacteria

* Correspondence: Ljxer64@qq.com; pangyupound@163.com
†Yaoju Tan and Biyi Su contributed equally to this work.
[1]Department of Clinical Laboratory, Guangzhou Chest Hospital, State Key Laboratory of Respiratory Disease, No. 62, Hengzhigang Road, Yuexiu District, Guangzhou, Guangdong Province 510095, People's Republic of China
[2]National Clinical Laboratory on Tuberculosis, Beijing Key laboratory on Drug-resistant Tuberculosis Research,, Beijing Chest Hospital, Beijing Tuberculosis and Thoracic Tumor Institute, No. 9, Beiguan Street, Tongzhou District, Beijing 101149, People's Republic of China

cultures [7]; consequently, the exact distribution of mycobacteria species among patients is not well known, especially in high-TB-burden settings.

Although China has achieved impressive reductions in TB prevalence and mortality over the past 20 years [8], NTM infections have become a serious issue, accounting for about one quarter of mycobacterial patient isolates according to the national population-based data [9], triggering public health concerns. More importantly, NTM prevalence varies greatly across China, and Southern China has a significantly higher proportion of NTM infection [1]. In addition, national epidemiological data have revealed that NTM species distribution differs significantly by region, reflecting the diversity of species distribution in the local environment [3]. Given that NTM species differ significantly in pathogenicity and drug susceptibility profiles, understanding this regional diversity is a major priority for optimizing appropriate treatment regimen. Unfortunately, previous reports regarding this issue are lacking, and few laboratory data were mainly on the basis of NTM isolates from microbiology laboratory, which made it difficult to differentiate NTM diseases from host respiratory colonization [1, 10]. Furthermore, information is limited regarding risk factors associated with this disease, thereby hampering attempts to implement effective infection control programmes. The objective of this study was to describe the prevalence of NTM species among pulmonary NTM patients in regional tuberculosis clinical centre in Southern China between 2013 and 2016. We also aimed to identify demographic and clinical factors associated with pulmonary NTM diseases between slowly growing mycobacteria (SGM) and rapidly growing mycobacteria (RGM).

Methods

Study design and population

This study was conducted at the Guangzhou Chest Hospital, an 800-bed regional tuberculosis clinical centre in Southern China. We retrospectively reviewed the medical records of pulmonary NTM patients registered in the hospital with positive mycobacterial cultures during 2013–2016. Factors that were assessed in this study included demographic and clinical characteristics, such as sex, age, residence, treatment history, laboratory examination results and comorbidities. The definition of NTM lung disease met the criteria established by the American Thoracic Society (ATS) in 2007 [11], including clinical symptoms and abnormal chest radiograph suggestive of pulmonary TB or NTM diseases; isolation of the same NTM species from more than two sputum specimens collected at different time points; and exclusion of other differential diagnoses. In addition, the residents were defined as individuals with the local household registration of Guangzhou, while the migrants were defined as individuals without local household registration of Guangzhou.

Laboratory examination

Media supplied with paranitrobenzoic acid was used for differential identification of *Mycobacterium tuberculosis* (MTB) complex and NTM. The NTM strains identified by conventional biochemical method were subcultured on the Löwenstein-Jensen (L-J) medium [1]. Colonies were scraped from the surface of L-J medium, and transferred to 500 μL Tris-EDTA (TE) buffer. The was heated at 95 °C for 30 min in a water bath, and the supernatant was used as DNA template for PCR amplification. The commercial Biochip test was performed for species identification of mycobacterium according to the manufacturer's instructions [12]. In addition, the isolates identified as *Mycobacterium chelonae-Mycobacterium abscessus* group by Biochip were further divided into subspecies with the sequencing of multiple genes, including 16S rRNA, *hsp65*, *rpoB*, and 16S–23S rRNA internal transcribed spacer (ITS) sequence as previously reported [9]. The PCR products were sent to Ruibo Company (Beijing, China) for DNA sequencing service. Nucleotide sequences were aligned with the homologous sequences of the reference mycobacteria strains by using multiple sequence alignments via the BLAST web pages (http://www.ncbi.nlm.nih.gov/BLAST).

Drug susceptibility testing

The in vitro drug susceptibility of *M. abscessus* complex was determined with a broth microdilution method based on the guidelines from the Clinical and Laboratory Standards Institute (CLSI) [13]. Eight antimicrobial agents were enrolled in this study, including amikacin, clarithromycin, linezolid, tobramycin, cefoxitin, ciprofloxacin, doxycycline and imipenem. The breakpoint values to distinguish susceptibility and resistance for drugs were followed as recommendation from CLSI [13]. For *M. avium* and *M. intracellulare* isolates, three agents were selected for MIC assessment, including clarithromycin, moxifloxacin and linezolid. The in vitro drug susceptibility for these drugs were evaluated with a broth microdilution method, and their breakpoint values were followed the recommendation from CLSI [13].

Statistical analysis

All collected data were entered using Epi Data version 3.1 (EpiData Association, Odense, Denmark). Each entry was cross checked independently to ensure the data quality. The predictor variables of age, sex, residence, previous history for tuberculosis, and comorbidity were tested for association with various NTM diseases using univariate and multivariate logistic analysis. The level of significance of univariate analysis was 0.05, and that for inclusion in the multivariate model was 0.15. Association between NTM diseases and predictor variables was calculated using adjusted odds ratio and 95% confidence interval. In addition, comparison of rate of drug resistance between different NTM species was evaluated by chi-square and Fisher's exact tests. Differences were considered to be statistically significant at $P < 0.05$. We conducted analyses by using SPSS version 20.0 (SPSS Inc., Chicago, USA).

Results

Proportion of different NTM species

A total of 607 pulmonary NTM patients were enrolled during January 1, 2013-December 31, 2017. Among the 607 NTM cases, the most prevalent species were *M. avium* complex (MAC, 270 isolates, 44.5%), *M. abscessus* complex (MABC, 246 isolates, 40.5%), *M. kansasii* (61 isolates, 10.0%) and *M. fortuitum* (17 isolates, 2.8%). These four groups accounted for 97.9% of all mycobacteria identified. Of 270 *M. avium* complex isolates, there were 171 *M. intracellulare* (63.3%, 171/270) and 99 *M. avium* (36.7%, 99/270) isolates, respectively. In addition, 58.9% (145/246) of *M. abscessus* complex isolates were *M. abscessus* subspecies *abscessus*, and the remining 41.1% (101/246) belonged to *M. abscessus* subspecies *massiliense* (Fig. 1).

Factors associated with SGM and RGM infections

Comparison in demographic and clinical characteristics of NTM patients between SGM and RGM is summarized in Table 1. The male:female ratio was significantly lower among patients infected with RGM than among those with SGM [adjusted odds ratio (aOR): 0.526, 95% confidence interval (95% CI): 0.429–0.862; $P = 0.005$]. In addition, the risk of developing RGM disease significantly decreased with advancing age. Compared with patients with SGM, the adjusted odds ratios were 0.488 (95% CI: 0.287–0.827) for 40–60 years group and 0.395 (95% CI: 0.235–0.666) for > 60 years group, respectively. We also found that the prevalence of infection caused by RGM and SGM differed significantly in resident and migrant population, and pulmonary RGM diseases were more common in migrant population than resident population (aOR: 1.551; 95% CI: 1.092–2.202; $P = 0.014$). Notably, patients with pulmonary RGM diseases were significantly more likely to have bronchiectasis underlying noted than those with SGM diseases (aOR: 1.521; 95% CI: 1.064–2.176; $P = 0.021$). In contrast, there were no other differences regarding TB history or comorbidities noted between SGM and RGM, respectively ($P > 0.05$).

In vitro drug susceptibility profiles of MAC and MABC

We further analysed the in vitro drug susceptibility profiles of *M. avium* complex and *M. abscessus* complex. As shown in Table 2, clarithromycin was the most highly active agent against *M. avium* complex, and the percentages of resistant strains were 4.2% (4/95) for *M. avium* and 3.8% (6/159) for *M. intracellulare*, respectively. Moxifloxacin and linezolid also showed potent activity against *M. avium* complex. There were 5 (5.3%) *M. avium* isolates and 8 (5.0%) *M. intracellulare* isolates resistant to moxifloxacin. For linezolid, the proportions of resistant isolates were 11.6% (11/95) for *M. avium* and 8.2% (13/159) for *M. intracellulare*, respectively. Of the antimicrobial agents tested, amikacin, clarithromycin, linezolid and tobramycin showed highly active against *M. abscessus* complex, and less than 5% of *M.*

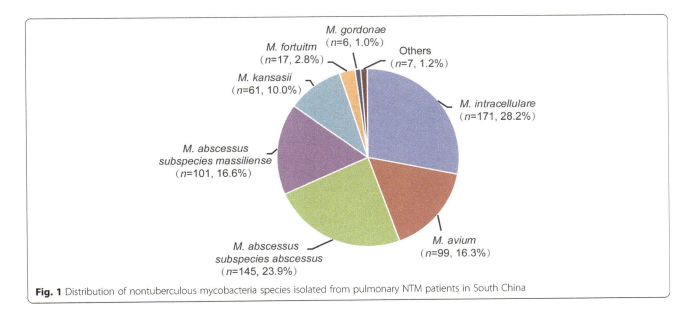

Fig. 1 Distribution of nontuberculous mycobacteria species isolated from pulmonary NTM patients in South China

Table 1 Comparison in demographic and clinical characteristics of NTM patients between slowly growing mycobacteria and rapidly growing mycobacteria at Guangzhou Chest Hospital, China, January 1, 2013 to December 31, 2017

Characteristics	No. of pulmonary NTM cases (%)		Univariate analysis		Multivariate analysis	
	SGM ($n = 344$)	RGM ($n = 263$)	OR (95% CI)	P value	OR (95% CI)	P value
Gender						
Female	170 (49.4)	171 (65.0)	0.526 (0.378–0.731)	< 0.001	0.608 (0.429–0.862)	0.005
Male	174 (50.6)	92 (35.0)	1.000	–	1.000	–
Age group (years)						
18–40	34 (9.9)	53 (20.2)	1.000	–	1.000	–
40–60	122 (35.5)	106 (40.3)	0.557 (0.337–0.922)	0.023	0.488 (0.287–0.827)	0.008
> 60	188 (54.7)	104 (39.5)	0.355 (0.217–0.581)	< 0.001	0.395 (0.235–0.666)	< 0.001
TB history						
No	149 (43.8)	96 (36.5)	1.000	–		
Yes	195 (57.4)	167 (63.5)	1.329 (0.953–1.852)	0.093		
Population						
Residence	168 (48.8)	89 (33.8)	1.000	–	1.000	–
Migration	176 (51.2)	174 (66.2)	1.855 (1.331–2.585)	< 0.001	1.551 (1.092–2.202)	0.014
Diabetes						
No	328 (95.3)	252 (95.8)	1.000	–		
Yes	16 (4.7)	11 (4.2)	0.895 (0.408–1.962)	0.895		
Bronchiectasis						
No	158 (45.9)	93 (35.4)	1.000	–	1.000	–
Yes	186 (54.1)	170 (64.6)	1.553 (1.116–2.16)	0.009	1.521 (1.064–2.176)	0.021
COPD						
No	326 (94.8)	256 (97.3)	1.000	–		
Yes	18 (5.2)	7 (2.7)	0.495 (0.204–1.204)	0.121		
Tumor						
No	321 (93.3)	251 (95.4)	1.000	–		
Yes	23 (6.7)	12 (4.6)	0.667 (0.326–1.367)	0.269		

SGM slowly growing mycobacteria, *RGM* rapidly growing mycobacteria, *COPD* chronic obstructive pulmonary disease, *OR* odds ratio, *95% CI* 95% confidence interval

avium and *M. intracellulare* were resistant to each drug, respectively. In addition, cefoxitin had moderate activity against *M. abscessus* complex, and the percentages of cefoxitin-resistance were observed in 33.8% (46/136) of *M. abscessus subspecies abscessus* and 25.3% (24/95) of *M. abscessus subspecies massiliense* isolates. Statistical analysis revealed that there were no significant differences in the drug resistant rate between *M. abscessus subspecies abscessus* and *M. abscessus subspecies massiliense* ($P > 0.05$) (Table 3).

Table 2 Comparison of in vitro drug susceptibility profiles between *M. intracellulare* and *M. avium* isolates

Antimicrobial agents	No. of resistant isolates (%)		P value
	M. avium ($n = 95$)	*M. intracellulare* ($n = 159$)	
Clarithromycin	4 (4.2)	6 (3.8)	1.000
Moxifloxacin	5 (5.3)	8 (5.0)	1.000
Linezolid	11 (11.6)	13 (8.2)	0.370

The breakpoints to establish susceptibility and resistance for clarithromycin, moxifloxacin and linezolid were followed as recommendation from Clinical and Laboratory Standards Institute (CLSI-M24-A2)

Discussion

Pulmonary NTM disease is of increasing public health concern worldwide [6]. This study firstly describes the demographic and clinical characteristics of patients with pulmonary NTM disease in Southern China. Our study has demonstrated that the most common NTM that causes pulmonary disease in Southern China is *M. avium* complex, accounting for 44.5% of pulmonary NTM disease burden in this study, which is consistent with its predominance in other parts of the world, including the United States (85%) [14], Denmark (81%)

Table 3 Comparison of in vitro drug susceptibility profiles between M. abscessus subspecies abscessus and M. abscessus subspecies massiliense isolates

Antimicrobial agents	No. of resistant isolates (%)		P value
	M. abscessus subspecies abscessus (n = 136)	M. abscessus subspecies massiliense (n = 95)	
Amikacin	3 (2.2)	2 (2.1)	1.000
Clarithromycin	6 (4.4)	3 (3.2)	0.740
Linezolid	6 (4.4)	2 (2.1)	0.476
Tobramycin	6 (4.4)	2 (2.1)	0.476
Cefoxitin	46 (33.8)	24 (25.3)	0.164
Ciprofloxacin	86 (63.2)	68 (71.6)	0.186
Doxycycline	127 (93.4)	94 (98.9)	0.050
Imipenem	134 (98.5)	95 (100.0)	1.000

The breakpoints to establish susceptibility and resistance for drugs were followed as recommendation from Clinical and Laboratory Standards Institute (CLSI-M24-A2)

[15] and South Korea (48%) [16]. The second most frequently identified NTM specie is *M. abscessus* complex. Despite occurring less frequently in Northern America and Europe [14, 15], this species was found to generally cause > 30% of pulmonary NTM infections in India [17], Taiwan [18] and South Korea [16]. The marked geographic variation in mycobacteria species could reflect the diversity of species composition of NTM in environmental niches [3]. Interestingly, all the regions with high isolation frequency of *M. abscessus* are in Asia; we thus speculate that Asian persons may also be more susceptible to *M. abscessus* infection. In line with our hypothesis, Adjemian and colleagues found that Asian persons have an increased risk for infection with *M. abscessus* than other ethnics [19]. Hence, the ethnic factors contributing to susceptibility to different NTM species may also play an important role in the diverse geographic NTM patterns across world regions.

Another interesting finding of this study is that the frequency of NTM species from pulmonary patients differs significantly from the observations from a recent laboratory-based study in Guangzhou [1]. First, *M. avium* complex exceeds *M. abscessus* complex as the predominant causative agent of pulmonary NTM disease, which reflects the inherent difference in NTM prevalence between pulmonary diseases and colonization. The species difference of pulmonary NTM colonization may partly determine the frequency and manifestations of pulmonary NTM disease [3]. However, the variation of pathogenicity among distinct NTM species could greatly contribute to the prevalence of diseases due to NTM species [20]. A population-based study of patients with respiratory NTM isolates from the Netherlands revealed that differences in clinical relevance exist among NTM species [20]. Similar results were noted in a systematic review in Eastern Asian that *M. avium* complex was clinically more relevant than *M. abscessus* complex among patients meeting the ATS diagnostic criteria [21]. Although experimental evidences are limited, there is no doubt that the relative greater pathogenicity of *M. avium* complex compared with *M. abscessus* complex would increase the risk from NTM colonization to active disease in respiratory tract.

Second, *M. gordonae* was the third frequently isolates species in South China on the basis of previous data, accounting for 22.5% of NTM isolates [1]. In contrast, only 1% of pulmonary NTM diseases was caused by *M. gordonae* in the present study. This finding confirms that this species is a rarely isolated weak pathogen, majorly contributing to patient colonization and culture contamination rather than patient disease [3].

Third, several rare geographically restricted NTM species identified by previous study was not associated with NTM diseases [1]. Although for these species the small number of isolates decrease the reliability of conclusions, the disappearance of previous laboratory isolation of these rare species among NTM patients may reflect NTM colonization due to their weak pathogenicity for human individuals. Therefore, the significant change in the prevalence of NTM species between pulmonary diseases and colonization indicates that the pathogenicity differs by species, thereby leading to the difference in clinical relevance of the various NTM species, which should be taken into consideration in formulating the diagnostic criteria for pulmonary NTM diseases.

Pulmonary NTM disease is not uncommon, particularly among elderly females [22]. Our results demonstrate that female is more likely to be associated with the acquisition of NTM diseases caused by RGM than SGM. In agree with our observation, an early study from the United States suggested that *M. avium* complex lung disease was more common among males than females

[23]. The gender difference in the NTM diseases may reflect differences in the immune responses during infection between RGM and SGM [24]. Generally, females exhibit greater cell-mediated immune responses to infection and vaccination than males [25], which is also important in host defense against mycobacteria. We therefore hypothesize that this instinct immunological difference may affect in SGM infections more than RGM infections.

Numerous studies have documented that pulmonary NTM infection more frequently affect elderly patients [6, 25]. In this study, we found that the prevalence of SGM increased significantly with advancing age. Furthermore, half of SGM diseases occurred in patients > 60 years of age. On one hand, the immunity in elderly persons is less able to produce an effective immune response after challenges with mycobacteria than the young [26]. This condition would result in greater incidence or reactivation of mycobacteria. On the other hand, the high incidence of co-morbidities presumed to affect the immune response in this population, such as diabetes, kidney failure, and immunosuppressive therapy, may favor the progression of pulmonary NTM infection. More studies are need to evaluate the relative contribution of each factor to the increased risk of pulmonary SGM diseases.

The association between bronchiectasis and NTM disease has been described by several reports [27–29]. We found that the presence of bronchiectasis appears to be more closely associated with RGM than SGM. It has been hypothesized that the impaired secretion clearance due to bronchiectasis enables NTM airway colonization and increases the risk of infection [29]. A recent report by Williams et al. compared the biofilm formation between RGM and SGM, demonstrating that *M. avium* complex is better equipped to grow in low-nutrient conditions than RGM by the development of more culturable biofilm [30]. Although the exact reason remains unknown, the reduced capability in the synthesis of biofilm of RGM allows these species prefer to inhabit in architectural-defected airway rather than normal airway, offering an explanation for the greater occurrence of bronchiectasis among pulmonary RGM cases.

This study is subject to several limitations. First, HIV infection has been regarded as an independent risk factor for NTM infections [31], while the HIV-positive patients were not included in this study because the HIV-positive patients with were transferred to another hospital receiving antiviral treatment. Given that *M. avium* infections are frequently encountered in AIDS patients [31], we may underestimate the prevalence of *M. avium* isolates in Southern China. Second, the clinical outcomes of pulmonary NTM patients were not collected in this study, because patients are not under follow-up for NTM diseases in China. As a consequence, we only analysed in vitro antibiotic susceptibility of NTM isolates rather than its correlation with treatment results. Therefore, further study is urgently needed to investigate the correlation between in vitro drug susceptibility and clinical outcomes among NTM patients. Third, another important explanation for poor response to macrolide-based chemotherapy for *M. abscessus* infections is the inducible macrolide resistance phenotype. Unfortunately, the routine detection of drug susceptibility for RGM only incubates 96-well microtiter plates for 3 days, whereas the detection of inducible resistance requires an extended incubation of plates with reading after 14 days of incubation. As a consequence, the resistance to clarithromycin for *M. abscessus* would be underestimated. Fourth, although cavitary is another major category regarding NTM pulmonary diseases, the radiological characteristics were not collected in this study due to the limited information in the medical records of patients. Nevertheless, this study provides important hints to help clinicians interpret laboratory results and recognize the risk factors associated with various NTM species.

Conclusion

In conclusion, our data illustrate that the *M. avium* complex is the most predominate causative agent of pulmonary NTM disease in Southern China. Female, migrant population, the presence of bronchiectasis are independent risk factors for pulmonary diseases due to RGM. In addition, the prevalence of SGM increases significantly with advancing age. In view of the growing public health concern, further studies will be carried out to determine the association between in vitro susceptibility and treatment outcome among these NTM patients, which is essential to help clinicians select effective regimens for the treatment of NTM infections.

Acknowledgments
We thank all staffs from Guangzhou Chest Hospital for their help in carrying out this study.

Funding
This research was supported by the Guangzhou Collaborative Innovation Major Project on Health and Medicine (201604020019), National Key Project (2015ZX10003003) and the Beijing Municipal Administration of Hospitals' Youth Programme (QML20171601).

Authors' contributions
YT, BS, WS, XC, SK, HK, JL, and YP: Substantial contributions to conception and design of, or acquisition of data or analysis and interpretation of data. YT, BS, JL, and YP: Drafting the article or revising it critically for important intellectual content. All authors read and approved the final manuscript.

Competing interests
The authors declare that they have no competing interests.

References

1. Pang Y, Tan Y, Chen J, Li Y, Zheng H, Song Y, Zhao Y. Diversity of nontuberculous mycobacteria in eastern and southern China: a cross-sectional study. Eur Respir J. 2017;49(3):1601429.
2. Falkinham JO III. Epidemiology of infection by nontuberculous mycobacteria. Clin Microbiol Rev. 1996;9(2):177–215.
3. Hoefsloot W, van Ingen J, Andrejak C, Angeby K, Bauriaud R, Bemer P, Beylis N, Boeree MJ, Cacho J, Chihota V, et al. The geographic diversity of nontuberculous mycobacteria isolated from pulmonary samples: an NTM-NET collaborative study. Eur Respir J. 2013;42(6):1604–13.
4. Bryant JM, Grogono DM, Greaves D, Foweraker J, Roddick I, Inns T, Reacher M, Haworth CS, Curran MD, Harris SR, et al. Whole-genome sequencing to identify transmission of Mycobacterium abscessus between patients with cystic fibrosis: a retrospective cohort study. Lancet. 2013;381(9877):1551–60.
5. Grubek-Jaworska H, Walkiewicz R, Safianowska A, Nowacka-Mazurek M, Krenke R, Przybylowski T, Chazan R. Nontuberculous mycobacterial infections among patients suspected of pulmonary tuberculosis. Eur J Clin Microbiol Infect Dis. 2009;28(7):739–44.
6. McShane PJ, Glassroth J. Pulmonary disease due to nontuberculous mycobacteria: current state and new insights. Chest. 2015;148(6):1517–27.
7. Hernandez-Garduno E, Elwood RK. Increasing incidence of nontuberculous mycobacteria, Taiwan, 2000-2008. Emerg Infect Dis. 2010;16(6):1047 author reply 1047-1048.
8. Wang L, Zhang H, Ruan Y, Chin DP, Xia Y, Cheng S, Chen M, Zhao Y, Jiang S, Du X, et al. Tuberculosis prevalence in China, 1990-2010; a longitudinal analysis of national survey data. Lancet. 2014;383(9934):2057–64.
9. Zhang Z, Pang Y, Wang Y, Cohen C, Zhao Y, Liu C. Differences in risk factors and drug susceptibility between Mycobacterium avium and Mycobacterium intracellulare lung diseases in China. Int J Antimicrob Agents. 2015;45(5):491–5.
10. Shao Y, Chen C, Song H, Li G, Liu Q, Li Y, Zhu L, Martinez L, Lu W. the epidemiology and geographic distribution of nontuberculous mycobacteria clinical isolates from sputum samples in the eastern region of China. PLoS Negl Trop Dis. 2015;9(3):e0003623.
11. Griffith DE, Aksamit T, Brown-Elliott BA, Catanzaro A, Daley C, Gordin F, Holland SM, Horsburgh R, Huitt G, Iademarco MF, et al. An official ATS/IDSA statement: diagnosis, treatment, and prevention of nontuberculous mycobacterial diseases. Am J Respir Crit Care Med. 2007;175(4):367–416.
12. Zhu L, Jiang G, Wang S, Wang C, Li Q, Yu H, Zhou Y, Zhao B, Huang H, Xing W, et al. Biochip system for rapid and accurate identification of mycobacterial species from isolates and sputum. J Clin Microbiol. 2010; 48(10):3654–60.
13. Clinical and Laboratory Standards Institute. Susceptibility testing of mycobacteria, nocardia, and other aerobic actinomycetes; approved standard, 2nd ed; CLSI document M24-A2. Clinical and Laboratory Standards Institute, Wayne. (2011).
14. Cassidy PM, Hedberg K, Saulson A, McNelly E, Winthrop KL. Nontuberculous mycobacterial disease prevalence and risk factors: a changing epidemiology. Clin Infect Dis. 2009;49(12):e124–9.
15. Andrejak C, Thomsen VO, Johansen IS, Riis A, Benfield TL, Duhaut P, Sorensen HT, Lescure FX, Thomsen RW. Nontuberculous pulmonary mycobacteriosis in Denmark: incidence and prognostic factors. Am J Respir Crit Care Med. 2010;181(5):514–21.
16. Koh WJ, Kwon OJ, Jeon K, Kim TS, Lee KS, Park YK, Bai GH. Clinical significance of nontuberculous mycobacteria isolated from respiratory specimens in Korea. Chest. 2006;129(2):341–8.
17. Prevots DR, Marras TK. Epidemiology of human pulmonary infection with nontuberculous mycobacteria: a review. Clin Chest Med. 2015;36(1):13–34.
18. Chien JY, Lai CC, Sheng WH, Yu CJ, Hsueh PR. Pulmonary infection and colonization with nontuberculous mycobacteria, Taiwan, 2000-2012. Emerg Infect Dis. 2014;20(8):1382–5.
19. Adjemian J, Frankland TB, Daida YG, Honda JR, Olivier KN, Zelazny A, Honda S, Prevots DR. Epidemiology of nontuberculous mycobacterial lung disease and tuberculosis, Hawaii. USA Emerg Infect Dis. 2017;23(3):439–47.
20. van Ingen J, Bendien SA, de Lange WC, Hoefsloot W, Dekhuijzen PN, Boeree MJ, van Soolingen D. Clinical relevance of non-tuberculous mycobacteria isolated in the Nijmegen-Arnhem region. The Netherlands Thorax. 2009;64(6):502–6.
21. Simons S, van Ingen J, Hsueh PR, Van Hung N, Dekhuijzen PN, Boeree MJ, van Soolingen D. Nontuberculous mycobacteria in respiratory tract infections. eastern Asia Emerg Infect Dis. 2011;17(3):343–9.
22. Winthrop KL, McNelley E, Kendall B, Marshall-Olson A, Morris C, Cassidy M, Saulson A, Hedberg K. Pulmonary nontuberculous mycobacterial disease prevalence and clinical features: an emerging public health disease. Am J Respir Crit Care Med. 2010;182(7):977–82.
23. O'Brien RJ, Geiter LJ, Snider DE Jr. The epidemiology of nontuberculous mycobacterial diseases in the United States. Results from a national survey Am Rev Respir Dis. 1987;135(5):1007–14.
24. vom Steeg LG, Klein SL. SeXX matters in infectious disease pathogenesis. PLoS Pathog. 2016;12(2):e1005374.
25. Klein SL, Jedlicka A, Pekosz A. The Xs and Y of immune responses to viral vaccines. Lancet Infect Dis. 2010;10(5):338–49.
26. Solana R, Pawelec G, Tarazona R. Aging and innate immunity. Immunity. 2006;24(5):491–4.
27. Fowler SJ, French J, Screaton NJ, Foweraker J, Condliffe A, Haworth CS, Exley AR, Bilton D. Nontuberculous mycobacteria in bronchiectasis: prevalence and patient characteristics. Eur Respir J. 2006;28(6):1204–10.
28. Reich JM. Genesis of the nodular bronchiectasis phenotype of pulmonary disease due to nontuberculous mycobacteria. Chest. 2016;149(4):1113.
29. Cook JL. Nontuberculous mycobacteria: opportunistic environmental pathogens for predisposed hosts. Br Med Bull. 2010;96:45–59.
30. Williams MM, Yakrus MA, Arduino MJ, Cooksey RC, Crane CB, Banerjee SN, Hilborn ED, Donlan RM. Structural analysis of biofilm formation by rapidly and slowly growing nontuberculous mycobacteria. Appl Environ Microbiol. 2009;75(7):2091–8.
31. Guthertz LS, Damsker B, Bottone EJ, Ford EG, Midura TF, Janda JM. Mycobacterium avium and Mycobacterium intracellulare infections in patients with and without AIDS. J Infect Dis. 1989;160(6):1037–41.

Intratracheal administration of adipose derived mesenchymal stem cells alleviates chronic asthma in a mouse model

Ranran Dai[1†], Youchao Yu[1†], Guofeng Yan[2], Xiaoxia Hou[1], Yingmeng Ni[1] and Guochao Shi[1*]

Abstract

Background: Adipose-derived mesenchymal stem cell (ASCs) exerts immunomodulatory roles in asthma. However, the underlying mechanism remains unclear. The present study aimed to explore the effects and mechanisms of ASCs on chronic asthma using an ovalbumin (OVA)-sensitized asthmatic mouse model.

Methods: Murine ASCs (mASCs) were isolated from male Balb/c mice and identified by the expression of surface markers using flow cytometry. The OVA-sensitized asthmatic mouse model was established and then animals were treated with the mASCs through intratracheal delivery. The therapy effects were assessed by measuring airway responsiveness, performing immuohistochemical analysis, and examining bronchoalveolar lavage fluid (BALF). Additionally, the expression of inflammatory cytokines and IgE was detected by CHIP and ELISA, respectively. The mRNA levels of serum indices were detected using qRT-PCR.

Results: The mASCs grew by adherence with fibroblast-like morphology, and showed the positive expression of CD90, CD44, and CD29 as well as the negative expression of CD45 and CD34, indicating that the mASCs were successfully isolated. Administering mASCs to asthmatic model animals through intratracheal delivery reduced airway responsiveness, the number of lymphocytes ($P < 0.01$) and the expression of IgE ($P < 0.01$), IL-1β ($P < 0.05$), IL-4 ($P < 0.001$), and IL-17F ($P < 0.001$), as well as increased the serum levels of IL-10 and Foxp3, and the percentage of CD4 + CD25 + Foxp3+ Tregs in the spleen, and reduced the expression of IL-17 ($P < 0.05$) and RORγ.

Conclusions: Intratracheal administration of mASCs alleviated airway inflammation, improved airway remodeling, and relieved airway hyperresponsiveness in an OVA-sensitized asthma model, which might be associated with the restoration of Th1/Th2 cell balance by mASCs.

Keywords: Chronic asthma, Airway hyperresponsiveness, Mesenchymal stem cells, Regulatory T cells

Background

As a common chronic respiratory disease, the prevalence of asthma keeps increases every year [1]. The characteristics of asthma include bronchial hyperreactivity and symptoms of airway obstruction [2]. The combination of corticosteroids and long-acting β2-adrenoceptor agonists is widely used to control asthma in most patients [3]. However, asthma is not yet cured and clinical symptoms are still difficult to alleviate [2]. Therefore, it is necessary to explore novel therapies and their mechanisms.

Multiple types of cells are involved in asthma pathology, including eosinophils, mast cells, T lymphocytes, invariant NKT cells, basophils, type 2 innate lymphoid cells (ILC2s) and others [4]. An imbalance of Th1 lymphocytes/Th2 lymphocytes (Th1/Th2) is thought to be involved in asthma pathogenesis of asthma [5], but this imbalance cannot fully explain the pathological mechanism of asthma. Regulatory T cells (Tregs), including natural regulatory T cells (nTregs) and inducible/adaptive regulatory T cells (iTregs or Tregs), play a more critical role in autoimmune diseases and allergic diseases through regulating helper T cells [6]. The

---

* Correspondence: GreadS567@163.com
†Ranran Dai and Youchao Yu contributed equally to this work.
[1]Department of Pulmonary and Critical Care Medicine, Ruijin Hospital, Shanghai Jiaotong University, School of Medicine, NO.197, Ruijin Er Road, Shanghai 200025, China
Full list of author information is available at the end of the article

phenotype of Tregs is characterized by constitutively high expression of cell surface molecules, such as CD25/GITR/CTLA4 and the transcription factor Foxp3 [5]. The role of Tregs in asthma has been demonstrated in both human and animal studies [7–9]. Shi et al. found that the Th2 response is associated with a deficiency of CD4 + CD25 + Tregs in patients with asthma [5]. Tao et al. revealed that Tregs are significantly less abundant in children with allergic rhinitis (AR) accompanyied by bronchial asthma (BA) than those with AR or BA alone or control subjects [10]. In a mouse asthma model of asthma, infusing CD4+ CD25+ Tregs can alleviate airway inflammation and airway hyperresponsiveness through increasing the serum level of IL-10 [9].

Mesenchymal stem cells (MSCs), pluripotent cells derived from early mesoderm, can differentiate into fat, bone, cartilage, epithelial cells and endothelial cells [11]. Many studies have reported that MSCs are beneficial to the remission of asthma remission [12–14]. It has been demonstrated that when MSCs are infused into mice with ovalbumin (OVA)-sensitized asthma, the serum IgE level is significantly downregulated and airway inflammation is markedly relieved [15, 16]. Importantly, adipose-derived mesenchymal stem cells (ASCs) reduce inflammation and induce Tregs in immune disorders such as rheumatoid arthritis [17]. However, the effects and mechanisms of ASCs in asthma have rarely been reported.

In the present study, mouse ASCs (mASCs) were intratracheally applied into mice in an OVA-sensitized chronic asthma model, and then the clinical symptoms of mouse asthma were extensively investigated. The underlying mechanisms were also revealed.

Methods

Animal preparation

The Ethics Committee of Shanghai Jiaotong University (Shanghai, China) approved this study. Ten male and eighty female Balb/c mice of 6–8 weeks age and 16–18 g weight were provided by Shanghai Silaike Laboratory Animal Co., Ltd. (Shanghai, China) and fed in the animal experimental center of school of Medicine, Shanghai Jiao Tong University at suitable environment. The male mice were fed with high fat diet for 4 weeks while the female mice were provided normal food and water under a 12 h/12 h light/dark cycle.

Isolation and culture of murine ASCs

The male Balb/c mice were sacrificed via cervical dislocation and immersed into 75% alcohol for 2 min. Then, the groin subcutaneous fat tissues were aseptically removed and minced with scissors, followed by washing with phosphate buffer saline (PBS) and digestion with collagenase I [18]. The mASCs were obtained after the floating fat and undigested tissues were centrifuged. Next, the mASCs were resuspended in serum-free medium, inoculated into a T75 flask and cultured in a 37°C incubator with 5% CO_2.

Flow cytometry

The expression of CD90, CD44, CD29, CD34 and CD45 on mASCs was detected using flow cytometry (FACS, Epics Altra, Coulter, Beckman, USA). When the confluency of mASCs reached 80–90%, the cell density was adjusted to 1×10^6/ml. Then the cell suspensions were acquired from mASCs of the mice, respectively. The FACS was conducted after incubation with antibodies against CD90-PE, CD44-PE, CD29-PE, CD34-PE, and CD45-PE (BD Pharmingen, San Diego, USA).

Animal model, grouping and administration

Female Balb/c mice were randomly divided into four groups containing ten mice each group: PBS + PBS group, PBS + mASCs group, OVA + PBS group, and OVA+ mASCs group. An OVA-sensitized allergic asthma model was established following a previously described procedure [19]. Briefly, the mice in the PBS + PBS and PBS + mASCs groups were intraperitoneally injected with 100 μl PBS while the mice in the OVA + PBS and OVA + mASCs groups were intraperitoneally injected with 100 μl of 0.1% OVA (Sigma-Aldrich, Saint Louis, Missouri, USA) at Days 0, 7, and 14. Then, the mice were anesthetized by injecting 30 μl chloral hydrate and fixed in the operation panel. The mouse headswere lift, keeping an angle of 30° between the head and the ground. Mouse tongues were pulled out with wide-nose pliers, and the trace syringe was inserted into the trachea directly by the laryngeal glottis under laryngoscopy. In total, 30 μl of PBS were intratracheally injected into the mice of the PBS + PBS and OVA + PBS groups at Day 21 via endotracheal instillation. At the same time, 1×10^6 mASCs in 30 μl PBS were intratracheally injected into the mice of the PBS + mASCs and OVA + mASCs groups. Thirty minutes after the transplantation, the mice were maintained in a chamber filled with 2.5% atomized-OVA for an extra 30 min. All the mice were challenged for 30 min with 2.5% atomized-OVA 3 times a week for 8 consecutive weeks. All female Balb/c mice were sacrificed within 24 h after the last atomized-OVA challenge through intraperitoneal injection of 300 mg/kg pentobarbital sodium.

Airway hyperresponsiveness test

The mice were anesthetized by injecting 5 mg/kg midazolam and 100 mg/kg alcidione. Then airway responsiveness was determined with an EMMS system (EMMS, Hampshire, UK) by measuring lung resistance (R_L) in response to inhaled methacholine (MCh; Sigma-Aldrich) at concentrations of 4 to 256 mg/mL for 20 s. The provocative challenge 100 (PC100) was calculated from the dose of MCh at which R_L was 100% above the baseline level.

Preparation of bronchoalveolar lavage fluid
BALF was obtained by lavaging the trachea with cold PBS three times [20]. After centrifugation, the supernatants were used for cytokine analysis. The cell pellets were resuspended in PBS. The total number of cells was calculated under a microscope after Trypan blue staining, and the number of neutrophils, eosinophils, macrophages, and lymphocytes was determined after staining with Wright and Giemsa solutions.

Immunohistochemical analysis
The left lung was fixed with 10% formalin solution for 24 h and embedded in paraffin. Then the samples were prepared using a standard protocol. The 5-μm-thick sections were subjected to HE, MASSON and AB-PAS staining according to previously described methods [21]. Besides, the expression of Muc5AC was visualized by immunohistochemical analysis after adding an anti-Muc5AC antibody (Abcam, Cambridge, UK).

The percentage of CD4 + CD25 + Foxp3+ Tregs in spleen
The cells were filtrated after the spleen was fully ground and red blood cells were removed with erythrocyte lysis buffer. After washing twice with PBS, spleen cells were stained with anti-mouse CD4-FITC, CD25-APC, and Foxp3-PE antibodies (eBioscience, San Diego, CA, USA). The percentage of CD4 + CD25 + Foxp3+ Tregs was analyzed by flow cytometry (Epics Altra, Coulter, Beckman, USA).

Quantitative real-time PCR (qRT-PCR) analysis
Total RNA of right lung tissues was extracted using Trizol (Invitrogen, Carlsbad, California, USA) and cDNA samples were prepared by a first strand cDNA synthesis kit (Promega, Wisconsin, Madison, USA) thereafter. The sequences of the primers were as follows: Foxp3, forward-5′-GCCTTCAGACGAGACTTG-3′, reverse – 5′-CATTGGGTTCTTGTCAGAG-3′; RORγt, forward-5′-CAGGAG CATGGAAGT-CGTC-3′, reverse-5′-CCG TGTAGAGGGCAATCTCA-3′; IL-10, forward-5′-CCC TT-TGCTATGGTGTCCT-3′, reverse-5′-GGATCTCCC TGGTTTCTCTT-3′; IL-17F, forward-5′-AGGGAAGAA GCAGCCATT-3′, reverse-5′-CCAACATCAACAGT AG-CAAA-3′; and β-actin, forward-5′-CAGAAGGAC TCCTACGTG-3′, reverse-5′-GCTCGGTCAGGATC TTCATG-3′. β-actin was measured as an internal control. The relative expression of mRNA was normalized to expression of β-actin.

Measurement of inflammatory cytokines in serum and BALF
Serum samples were obtained from mice in the four groups. Firstly, the mice were fixed in a supine position and the hair of the anterior chest was cut. After the skin was disinfected, 800 μl of blood was extracted from the area with the strongest heart beat using the cardiac puncture method. Then, the blood samples were centrifuged and the serum samples were obtained. Protein was extracted from the serum and BALF samples. In total, 50 μl of protein samples were acquired and normalized to the standard samples gradient elution on a slide. Fluorescein was measured as a detection signal. The expression of IL-1β, IL-4, IL-10 and IL-17F was quantified using CHIP by comparing the signal of these genes with those of the standard samples, respectively. Additionally, protein expression of IgE was measured by ELISA kits (eBioscience, San Diego, CA, USA) according to the manufacturer's instructions.

Statistical analysis
Data were analyzed by SPSS21.0 software and presented as mean ± standard deviation. A normality test and homogeneity variance analysis were first conducted to analyze the data. Then, the differences among multiple groups were determined using one-way ANOVA followed by the Fishers least significant difference (LSD) method. $P < 0.05$ was considered to be statistically significant.

Results
The morphological observation of mASCs and the expression of their surface markers
The mASCs grew adherent with a fibroblast-like morphology, which gradually transformed to an irregular star shape with further passaging (Fig. 1a). FACS analysis showed that the surface expression of CD90, CD44, and CD29 on mASCs was high, while the expression of CD34 and CD45 was relatively low (Fig. 1b). These data demonstrated that mASCs isolation was successful.

Effect of mASCs on the pathomorphology of lung tissue in OVA-induced asthma model mice
Compared to control mice, OVA-challenged mice showed abnormal lung structure by HE staining, including inverted bronchial mucosa cilia, wall thickening, and swelled mucous membrane, while treatment with mASCs in the OVA group markedly reduced the number of inflammatory cells (Fig. 2a-d). To determine differences in tissue composition of the experimental groups, MASSON staining was conducted. The results found that the manifestation of the tissues in the four groups was not significantly different, and fibrosis was not observed (Fig. 2e-f). In addition, the tissues of mice in the OVA + mASCs group had only slight fibrosis, indicating that the transplantating mASCs could relieve

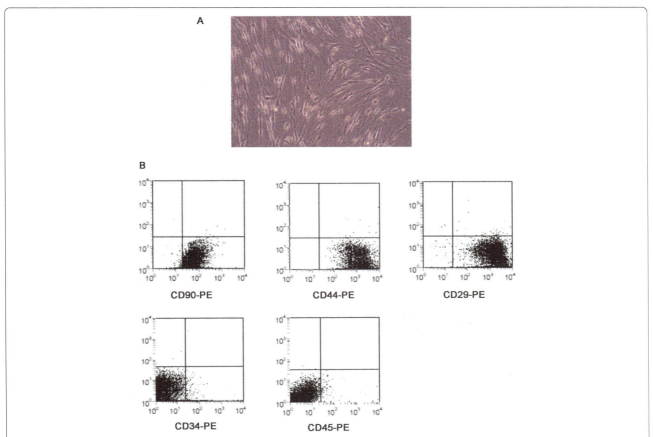

Fig. 1 The identification of adipose-derived mesenchymal stem cells of mice (mASCs). **a** The morphology of mASCs under A microscope (400X); **b** The expression of CD90, CD44, CD29, CD34 and CD45 on the surface of mASCs by flow cytometry

fibrosis in the mice with chronic asthma (Fig. 2g-h). According to the AB-PAS staining, the tissues of mice in the PBS + PBS and PBS + mASCs groups were not significantly different. No mucus in the lumen and no goblet cell hyperplasia were observed in the PBS + PBS and PBS + mASCs groups (Fig. 2i-j). However, mice in the OVA+ PBS group exhibited goblet cell hyperplasia and increased blue mucus, but goblet cell hyperplasia was relieved and blue mucus was reduced in the OVA + mASCs group (Fig. 2k-l). Furthermore, immunohistochemical analysis indicated that Muc5ac secretion was low and similar in the PBS + PBS and PBS + mASCs groups (Fig. 2m-n), but was high in the OVA + PBS group. At the same time, in the OVA + mASCs group, the secretion of Muc5ac protein was obviously reduced compared with the level in the OVA + PBS group (Fig. 2o-p, $P < 0.001$). The quantitative results of Muc5ac are shown in Fig. 2q.

Effect of mASCs on lung function and airway hyperresponsiveness in OVA-induced asthma model mice

A pulmonary function test was conducted to evaluate whether the application of mASCs could restore lung function to some extent. For normal mice, changes to R_L in mASCs-treated mice were not significantly different from that of PBS-treated mice (Fig. 3a). However, the R_L in OVA-challenged mice kept increasing as methacholine concentration increased, indicating that the asthma model was established successfully. After intratracheal administration of mASCs, changes to R_L in the asthma model significantly declined when methacholine concentration was set to 64 mg/mL, 128 mg/mL and 256 mg/mL, respectively ($P < 0.01$, Fig. 3a). Further analysis of –log [PC100] among all these four groups showed that the inhalation of OVA significantly increased airway resistance while intratracheal transplantation mASCs could reduce airway responsiveness ($P < 0.01$, Fig. 3b).

Effect of mASCs on the percentage of CD4 + CD25 + Foxp3 + Tregs in spleen in OVA-induced asthma model mice

The percentage of CD4 + CD25 + Foxp3 + Tregs in spleen of control mice was similar regardless of mASCs while the percent of Tregs significantly decreased in OVA-challenged mice compared with control mice ($P < 0.05$, Fig. 4). Although the transplantation of mASCs through trachea in an asthma model promoted the percentage of Tregs in the

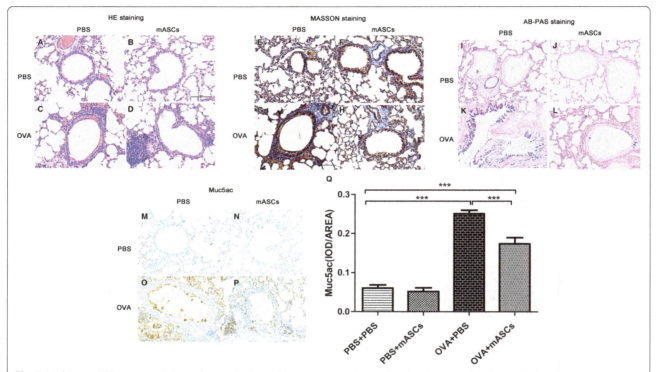

Fig. 2 Applying mASCs improved the pathomorphology of lung tissues in OVA-induced asthma model mice. **a-d**, The HE staining of lung tissues in the PBS + PBS group, PBS + mASCs group, OVA + PBS group, and OVA+ mASCs group, respectively; **e-h** The fibrosis of lung tissues in the PBS + PBS group, PBS + mASCs group, OVA + PBS group, and OVA+ mASCs group, respectively, by MASSON staining; **i-l** The mucus of lung tissues in the PBS + PBS group, PBS + mASCs group, OVA + PBS group, and OVA+ mASCs group, respectively, by AB-PAS staining; **m-p** The Muc5ac expression of lung tissues in the PBS + PBS group, PBS + mASCs group, OVA + PBS group, and OVA+ mASCs group, respectively, by immunohistochemical analysis. Bar = 100 μm. mASCs, mouse adipose-derived mesenchymal stem cells; PBS, phosphate buffered saline; OVA, ovalbumin. **q** The quantitative results of Muc5ac in figure 2m-p

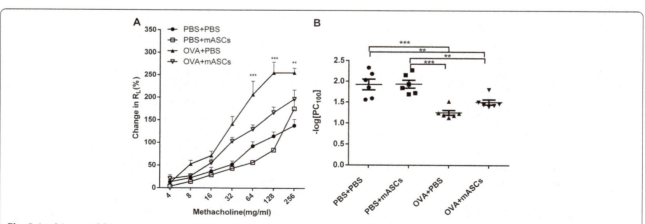

Fig. 3 Applying mASCs improved lung function and airway hyperresponsiveness in OVA-induced asthma model mice. **a** The lung resistance (R_L) in response to inhaled methacholine by airway responsiveness test; **b** The provocative challenge 100 (PC100) by airway responsiveness test. **$P < 0.01$, and ***$P < 0.001$. mASCs, mouse adipose-derived mesenchymal stem cells; PBS, phosphate buffer saline; OVA, ovalbumin

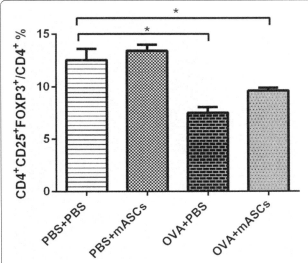

Fig. 4 The percentage of CD4+ CD25+ Foxp3+ Tregs in spleen in the PBS + PBS group, PBS + mASCs group, OVA + PBS group, and OVA+ mASCs group, respectively, by flow cytometry analysis. *$P < 0.05$. mASCs, mouse adipose-derived mesenchymal stem cells; PBS, phosphate buffered saline; OVA, ovalbumin

spleen, the difference was not statistically significant (Fig. 4).

Effect of mASCs on cell count and subsets in BALF in OVA-induced asthma model mice

In the control mice, the administration of mASCs did not change the total cell number in BALF nor the cell subsets. However, the total cell number and lymphocytes were significantly higher in asthma model mice than that in control mice ($P < 0.01$, Fig. 5). In addition, eosinophils and neutrophils were significantly higher in asthma model mice than that in control mice ($P < 0.05$, Fig. 5).

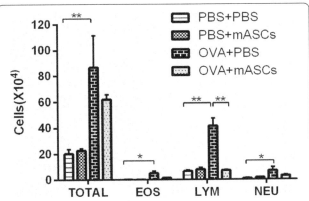

Fig. 5 Cell counts and subsets in bronchoalveolar lavage fluid (BALF) samples in the PBS + PBS group, PBS + mASCs group, OVA + PBS group, and OVA+ mASCs group, respectively. *$P < 0.05$ and **$P < 0.01$. mASCs, mouse adipose-derived mesenchymal stem cells; PBS, phosphate buffered saline; OVA, ovalbumin

Compared with mice exposed to OVA challenge alone, applying mASCs in OVA-challenged mice reduced the number of cell subsets, eosinophils, neutrophils, and lymphocytes, while only the alteration of lymphocytes was statistically different ($P < 0.01$, Fig. 5).

Effect of mASCs on inflammatory cytokines in OVA-induced asthma model mice

The expression of serum IL-1β, IL-4, and IL-17F were all significantly increased in the asthma model animals when compared with levels in mice from the PBS + PBS group ($P < 0.05$, $P < 0.01$, and $P < 0.001$, respectively, Fig. 6a). However, the secretion of all these three cytokines drastically decreased after intratracheal transplantation of mASCs when compared with those in the asthma model group ($P < 0.05$, $P < 0.001$, and $P < 0.001$, respectively, Fig. 6a). The expression of serum IgE was determined by ELISA, and the results showed that IgE level in OVA-sensitized mice was dramatically elevated when compared with the level in the PBS + PBS group ($P < 0.01$, Fig. 6a). However, intratracheal administration of mASCs in OVA challenge mice could inhibit serum IgE level, which was significantly different when compared with OVA + PBS group ($P < 0.01$, Fig. 6a). A similar trend was found in the BALF level of both IL-4 and IL17F, which were significantly enhanced after OVA-challenged (all $P < 0.001$, Fig. 6b) but decreased after administration of mASCs (all $P < 0.001$, respectively, Fig. 6b). However, the level of IL-10 decreased OVA challenge but increased after administration of mASCs ($P < 0.05$). In addition, in the lung tissues, the mRNA levels of IL-10 and Foxp3 in OVA-treated mice was significantly reduced ($P < 0.01$ and $P < 0.001$, Fig. 6c), while the expression of IL-17 and RORγ was increased compared with expression in the PBS + PBS group (all $P < 0.001$, Fig. 6c).

Discussion

Asthma is an airway chronic inflammatory disease of the airway involving a variety of cells and components. This chronic inflammation is associated with airway hyperresponsiveness. The mouse asthma model used in the present study perfectly mimicked the pathophysiological characteristics of human asthma. The results demonstrated that intratracheal administration of mASCs could not only reduce airway hyperresponsiveness, inflammatory cell infiltration, and Muc5ac secretion, but also improve airway remodeling.

Th1/Th2 cell imbalance is involved in asthma pathogenesis [22]. Th1 cells exert a protective effect on asthma through releasing IFN-γ and IL-2, while Th2 cells mainly secrete IL-4, IL-5, and IL-13, and then promote the development of asthma [23, 24]. IL-4 can

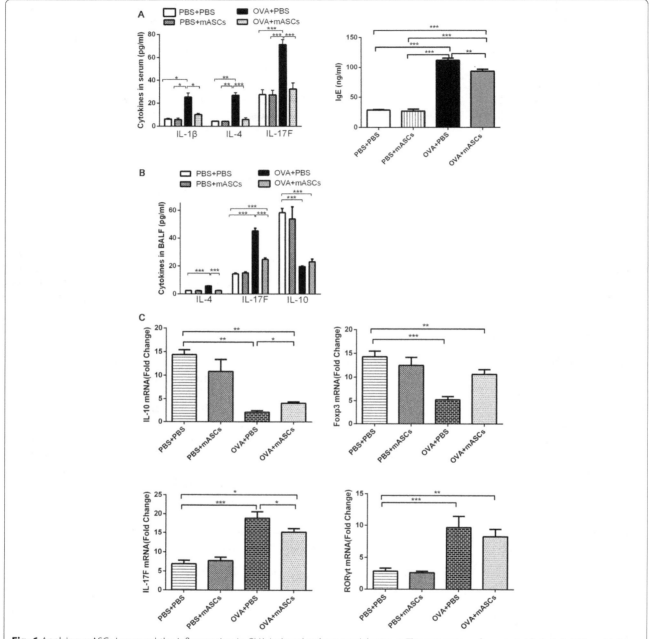

Fig. 6 Applying mASCs improved the inflammation in OVA-induced asthma model mice. **a** The expression of serum IL-1β, IL-4, IL-17F, and IgE in the PBS + PBS group, PBS + mASCs group, OVA + PBS group, and OVA+ mASCs group, respectively, by CHIP and ELISA; **b** The expression of IL-4, IL-17F, and IL-10 in BALF in the PBS + PBS group, PBS + mASCs group, OVA + PBS group, and OVA+ mASCs group, respectively, by CHIP; **c** The mRNA levels of IL-10, Foxp3, IL-17, and RORγ in the lung tissues of PBS + PBS group, PBS + mASCs group, OVA + PBS group, and OVA+ mASCs group, respectively, by qRT-PCR. *$P < 0.05$, **$P < 0.01$ and ***$P < 0.001$. mASCs, mouse adipose-derived mesenchymal stem cells; PBS, phosphate buffered saline; OVA, ovalbumin; BALF, bronchoalveolar lavage fluid

promote the secretion of IgE and increase the secretion of Muc5ac protein in the airway, which leads to high airway response [23, 24]. In this study, we found that Th1 cell secretion was insufficient while Th2 cell secretion was excessive in a chronic asthma mouse model. Furthermore, the expression of serum IL-1β, IL-4 and IL-17F was higher in the asthmatic model compared to those being transplanted by mASCs, indicating that cell therapy might improve the degree of asthma airway inflammation and airway remodeling through regulating the Th1/Th2 ratio. Our results were similar with those of a study by Nemeth [25].

The malfunction of Tregs is another important mechanism of asthma. Growing evidences shows that asthma is closely related to Tregs [26]. The decline in the number of Tregs as well as their function in asthma is an important manifestation of an immune disorders [27]. A previous study showed that human and mouse MSCs could be induced into CD4 + CD25+ Tregs both in vitro and in vivo, and the immune regulation mediated by MSCs was associated with an increase in number of T cells and the associated cytokine levels [28]. In the present study, the ratio of Tregs to CD4+ T lymphocytes in spleen of asthma model animals was significantly lower than that of the normal group, while the administration of mASCs improved the percentage of Tregs, and reduced the degree of infiltration of inflammatory cells in small bronchial and vascular submucosal tissues in chronic asthmatic mice. Importantly, the transplantation of mASCs showed no influence on normal lung tissue.

As pro-inflammatory cells, Th17 cells can induce the occurrence of asthma and autoimmune diseases by secreting inflammatory factors such as IL-17A, IL-17F, IL-6 and tumor necrosis factor-α [29]. RORγt is the key transcription factor regulating Th17 cell differentiation [30]. In the present study, the IL-17F level in serum and BALF was higher in asthmatic model than that in normal mice, while the IL-10 level was lower in asthmatic model animals. Applying mASCs could downregulate IL-17 and RORγ in asthmatic mice, and upregulate IL-10 and FOXP3, implying that cell therapy could restore the balance of Th17/Treg cells through suppressing the differentiation of Th17 cells and inducing the transcription of Foxp3, which ultimately alleviated airway inflammation and remodeling.

Conclusions

In conclusion, intratracheal administration of mASCs could alleviate the airway inflammation of lung tissue in an OVA-sensitized mouse asthma model, improve airway remodeling and relieve airway hyperresponsiveness. The mechanism might be associated with the restoration of Th1/Th2 cell balance by mASCs.

Abbreviations
ASCs: Adipose-derived mesenchymal stem cell; BALF: Bronchoalveolar lavage fluid; LSD: Least significant difference; MSCs: Mesenchymal stem cells; OVA: Ovalbumin; PBS: Phosphate buffer saline; TH1/TH2: Th1 lymphocytes/ Th2 lymphocytes

Acknowledgements
This work was supported by National Nature Science Foundation of China (Program No. 81470216) and Shanghai Municipal Planning Commission of science and Research Fund.

Funding
This work was supported by National Nature Science Foundation of China (Program No. 81470216) and Shanghai Municipal Planning Commission of science and Research Fund.

Authors' contributions
Conception and design of the research: RD and GS. Acquisition of data: GY. Analysis and interpretation of data: RD and XH. Statistical analysis: RD and YN. Obtaining funding: GS and RD. Drafting the manuscript: YY. Revision of manuscript for important intellectual content: GS and RD. All authors read and approved the final manuscript.

Competing interests
The authors declare that they have no competing interests.

Author details
[1]Department of Pulmonary and Critical Care Medicine, Ruijin Hospital, Shanghai Jiaotong University, School of Medicine, NO.197, Ruijin Er Road, Shanghai 200025, China. [2]School of Medicine, Shanghai Jiaotong University, Shanghai 200025, China.

References
1. Barnes PJ. New therapies for asthma: is there any progress? Trends Pharmacol Sci. 2010;31(7):335–43.
2. Braman SS. The global burden of asthma. Chest J. 2006;130(1_suppl):4S–12S.
3. Chung KF, Adcock IM. Combination therapy of long-acting β2-adrenoceptor agonists and corticosteroids for asthma. Treat Respir Med. 2004;3(5):279–89.
4. Barnes PJ. Immunology of asthma and chronic obstructive pulmonary disease. Nat Rev Immunol. 2008;8(3):183.
5. Shi Y, Shi G, Wan H, Jiang L, Ai X, Zhu H, Tang W, Ma J, Jin X, Zhang B. Coexistence of Th1/Th2 and Th17/Treg imbalances in patients with allergic asthma. Chin Med J. 2011;124(13):1951–6.
6. Lloyd CM, Hawrylowicz CM. Regulatory T cells in asthma. Immunity. 2009;31(3):438–49.
7. Kearley J, Barker JE, Robinson DS, Lloyd CM. Resolution of airway inflammation and hyperreactivity after in vivo transfer of CD4+ CD25+ regulatory T cells is interleukin 10 dependent. J Exp Med. 2005;202(11):1539–47.
8. Lewkowich IP, Herman NS, Schleifer KW, Dance MP, Chen BL, Dienger KM, Sproles AA, Shah JS, Köhl J, Belkaid Y. CD4+ CD25+ T cells protect against experimentally induced asthma and alter pulmonary dendritic cell phenotype and function. J Exp Med. 2005;202(11):1549–61.
9. Boudousquie C, Pellaton C, Barbier N, Spertini F. CD4+ CD25+ T cell depletion impairs tolerance induction in a murine model of asthma. Clin Exp Allergy. 2009;39(9):1415–26.
10. Tao B, Ruan G, Wang D, Li Y, Wang Z, Yin G. Imbalance of peripheral Th17 and regulatory T Cells in children with allergic Rhinitis AND bronchial asthma. Iran J Allergy Asthma Immunol. 2015;14(3):273.
11. Charbord P. Bone marrow mesenchymal stem cells: historical overview and concepts. Hum Gene Ther. 2010;21(9):1045–56.
12. Ge X, Bai C, Yang J, Lou G, Li Q, Chen R. Effect of mesenchymal stem cells on inhibiting airway remodeling and airway inflammation in chronic asthma. J Cell Biochem. 2013;114(7):1595–605.
13. Mathias LJ, Khong SM, Spyroglou L, Payne NL, Siatskas C, Thorburn AN, Boyd RL, Heng TS. Alveolar macrophages are critical for the inhibition of allergic asthma by mesenchymal stromal cells. J Immunol. 2013;191(12):5914–24.
14. Ou-Yang H-F, Huang Y, Hu X-B, Wu C-G. Suppression of allergic airway inflammation in a mouse model of asthma by exogenous mesenchymal stem cells. Exp Biol Med. 2011;236(12):1461–7.
15. Sun YQ, Deng MX, He J, Zeng QX, Wen W, Wong DS, Tse HF, Xu G, Lian Q, Shi J. Human pluripotent stem cell-derived mesenchymal stem cells prevent allergic airway inflammation in mice. Stem Cells. 2012;30(12):2692–9.
16. Temelkovski J, Hogan SP, Shepherd DP, Foster PS, Kumar RK. An improved murine model of asthma: selective airway inflammation, epithelial lesions and increased methacholine responsiveness following chronic exposure to aerosolised allergen. Thorax. 1998;53(10):849–56.
17. Gonzalez-Rey E, Gonzalez MA, Varela N, O'Valle F, Hernandez-Cortes P, Rico L, Büscher D, Delgado M. Human adipose-derived mesenchymal stem cells reduce inflammatory and T cell responses and induce regulatory T cells in vitro in rheumatoid arthritis. Ann Rheum Dis. 2010;69(1):241–8.
18. Cho KS, Park HK, Park HY, Jung JS, Jeon SG, Kim YK, Roh HJ. IFATS collection: immunomodulatory effects of adipose tissue-derived stem cells

in an allergic rhinitis mouse model. Stem Cells. 2009;27(1):259-65.
19. Kianmeher M, Ghorani V, Boskabady MH. Animal model of asthma, various methods and measured parameters: a methodological review. Iran J Allergy Asthma Immunol. 2016;15(6):445.
20. Feizpour A, Boskabady MH, Ghorbani A. Adipose-derived stromal cell therapy affects lung inflammation and tracheal responsiveness in Guinea pig model of COPD. PLoS One. 2014;9(10):e108974.
21. Mohammadian M, Boskabady MH, Kashani IR, Jahromi GP, Omidi A, Nejad AK, Khamse S, Sadeghipour HR. Effect of bone marrow derived mesenchymal stem cells on lung pathology and inflammation in ovalbumin-induced asthma in mouse. Iran J Basic Med Sci. 2016;19(1):55-63.
22. Mazzarella G, Bianco A, Catena E, De Palma R, Abbate G. Th1/Th2 lymphocyte polarization in asthma. Allergy. 2000;55(s61):6-9.
23. H-j P, Lee C-M, Jung ID, Lee JS, Y-i J, Chang JH, Chun S-H, Kim M-J, Choi I-W, Ahn S-C. Quercetin regulates Th1/Th2 balance in a murine model of asthma. Int Immunopharmacol. 2009;9(3):261-7.
24. Kidd P. Th1/Th2 balance: the hypothesis, its limitations, and implications for health and disease. Altern Med Rev. 2003;8(3):223-46.
25. Nemeth K, Keane-Myers A, Brown JM, Metcalfe DD, Gorham JD, Bundoc VG, Hodges MG, Jelinek I, Madala S, Karpati S. Bone marrow stromal cells use TGF-β to suppress allergic responses in a mouse model of ragweed-induced asthma. Proc Natl Acad Sci. 2010;107(12):5652-7.
26. Yun L, Xin-sheng F, Jing-hua Y, Li X, Shan-shan W. CD4+ CD25+ FOXP3+ T cells, Foxp3 gene and protein expression contribute to antiasthmatic effects of San'ao decoction in mice model of asthma. Phytomedicine. 2014;21(5):656-62.
27. Poon AH, Chouiali F, Tse SM, Litonjua AA, Hussain SN, Baglole CJ, Eidelman DH, Olivenstein R, Martin JG, Weiss ST. Genetic and histological evidence for autophagy in asthma pathogenesis. J Allergy Clin Immunol. 2012;129(2):569.
28. Svobodova E, Krulova M, Zajicova A, Pokorna K, Prochazkova J, Trosan P, Holan V. The role of mouse mesenchymal stem cells in differentiation of naive T-cells into anti-inflammatory regulatory T-cell or proinflammatory helper T-cell 17 population. Stem Cells Dev. 2011;21(6):901-10.
29. Yang J, Sundrud MS, Skepner J, Yamagata T. Targeting Th17 cells in autoimmune diseases. Trends Pharmacol Sci. 2014;35(10):493-500.
30. Yang XO, Pappu BP, Nurieva R, Akimzhanov A, Kang HS, Chung Y, Ma L, Shah B, Panopoulos AD, Schluns KS. T helper 17 lineage differentiation is programmed by orphan nuclear receptors RORα and RORγ. Immunity. 2008;28(1):29-39.

Change in the prevalence asthma, rhinitis and respiratory symptom over a 20 year period: associations to year of birth, life style and sleep related symptoms

Christer Janson[1*], Ane Johannessen[2], Karl Franklin[3], Cecilie Svanes[4], Linus Schiöler[5], Andrei Malinovschi[6], Thorarinn Gislason[7,8], Bryndis Benediktsdottir[7,8], Vivi Schlünssen[9,10], Rain Jõgi[11], Deborah Jarvis[12] and Eva Lindberg[1]

Abstract

Background: The aim of this investigation was to study change in adults over a 20 year period in the prevalence of respiratory symptoms and disorders and its association to year of birth, life style and sleep related variables.

Method: Adults 20–44 years of age, 6085 women and 5184 men, were randomly selected from seven centres in Northern Europe and followed for 20 years. The number of participants in the first survey was 21,595 and 11,269 participated in all three surveys. The participants were divided into three birth cohorts: 1944–1955, 1956–1965 and 1966–1975.

Results: During the 20 year period the prevalence of wheeze decreased (− 2%) and the prevalence of asthma (+ 4%) and allergic rhinitis (+ 5%) increased, whereas the prevalence of nocturnal respiratory symptoms was relatively unchanged. The increase in allergic rhinitis was largest in those born 1966 to 1975 except in Estonia. There was large decrease in smoking (− 20%), increase in obesity (+ 7%) and snoring (+ 6%) during the study period. Smoking, obesity, snoring and nocturnal gastroesophageal reflux (nGER) were related to a higher risk of all symptoms. Obesity, snoring and nGER were also independently related to asthma.

Conclusion: We conclude that as our participants got older there was a decrease in wheeze, no change in nocturnal symptoms and an increase in reported asthma and allergic rhinitis. These changes in prevalence are probably related to a decrease in smoking being counteracted by an increase in allergy, obesity and sleep related disorders.

Keywords: Asthma, Allergic rhinitis, Obesity, Smoking, Gastroesophageal reflux

Background

Studies investigating time trends in asthma and respiratory symptoms by repeated cross sectional analyses have shown a decrease in the prevalence of some respiratory symptoms, a moderate increase of self-reported asthma and a sharp increase in the prevalence of allergic rhinitis in the last two decades [1–3]. There is, however, limited information available on how the prevalence of respiratory symptoms, asthma and allergic rhinitis changes with age. In the follow up of the European Community Respiratory Health Survey (ECRHS II) 11,000 young adults were followed for 10 years [4]. No large change in respiratory symptoms was found with age, but the prevalence of self-reported asthma and allergic rhinitis increased. The greater change in prevalence of allergic rhinitis was found in the youngest age group. In the second follow-up (ECRHS III), we see a decrease in the prevalence of wheeze while the prevalence of reported asthma continued to increase [5]. Other longitudinal studies of adults have shown diverging results with an increase in wheeze and cough with age in an English and a Canadian study [6, 7] and a decrease in the prevalence of wheeze in a German study [8].

* Correspondence: christer.janson@medsci.uu.se
[1]Department of Medical Sciences, Respiratory, Allergy and Sleep Medicine, Uppsala University, Uppsala, Sweden
Full list of author information is available at the end of the article

Subsequent analyses of data from ECRHS II has shown an increase in obesity [9] and a sharp decrease in smoking [10]. Obesity was a strong risk factor for onset of respiratory symptoms in the Respiratory Health In Northern Europe study (RHINE) which is a 10 year follow-up of participants in the ECRHS from the Nordic countries [11]. It is possible that lack of change in the prevalence of respiratory symptoms with age in the ECRHS II [4], was related to the decrease in smoking and increase in obesity counteracting each other. In the RHINE study we also found that onset of respiratory symptoms and self-reported asthma was related to sleep related variables such as snoring and nocturnal gastro-esophageal reflux (nGER) [11].

In 2010–2012 we conducted a second follow-up of the RHINE population (RHINE III) [12]. This follow-up also included information on body mass index (BMI), smoking, snoring and nGER. It is therefore now possible to investigate change in respiratory health by age and factors related to this change over a 20 year period. The aim of this investigation was to study change in the prevalence of respiratory symptoms and its association to year of birth, smoking, obesity, snoring and nGER.

Methods

ECRHS stage I took place in 1990–1994. In stage I of the ECRHS, males and females aged 20–44 years were randomly selected from the population register in the participating centres [13]. A postal questionnaire was sent to 3000–4000 subjects at each centre. From those who responded, a random sample was selected to undergo a more detailed clinical examination (stage 2). In addition a "symptomatic sample", reporting symptoms of waking with shortness of breath, asthma attacks or using asthma medication in stage 1 were also studied. The clinical examination included a structured interview where the subjects were asked about symptoms, respiratory disorders, smoking and other types of exposure [13]. The examination also included allergy testing, spirometry and measuring height and weight. In some centres an additional questionnaire collecting data on sleep disturbances was used [14].

RHINE II is a follow-up study of participants from ECRHS stage 1 from seven Northern European centres: Reykjavik (Iceland); Bergen (Norway); Aarhus (Denmark); Gothenburg, Uppsala, Umea (Sweden); and Tartu (Estonia) [11]. RHINE II consisted of a postal questionnaire sent in 1999–2001. In 2010–2012 a second follow-up by postal questionnaire was performed in the same centres (RHINE III) [12, 15]. The questionnaire was once again sent out to all participants of ECRHS stage 1. A summary of the number of participant and the data collected is presented in Table 1.

Informed consent was obtained from each participant and the study was approved by regional committees of medical research ethics in each country.

Respiratory health

In all three surveys identical yes/no-questions were posed about presence of respiratory symptoms at any time in the last 12 months: wheezing, nocturnal chest tightness, nocturnal shortness of breath and nocturnal cough. Subjects were considered to have asthma if they reported that they currently were using medication against asthma or have had an attack of asthma with the last 12 months [16]. Allergic rhinitis was defined as a positive answer to the question "Do you have any nasal allergies including allergic rhinitis?". In some of the analyses nocturnal chest tightness and nocturnal shortness of breath were combined and labeled nocturnal dyspnea [11].

Year of birth

The participants were divided into three birth cohorts: 1944–1955, 1956–1965 and 1966–1975.

Life style factors
Smoking

Questions on smoking were not included in the first survey in all centres. The second and third survey did, however, include questions on ex- and current smoking as well as age of starting and stopping to smoke. This information was used to estimate whether or not a participant was a smoker at the first survey or not. The question: "Are you a smoker?" was used to define current smokers in the second and third survey.

Body mass index

Body mass index (BMI) was calculated for each subject as weight in kilograms divided by the squared height in meters (kg/m^2). Subjects with BMI ≥30 were classified as being obese. Information on height and weight was only collected from one centre in the first postal survey (Bergen). In the other centres data on height and weight collected on the subsample that underwent the clinical investigation (stage 2) was used for the first time period. In the second and third survey information on height and weight were collected from questionnaires in the same way in all centres.

Sleep related variables

The postal questionnaire in survey two and three contained several multiple-choice questions in which the subjects were asked to estimate the frequency of various sleep related symptoms on a 5-points scale: never; less than once a week; one to two nights a week; three to five nights a week and almost every night [11]. For the first survey similar information was only available from the

Table 1 Number of participants with available data

	Respiratory symptoms	Smoking	BMI	Sleep related
1990–1994	21,595	14,780	6604	1867
1999–2001	16,049	15,930	15,930	15,762
2010–2012	13,093	12,738	12,930	12,811
≥ 2 surveys	17,711	13,117	12,504	11,338
All three surveys	11,269	10,858	3669	1143

subsample that underwent the clinical examination in three of the centres: Reykjavik, Gothenburg and Uppsala.

The question asked regarding nocturnal gastroesophageal reflux was: "Do you have heartburn or belching when you have gone to bed?" Subjects reporting these symptoms 1 to 2 nights per week or more, are in this study referred to as reporting nGER [11]. The question asked regarding snoring was: "Do you snore loudly and disturbingly?" Subjects reporting such snoring 3 to 5 times per week or more are referred to as reporting habitual snoring [17].

Statistics

Absolute net change in symptom and disease status between the surveys was estimated using population averaged, generalised estimating equations for a binomial outcome with identity link, with participants identified as the clustering factor and the number of the survey as an independent variable. Results were expressed as net between the surveys. The Wald test was used to examine differences in change of prevalence by birth cohort.

The influence of year of birth, life style (smoking and BMI) and sleep related variables (snoring and nGER) on respiratory health was analysed using mixed effects logistic regression in order to take into account that number of times information on risk factors was available varied between the participants.

Estimates of the influence of birth year on allergic rhinitis by centre were examined for heterogeneity and combined using random effects meta-analysis.

Results

The prevalence of respiratory symptoms, asthma and allergic rhinitis for those 11,269 subjects (6085 women and 5184 men, mean age (±SD) in first survey 32.2 ± 7.1 years) that participated in all three studies is presented in Table 2. There was a clear decrease in the prevalence of wheeze and an increase in the prevalence of asthma and allergic rhinitis, whereas the prevalence of nocturnal respiratory symptoms was relatively unchanged. Change in the prevalence of wheeze, asthma and allergic rhinitis by centre is presented in fig. 1. Overall the trends were the same in all centres except for wheeze where the prevalence did not decrease in two of the seven centres (Reykjavik and Tartu). There was a large decrease in the prevalence of smoking while an increase in obesity and snoring was found when comparing the second and third survey where data was available for a larger proportion of the population (Table 2).

The prevalence of symptoms, asthma and rhinitis in the three surveys relation to year of birth is presented in figs. 2 and 3. The youngest group (born 1966–1975) had the highest decrease in wheeze and nocturnal dyspnea, the lowest increase in asthma and the highest increase in allergic rhinitis.

Table 2 Prevalence of symptoms, disorders and lifestyle and sleep related variables for subjects who participated in all three surveys (%, n = 11,269)

	Prevalence %			Change in prevalence % (95% CI)	
	1990–94	1999–2001	2010–2012	1990–2012	p-value
Wheeze	20.4	19.5	18.6	−2.2 (−3.0, −1.5)	< 0.0001
Nocturnal chest tightness	11.1	11.3	10.3	−0.6 (−1.2, 0.1)	0.08
Nocturnal breathlessness	4.7	4.6	5.3	0.4 (−0.1, 0.8)	0.10
Nocturnal dyspnea	11.1	11.3	10.6	−0.7 (−1.2, −0.01)	0.02
Nocturnal cough	26.6	28.2	26.9	0.2 (−0.6, 1.1)	0.55
Asthma attacks	2.8	3.3	3.5	0.9 (0.5, 1.2)	< 0.0001
Asthma medication	3.6	5.5	7.6	4.1 (3.7, 4.5)	< 0.0001
Asthma	4.5	6.4	8.3	4.0 (3.5, 4.5)	< 0.0001
Allergic rhinitis	19.7	23.1	24.7	5.1 (4.5, 5.8)	< 0.0001
Smoking	37.7	25.7	16.4	−19.6 (−20.2, −18.9)	< 0.0001
Obesity (BMI > 30 kg/m2)		7.9	14.9	6.9.5 (6.4, 7.5)	< 0.0001
Snoring		17.8	24.2	6.3 (5.6, 7.2)	< 0.0001
Gastroesophageal reflux		7.0	7.3	0.2 (−0.4, 0.6)	0.57

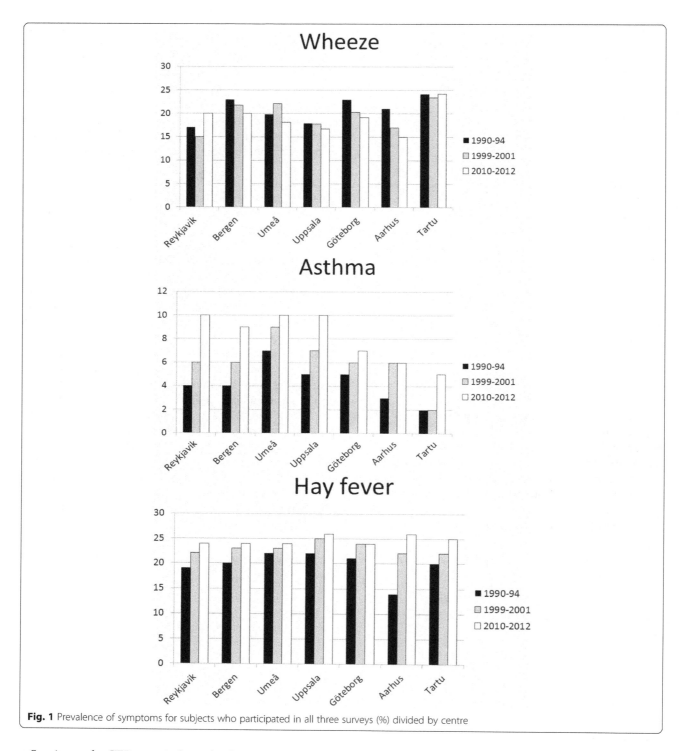

Fig. 1 Prevalence of symptoms for subjects who participated in all three surveys (%) divided by centre

Snoring and nGER were independently related to all respiratory symptoms, asthma and allergic rhinitis (Table 3). BMI was associated with all symptoms and asthma but not to allergic rhinitis. Smoking was related to a higher risk of all symptoms but not asthma and allergic rhinitis. Women had a much higher risk than men of nocturnal cough but also of all other symptoms and disorders except wheeze.

The risk of allergic rhinitis was higher in those born 1966 or later than in those born before 1956 (Table 3). This association was also studied by centre (Fig. 4). A strong association between belonging to the younger age group and allergic rhinitis was seen in all centres except Tartu and a borderline centre heterogeneity was found for this association ($p = 0.07$).

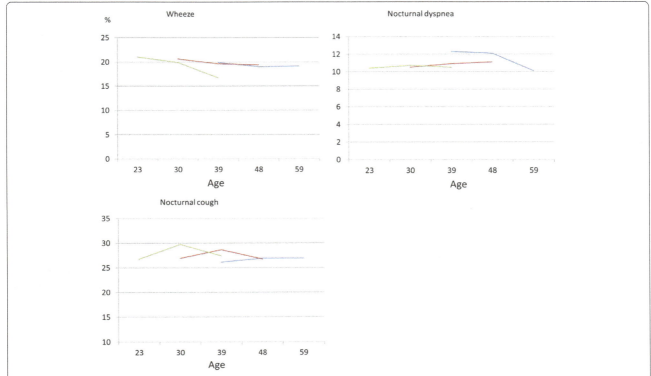

Fig. 2 The prevalence of respiratory symptoms in relation to mean age at the three surveys for participants born 1945–1955 (blue), 1956–1965 (red) and 1966–1975 (green), respectively

Discussion

The main result of this longitudinal study is that wheeze decrease, nocturnal respiratory symptoms remain unchanged and asthma and allergic rhinitis increases with age. The increase in allergic rhinitis was particularly strong in participants born after 1965 except in Estonia. Part of these changes in symptoms and disorders may be related to changes in life style (smoking, diet and exercise) and sleep related factors with a large decrease in smoking but an increase in obesity and snoring with age [9].

Our finding of a decrease in wheeze is in accordance with the results of analyses of repeated cross sectional studies in Northern Europe [1, 2]. An increase in self-reported asthma was found in the 10 and 20-year follow up of the ECRHS [4](ref) and in one Swedish repeated cross sectional studies [1], while an increase in allergic rhinitis has been found in a large number of studies [1–3, 18].

The increase in allergic rhinitis was largest in the youngest birth cohort – those born between 1966 and 1975. Analyses of risk factors also showed that belonging

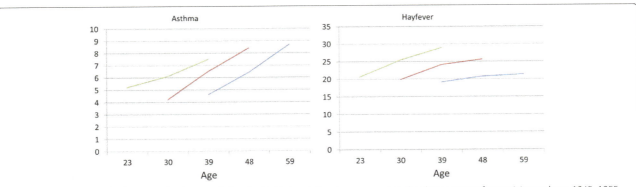

Fig. 3 The prevalence of self-reported asthma and allergic rhinitis in relation to mean age at the three surveys for participants born 1945–1955 (blue), 1956–1965 (red) and 1966–1975 (green), respectively

Table 3 Year of birth, gender, life style and sleep related variables in association with respiratory symptoms and disorder (adjusted[a] odds ratio (95% CI))

	Wheeze	Nocturnal dyspnea	Nocturnal cough	Asthma	Allergic rhinitis
Born 1945–1955	1	1	1	1	1
1956–1965	1.04 (0.92–1.18)	0.93 (0.82–1.05)	1.03 (0.93–1.14)	1.03 (0.84–1.27)	1.62 (1.32–1.99)
1966–1975	1.14 (0.99–1.33)	0.95 (0.81–1.10)	1.11 (0.99–1.25)	1.05 (0.82–1.34)	2.36 (1.85–3.01)
Women	1.09 (0.97–1.22)	1.26 (1.13–1.41)	2.35 (2.14–2.57)	1.66 (1.38–2.01)	1.58 (1.32–1.89)
Smokers	5.65 (5.00–6.38)	1.68 (1.49–1.89)	2.04 (1.86–2.25)	0.98 (0.81–1.18)	0.60 (0.51–0.72)
Obesity	2.97 (2.55–3.45)	1.69 (1.45–1.96)	1.78 (1.57–2.02)	2.05 (1.62–2.60)	0.86 (0.68–1.09)
Snoring	1.85 (1.64–2.09)	1.71 (1.51–1.94)	1.56 (1.41–1.72)	1.61 (1.33–1.95)	1.42 (1.19–1.70)
Gastroesophageal reflux	2.85 (2.41–3.37)	3.67 (3.13–4.31)	2.50 (2.17–2.88)	2.78 (2.17–3.57)	1.73 (1.34–2.23)

[a] adjusted for centre and all the variables in the table

to the youngest birth cohort increased the likelihood of having allergic rhinitis more than two fold. This risk association was found in all centres except in Tartu in Estonia. This result fits well with data from the ECRHS showing a lower prevalence of atopy in the eastern part of Germany [19] and a corresponding difference between Estonia and Sweden [20]. In both these studies difference in atopy was larger in the younger than the older birth cohorts. Corresponding geographical differences have also been reported from a number of studies on children [21, 22]. The lack of age association with allergic rhinitis in Tartu is probably related to the fact that Estonia during the cold war period underwent less environmental changes than those that occurred in the Scandinavian countries.

Smoking and obesity were as expected associated with respiratory symptom [11, 23–26]. Obesity was also associated with self-reported asthma whereas this was not the case for smoking. During the follow up there was a large decrease in smoking and an increase in obesity. Other cohort studies. Have also found a clear positive association between incidence of wheeze and smoking [6, 7, 27]. We have previously found that smoking cessation and weight gain counteract each other when it comes to the effect of change in lung function [9]. It is therefore probably that the relative stability found in the

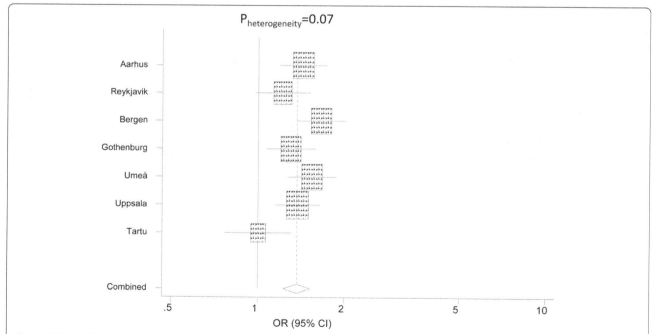

Fig. 4 Odds ratio for allergic rhinitis in those born after 1965 compared to those born before 1956 by study centre. The odds ratio is adjusted for sex, smoking, body mass index, gastro-esophageal reflux and centre. The area of each square is proportional to the reciprocal of the variance of the estimate for the country. The combined random effects estimate is shown by the dashed line, the diamond having the width of its 95% confidence interval

prevalence of all respiratory symptoms except wheeze is related to the beneficial effect of less smoking being balanced by the negative effect of increasing obesity.

Snoring was as in previous studies found to be associated with wheeze and nocturnal symptoms [11, 28]. In accordance to previous studies we also found an association between nGER and respiratory symptoms and disorders [11, 29–31]. Snoring became more prevalent as our population got older. This may partly be related to weight gain and may together with increasing obesity explain why there was no change in nocturnal respiratory symptoms despite a large decrease in smoking.

The strengths of this study are the large population size and the long follow-up time. The questions used are standardized and have been used in a large number of previous studies [32, 33]. The response rate is acceptable given the long follow-up time and the long term responders were fairly similar to non-responders in term of symptomatology [12]. A draw-back is that our results are only based on self-reported data and that there was a variation in the amount of data that was available at the different surveys.

Conclusion

We conclude that as our participants got older there was a decrease in wheeze, no change in nocturnal symptoms and an increase in reported asthma and allergic rhinitis. The increase in allergic rhinitis was particularly strong in younger adults except in Estonia. These changes in prevalence are probably related to a decrease in smoking being counteracted by an increase in allergy, obesity and sleep related disorders. Measures targeting obesity and sleep disordered breathing maybe important in order to reduce the burden of respiratory disorders in the society.

Abbreviations
BMI: Body mass index; ECRHS: European Community Respiratory Health Survey; nGER: nocturnal gastroesophageal reflux; RHINE: Respiratory Health In Northern Europe study

Funding
The study was funded by the Swedish Heart and Lung Foundation, the Swedish Association Against Asthma and Allergy, the Swedish Association against Heart and Lung Disease, the Swedish Council for Working Life and Social Research, the Bror Hjerpstedt Foundation, The Faculty of Health, Aarhus University, Denmark (Project No. 240008), The Wood Dust Foundation (Project No. 444508795), The Danish Lung Association,, The Norwegian Research Council project 135773/330, The Norwegian Asthma and Allergy Association, The Icelandic Research Council and the Estonian Science Foundation (Grant No. 4350).Vivi Schlünssen, Thorarinn Gislason and Cecilie Svanes are members of the COST BM1201 network.

Authors' contributions
The manuscript was drafted b CJ, CJ and LS analysed the data. All authors collected data, contributed with feedback on the analyses and manuscript, and approved the manuscript.

Competing interests
The authors declare that they have no competing interests.

Author details
[1]Department of Medical Sciences, Respiratory, Allergy and Sleep Medicine, Uppsala University, Uppsala, Sweden. [2]Centre for Clinical Research, Haukeland University Hospital, Bergen, Norway. [3]Dept. of Surgical and Perioperative Sciences, Surgery, Umea University, Umea, Sweden. [4]Institute of Clinical Science, University of Bergen, Bergen, Norway. [5]Department of Occupational and Environmental Medicine, Sahlgrenska University Hospital, Gothenburg, Sweden. [6]Department of Medical Sciences, Clinical Physiology, Uppsala University, Uppsala, Sweden. [7]Department of Respiratory Medicine and Sleep, the National University Hospital of Iceland, Reykjavik, Iceland. [8]Faculty of Medicine, University of Iceland, Reykjavik, Iceland. [9]Department of Public Health, Section for Environment, Occupation and Health, Aarhus University, Aarhus, Denmark. [10]National Research Center for the Working Environment, Copenhagen, Denmark. [11]Lung Clinic, Tartu University Clinics, Tartu, Estonia. [12]Respiratory Epidemiology, Occupational Medicine and Public Health, National Heart and Lung Institute, Imperial College, London, UK.

References
1. Bjerg A, Ekerljung L, Middelveld R, Dahlen SE, Forsberg B, Franklin K, Larsson K, Lotvall J, Olafsdottir IS, Toren K, et al. Increased prevalence of symptoms of rhinitis but not of asthma between 1990 and 2008 in Swedish adults: comparisons of the ECRHS and GA(2)LEN surveys. PLoS One. 2011;6:e16082.
2. Lötvall J, Ekerljung L, Rönmark EP, Wennergren G, Lindén A, Rönmark E, Torén K, Lundbäck B. West Sweden asthma study: prevalence trends over the last 18 years argues no recent increase in asthma. Respir Res. 2009;10:94.
3. Verlato G, Corsico A, Villani S, Cerveri I, Migliore E, Accordini S, Carolei A, Piccioni P, Bugiani M, Lo Cascio V, et al. Is the prevalence of adult asthma and allergic rhinitis still increasing? Results of an Italian study. J Allergy Clin Immunol. 2003;111:1232–8.
4. Chinn S. Increase in diagnosed asthma but not in symptoms in the European Community respiratory health survey. Thorax. 2004;59:646–51.
5. Jarvis D, Newson R, Janson C, Corsico A, Heinrich J, Anto JM, Abramson MJ, Kirsten AM, Zock JP, Bono R, et al. Prevalence of asthma-like symptoms with ageing. Thorax. 2017;
6. Frank PI, Hazell ML, Morris JA, Linehan MF, Frank TL. A longitudinal study of changes in respiratory status in young adults, 1993-2001. Int J Tuberc Lung Dis. 2007;11:338–43.
7. Karunanayake CP, Rennie DC, Pahwa P, Chen Y, Dosman JA. Predictors of respiratory symptoms in a rural Canadian population: a longitudinal study of respiratory health. Can Respir J. 2011;18:149–53.
8. Schaper C, Glaser S, Obst A, Schmidt CO, Volzke H, Felix SB, Ewert R, Koch B. Symptoms and diagnosis of asthma in a general population – longitudinal results from the SHIP database. J Asthma. 2010;47:860–4.
9. Chinn S, Jarvis D, Melotti R, Luczynska C, Ackermann-Liebrich U, Antó JM, Cerveri I, de Marco R, Gislason T, Heinrich J, et al. Smoking cessation, lung function, and weight gain: a follow-up study. Lancet. 2005;365:1629–35.
10. Janson C, Kunzli N, de Marco R, Chinn S, Jarvis D, Svanes C, Heinrich J, Jogi R, Gislason T, Sunyer J, et al. Changes in active and passive smoking in the European Community respiratory health survey. Eur Respir J. 2006;27:517–24.
11. Gunnbjornsdottir MI, Omenaas E, Gislason T, Norrman E, Olin AC, Jogi R, Jensen EJ, Lindberg E, Bjornsson E, Franklin K, et al. Obesity and nocturnal gastro-oesophageal reflux are related to onset of asthma and respiratory symptoms. Eur Respir J. 2004;24:116–21.
12. Johannessen A, Verlato G, Benediktsdottir B, Forsberg B, Franklin K, Gislason T, Holm M, Janson C, Jogi R, Lindberg E, et al. Longterm follow-up in European respiratory health studies - patterns and implications. BMC Pulm Med. 2014;14:63.
13. Burney PG, Luczynska C, Chinn S, Jarvis D. The European Community respiratory health survey. Eur Respir J. 1994;7:954–60.
14. Janson C, De Backer W, Gislason T, Plaschke P, Björnsson E, Hetta J, Kristbjarnarson H, Vermeire P, Boman G. Increased prevalence of sleep disturbances and daytime sleepiness in subjects with bronchial asthma: a population study of young adults in three European countries. Eur Respir J. 1996;9:2132–8.

15. Timm S, Svanes C, Janson C, Sigsgaard T, Johannessen A, Gislason T, Jogi R, Omenaas E, Forsberg B, Toren K, et al. Place of upbringing in early childhood as related to inflammatory bowel diseases in adulthood: a population-based cohort study in northern Europe. Eur J Epidemiol. 2014;29:429–37.
16. Variations in the prevalence of respiratory symptoms, self-reported asthma attacks, and use of asthma medication in the European Community Respiratory Health Survey (ECRHS). Eur Respir J. 1996;9:687–95.
17. Franklin KA, Gislason T, Omenaas E, Jogi R, Jensen EJ, Lindberg E, Gunnbjornsdottir M, Nystrom L, Laerum BN, Bjornsson E, et al. The influence of active and passive smoking on habitual snoring. Am J Respir Crit Care Med. 2004;170:799–803.
18. de Marco R, Cappa V, Accordini S, Rava M, Antonicelli L, Bortolami O, Braggion M, Bugiani M, Casali L, Cazzoletti L, et al. Trends in the prevalence of asthma and allergic rhinitis in Italy between 1991 and 2010. Eur Respir J. 2012;39:883–92.
19. Nowak D, Heinrich J, Jorres R, Wassmer G, Berger J, Beck E, Boczor S, Claussen M, Wichmann HE, Magnussen H. Prevalence of respiratory symptoms, bronchial hyperresponsiveness and atopy among adults: west and East Germany. Eur Respir J. 1996;9:2541–52.
20. Jogi R, Janson C, Bjornsson E, Boman G, Bjorksten B. Atopy and allergic disorders among adults in Tartu, Estonia compared with Uppsala, Sweden. Clin Exp Allergy. 1998;28:1072–80.
21. von Mutius E, Fritzsch C, Weiland SK, Roll G, Magnussen H. Prevalence of asthma and allergic disorders among children in united Germany: a descriptive comparison. BMJ. 1992;305:1395–9.
22. Braback L, Breborowicz A, Dreborg S, Knutsson A, Pieklik H, Bjorksten B. Atopic sensitization and respiratory symptoms among polish and Swedish school children. Clin Exp Allergy. 1994;24:826–35.
23. Ronmark E, Andersson C, Nystrom L, Forsberg B, Jarvholm B, Lundback B. Obesity increases the risk of incident asthma among adults. Eur Respir J. 2005;25:282–8.
24. Beuther DA, Sutherland ER. Overweight, obesity, and incident asthma: a meta-analysis of prospective epidemiologic studies. Am J Respir Crit Care Med. 2007;175:661–6.
25. Uddenfeldt M, Janson C, Lampa E, Leander M, Norback D, Larsson L, Rask-Andersen A. High BMI is related to higher incidence of asthma, while a fish and fruit diet is related to a lower- Results from a long-term follow-up study of three age groups in Sweden. *Respir Med.* 2010;104:972–80.
26. Accordini S, Janson C, Svanes C, Jarvis D. The role of smoking in allergy and asthma: lessons from the ECRHS. Curr Allergy Asthma Rep. 2012;12:185–91.
27. Eagan TM, Bakke PS, Eide GE, Gulsvik A. Incidence of asthma and respiratory symptoms by sex, age and smoking in a community study. Eur Respir J. 2002;19:599–605.
28. Ekici A, Ekici M, Kurtipek E, Keles H, Kara T, Tunckol M, Kocyigit P. Association of asthma-related symptoms with snoring and apnea and effect on health-related quality of life. Chest. 2005;128:3358–63.
29. Emilsson OI, Bengtsson A, Franklin KA, Toren K, Benediktsdottir B, Farkhooy A, Weyler J, Dom S, De Backer W, Gislason T, Janson C. Nocturnal gastro-oesophageal reflux, asthma and symptoms of OSA: a longitudinal, general population study. Eur Respir J. 2013;41:1347–54.
30. Emilsson OI, Janson C, Benediktsdottir B, Juliusson S, Gislason T. Nocturnal gastroesophageal reflux, lung function and symptoms of obstructive sleep apnea: results from an epidemiological survey. Respir Med. 2012;106:459–66.
31. Gislason T, Janson C, Vermeire P, Plaschke P, Bjornsson E, Gislason D, Boman G. Respiratory symptoms and nocturnal gastroesophageal reflux: a population-based study of young adults in three European countries. Chest. 2002;121:158–63.
32. Janson C, Anto J, Burney P, Chinn S, de Marco R, Heinrich J, Jarvis D, Kuenzli N, Leynaert B, Luczynska C, et al. The European Community respiratory health survey: what are the main results so far? European Community Respiratory Health Survey II. *Eur Respir J.* 2001;18:598–611.
33. Omenaas E, Svanes C, Janson C, Toren K, Jogi R, Gislason T, Franklin KA, Gulsvik A. What can we learn about asthma and allergy from the follow-up of the RHINE and the ECRHS studies? Clin Respir J. 2008;2(Suppl 1):45–52.

Erlotinib versus gefitinib for brain metastases in Asian patients with exon 19 EGFR-mutant lung adenocarcinoma: a retrospective, multicenter study

Ye Jiang[1†], Jing Zhang[2†], Juanjuan Huang[3†], Bo Xu[4], Ning Li[1], Lei Cao[3] and Mingdong Zhao[5*]

Abstract

Background: The purpose of this study was to compare clinical outcomes of Erlotinib versus Gefitinib in the treatment of Asian patients with exon 19 EGFR-mutant lung adenocarcinoma and newly diagnosed brain metastases.

Methods: Consecutive Asian patients with exon 19 EGFR-mutant lung adenocarcinoma and newly diagnosed brain metastases were identified and initially received peroral administration of 150 mg/d erlotinib or 250 mg/d gefitinib during 2009–2015. Overall survival (OS) was the primary endpoint. Progression-free survival (PFS) was the second endpoint.

Results: The cohort consisted of 227 Asian patients (erlotinib-treated cohort: $n = 112$, mean age = 58.5 years [SD: 20.13]; gefitinib-treated cohort: $n = 115$, mean age = 58.4 years [SD: 19.52]). In a multivariate analysis controlling for age, sex and time span of smoking history, significant difference was detected in the 36-month OS between erlotinib and gefitinib groups (58.3% vs. 49.1%, $p = 0.012$). There was also significant difference in the 36-month PFS between erlotinib and gefitinib groups (64% vs. 53%, $p = 0.013$).

Conclusion: For Asian patients with exon 19 EGFR-mutant lung adenocarcinoma and brain metastases, erlotinib was associated with a significantly longer OS and a more prolonged PFS and compared with gefitinib.

Keywords: Erlotinib, Gefitinib, Lung adenocarcinoma, Overall survival

Background

Based on previous studies [1–4], gefitinib or erlotinib, epidermal growth factor receptor mutation - tyrosine kinase inhibitor (EGFR-TKI), has been a successful regimen managing advanced non-small cell lung cancer (NSCLC). Furthermore, the data from randomized controlled trials(RCTs) and other investigations have also indicated that EGFR-TKI has advantageous when used as an initial treatment for Asian patients with EGFR-mutant lung adenocarcinoma and brain metastases [5–7]. Yet overall survival (OS) and progression-free survival (PFS) remain controversial for Asian patients with exon 19 EGFR-mutant lung adenocarcinoma and brain metastases [8–14].

We therefore conducted a retrospective review of Asian patients with exon 19 EGFR-mutant lung adenocarcinoma and brain metastases. To our knowledge, this is the first analysis that directly compares gefitinib against erlotinib as initial treatment for brain metastases following exon 19 EGFR-mutant lung adenocarcinoma. We hypothesized that there would be differences in both OS and PFS between patients treated with gefitinib vs. erlotinib.

Materials and methods

Study population and end points

The clinical and molecular characteristics and outcome data for 335 Asian patients with exon 19 EGFR-mutant lung adenocarcinoma and newly diagnosed brain metastases retrieved from a registry database were identified at the 4 medical centres between January 2009 and January

* Correspondence: zhaonissann@163.com
†Ye Jiang, Jing Zhang and Juanjuan Huang contributed equally to this work.
[5]Department of Orthopaedics, Jinshan Hospital, Fudan University, Longhang Road No. 1508, Jinshan District, Shanghai City 201508, China
Full list of author information is available at the end of the article

2015. Information regarding erlotinib or gefitinib delivery, disease status and survival was obtained from the medical record. Inclusion criteria: age range: 50~ 70 years; patients harbouring exon 19 EGFR mutation; all patients with stage IV lung adenocarcinoma at initial diagnosis; patients initially receiving peroral administration of 150 mg/d erlotinib or 250 mg/d gefitinib; EGFR mutation testing performed in all patients by the molecular diagnostic core laboratory of the Department of Pathology. Exclusion criteria: patients with de novo EGFR-TKI resistance mutations; previous chemotherapy or radiotherapy; no pre-treatment imaging; discontinuation or interruption of erlotinib or gefitinib; death; refusal; organ failure; severe infectious diseases (e.g., systemic inflammatory response syndrome); mental illness; cognitive dysfunction; uncontrolled diabetes mellitus or hypertension. OS was the primary endpoint. PFS was the second endpoint.

Definitions of the descriptive variables

OS was defined as the period from treatment initiation to the date of death from any cause. PFS was defined as the period from treatment initiation to the date of disease progression. Lung adenocarcinoma staging was performed according to the 7th edition of the Lung Cancer Stage Classification System [15]. For EGFR mutation testing, tumour specimens from primary lung adenocarcinoma were obtained by either needle biopsy/aspiration prior to EGFR-TKI therapy. Imaging examination was carried out every 2 months to assess the drug-related patient's response. Lung adenocarcinoma response was assessed in accordance with the Response Evaluation Criteria in Solid Tumours (RECIST) by imaging procedure 1 month after treatment and then every 2 months thereafter or when clinically indicated. Responses to EGFR-TKI were conducted by independent radiological reviews. For OS analyses, patients who were still alive or not lost to follow-up at the primary analysis cut-off date were noted at the final follow-up. Living patients were censored at the date of last contact. DNA which was extracted from formalin-fixed, paraffin-embedded tumour tissue was tested with polymerase chain reaction-based assays, as described by Pan et al. [16].

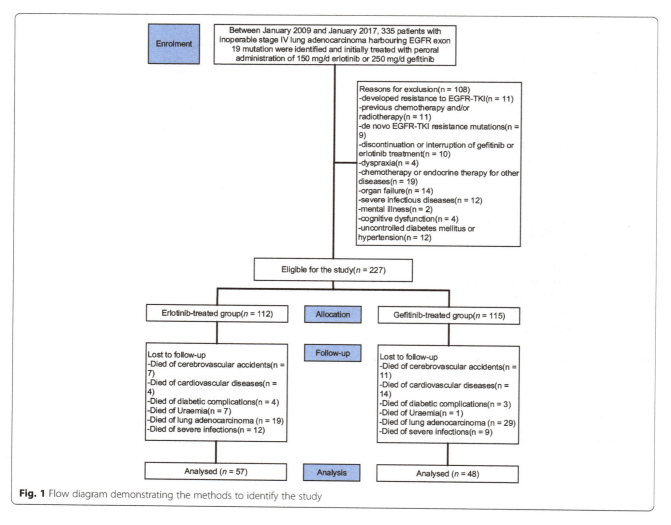

Fig. 1 Flow diagram demonstrating the methods to identify the study

Statistical analysis

Categorical variables expressed as the count and percentage were analysed using χ^2-test or the Mann–Whitney U-test. Continuous numeric variables expressed as the mean and SD were analysed with Student's t-test. Survival probabilities estimated using the Kaplan-Meier method were compared between groups by the log-rank test. Cox regression analyses were executed to adjust for age, sex and time span of smoking history. Statistical analyses were performed using SPSS (version 24.0; IBM, Inc., Chicago, IL, USA) software. A value of $p < 0.05$ was considered statistically significant.

Results

Patient characteristics

In total, 227 Asian patients with exon 19 EGFR-mutant lung adenocarcinoma and brain metastases were included (erlotinib: $n = 112$, mean age = 58.5 years [SD: 20.13]; gefitinib: $n = 115$, mean age = 58.4 years [SD: 19.52]), as summarized in Fig. 1. The comparisons of the demographic characteristics are presented in Table 1. The median follow-up at the primary analysis cut-off date was 36 months (IQR: 14.5–39.6) for the erlotinib group and 36 months (IQR: 13.3–39.2) for the gefitinib group. The time to occurrence of the progression of brain tumours was significantly prolonged after erlotinib compared with gefitinib. No between-group significant differences were detected in regard to drug-related toxicity or intolerable adverse reactions.

Survival analysis

Deaths occurred in the erlotinib and gefitinib groups (44.6 and 58.3%, respectively), as presented in Table 2. Twenty-seven cases had recurrences, 9 of which received the conversion from gefitinib to erlotinib, and no significant increase in brain metastases; 5 continued to receive gefitinib, and brain metastases further worsen until they nearly died; 2 terminated the treatment of gefitinib and eventually died; the therapy of 11 cases was unidentified. There were more than 3 metastases (the sites included the brain, bone, lung, liver, and lymph nodes) in 70 patients in the two groups (28 vs. 42 for erlotinib and gefitinib groups, respectively, $p = 0.06$). All tumours detected were histopathologically parallel to lung adenocarcinoma with identical exon 19 EGFR mutation, excluding a second lung tumour as a possibility.

Median PFS and median OS of erlotinib-treated patients were 10.8 months (95% CI: 4 to 16) and 28.3 months (95% CI: 3 to NA), respectively. Median PFS and median OS of gefitinib-treated patients were 8.4 months (95% CI: 4 to 13) and 25.0 months (95% CI: 5 to NA), respectively, as presented in Figs. 2 and 3. A statistically significant difference was detected in median PFS and median OS between groups. Multivariate analysis, after adjusting for age, sex and time span of smoking history, indicated that erlotinib-treated patients had a 36-month PFS rate of 64% compared with 53% for gefitinib-treated patients (HR = 0.28; 95% CI: 0.17–0.41; $p = 0.013$); erlotinib-treated patients had a 36-month OS of 58.3% compared with 49.1% for gefitinib-treated patients (HR: 0.21; 95% CI: 0.15 to 0.37; $p = 0.012$).

Table 1 Baseline characteristics between groups

Variable	Erlotinib ($n = 112$)	Gefitinib ($n = 115$)	p - value
Age at onset (years)	58.4 ± 19.52	58.5 ± 20.13	0.212[a]
Sex			0.846[b]
Female	85	86	
Male	27	29	
Smoking status			0.644[c]
Never a smoker	67	65	
Former smokers	23	26	
Current smokers	22	24	
Largest size of brain metastasis			0.841[c]
≤ 10 mm	26	28	
> 10 mm	86	87	
Number of brain metastasis			0.764[c]
≤ 3	65	69	
> 3	47	46	
ECOG performance status			0.838[c]
0	33	35	
1	46	43	
2	25	27	
3	8	10	
Neurological symptoms before the initiation of TKIs			0.352[c]
Nausea	6	5	
Headache	3	3	
Depressed level of consciousness	2	2	
Gait disturbance	1	0	
Muscle weakness	0	1	
Dizziness	1	1	
Urinary retention	1	1	
Cognitive disturbance	2	2	
Memory impairment	1	2	
Blurred vision	2	1	

[a]Analysed using independent-samples t-test. [b]Analysed using chi-squared test. [c]Analysed using the Mann-Whitney test. *ECOG* Eastern Cooperative Oncology Group. *TKIs* Tyrosine kinase inhibitors

Table 2 Survival analysis at final follow-up

Variable	Erlotinib (n = 112)	Gefitinib (n = 115)	p - value
median PFS (months)	10.8(range, 0–21.3)	8.4(range, 0–20.5)	0.014*a
median OS (months)	28.3(range, 3.6–36.2)	25.0(range, 3.3–36.3)	0.033*a
Deaths, No.	50	67	0.04*b
Age(y)	68.1 ± 8.73	67.7 ± 9.34	0.175c
Sex			0.133b
Female	30	49	
Male	20	18	
Smoking status			0.770d
Never a smoker	30	44	
Former smokers	13	10	
Current smokers	7	13	
Largest size of brain metastasis			0.326d
≤ 10 mm	11	10	
> 10 mm	39	57	
Number of brain metastasis			0.467d
≤ 3	22	25	
> 3	28	42	
ECOG performance status			0.177d
0	6	8	
1	15	30	
2	21	22	
3	8	7	

*Statistically significant. aAnalysed using the log-rank test; bAnalysed using independent-samples t-test; cAnalysed using chi-squared test; dAnalysed using the Mann-Whitney test. *PFS* progression-free disease-free survival; *OS* overall survival; *ECOG* Eastern Cooperative Oncology Group

Discussion

In the current study, Asian patients with positive exon 19 EGFR-mutant lung adenocarcinoma and newly diagnosed brain metastases who initially received peroral administration of 150 mg/d erlotinib or 250 mg/d gefitinib were followed for a mean of 36 months, and the most important finding was that erlotinib was associated with a significantly longer OS and more prolonged PFS than gefitinib.

This has increasingly become a consensus that the supreme benefit of EGFR-TKI therapy occurred in patients with EGFR-mutant lung adenocarcinoma and brain metastases [11, 15–19]. The evidence in the previous literature regarding the optimal treatment strategy for the initial management of Asia patients with metastatic EGFR-mutant lung adenocarcinoma was questionable [5, 6, 17], although there are limited randomized trials directing this therapy. To date, there was no solid evidence that gefitinib or erlotinib had less efficacy than afatinib in first-line treatment of patients with EGFR-mutant lung adenocarcinoma and brain metastases [1–4, 12]. Several studies indicated that gefitinib may be superior to erlotinib, but the finding was based on low event numbers and small sample sizes [20–22]. Our findings were in line with previous prospective trials that the response rates to EGFR-TKI therapy in stage IV lung adenocarcinoma patients harbouring exon 19 EGFR mutation ranged from 60 to 70% [13, 22]. Moreover, more studies that compared both OS and PFS between erlotinib and gefitinib in stage IV exon 19 EGFR-mutant lung adenocarcinoma patients after completion of all standard adjuvant chemotherapy and/or radiation therapy also showed similar outcomes [5, 12, 21]. Previous studies established erlotinib was superior to gefitinib in advanced EGFR-mutated patients with leptomeningeal metastases from lung adenocarcinomas that progressed during gefitinib therapy but responded to erlotinib [3, 15, 20, 21].

A retrospective multicenter study by Fan et al. [5] exhibited that median PFS of gefitinib and erlotinib groups was 3.6 and 4.6 months, respectively ($p < 0.027$). Median OS of gefitinib and erlotinib groups was 9.6 and 10.7 months, respectively ($p < 0.013$). Nevertheless, a previous meta-analysis reported by Normando et al. [23] demonstrated no significant difference in the PFS and OS of erlotinib or gefitinib in patients with EGFR-mutant lung adenocarcinoma and brain metastases. Recent studies [20, 24] exhibited that the PFS and OS of gefitinib-treated patients was significantly lower than that of erlotinib-treated patients. In exploratory analysis of EGFR-mutated patients, gefitinib failed to generate a PFS or OS benefit [6, 25]. Considering this was an underpowered study that was terminated early with some cases undergoing a short treatment time, the results did not seem to draw conclusions about the impact of erlotinib or gefitinib. Nevertheless, evidence-based medicine analysis [26] exhibited that the PFS and OS of erlotinib-treated young patients (45–55 years old) failed to be superior to gefitinib-treated young patients. Several studies have reported that gefitinib might be a soothing choice for the initial treatment of patients with EGFR-mutant lung adenocarcinoma and newly diagnosed brain metastases [5, 27, 28]. However, another considered problem is that the results after a failed erlotinib or gefitinib are relatively controversial [4]. Currently, there is no consensus about which drug to use in Asian patients with EGFR-mutant lung adenocarcinoma and brain metastases [29]. In China, 80% of patients prefer receiving gefitinib over erlotinib for brain metastases following EGFR-mutant lung adenocarcinoma. The main reason is that gefitinib has a price advantage, and medical insurance can be reimbursed. Only when gefitinib resistance occur are they willing to accept erlotinib treatment. Thus, further study is

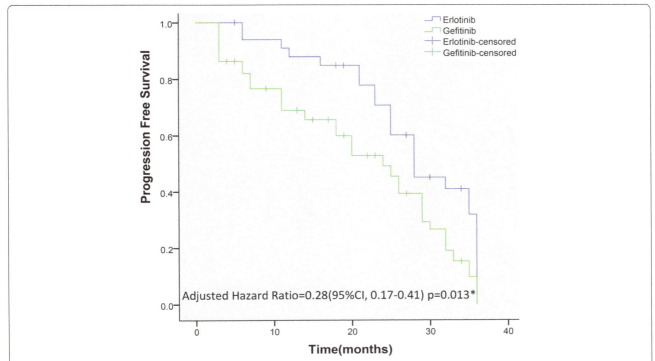

Fig. 2 Kaplan–Meier Curves for PFS. The median PFS was 10.8 months (range, 0–21.3 months) in the erlotinib group and 8.4 months (range, 0–20.5 months) in the gefitinib group. A statistically significant difference was detected in PFS between groups. *The hazard ratio was calculated using the Cox proportional hazards model, with age, sex and time span of smoking history as covariates and gefitinib/erlotinib therapy as the time-dependent factor. With respect to PFS, the results were analysed using the log-rank test ($p = 0.014$)

compulsory on the effects of familial exon 19 EGFR mutation on Asian ethnicity. Consequently, whether erlotinib is superior to gefitinib in the treatment of young patients with brain metastases following EGFR-mutant lung adenocarcinoma, a prospective randomized controlled study of larger samples is required for clarification. Noteworthy, any data from EGFR-TKI trials that fail to select patients based on molecular and clinical characteristics and EGFR-mutant presence may be misrepresentative.

Erlotinib, a specific EGFR-TKI, has been shown to improve PFS compared with chemotherapy when given as first-line treatment for Asian patients with NSCLC with activating EGFR mutations [12, 30]. A multicentre, open-label, randomised phase 3 trial (EURTAC) [30] which is the first prospective head-to-head phase 3 study has shown that erlotinib had longer PFS and milder side-effects than standard chemotherapy in non-Asian patients with advanced NSCLC and EGFR mutations. A randomised, phase III study(OPTIMAL, CTONG-0802) [31] comparing erlotinib with chemotherapy as first-line treatment of EGFR mutation-positive advanced NSCLC showed erlotinib should be considered standard first-line treatment of patients with advanced NSCLC and EGFR mutations. Our findings were consistent with the OPTIMAL. In our study, some statistical results could not be obtained when comparing the OS and PFS between groups. One potential explanation may be attributed to that the treatment period of some patients was less than 6 months, related to premature death.

As an EGFR-targeted drug for effective treatment of advanced NSCLC, erlotinib's main drug-related toxicity was rash, mostly mild to moderate [32]. The rashes in most patients in this study were comparable to those in previous studies [11, 31], and the symptoms tended to improve after appropriate treatment. The incidence of grade 3 or 4 adverse events was low. No patient reduced or discontinued treatment due to intolerable adverse reactions.

This study should be interpreted considering important limitations. Firstly, the most important limitation is the retrospective nature, which limits the level of evidence. Many cases were excluded from the analysis owing to lack of baseline data. The excluded cases may introduce bias which is scarcely possible to account for and fails to be representative of the larger sample. Secondly, our findings were also limited by the frequency and length of follow-up. Thirdly, although potential confounders were adjusted by us, other unpredictable factors may also be relevant.

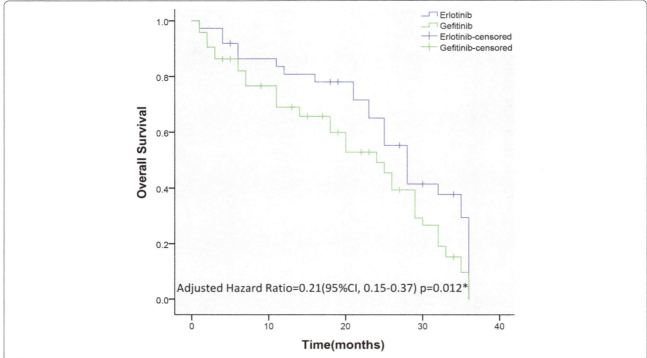

Fig. 3 Kaplan–Meier Curves for OS. The median OS was 28.3 months (range, 3.6–36.2 months) in the erlotinib group and 25.0 months (range, 3.3–36.3 months) in the gefitinib group. There was a statistically significant difference in OS between groups. *The hazard ratio was calculated using the Cox proportional hazards model, with age, sex and time span of smoking history as covariates and gefitinib/erlotinib therapy as the time-dependent factor. With respect to the OS, the results were analysed using the log-rank test ($p = 0.033$)

Conclusion

For Asian patients with EGFR-mutant lung adenocarcinoma and brain metastases, erlotinib was associated with a more prolonged PFS and a significantly longer OS compared with gefitinib. Patients with gefitinib-resistant brain metastases appear to be more suitable for treatment with erlotinib. In addition, if gefitinib or erlotinib were to be assessed again in the adjuvant setting, the proper duration of drug use to maximise efficacy but minimise adverse reaction should not be disregarded. Further follow-up is deserved to verify whether previous findings persist over a longer period.

Abbreviations
CI: confidence interval; ECOG: Eastern Cooperative Oncology Group; EGFR: epidermal growth factor receptor; HR: hazard ratio; IQR: interquartile range; NSCLC: non-small cell lung cancer; OS: overall survival; PFS: progression-free survival; RCTs: randomized controlled trials; SD: standard deviation; TKIs: tyrosine kinase inhibitors

Acknowledgements
The authors would like to acknowledge Dr. Huihan Wang for her assistance with the technical help.

Funding
Funding for this research was received from the Shanghai Municipal Health and Family Planning Commission Fund Project (Grant No. 201640057), and the National Natural Science Foundation of China (Grant No. 81600065; 81270011; 81472125).

Authors' contributions
YJ: Planning and study design, study execution, writing–initial draft, and writing–final revision. JZ and JH: Statistical analysis/interpretation, writing–initial draft, and writing–final revision. BX: Planning and study design. NL and LC: Study execution. MZ: Study execution. JZ and LC: Data collection and study execution. YJ and MZ: Writing–initial draft, and writing–final revision. Each author contributed important intellectual content during the drafting or revision of the article and accepts accountability for the overall work by ensuring that questions pertaining to the accuracy or integrity of any portion of the work were appropriately investigated and resolved. All authors read and approved the final manuscript.

Competing interests
The authors declare that they have no competing interests.

Author details
[1]Department of Neurology, The Affiliated hospital of Hebei University, Yuhua East Road No. 212, Baoding 071000, Hebei, China. [2]Department of Respiratory Medicine, The First Affiliated Hospital, Sun Yat-sen University, No. 58, Zhongshan 2nd Road, Yuexiu District, Guangzhou 510080, China. [3]Department of Anesthesiology, The Central Hospital of Wuhan, Tongji Medical College, Huazhong University of Science and Technology, Gusao Road No. 16, Jianghan District, Wuhan 430014, Hubei, China. [4]Department of Thoracic surgery, The First Affiliated Hospital, Sun Yat-sen University, No. 58, Zhongshan 2nd Road, Yuexiu District, Guangzhou 510080, China. [5]Department of Orthopaedics, Jinshan Hospital, Fudan University, Longhang Road No. 1508, Jinshan District, Shanghai City 201508, China.

References

1. Yomo S, Oda K. Impacts of EGFR-mutation status and EGFR-TKI on the efficacy of stereotactic radiosurgery for brain metastases from non-small cell lung adenocarcinoma: a retrospective analysis of 133 consecutive patients. Lung Cancer. 2018;119:120–6.
2. Urata Y, Katakami N, Morita S, Kaji R, Yoshioka H, Seto T, et al. Randomized phase III study comparing Gefitinib with Erlotinib in patients with previously treated advanced lung adenocarcinoma: WJOG 5108L. J Clin Oncol. 2016; 34(27):3248.
3. Ostoros G, Sarosi V, Mandoky L, Pinter F, Schwab R, Petak I, et al. Effectiveness of erlotinib in lung adenocarcinomas with classic and alternative EGFR mutations detected by Roche 454 GS-FLX next-generation sequencing (NGS). J Clin Oncol. 2013;31(15).
4. Lee CN, Chen HY, Liu HE. Favorable response to Erlotinib in a lung adenocarcinoma with both epidermal growth factor receptor exon 19 deletion and K-ras G13D mutations. J Clin Oncol. 2010;28(7):E111–E2.
5. Fan WC, Yu CJ, Tsai CM, Huang MS, Lai CL, Hsia TC, et al. Different efficacies of Erlotinib and Gefitinib in Taiwanese patients with advanced non-small cell lung Cancer a retrospective multicenter study. J Thorac Oncol. 2011;6(1):148–55.
6. Janjigian YY, Park BJ, Kris MG, Miller VA, Riely GJ, Zheng J, et al. Impact on disease-free survival of adjuvant erlotinib or gefitinib in patients with resected lung adenocarcinomas that harbor epidermal growth factor receptor (EGFR) mutations. J Clin Oncol. 2009;27(15).
7. Kashima J, Okuma Y, Miwa M, Hosomi Y. Retrospective analysis of survival in patients with leptomeningeal carcinomatosis from lung adenocarcinoma treated with erlotinib and gefitinib. Jpn J Clin Oncol. 2017;47(4):357–62. https://doi.org/10.1093/jjco/hyw206.
8. Gerber NK, Yamada Y, Rimner A, Shi WJ, Riely GJ, Beal K, et al. Erlotinib versus radiation therapy for brain metastases in patients with EGFR-mutant lung adenocarcinoma. Int J Radiat Oncol Biol Phys. 2014;89(2):322–9.
9. Zhuang H, Yuan Z, Wang J, Zhao L, Wang P. Phase II study of WBRT with or without concurrent Erlotinib for patients with brain metastases from lung adenocarcinoma. Int J Radiat Oncol Biol Phys. 2012;84(3):S102.
10. Zhuang HQ, Yuan ZY, Wang J, Zhao LJ, Pang QS, Wang P. Phase II study of whole brain radiotherapy with or without erlotinib in patients with multiple brain metastases from lung adenocarcinoma. Drug Des Dev Ther. 2013;7:1179–86.
11. Janjigian YY, Park BJ, Zakowski MF, Ladanyi M, Pao W, D'Angelo SP, et al. Impact on disease-free survival of adjuvant Erlotinib or Gefitinib in patients with resected lung adenocarcinomas that harbor EGFR mutations. J Thorac Oncol. 2011;6(3):569–75.
12. Yang CJ, Hung JY, Tsai MJ, Wu KL, Liu TC, Chou SH, et al. The salvage therapy in lung adenocarcinoma initially harbored susceptible EGFR mutation and acquired resistance occurred to the first-line gefitinib and second-line cytotoxic chemotherapy. BMC Pharmacol Toxicol. 2017;18.
13. Bean J, Brennan C, Shih JY, Riely G, Viale A, Wang L, et al. MET amplification occurs with or without T790M mutations in EGFR mutant lung tumors with acquired resistance to gefitinib or erlotinib. Mol Cancer Ther. 2007;6(12):3333S–4S.
14. Asami K, Kawahara M, Atagi S, Kawaguchi T, Okishio K. Duration of prior gefitinib treatment predicts survival potential in patients with lung adenocarcinoma receiving subsequent erlotinib. Lung Cancer. 2011;73(2):211–6.
15. Cardona AF, Arrieta O, Zapata MI, Rojas L, Wills B, Reguart N, et al. Acquired resistance to Erlotinib in EGFR mutation-positive lung adenocarcinoma among Hispanics (CLICaP). Target Oncol. 2017;12(4):513–23.
16. Pan QL, Pao W, Ladanyi M. Rapid polymerase chain reaction-based detection of epidermal growth factor receptor gene mutations in lung adenocarcinomas. J Mol Diagn. 2005;7(3):396–403.
17. Pao W, Wang TY, Riely GJ, Miller VA, Pan QL, Ladanyi M, et al. KRAS mutations and primary resistance of lung adenocarcinomas to gefitinib or erlotinib. PLoS Med. 2005;2(1):57 61.
18. Sholf LM, Janne PA, Jackman DM, Joshi VA. Lindeman NI. EGFR kinase domain mutations, but not copy number, predict response to erlotinib and gefitinib in patients with advanced lung adenocarcinoma. J Mol Diagn. 2007;9(5):692.
19. Tanaka K, Hida T, Oya Y, Oguri T, Yoshida T, Shimizu J, et al. EGFR mutation impact on definitive concurrent Chemoradiation therapy for inoperable stage III adenocarcinoma. J Thorac Oncol. 2015;10(12):1720–5.
20. Yang JJ, Zhou Q, Yan HH, Zhang XC, Chen HJ, Tu HY, et al. A phase III randomised controlled trial of erlotinib vs gefitinib in advanced non-small cell lung cancer with EGFR mutations. Br J Cancer. 2017;116(5):568–74.
21. Tetsumoto S, Osa A, Kijima T, Minami T, Hirata H, Takahashi R, et al. Two cases of leptomeningeal metastases from lung adenocarcinoma which progressed during gefitinib therapy but responded to erlotinib. Int J Clin Oncol. 2012;17(2):155–9.
22. Xu Y, Liu HY, Chen J, Zhou QH. Acquired resistance of lung adenocarcinoma to EGFR-tyrosine kinase inhibitors gefitinib and erlotinib. Cancer Biol Ther. 2010; 9(8):572–82.
23. Normando SRC, Cruz FM, del Giglio A. Cumulative meta-analysis of epidermal growth factor receptor-tyrosine kinase inhibitors as first-line therapy in metastatic non-small-cell lung cancer. Anti-Cancer Drugs. 2015;26(9):995–1003.
24. Shen YC, Tseng GC, Tu CY, Chen WC, Liao WC, Chen WC, et al. Comparing the effects of afatinib with gefitinib or Erlotinib in patients with advanced-stage lung adenocarcinoma harboring non-classical epidermal growth factor receptor mutations. Lung Cancer. 2017;110:56–62.
25. Katayama T, Shimizu J, Suda K, Onozato R, Fukui T, Ito S, et al. Efficacy of Erlotinib for brain and leptomeningeal metastases in patients with lung adenocarcinoma who showed initial good response to Gefitinib. J Thorac Oncol. 2009;4(11):1415–9.
26. Wu SG, Shih JY, Yu CJ, Yang PC. Lung adenocarcinoma with good response to erlotinib after gefitinib treatment failure and acquired T790M mutation. J Thorac Oncol. 2008;3(4):451–2.
27. Yu SF, Wang Y, Li JL, Hao XZ, Wang B, Wang ZP, et al. Gefitinib versus erlotinib as salvage treatment for lung adenocarcinoma patients who benefited from the initial gefitinib: a retrospective study. Thorac Cancer. 2013;4(2):109–16.
28. Xing PY, Li JL, Shi YK, Zhang XR. Recurrent response to advanced lung adenocarcinoma with erlotinib developing leptomeningeal metastases during gefitinib therapy and two case reports. Thorac Cancer. 2014;5(1):38–42.
29. Chang CH, Lee CH, Wang JY. Gefitinib or Erlotinib for previously treated lung adenocarcinoma: which is superior? J Clin Oncol. 2017;35(12):1374.
30. Rosell R, Carcereny E, Gervais R, Vergnenegre A, Massuti B, Felip E, et al. Erlotinib versus standard chemotherapy as first-line treatment for European patients with advanced EGFR mutation-positive non-small-cell lung cancer (EURTAC): a multicentre, open-label, randomised phase 3 trial. Lancet Oncol. 2012;13(3):239–46.
31. Zhou C, Wu YL, Chen G, Feng J, Liu XQ, Wang C, et al. Final overall survival results from a randomised, phase III study of erlotinib versus chemotherapy as first-line treatment of EGFR mutation-positive advanced non-small-cell lung cancer (OPTIMAL, CTONG-0802). Ann Oncol. 2015;26(9):1877–83.
32. Fukui T, Otani S, Hataishi R, Jiang SX, Nishii Y, Igawa S, et al. Successful rechallenge with erlotinib in a patient with EGFR-mutant lung adenocarcinoma who developed gefitinib-related interstitial lung disease. Cancer Chemother Pharmacol. 2010;65(4):803–6.

Lymphatic vessel density as a prognostic indicator in Asian NSCLC patients

Shuanglan Xu[1], Jiao Yang[2], Shuangyan Xu[3], Yun Zhu[4], Chunfang Zhang[1], Liqiong Liu[1], Hao Liu[4], Yunlong Dong[4], Zhaowei Teng[4] and Xiqian Xing[1]*

Abstract

Background: To determine the association of lymphatic vessel density (LVD) with the prognosis of Asian non-small cell lung cancer (NSCLC) patients via a meta-analysis.

Methods: Eligible studies were selected by searching PubMed and EMBASE from inception to July 25, 2017. The reference lists of the retrieved articles were also consulted. The information was independently screened by two authors. When heterogeneity was significant, a random-effects model was used to determine overall pooled risk estimates.

Results: A total of 15 studies with 1075 patients were finally included in the meta-analysis. LVD was positively associated with the prognosis of NSCLC in the overall analysis (hazard ratio (HR) 1.14, 95% confidence interval (95% CI): 1.02–1.27, $p = 0.000$, $I^2 = 73.2\%$). Subgroup analyses were performed on 5 VEGFR-3 groups ($p = 0.709$, $I^2 = 0.0\%$), 3 LYVE-1 groups ($p = 0.01$, $I^2 = 86.4\%$), 5 D2–40 groups ($p = 0.019$, $I^2 = 66.2\%$), and 2 podoplanin groups ($p = 0.094$, $I^2 = 64.5\%$). Sensitivity analysis indicated robust results. There was no publication bias.

Conclusions: LVD is an indicator of poor prognosis in Asian NSCLC patients.

Keywords: NSCLC, Lymphatic vessel density, LVD, Prognostic, Meta-analysis

Background

Lung cancer is a malignant disease associated with the highest mortality rate (18.2%) among all types of cancer worldwide [1, 2]. Non-small cell lung cancer (NSCLC) represents the majority (~ 85%) of all lung cancer cases, with lung adenocarcinoma (ADC) and squamous cell carcinoma (SCC) being the most frequently diagnosed histological types [3]. Approximately half of all NSCLC patients have metastasis, and this type of cancer is usually diagnosed at advanced stages. Despite great progress in treatment modalities (such as surgical resection, chemotherapy, radiotherapy, targeted therapy, biotherapy, and cellular immunotherapy), the prognosis of NSCLC remains poor, and the long-term survival of NSCLC patients is still dismal [4]. Thus, it is important to find novel prognostic therapeutic targets and precise prognostic markers for this type of cancer.

Cancer relapse and metastasis lead to poor prognosis. The most common mode of metastasis is lymph node metastasis. During the early stages of tumor dissemination, malignant cells spread from primary sites to regional lymph nodes. Therefore, the lymphatic system plays an important role in cancer biology [5]. The formation of new lymphatic vessels (lymphangiogenesis) occurs through several steps, including the migration, proliferation and sprouting of lymphatic endothelial cells, which are triggered by vascular endothelial growth factor receptor (VEGFR)-3, VEGF-C or VEGF-D [6]. The lymphatic vessel density (LVD) is the parameter that is most frequently used to quantify tumor lymphangiogenesis, especially for melanoma [7], oral squamous cell carcinoma [8], thyroid carcinoma [9], colorectal cancer [10], breast cancer [11], and lung cancer [12].

---

* Correspondence: xingxiqiankm@163.com
[1]First Department of Respiratory Medicine, Yan'an Hospital Affiliated to Kunming Medical University, No. 245, East Renmin Road, Kunming 650051, Yunnan, China
Full list of author information is available at the end of the article

Previous studies have identified novel molecular markers of the lymphatic endothelium that have been used to study tumor-associated lymphangiogenesis via immunochemistry. These markers include VEGFR-3, Lymphatic vessel endothelial hyaluronan receptor-1 (LYVE-1), D2–40, podoplanin, Prox-1 and desmoplakin, among others [13–16]. VEGFR-3, also known as Flt4, is a member of the fms-like tyrosine kinase family, and it specifically binds VEGF-C and VEGF-D. LYVE-1 is a homolog of the vascular endothelium-specific hyaluronan receptor CD44 [17]. The antibody against D2–40 has been shown to specifically recognize the M2A antigen and podoplanin [18, 19]. Podoplanin is a glomerular podocyte membrane mucoprotein [20]. The transcription factor prox-1 is a homolog of the *drosophila* homeobox gene product that is involved in the regulation of early lymphatic development [21]. Desmoplakin, also known as desmosome-related transmembrane protein, is a desmosomal protein expressed at intercellular junctions. Some studies have shown that lymphatic endothelium markers can be used to predict poor prognoses in NSCLC patients [22–24], but other studies have refuted this view [25–27]. Therefore, whether LVD is a prognostic biomarker for the survival of NSCLC patients remains controversial. The aim of this meta-analysis was to examine whether LVD can predict the prognosis of Asian NSCLC patients.

Methods

Search strategy

PubMed and EMBASE were searched from inception to July 25, 2017, to find related studies. The search terms used were 1) "Non-small cell lung cancer", "Non-small cell lung carcinoma", "NSCLC", "lung adenocarcinoma", "adenocarcinoma of lung", "lung squamous cell cancer", "squamous cell cancer of the lung", "lung squamous cell carcinoma", "squamous cell carcinoma of the lung", "lung large cell cancer", "large cell cancer of the lung", "lung large cell carcinoma", and "lung large cell carcinoma"; 2) "Lymphangiogenesis", "Lymphangiogeneses", "Lymphatic microvessel density", "Lymphatic vessel density", "Lymphatic microvessel", and "Lymphatic vessel"; and 3) "prognostic", "prognosis", and "survival".

Study selection

The inclusion criteria were as follows: 1) a cohort study; 2) an Asian study population; 3) diagnosis of NSCLC based on lung histology, with the most important histological types being ADC, SCC and large cell cancer (LCC); 4) evaluation of the association between LVD and the prognosis of NSCLC patients; 5) analysis of lymph microvessel markers by immunohistochemistry; and 6) the presence of sufficient data to calculate the adjusted hazard ratio (HR) or risk ratio (RR) and the corresponding 95% confidence intervals (CIs). Studies were excluded if they had non-human study subjects. If the data were duplicated or the same population was used in more than one study, we chose the most recent or complete study.

Data extraction

The eligible studies selected for our meta-analysis were independently evaluated by two reviewers (XXQ and XSL) based on the aforementioned selection criteria. The following information was extracted from the eligible studies: the name of the first author, publication year, study period, country, sample number, sex of patients, median follow-up period, mean age or age range of patients, histology, histological type, TNM stage, and lymphatic endothelium markers (in Table 1). In addition, HR and 95% CIs were evaluated. Two authors (TZW and XSY) summarized the extracted data. Any disagreements were resolved by discussion.

Statistical analyses

To compute a pooled HR with a 95% CI, the Q-test and the I^2 test were used to assess heterogeneity among the studies [28]. We also calculated P values for the Q-test, which represented heterogeneity; heterogeneity was present if the P value was less than 0.10. The random-effects model was applied when $I^2 > 50\%$ [29]; otherwise, the fixed-effects model was applied [30]. Subgroup analyses based on lymphatic endothelium markers were performed to further explore the source of heterogeneity. Additionally, Begg's rank correlation test and Egger's linear regression test were conducted to assess the extent of potential publication bias [31]. Finally, a sensitivity analysis was performed by sequentially omitting one study per cycle to evaluate the stability of the results [32]. The data analyses were conducted using the STATA statistical software version 12.0 (STATA Corp. LLC, College Station, TX, USA).

Results

Literature search and study characteristics

Using the predefined search strategy and inclusion criteria, 15 studies [22–27, 33–41] involving 1075 participants were ultimately included in this meta-analysis. The detailed study selection process is presented in Fig. 1. In total, 251 articles (108 from PubMed and 143 from EMBASE) were retrieved. Among these articles, 236 articles were excluded after eliminating duplicates, screening the titles and abstracts, and reviewing the full text. Finally, 15 articles were included in our analysis.

The characteristics of the 15 eligible studies are shown in Table 1. These studies included 1075 participants from Asia, including Japan and China; a total of 11 studies investigated NSCLC, 3 studies investigated ADC, and 1 study investigated lung cancer. All studies used immunohistochemistry

Table 1 Characteristics of the 15 studies

Author-year (study period) Country	Sample number	Sex Males	Sex Females	Median follow-up period (months)	Age: mean age or range	Histology	Histological type ADC	SCC	LCC	Others	TNM stage	Lymphatic endothelium markers
Kitano-2017 (1988–2010) Japan [33]	89	64	25	range 10–153	< 60 y 25 ≥60 y 64	NSCLC	53	36	0	0	II 40 III + IV 49	VEGFR-3
Nunomiya-2014 (2008–2011) Japan [25]	58	50	8	ND	71.3 y	NSCLC 40 SCLC 14 Others 4	ND	ND	ND	ND	I + II 20 III + IV 37	LYVE-1
Hao-2014 (2004–2012) China [34]	140	72	68	ND	≤65 y 56 > 65 y 84	NSCLC	36	39	28	4	I–IIIA	LYVE-1
Zhang-2012 (2003–2006) China [22]	65	38	27	ND	51.5 y (range 32–76 y) < 55 y 26 ≥55 y 39	ADC	65	0	0	0	I + II 38 III + IV 27	D2–40
Dai-2011 (1999–2003) China [35]	98	ND	ND	37.53 ± 4.05	ND	NSCLC	59	39	0	0	ND	Podoplanin
Yamashita-2010 (1993–2000) Japan [36]	117	77	40	68.7	67.8 y (range 47–85 y) < 68 y 67 ≥68 y 50	Stage I NSCLC	78	31	6	2	IA 58 IB 59	VEGFR-3
Chen-2010 (1999–2001) China [37]	52	41	11	ND	51.9 y (range 29–77 y) < 60 y 31 ≥60 y 21	NSCLC	16	23	0	13	I + II 33 III 19	LYVE-1
Sun-2009 (1995–2004) China [38]	82	63	19	ND	< 55 y 40 ≥55 y 42	NSCLC	41	31	10	0	I + II 48 III + IV 34	D2–40
Iwakiri-2009 (1998–1990) Japan [39]	215	159	56	ND	63.0 y (range 53–71.8 y) < 63 y 109 ≥63 y 106	NSCLC	116	82	10	7	I + II 147 IIIA 68	D2–40
Kitano-2009 (ND) Japan [23]	82	45	37	ND	65 y	ADC	82	0	0	0	I + II 65 III + IV 17	Podoplanin
Kadota-2008 (1998–2002) Japan [24]	147	100	47	ND	67 y (range 35–82 y)	NSCLC	93	49	5	0	I + II 108 III 39	D2–40
Ohta-2006 (1981–2004) Japan [40]	44	23	21	20	64.4 y	NSCLC	25	17	0	2	IIIA 35 IIIB 9	D2–40
Kojima-2005 (1981–1998) Japan [26]	129	62	67	69.9	61 y (range 38–78 y)	ADC	129	0	0	0	ND	VEGFR-3
Chen-2004 (1985–1990) Japan [41]	206	148	58	ND	< 64 y 101 ≥64 y 105	NSCLC	116	75	10	5	I + II 144 IIIA 62	VEGFR-3
Arinaga-2003 (1990–1996) Japan [27]	180	133	47	54.6	65 y (range 35–84 y)	NSCLC	65	101	0	14	I + II 130 III 41	VEGFR-3

NSCLC non-small cell lung carcinoma, *SCLC* small cell lung carcinoma, *ADC* adenocarcinoma, *SCC* squamous cell cancer, *LCC* large cell cancer, *VEGFR-3* vascular endothelial growth factor receptor-3, *LYVE-1* lymphatic vessel endothelial receptor 1, *y* year, *ND* no data

to assess LVD using different lymphatic endothelium markers, including VEGFR-3 in 5 studies, LYVE-1 in 3 studies, D2–40 in 5 studies, podoplanin in 2 studies.

Main analysis

LVD was positively associated with the prognosis of NSCLC in the overall analysis (HR 1.14, 95% CI: 1.02–1.27) (Fig. 2). However, significant heterogeneity was detected across studies ($I^2 = 73.2\%$; $P = 0.000$).

Subgroup meta-analysis

The results of subgroup analyses using the lymphatic endothelium markers that were selected to evaluate LVD via immunohistochemistry support our findings. A positive relationship was observed between the expression of lymphatic endothelium markers and the prognoses of NSCLC patients ($p = 0.000$, $I^2 = 73.2\%$). No statistically significant heterogeneity was observed in the 5 VEGFR-3 group ($p = 0.709$, $I^2 = 0.0\%$); however, there was considerable heterogeneity in the 3 LYVE-1 groups ($p = 0.01$, $I^2 = 86.4\%$),

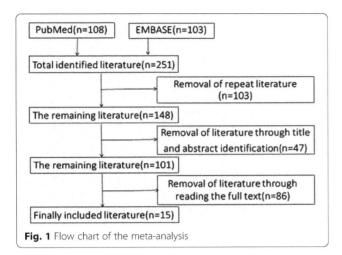

Fig. 1 Flow chart of the meta-analysis

the 5 D2–40 groups ($p = 0.019$, $I^2 = 66.2\%$) and the 2 podoplanin groups ($p = 0.094$, $I^2 = 64.5\%$) (Fig. 3). Nevertheless, the data were not sufficient to determine the prognostic value of LVD among Asian populations based on sex, median follow-up period, mean age or age range, histological type, or TNM stage.

Sensitivity analysis
To evaluate the robustness of our analysis, we conducted a sensitivity analysis by recalculating the pooled results from the primary analyses after excluding one study per iteration. None of the studies when excluded altered the overall combined results (Fig. 4).

Publication bias
No evidence of publication bias was found based on the Begg's rank correlation test ($p > |z| = 0.488$) or Egger's linear regression test ($p > |z| = 0.133$) (Figs. 5 and 6).

Discussion
NSCLC is the most common subtype of lung cancer, with a high incidence, high mortality, low survival rate, low diagnosis rate and treatment rate. It has been challenging to improve survival rates due to the lack of precise prognostic markers. To overcome this problem, a comprehensive understanding of lymphatic endothelium markers is needed. It is important to examine whether LVD can be an indicator of the prognosis in Asian NSCLC patients.

In our present meta-analysis, LVD was positively associated with the prognosis of NSCLC (HR: 1.14, 95% CI: 1.02–1.27), indicating that high LVD indeed predicts poor survival in Asian NSCLC populations. To date, only Wang and colleagues [42] have described the relationship between LVD and the prognoses of NSCLC patients worldwide. Nevertheless, there was considerable heterogeneity among the included studies, which may make the results unreliable. However, sensitivity analysis did not reveal the source of heterogeneity. Furthermore, subgroup analyses were conducted using lymphatic endothelium markers. Additionally, publication bias was detected. Our study only focused on Asian patients, and thus our results are applicable for Asian populations. Although heterogeneity was also observed, the findings

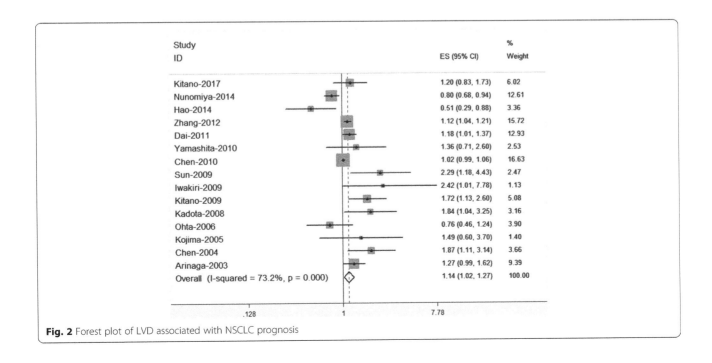

Fig. 2 Forest plot of LVD associated with NSCLC prognosis

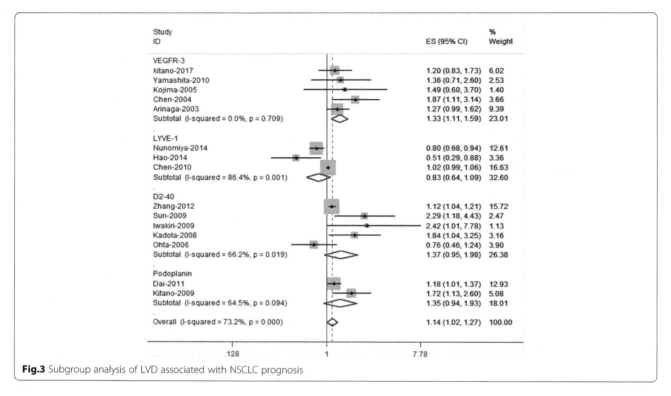

Fig.3 Subgroup analysis of LVD associated with NSCLC prognosis

were stable and robust based on our sensitivity analysis. In addition, subgroup analyses were performed based on the four lymphatic endothelium markers to further explore the origin of heterogeneity. Except VEGFR-3, the other three markers gave rise to considerable heterogeneity. Our meta-analysis included five additional studies that were more recent than those included in the study by Wang and colleagues. Moreover, no publication bias was observed in our study. The study by Zheng and colleagues [43] showed that the VEGF family is important for tumorigenesis and metastasis and that high VEGF and/or VEGFR expression, especially VEGF-C/VEGFR-3 co-expression, is indicative of poor survival in patients with NSCLC. However, that study did not evaluate other lymphatic endothelium markers, which were included in subgroup analyses in our study.

The role of LVD as a prognostic predictor in NSCLC remains controversial. Kajita and colleagues were the first to report VEGFR-3 expression in lung cancer cells, but they did not evaluate its impact on the prognosis or

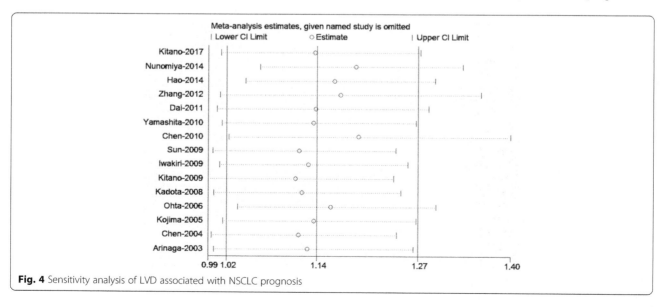

Fig. 4 Sensitivity analysis of LVD associated with NSCLC prognosis

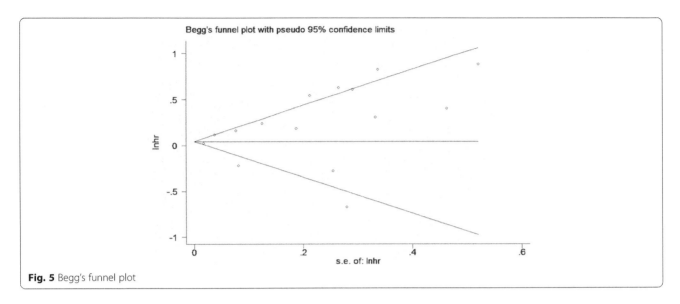

Fig. 5 Begg's funnel plot

the correlation of VEGFR-3 expression with clinicopathologic features in patients with NSCLC [44]. Later, many studies demonstrated that VEGF-C, VEGF-D, VEGFR-3 and other markers are independent markers of poor prognostic in patients with NSCLC. Thus, these markers may be ideal targets for diagnosis or therapy to improve the prognosis of NSCLC patients [34]. The study by Arinaga demonstrated that the combined expression of VEGF-C and VEGFR-3 has a negative impact on the prognosis of patients with NSCLC [27]. In addition, the study by Zhang and colleagues revealed that D2–40-positive peritumoral LVD may be an independent prognostic factor for lung adenocarcinoma. Thus, D2–40-positivity may be used to predict patient prognosis in lung adenocarcinoma. Moreover, the reduction of peritumoral lymphangiogenesis has been suggested to inhibit the metastasis of lung adenocarcinoma [22]. However, some studies have claimed that high LVD may be a marker for good prognosis. The study by Nunomiya and colleagues showed that lung cancer patients with lower LYVE-1 levels have poorer prognoses than patients with higher LYVE-1 levels [25]. Yang and his team demonstrated the role of the epigenetic regulation of desmoplakin in increasing the sensitivity of cancer cells to anticancer drug-induced apoptosis, implying the clinical value of desmoplakin for the treatment of patients with lung cancer [45]. Nevertheless, more studies are needed in the near future to verify whether LVD is indicative of good or bad prognosis in NSCLC patients.

VEGFR-3, D2–40, LYVE-1 and podoplanin are widely used and extremely valuable markers of lymphatic vessels. However, one study has reported that lymphatic

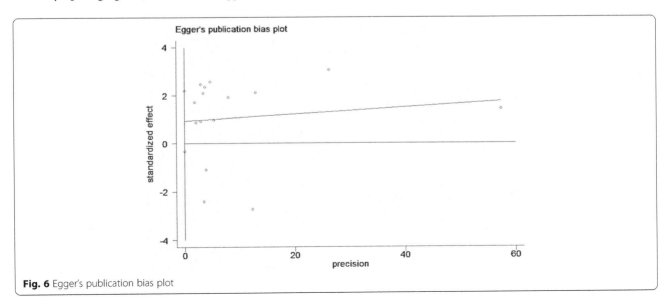

Fig. 6 Egger's publication bias plot

endothelium markers are not only expressed on lymphatic vessels but also expressed on blood vessels, tumor cells or in normal tissues [13]. One of the major drawbacks is the lack of specific markers for the lymphatic endothelium. One study [46] indicated that LYVE-1 and Prox-1 are molecular markers of lymphangiogenesis in NSCLC and that they can be used as important markers for the evaluation of lymphatic metastasis and prognoses in patients with NSCLC. Another study [43] showed that high VEGF and/or VEGFR expression is indicative of poor survival in patients with NSCLC and that VEGF-C/VEGFR-3 co-expression is a better prognostic indicator than other markers. Therefore, the evaluation of co-expressed markers may be useful to determine LVD.

Irrespective of its strengths, the meta-analysis also has certain limitations. First, although we searched all retrospective studies for the association between LVD and the prognosis of NSCLC, the eligible studies were restricted to those published in English or Chinese. Because of linguistic barrier, some non-English or non-Chinese studies were excluded. In addition, we also missed some studies that may have been published in books or journals that were not available in the online databases. Additionally, studies with negative data may not have been submitted by investigators, or studies with nonsignificant results may have been rejected by journals. Nevertheless, there was no significant publication bias in our study, although we could not completely rule out publication bias. Second, few studies did not present clear or complete data, making data analysis difficult. When we could not obtain original data from the authors via email or other means, we had to exclude those studies. Third, because of the small number of eligible articles, our study was not the most comprehensive. Fourth, our results cannot be generalized to populations worldwide, especially non-Asian populations. Thus, more comprehensive and higher quality analyses are still required in the future.

Conclusions

In summary, this meta-analysis indicated that LVD is an indicator of the prognosis of Asian NSCLC patients. However, higher quality and more comprehensive analyses are still needed as more data are published in the future.

Abbreviations
95% CI: 95% confidence interval; ADC: Adenocarcinoma; HR: Hazard ratio; LCC: Large cell cancer; LVD: Lymphatic vessel density; LYVE-1: Lymphatic vessel endothelial hyaluronan receptor-1; NSCLC: Non-small cell lung cancer; SCC: Squamous cell carcinoma; VEGFR: Vascular endothelial growth factor receptor

Acknowledgments
We appreciate the contribution of all patients, their families, the investigators and the medical staff. We are grateful to all authors.

Funding
This study was supported by grants from the National Natural Science Foundation of China (No. 81560694 and 81760015), the Young Academic and Technical Leaders of Yunnan Province (No. 2017HB053), and the Medical Science Leaders of Yunnan Province (No. 201627).

Authors' contributions
XSL and XXQ were responsible for the initial plan, study design, data collection, data extraction, data interpretation, manuscript drafting, statistical analysis, and performance of the study. TZW and XSY were responsible for critical revision of the manuscript. YJ, ZY, ZCF, LLQ, LH and DYL were responsible for data interpretation, manuscript drafting, supervision, and critical revision of the manuscript. XSL and TZW act as the guarantors for this article and take full responsibility for this study. All authors have read and approved the final manuscript.

Competing interests
The authors declare that they have no competing interests.

Author details
[1]First Department of Respiratory Medicine, Yan'an Hospital Affiliated to Kunming Medical University, No. 245, East Renmin Road, Kunming 650051, Yunnan, China. [2]First Department of Respiratory Medicine, The First Affiliated Hospital of Kunming Medical University, Kunming 650032, Yunnan, China. [3]Department of Dermatology, The Second Affiliated Hospital of Kunming Medical University, Kunming 650032, Yunnan, China. [4]The People's Hospital of Yuxi City, The 6th Affiliated Hospital of Kunming Medical University, Yuxi 653100, Yunnan, China.

References
1. Siegel RL, Miller KD, Jemal A. Cancer statistics, 2017. CA Cancer J Clin. 2017; 67:7–30.
2. Torre LA, Bray F, Siegel RL, Ferlay J, Lortet-Tieulent J, Jemal A. Global cancer statistics, 2012. CA Cancer J Clin. 2015;65:87–108. https://doi.org/10.3322/caac.21262. (Epub 2015 Feb 4)
3. Li J, Li D, Wei X, Su Y. In silico comparative genomic analysis of two non-small cell lung cancer subtypes and their potentials for cancer classification. Cancer Genomics Proteom. 2014;11:303–10.
4. Tang Z, Li J, Shen Q, Feng J, Liu H, Wang W, et al. Contribution of upregulated dipeptidyl peptidase 9 (DPP9) in promoting tumoregenicity, metastasis and the prediction of poor prognosis in non-small cell lung cancer (NSCLC). Int J Cancer. 2017;140:1620–32. https://doi.org/10.1002/ijc.30571. (Epub 2017 Feb 2)
5. Dai C, Ren Y, Xie D, Zheng H, She Y, Fei K, et al. Does lymph node metastasis have a negative prognostic impact in patients with NSCLC and M1a disease? J Thorac Oncol Off Publ Int Assoc Study Lung Cancer. 2016;11: 1745–54. https://doi.org/10.1016/j.jtho.2016.06.030. (Epub 2016 Aug 24)
6. Pérez-Guijarro E, Merlino G. Lymphangiogenesis: from passive disseminator to dynamic metastatic enabler. Pigment Cell Melanoma Res. 2017;30:509–10. https://doi.org/10.1111/pcmr.12621. (Epub 2017 Oct 16)
7. Špirić Z, Eri Ž, Erić M. Lymphatic vessel density and VEGF-C expression as independent predictors of melanoma metastases. J Plast Reconstr Aesthet Surg JPRAS. 2017;70:1653–9. https://doi.org/10.1016/j.bjps.2017.06.040. (Epub 2017 Sep 13)
8. Abdul-Aziz MA, Amin AK, El-Rouby DH, Shaker OG. Lymphangiogenesis in oral squamous cell carcinoma: correlation with VEGF-C expression and lymph node metastasis. Int J Dent. 2017;2017:7285656. https://doi.org/10.1155/2017/7285656. (Epub 2017 Jun 7)
9. Pereira F, Pereira SS, Mesquita M, Morais T, Costa MM, Quelhas P, et al. Lymph node metastases in papillary and medullary thyroid carcinoma are independent of intratumoral lymphatic vessel density. Eur Thyroid J. 2017;6: 57–64. https://doi.org/10.1159/000457794. (Epub 2017 Mar 17)
10. Pappas A, Lagoudianakis E, Seretis C, Koronakis N, Keramidaris D, Grapatsas K, et al. Role of lymphatic vessel density in colorectal cancer: prognostic significance and clinicopathologic correlations. Acta Gastroenterol Belg. 2015;78:223–7.

11. Niemiec JA, Adamczyk A, Ambicka A, Mucha-Małecka A, Wysocki WM, Biesaga B, et al. Prognostic role of lymphatic vessel density and lymphovascular invasion in chemotherapy-naive and chemotherapy-treated patients with invasive breast cancer. Am J Transl Res. 2017;9:1435–47.
12. Wang G, Wang Z, Li C, Wang P, Chai D, Cheng Z. Relationship among the expression of lymphatic vessel density, microvessel density, carcinoembryonic antigenic mRNA, KAI1, and Kiss-1, and prognosis in patients with non-small cell lung cancer. Zhongguo Fei Ai Za Zhi. 2012;15: 348–54. https://doi.org/10.3779/j.issn.1009-3419.2012.06.05.
13. Cueni LN, Detmar M. New insights into the molecular control of the lymphatic vascular system and its role in disease. J Invest Dermatol. 2006; 126:2167–77.
14. Waś H. Characterization of markers and growth factors for lymphatic endothelium. Postepy Biochem. 2005;51:209–14.
15. Lingtong W, Qiangxiu W. Lymphatic endothelium-specific markers: A Systematic Review. Shandong Med. 2008;48:114–5.
16. YU S, Binquan W. Lymphatic endothelium-specific markers. A Systematic Review. J Shanxi Med Univ 2007;03:274–77.
17. Banerji S, Ni J, Wang SX, Clasper S, Su J, Tammi R, et al. LYVE-1, a new homologue of the CD44 glycoprotein, is a lymph-specific receptor for hyaluronan. J Cell Biol. 1999;144:789–801.
18. Kahn HJ, Bailey D, Marks A. Monoclonal antibody D2-40, a new marker of lymphatic endothelium, reacts with Kaposi's sarcoma and a subset of angiosarcomas. Mod Pathol. 2002;15:434–40.
19. Van den Eynden GG, Van der Auwera I, Van Laere SJ, Huygelen V, Colpaert CG, van Dam P, et al. Induction of lymphangiogenesis in and around axillary lymph node metastases of patients with breast cancer. Br J Cancer. 2006;95: 1362–6.
20. Breiteneder-Geleff S, Soleiman A, Kowalski H, Horvat R, Amann G, Kriehuber E, et al. Angiosarcomas express mixed endothelial phenotypes of blood and lymphatic capillaries: podoplanin as a specific marker for lymphatic endothelium. Am J Pathol. 1999;154:385–94.
21. Wigle JT, Oliver G. Prox1 function is required for the development of the murine lymphatic system. Cell. 1999;98:769–78.
22. Zhang BC, Guan S, Zhang YF, Yao GQ, Yang B, Zhao Y, et al. Peritumoral lymphatic microvessel density is related to poor prognosis in lung adenocarcinoma: a retrospective study of 65 cases. Exp Ther Med. 2012;3: 636–40.
23. Kitano H, Kageyama S, Hewitt SM, Hayashi R, Doki Y, Ozaki Y, et al. Podoplanin expression in cancerous stroma induces lymphangiogenesis and predicts lymphatic spread and patient survival. Arch Pathol Lab Med. 2010;134:1520–7. https://doi.org/10.1043/2009-0114-OA.1.
24. Kadota K, Huang CL, Liu D, Ueno M, Kushida Y, Haba R, et al. The clinical significance of lymphangiogenesis and angiogenesis in non-small cell lung cancer patients. Eur J Cancer. 2008;44:1057–67. https://doi.org/10.1016/j.ejca.2008.03.012. (Epub 2008 Apr 8)
25. Nunomiya K, Shibata Y, Abe S, Inoue S, Igarashi A, Yamauchi K, et al. Relationship between serum level of lymphatic vessel endothelial hyaluronan Receptor-1 and prognosis in patients with lung cancer. J Cancer. eCollection. 2014;2014(5):242–7. https://doi.org/10.7150/jca.8486.
26. Kojima H, Shijubo N, Yamada G, Ichimiya S, Abe S, Satoh M, et al. Clinical significance of vascular endothelial growth factor-C and vascular endothelial growth factor receptor 3 in patients with T1 lung adenocarcinoma. Cancer. 2005;104:1668–77.
27. Arinaga M, Noguchi T, Takeno S, Chujo M, Miura T, Uchida Y. Clinical significance of vascular endothelial growth factor C and vascular endothelial growth factor receptor 3 in patients with nonsmall cell lung carcinoma. Cancer. 2003;97:457–64.
28. Higgins JP, Thompson SG, Deeks JJ, Altman DG. Measuring inconsistency in meta-analyses. BMJ. 2003;327:557–60.
29. Higgins JP, Thompson SG. Quantifying heterogeneity in a meta-analysis. Stat Med. 2002;21:1539–58.
30. Leonard T, Duffy JC. A Bayesian fixed effects analysis of the mantel-Haenszel model applied to meta-analysis. Stat Med. 2002;21:2295–312.
31. Harbord RM, Egger M, Sterne JA. A modified test for small-study effects in meta-analyses of controlled trials with binary endpoints. Stat Med. 2006;25: 3443–57.
32. Chootrakool H, Shi JQ, Yue R. Meta-analysis and sensitivity analysis for multi-arm trials with selection bias. Stat Med. 2011;30:1183–98. https://doi.org/10.1002/sim.4143. (Epub 2011 Jan 16)
33. Kitano H, Chung JY, Noh KH, Lee YH, Kim TW, Lee SH, et al. Synaptonemal complex protein 3 is associated with lymphangiogenesis in non-small cell lung cancer patients with lymph node metastasis. J Transl Med. 2017;15:138. https://doi.org/10.1186/s12967-017-1241-5.
34. Hao S, Yang Y, Liu Y, Yang S, Wang G, Xiao J, et al. JAM-C promotes lymphangiogenesis and nodal metastasis in non-small cell lung cancer. Tumour Biol. 2014;35:5675–87. https://doi.org/10.1007/s13277-014-1751-1. (Epub 2014 Mar 2)
35. Dai X, Wang W, Shen-Tu Y, Zhang J. Expression and prognostic value of VEGF-C and lymphangeogenesis in lung adenocarcinoma and squamous cell carcinoma. Zhongguo Fei Ai Za Zhi. 2011;14:774–9. https://doi.org/10.3779/j.issn.1009-3419.2011.10.02.
36. Yamashita T, Uramoto H, Onitsuka T, Ono K, Baba T, So T, et al. Association between lymphangiogenesis-/micrometastasis- and adhesion-related molecules in resected stage I NSCLC. Lung Cancer. 2010;70:320–8. https://doi.org/10.1016/j.lungcan.2010.02.013. (Epub 2010 Apr 2)
37. Chen X, Wan J, Liu J, Xie W, Diao X, Xu J, et al. Increased IL-17-producing cells correlate with poor survival and lymphangiogenesis in NSCLC patients. Lung Cancer. 2010;69:348–54. https://doi.org/10.1016/j.lungcan.2009.11.013.
38. Sun JG, Wang Y, Chen ZT, Zhuo WL, Zhu B, Liao RX, et al. Detection of lymphangiogenesis in non-small cell lung cancer and its prognostic value. J Exp Clin Cancer Res. 2009;28:21. https://doi.org/10.1186/1756-9966-28-21.
39. Iwakiri S, Nagai S, Katakura H, Takenaka K, Date H, Wada H, et al. D2-40-positive lymphatic vessel density is a poor prognostic factor in squamous cell carcinoma of the lung. Ann Surg Oncol. 2009;16:1678–85. https://doi.org/10.1245/s10434-009-0432-6. (Epub 2009 Mar 28)
40. Ohta Y, Shimizu Y, Minato H, Matsumoto I, Oda M, Watanabe G. Results of initial operations in non-small cell lung cancer patients with single-level N2 disease. Ann Thorac Surg. 2006;81:427–33.
41. Chen F, Takenaka K, Ogawa E, Yanagihara K, Otake Y, Wada H, et al. Flt-4-positive endothelial cell density and its clinical significance in non-small cell lung cancer. Clin Cancer Res. 2004;10:8548–53.
42. Wang J, Li K, Wang B, Bi J. Lymphatic microvessel density as a prognostic factor in non-small cell lung carcinoma: a meta-analysis of the literature. Mol Biol Rep. 2012;39:5331–8. https://doi.org/10.1007/s11033-011-1332-y. (Epub 2011 Dec 14)
43. Zheng CL, Qiu C, Shen MX, Qu X, Zhang TH, Zhang JH, et al. Prognostic impact of elevation of vascular endothelial growth factor family expression in patients with non-small cell lung cancer: an updated meta-analysis. Asian Pac J Cancer Prev. 2015;16:1881–95.
44. Kajita T, Ohta Y, Kimura K, Tamura M, Tanaka Y, Tsunezuka Y, et al. The expression of vascular endothelial growth factor C and its receptors in non-small cell lung cancer. Br J Cancer. 2001;85:255–60.
45. Yang L, Chen Y, Cui T, Knösel T, Zhang Q, Albring KF, et al. Desmoplakin acts as a tumor suppressor by inhibition of the Wnt/beta-catenin signaling pathway in human lung cancer. Carcinogenesis. 2012;33:1863–70. https://doi.org/10.1093/carcin/bgs226. (Epub 2012 Jul 12)
46. Chang C, Wang P, Yang H, Li L, Zhang LB. Expression of LYVE-1 and Prox-1 in non-small cell lung cancer and the relationship with lymph node metastasis. Sichuan Da Xue Xue Bao Yi Xue Ban. 2011;42:174–8.

Permissions

All chapters in this book were first published in PM, by BioMed Central; hereby published with permission under the Creative Commons Attribution License or equivalent. Every chapter published in this book has been scrutinized by our experts. Their significance has been extensively debated. The topics covered herein carry significant findings which will fuel the growth of the discipline. They may even be implemented as practical applications or may be referred to as a beginning point for another development.

The contributors of this book come from diverse backgrounds, making this book a truly international effort. This book will bring forth new frontiers with its revolutionizing research information and detailed analysis of the nascent developments around the world.

We would like to thank all the contributing authors for lending their expertise to make the book truly unique. They have played a crucial role in the development of this book. Without their invaluable contributions this book wouldn't have been possible. They have made vital efforts to compile up to date information on the varied aspects of this subject to make this book a valuable addition to the collection of many professionals and students.

This book was conceptualized with the vision of imparting up-to-date information and advanced data in this field. To ensure the same, a matchless editorial board was set up. Every individual on the board went through rigorous rounds of assessment to prove their worth. After which they invested a large part of their time researching and compiling the most relevant data for our readers.

The editorial board has been involved in producing this book since its inception. They have spent rigorous hours researching and exploring the diverse topics which have resulted in the successful publishing of this book. They have passed on their knowledge of decades through this book. To expedite this challenging task, the publisher supported the team at every step. A small team of assistant editors was also appointed to further simplify the editing procedure and attain best results for the readers.

Apart from the editorial board, the designing team has also invested a significant amount of their time in understanding the subject and creating the most relevant covers. They scrutinized every image to scout for the most suitable representation of the subject and create an appropriate cover for the book.

The publishing team has been an ardent support to the editorial, designing and production team. Their endless efforts to recruit the best for this project, has resulted in the accomplishment of this book. They are a veteran in the field of academics and their pool of knowledge is as vast as their experience in printing. Their expertise and guidance has proved useful at every step. Their uncompromising quality standards have made this book an exceptional effort. Their encouragement from time to time has been an inspiration for everyone.

The publisher and the editorial board hope that this book will prove to be a valuable piece of knowledge for researchers, students, practitioners and scholars across the globe.

List of Contributors

Jürgen Schäfer
Department of Radiology, Division of Pediatric Radiology, University of Tübingen, Tübingen, Germany

Matthias Griese
Children's Hospital, University of Munich, Munich, Germany

Ravishankar Chandrasekaran and Sanjay H. Chotirmall
Lee Kong Chian School of Medicine, Nanyang Technological University, Singapore, Singapore

Dominik Hartl
Department of Pediatrics I, University of Tübingen, Tübingen, Germany
Roche Pharma Research and Early Development (pRED), Immunology, Inflammation and Infectious Diseases (I3) Discovery and Translational Area, Roche Innovation Center, Basel, Switzerland

Arielle S. Selya and Gaurav Mehta
Master of Public Health Program, Department of Population Health, University of North Dakota, 1301 North Columbia Rd. Stop 9037, Grand Forks, ND 58202, USA

Sunita Thapa
Master of Public Health Program, Department of Population Health, University of North Dakota, 1301 North Columbia Rd. Stop 9037, Grand Forks, ND 58202, USA
Department of Public Policy, Vanderbilt University School of Medicine, 2525 West End Ave, Suite 1200, Nashville, TN 37203, USA

Ravishankar Chandrasekaran, Micheál Mac Aogáin and Sanjay H. Chotirmall
Lee Kong Chian School of Medicine, Nanyang Technological University, Clinical Sciences Building, 11 Mandalay Road, Singapore 308232, Singapore

James D. Chalmers
Division of Molecular and Clinical Medicine, School of Medicine, Ninewells Hospital and Medical School, Dundee, UK

Stuart J. Elborn
Imperial College and Royal Brompton Hospital, London, UK
Queen's University Belfast, Belfast, UK

Xinlun Tian and Kai-Feng Xu
Department of Respiratory Medicine, Peking Union Medical College Hospital, Peking Union Medical College and Chinese Academy of Medical Sciences, Beijing 100730, China

Jingzhou Zhang
Department of Respiratory Medicine, Peking Union Medical College Hospital, Peking Union Medical College and Chinese Academy of Medical Sciences, Beijing 100730, China
Department of Epidemiology, Mailman School of Public Health, Columbia University, New York, NY, USA

Xiao Hu
Department of Respiratory Medicine, Peking Union Medical College Hospital, Peking Union Medical College and Chinese Academy of Medical Sciences, Beijing 100730, China
Yale School of Public Health, Yale University, New Haven, CT, USA

Lusmaia Damaceno Camargo Costa and Paulo Sérgio Sucasas da Costa
Pediatric Pulmonology Unit, University Hospital, Federal University of Goiás, Primeira Avenida, S/N. Setor Leste Universitária, Goiânia CEP: 746050-20, Brazil

Paulo Augusto Moreira Camargos
Pediatric Pulmonology Unit, University Hospital, Federal University of Minas Gerais, Belo Horizonte, Brazil

Paul L. P. Brand
Princess Amalia Children's Centre, Isala Hospital, Zwolle, and UMCG Postgraduate School of Medicine, University Medical Centre and University of Groningen, Groningen, the Netherlands

Fabíola Souza Fiaccadori, Menira Borges de Lima Dias e Souza, Divina das Dôres de Paula Cardoso and Ítalo de Araújo Castro
Human Virology Department, Public Health and Tropical Pathology Institute, Federal University of Goiás, Goiânia, Brazil

Ruth Minamisava
Faculty of Nursing, Universidade Federal de Goiás, Goiânia, GO, Brazil

Robin J. Green
Department of Paediatrics and Child Health, Faculty of Health Sciences, University of Pretoria, Pretoria, South Africa

Refiloe Masekela
Department of Paediatrics and Child Health, Faculty of Health Sciences, University of Pretoria, Pretoria, South Africa
Department of Maternal and Child Health, Nelson R Mandela School of Medicine, College of Health Sciences, University of KwaZulu-Natal, 719 Umbilo Road, Congella, Durban 4013, South Africa

Solize Vosloo, Stephanus N. Venter and Wilhelm Z. de Beer
Department of Microbiology and Plant Pathology, University of Pretoria, Pretoria, South Africa

Steven A. Cowman, Robert Wilson and Michael R. Loebinger
National Heart and Lung Institute, Imperial College London, London, UK
Host Defence Unit, Royal Brompton Hospital, London, UK

Joseph Jacob
National Heart and Lung Institute, Imperial College London, London, UK
Department of Radiology, Royal Brompton Hospital, London, UK

Sayed Obaidee
Cambridge Centre for Lung Infection, Papworth Hospital, Cambridge, UK

R. Andres Floto and Charles S. Haworth
Cambridge Centre for Lung Infection, Papworth Hospital, Cambridge, UK
Department of Medicine, University of Cambridge, Cambridge, UK

Ana Beatriz Valverde, Juliana M. Soares, Karynna P. Viana, Bruna Gomes and Claudia Soares
Latin America Medical Department – GlaxoSmithKline, Estrada dos Bandeirantes, Rio de Janeiro 8464, Brazil

Rogerio Souza
Pulmonary Hypertension Unit, Pulmonary Department – Heart Institute, University of Sao Paulo Medical School, Av. Dr. Eneas de Carvalho Aguiar, 44, Sao Paulo 05403-000, Brazil

El-Hassane Ouaalaya
Univ. Bordeaux, Inserm, Bordeaux Population Health Research Center, team EPICENE, UMR 1219, F-33000 Bordeaux, France

Chantal Raherison
Univ. Bordeaux, Inserm, Bordeaux Population Health Research Center, team EPICENE, UMR 1219, F-33000 Bordeaux, France
Pole cardiothoracique, Respiratory Diseases Department, CHU de Bordeaux, F-33000 Bordeaux, France
Univ. Bordeaux, Inserm, Bordeaux Population Health Research Center, team EPICENE, UMR 1219, 146 rue Leo Saignat, 33076 Cedex Bordeaux, France

Alain Bernady
Rehabiliation Center, Cambo-les-Bains, France

Julien Casteigt
Pneumology Clinic, St Medard en Jalles, France

Cecilia Nocent-Eijnani
General Hospital, Bayonne, France

Laurent Falque
Pneumology Clinic, Bordeaux, France

Frédéric Le Guillou
Pneumology Clinic, La Rochelle, France

Laurent Nguyen and Annaig Ozier
Pneumology Clinic, St Augustin, Bordeaux, France

Mathieu Molimard
U1219 Pharmaco-epidemiology, Bordeaux University, Bordeaux, France

Izumi Kitagawa
Department of General Internal Medicine, Shonan Kamakura General Hospital, 1370-1 Okamoto, Kamakura, Kanagawa, Japan

Sho Nishiguchi
Department of General Internal Medicine, Shonan Kamakura General Hospital, 1370-1 Okamoto, Kamakura, Kanagawa, Japan
Department of Internal Medicine, Hayama Heart Center, Hayama, Kanagawa, Japan
Unit of Public Health and Preventive Medicine, School of Medicine, Yokohama City University, Yokohama, Kanagawa, Japan

Shusaku Tomiyama
Department of General Medicine, Iizuka Hospital, Fukuoka, Japan

Yasuharu Tokuda
Muribushi Okinawa Project for Teaching Hospitals, Okinawa, Okinawa Prefecture, Japan

List of Contributors

Emily K. Dudgeon
Scottish Centre for Respiratory Research, University of Dundee, Ninewells Hospital and Medical School, Ninewells Drive, Dundee DD1 9SY, Scotland

Megan Crichton and James D. Chalmers
Division of Molecular and Clinical Medicine, University of Dundee, Dundee DD1 9SY, UK

Laureano Molins and Ángela Guirao
Respiratory Institute, Hospital Clinic, University of Barcelona, Barcelona, Spain
Institut d'investigacions Biomèdiques August Pi i Sunyer (IDIBAPS), Barcelona, Spain

Alejandra López-Giraldo, Sandra Cuerpo and Álvar Agustí
Respiratory Institute, Hospital Clinic, University of Barcelona, Barcelona, Spain
Institut d'investigacions Biomèdiques August Pi i Sunyer (IDIBAPS), Barcelona, Spain
CIBER Enfermedades Respiratorias(CIBERES), Instituto de Salud Carlos III, Madrid, Spain

Tamara Cruz
Institut d'investigacions Biomèdiques August Pi i Sunyer (IDIBAPS), Barcelona, Spain
CIBER Enfermedades Respiratorias(CIBERES), Instituto de Salud Carlos III, Madrid, Spain

Rosa Faner
Institut d'investigacions Biomèdiques August Pi i Sunyer (IDIBAPS), Barcelona, Spain
CIBER Enfermedades Respiratorias(CIBERES), Instituto de Salud Carlos III, Madrid, Spain
Barcelona, Spain

Adela Saco and Josep Ramirez
Institut d'investigacions Biomèdiques August Pi i Sunyer (IDIBAPS), Barcelona, Spain
Department of Pathology, Hospital Clinic, Barcelona, Spain

Naushad Hirani and Richard Leigh
Department of Medicine, Cumming School of Medicine, University of Calgary, Calgary, AB, Canada

Christopher H. Mody
Department of Medicine, Cumming School of Medicine, University of Calgary, Calgary, AB, Canada
Respiratory Health Strategic Clinical Network, Alberta Health Services, Edmonton, AB, Canada

Sachin R. Pendharkar
Department of Medicine, Cumming School of Medicine, University of Calgary, Calgary, AB, Canada
Department of Community Health Sciences, Cumming School of Medicine, University of Calgary, Calgary, AB, Canada
O'Brien Institute for Public Health, Cumming School of Medicine, University of Calgary, Calgary, AB, Canada
University of Calgary, TRW Building, Rm 3E23, 3280 Hospital Drive NW, Calgary, AB T2N 4Z6, Canada

Danielle A. Southern
O'Brien Institute for Public Health, Cumming School of Medicine, University of Calgary, Calgary, AB, Canada
W21C Research and Innovation Centre, Cumming School of Medicine, University of Calgary, Calgary, AB, Canada

Maria B. Ospina and Jim Graham
Respiratory Health Strategic Clinical Network, Alberta Health Services, Edmonton, AB, Canada

Peter Faris
Research Priorities and Implementation, Alberta Health Services, Calgary, AB, Canada

Mohit Bhutani and Michael K. Stickland
Division of Pulmonary Medicine, Department of Medicine, Faculty of Medicine and Dentistry, University of Alberta, Edmonton, AB, Canada

Katy L. M. Hester and Anthony De Soyza
Institute of Cellular Medicine, Newcastle University, Newcastle upon Tyne NE2 4HH, UK
Adult Bronchiectasis Service, Freeman Hospital, Newcastle upon Tyne NE7 7DN, UK

Julia Newton
Faculty of Medical Sciences, Newcastle University, Newcastle upon Tyne NE2 4HH, UK

Tim Rapley
Department of Social Work, Education and Community Wellbeing, Northumbria University, Newcastle upon Tyne NE7 7XA, UK

Giacomo Sgalla and Luca Richeldi
Division of Respiratory Medicine, University Hospital "A. Gemelli", Catholic University of Sacred Heart, Rome, Italy
National Institute for Health Research Southampton Respiratory Biomedical Research Unit and Clinical and Experimental Sciences, University of Southampton, Southampton, UK

Simon L. F. Walsh
King's College Hospital, London, UK

Nicola Sverzellati
University Hospital of Parma, Parma, Italy

Sophie Fletcher, Mark G. Jones and Donna Davies
National Institute for Health Research Southampton Respiratory Biomedical Research Unit and Clinical and Experimental Sciences, University of Southampton, Southampton, UK

Stefania Cerri and Fabrizio Luppi
Centre for Rare Lung Disease, University Hospital of Modena, Modena, Italy

Borislav Dimitrov
Medical Statistics, Faculty of Medicine, University of Southampton, Southampton, UK

Dragana Nikolic and Anna Barney
Institute for Sound and Vibration Research, University of Southampton, Southampton, UK

Fabrizio Pancaldi and Luca Larcher
DISMI, University of Modena and Reggio Emilia, Reggio Emilia, Italy

Albert Y. H. Lim, Akash Verma, Soon Keng Goh, Ser Hon Puah and John A. Abisheganaden
Department of Respiratory and Critical Care Medicine, Tan Tock Seng Hospital, 11 Jalan Tan Tock Seng, Singapore 308433, Singapore

Sanjay H. Chotirmall
Lee Kong Chian School of Medicine, Translational Respiratory Research laboratory, Nanyang Technological University, Clinical Sciences Building, 11 Mandalay Road, Singapore 308232, Singapore

Eric T. K. Fok
Yong Loo Lin School of Medicine, National University of Singapore, 12 Science Drive 2, Singapore 117549, Singapore

Partha P. De
Department of Laboratory Medicine, Tan Tock Seng Hospital, 11 Jalan Tan Tock Seng, Singapore 308433, Singapore

Daryl E. L. Goh
Dalhousie Medical School, Dalhousie University, 1459 Oxford Street, Halifax, NS B3H 4R2, Canada

Nora Drick, Benjamin Seeliger and Hendrik Suhling
Department of Respiratory Medicine, Hannover Medical School, Carl-Neuberg-Str.1, 30625 Hannover, Germany

Tobias Welte and Jan Fuge
Department of Respiratory Medicine, Hannover Medical School, Carl-Neuberg-Str.1, 30625 Hannover, Germany
Biomedical Research in End-Stage and Obstructive Lung Disease Hannover (BREATH), Member of the German Centre for Lung Research (DZL), Hannover, Germany

Xuejun Guo
Department of Respiratory Medicine, Xinhua Hospital, Shanghai Jiaotong University School of Medicine, 1665, Kongjiang Road, Shanghai 200092, China

Wei Xiong
Department of Respiratory Medicine, Xinhua Hospital, Shanghai Jiaotong University School of Medicine, 1665, Kongjiang Road, Shanghai 200092, China
Department of Cardiopulmonary Circulation, Shanghai Pulmonary Hospital, Tongji University School of Medicine, Shanghai, People's Republic of China

Bigyan Pudasaini and Jinming Liu
Department of Cardiopulmonary Circulation, Shanghai Pulmonary Hospital, Tongji University School of Medicine, Shanghai, People's Republic of China

Yunfeng Zhao
Department of Respiratory Medicine, Punan Hospital, Pudong New District, Shanghai, China

Mei Xu
Department of Pediatrics, Kongjiang Hospital, Yangpu District, Shanghai, China
Department of Pediatrics, Shanghai Dinghai Community Health Service Center, Tongji University School of Medicine, Yangpu District, Shanghai, China

Kyungjong Lee
Department of Medicine, Division of Pulmonary and Critical Care Medicine, Samsung Medical Center, Sungkyunkwan University School of Medicine, Seoul, South Korea

Hye Ok Kim, Hee Kyoung Choi and Gi Hyeon Seo
Health Insurance Review and Assessment Service, 60 Hyeoksin-ro (Bangok-dong), Wonju-si, Gangwon-do 26465, South Korea

Johannes Bickenbach, Daniel Schöneis and Gernot Marx
Department of Intensive Care Medicine, Medical Faculty, RWTH Aachen University, Pauwelsstr. 30, D-52074 Aachen, Germany

List of Contributors

Nikolaus Marx and Michael Dreher
Department of Cardiology, Pneumology, Angiology and Intensive Care Medicine, Medical Faculty, RWTH Aachen University, Aachen, Germany

Sebastian Lemmen
Department of Infection Control and Infectious Diseases, Medical Faculty, RWTH Aachen University, Aachen, Germany

Flynn Slattery, Hunter Bennett and Alan Crockett
Alliance for Research in Exercise, Nutrition and Activity, Sansom Institute for Health Research, School of Health Sciences, Universitiy of South Australia, Adelaide, Australia

Kylie Johnston
School of Health Sciences, Sansom Institute for Health Research, University of South Australia, Adelaide, Australia

Catherine Paquet
Centre for Population Health Research, Sansom Institute for Health Research, School of
Health Sciences, University of South Australia, Adelaide, Australia

Janet Lutale
Department of Internal Medicine, Muhimbili University of Health and Allied Sciences, P.O BOX 65001 Dar es Salaam, Tanzania
Department of Internal Medicine, Muhimbili National Hospital, Dar es Salaam, Tanzania

Festo K. Shayo
Department of Internal Medicine, Muhimbili University of Health and Allied Sciences, Dar es Salaam, Tanzania
Department of Internal Medicine, Muhimbili National Hospital, Dar es Salaam, Tanzania
Tokyo Medical and Dental University, 1-5-45 Yushima, Bunkyo-ku, Tokyo 113-8510, Japan

Constanze Brock and Petra Lichtenberger
Department of Pulmonology, Kepler University Hospital, Krankenhausstrasse 9, A4021, Linz, Austria

Magdalena Humenberger, Andreas Horner and Bernd Lamprecht
Department of Pulmonology, Kepler University Hospital, Krankenhausstrasse 9, A4021, Linz, Austria
Faculty of Medicine, Johannes-Kepler-University, Linz, Austria

Anna Labek and Bernhard Kaiser
Department of Health Economics, Upper Austrian Health Insurance, Linz, Austria

Rupert Frechinger
Department of Medical Controlling, Kepler University Hospital, Linz, Austria

Cho Sun Leem
Division of Pulmonary and Critical Care Medicine, Department of Internal Medicine, Seoul National University Bundang Hospital, 82, Gumi-ro 173 Beon-gil, Bundang-gu, Seongnam-si, Gyeonggi-do 13620, Republic of Korea

Jun Yeun Cho, Youlim Kim, Eun Sun Kim, Sang Hoon Lee, Yeon Joo Lee, Jong Sun Park, Young-Jae Cho, Jae Ho Lee, Choon-Taek Lee and Ho Il Yoon
Division of Pulmonary and Critical Care Medicine, Department of Internal Medicine, Seoul National University Bundang Hospital, 82, Gumi-ro 173 Beon-gil, Bundang-gu, Seongnam-si, Gyeonggi-do 13620, Republic of Korea
Department of Internal Medicine, Seoul National University College of
Medicine, Seoul, Republic of Korea

Yaoju Tan, Biyi Su, Xingshan Cai, Shaojia Kuang, Haobin Kuang and Jianxiong Liu
Department of Clinical Laboratory, Guangzhou Chest Hospital, State Key Laboratory of Respiratory Disease, No. 62, Hengzhigang Road, Yuexiu District, Guangzhou, Guangdong Province 510095, People's Republic of China

Wei Shu and Yu Pang
National Clinical Laboratory on Tuberculosis, Beijing Key laboratory on Drug-resistant Tuberculosis Research, , Beijing Chest Hospital, Beijing Tuberculosis and Thoracic Tumor Institute, No. 9, Beiguan Street, Tongzhou District, Beijing 101149, People's Republic of China

Ranran Dai, Youchao Yu, Xiaoxia Hou, Yingmeng Ni and Guochao Shi
Department of Pulmonary and Critical Care Medicine, Ruijin Hospital, Shanghai Jiaotong University, School of Medicine, NO.197, Ruijin Er Road, Shanghai 200025, China

Guofeng Yan
School of Medicine, Shanghai Jiaotong University, Shanghai 200025, China

Christer Janson and Eva Lindberg
Department of Medical Sciences, Respiratory, Allergy and Sleep Medicine, Uppsala University, Uppsala, Sweden

Ane Johannessen
Centre for Clinical Research, Haukeland University Hospital, Bergen, Norway

Karl Franklin
Dept. of Surgical and Perioperative Sciences, Surgery, Umea University, Umea, Sweden

Cecilie Svanes
Institute of Clinical Science, University of Bergen, Bergen, Norway

Linus Schiöler
Department of Occupational and Environmental Medicine, Sahlgrenska University Hospital, Gothenburg, Sweden

Andrei Malinovschi
Department of Medical Sciences, Clinical Physiology, Uppsala University, Uppsala, Sweden

Thorarinn Gislason and Bryndis Benediktsdottir
Department of Respiratory Medicine and Sleep, the National University Hospital of Iceland, Reykjavik, Iceland
Faculty of Medicine, University of Iceland, Reykjavik, Iceland

Vivi Schlünssen
Department of Public Health, Section for Environment, Occupation and Health, Aarhus University, Aarhus, Denmark
National Research Center for the Working Environment, Copenhagen, Denmark

Rain Jõgi
Lung Clinic, Tartu University Clinics, Tartu, Estonia

Deborah Jarvis
Respiratory Epidemiology, Occupational Medicine and Public Health, National Heart and Lung Institute, Imperial College, London, UK

Ye Jiang and Ning Li
Department of Neurology, The Affiliated hospital of Hebei University, Yuhua East Road No. 212, Baoding 071000, Hebei, China

Jing Zhang
Department of Respiratory Medicine, The First Affiliated Hospital, Sun Yat-sen University, No. 58, Zhongshan 2nd Road, Yuexiu District, Guangzhou 510080, China

Juanjuan Huang and Lei Cao
Department of Anesthesiology, The Central Hospital of Wuhan, Tongji Medical College, Huazhong University of Science and Technology, Gusao Road No. 16, Jianghan District, Wuhan 430014, Hubei, China

Bo Xu
Department of Thoracic surgery, The First Affiliated Hospital, Sun Yat-sen University, No. 58, Zhongshan 2nd Road, Yuexiu District, Guangzhou 510080, China

Mingdong Zhao
Department of Orthopaedics, Jinshan Hospital, Fudan University, Longhang Road No. 1508, Jinshan District, Shanghai City 201508, China

Shuanglan Xu, Chunfang Zhang, Liqiong Liu and Xiqian Xing
First Department of Respiratory Medicine, Yan'an Hospital Affiliated to Kunming Medical University, No. 245, East Renmin Road, Kunming 650051, Yunnan, China

Jiao Yang
First Department of Respiratory Medicine, The First Affiliated Hospital of Kunming Medical University, Kunming 650032, Yunnan, China

Shuangyan Xu
Department of Dermatology, The Second Affiliated Hospital of Kunming Medical University, Kunming 650032, Yunnan, China

Yun Zhu, Hao Liu, Yunlong Dong and Zhaowei Teng
The People's Hospital of Yuxi City, The 6th Affiliated Hospital of Kunming Medical University, Yuxi 653100, Yunnan, China

Index

A
Acinetobacter Baumanii, 160, 163
Aetiology, 18-22, 28-30, 114, 131
Airway Hyperresponsiveness, 214-215, 218-219, 221
Allergic Rhinitis, 215, 221-230
Antimicrobial Therapy, 5, 160
Arterial Hypertension, 65-66, 71-72, 104, 144-145, 148, 152-153, 192-193
Asthma, 1-2, 5, 9, 12-17, 20, 28, 31, 41-46, 76, 89-91, 96-97, 102-104, 115, 117, 119-121, 131, 135-143, 176, 186-187, 200, 214-230
Asthma Exacerbation, 41-46

B
Bacterial Diversity, 47-48, 50, 54
Bacterial Pneumonia, 160
Blood Eosinophils, 135, 138-140, 142
Brain Metastases, 231, 233-237
Bronchiectasis, 1-11, 18-31, 47-48, 50-58, 60-64, 73-74, 76-77, 79, 89-91, 93-97, 113-123, 125-126, 129, 131, 133-134, 141, 207, 209-210, 212-213
Bronchoalveolar Lavage Fluid, 9, 167, 214, 216, 219-220

C
Chronic Asthma, 214-215, 217, 220
Chronic Obstructive Pulmonary Disease, 1, 10, 16-17, 28, 61, 63, 73, 81, 98, 103-107, 111-112, 120-121, 141, 161, 163, 165-166, 188, 194-195, 199-200, 210
Cluster Analysis, 29, 53, 73-75, 77, 79-81, 142-143
Colorectal Cancer, 238, 244
Comorbidities, 29, 70, 73-81, 106, 109, 111, 114, 120, 136, 141, 154, 156-158, 160, 192, 194-195, 199, 207-208
Computed Tomography, 4-5, 10-11, 22, 28, 57, 63-64, 122, 127, 201, 204, 206
Cystic Fibrosis, 1-2, 8-11, 18, 20, 28-31, 47-48, 51-52, 55-56, 58, 64, 90, 97, 114-115, 117, 120-121, 134, 213

D
Delayed Isolation, 82-83, 86-87
Depression, 12-15, 17, 73, 76-77, 79-80, 114, 117, 119-120
Drosophila, 239
Dyspnea, 44, 74-75, 80-81, 86, 224-225, 228

E
Emphysema, 7, 62, 98, 106, 123, 125-127, 154, 165, 192
Eosinophilic Asthma, 135, 138, 140-143
Epidemiology, 8-9, 17-20, 22, 28, 39, 46, 65-66, 69, 71, 73, 81, 128-129, 134, 159, 207, 213, 229
Erlotinib Versus, 231, 237

F
Flow Cytometry, 98-101, 103, 214-217, 219
Forced Expiratory Volume, 5, 32, 35-37, 39-40, 61, 63, 81, 100, 137-140, 168-169, 181, 193, 199

G
Gastroesophageal Reflux, 223, 225, 228-230
Gefitinib, 231-237

H
Human Immunodeficiency Virus, 47, 64, 83, 130

I
Idiopathic Pulmonary Fibrosis, 122, 127-128
Immunofluorescence, 42, 98, 101, 103
Inflammation, 1-3, 5, 7-10, 12, 15, 18, 26, 28, 30, 42, 45, 48, 54-55, 74, 81, 97, 102, 104, 115, 120, 135, 140-142, 214-215, 219-222
Inhaled Therapy, 195-200
Interleukin, 2, 9, 28, 135, 142, 181, 186-187, 221

K
Klebsiella, 3, 24, 28

L
Latent Class Analysis, 57-60, 62, 64
Lung Adenocarcinoma, 206, 231-235, 237-239, 243, 245
Lung Cancer, 12, 16-17, 73, 99, 154-159, 201-202, 205-206, 231, 236-239, 241-245
Lung Cell, 104
Lung Function, 2-3, 5, 8-10, 17, 19, 21, 30-33, 35-40, 48, 50, 53-54, 58-59, 73-75, 80, 97, 99, 101, 104, 117, 133-136, 138-143, 158, 168-169, 173, 192, 194, 196, 199, 228-230
Lung Microbiome, 8, 18, 47-48, 54-55
Lung Parenchyma, 18, 98-99, 101-102, 126-127
Lung Repair, 98
Lymphangiogenesis, 238-239, 243-245
Lymphatic Metastasis, 201, 244
Lymphatic Vessel Density, 238, 244-245

M
Mechanical Ventilator Weaning, 160
Mepolizumab, 135-136, 138, 140-143
Mesenchymal Stem Cell, 214, 221
Microbiology, 2, 8, 18, 23, 27, 29-30, 47, 55
Microbiome, 2, 8, 18-19, 26-31, 47-48, 53-56

Multidrug Resistance, 160, 163, 166
Multimorbidity, 73
Murine, 214-215, 221-222, 245
Mycobacterium Abscessus, 2, 8, 28, 129, 131, 134, 207-208, 213
Mycobacterium Fortuitum, 129, 131, 207
Mycobiome, 2, 18, 26-27, 30-31

N
Neutrophil, 2-3, 9, 18-19, 61, 97, 143
Nicotine Dependence, 12, 16-17
Nodal Metastasis, 201-205, 245
Non-tuberculous Mycobacteria, 8, 30, 64, 129, 134

O
Ovalbumin, 214-215, 218-222

P
Paediatric, 3, 10-11, 18, 20-21, 23, 27, 30, 56, 72
Pathogenesis, 1-3, 7-8, 19, 21, 27, 29, 102, 141, 213-214, 222
Pneumonia, 20-21, 54-55, 86, 88, 110, 122-124, 127-128, 160-162, 164, 166-167

Podoplanin, 238-240, 243, 245
Prognostic Indicator, 238, 244
Pseudomonas Aeruginosa, 2, 8, 10, 18, 23, 26, 28, 30, 54-55, 91, 97, 114, 160, 166
Pulmonary Hypertension, 65, 69-72, 76, 79, 148, 152-153
Pulmonary Nontuberculous, 57, 134, 207, 213
Pulmonary Tuberculosis, 82, 88, 129, 131, 134, 213

R
Radiosurgery, 154, 237
Renal Disease, 106, 108-109, 191
Respiratory Infection, 46, 163-164
Respiratory Syncytial Virus, 41, 43, 45

S
Septic Pneumonic Shock, 160-161, 164
Severe Eosinophilic Asthma, 135, 138, 141-143
Spirometry, 10, 32-33, 35-40, 73-74, 98-100, 103, 111, 142, 168, 170-173, 181-182, 186-187, 189, 191, 195-199, 224

T
Thoracic Surgery, 102, 154, 159, 205, 236
Thyroid Carcinoma, 238, 244

CPSIA information can be obtained
at www.ICGtesting.com
Printed in the USA
BVHW051000230519
549125BV00003B/130/P